PRAISE FOR *SOCIAL DETERMINANTS OF HEALTH: CANADIAN PERSPECTIVES*

"[*Social Determinants of Health*] may not be light summer reading for the cottage or the beach, but it does shed a lot of light on the way we live now as Canadians. Edited by York University professor Dennis Raphael and with a thoughtful foreword by Roy Romanow, it's a collection of research and observations by academics and leading-edge thinkers (a whole new community, in a way, formed around this issue) about how social determinants of health play out in Canadian life.

"Raphael's book explores each of recognized social determinants that impact on health and well-being in Canada in the context of what exists 'on the ground'—how theory translates into real life. If a book can walk the walk as well as talk the talk, this one does. It's a significant resource for teachers, students, and researchers. But it's also a useful, important, and eye-opening reminder for all of us about how our political and societal choices determine the health—literally, the extent of illness, disease, disability, medical costs—of Canadians."

—Judy Gerstel, *The Toronto Star*

"This book makes a highly significant contribution to the field of Public Health in Canada. Aside from being well-researched and well-written, a major strength of the book is its focus on identifying clear policy directions to improve the health of Canadians by influencing each of the social determinants. Raphael's book is essential reading for university students, practitioners, program managers, and policy-makers in all of the human service sectors."

—Benita Cohen, University of Manitoba

"We finally have a Canadian book that we can refer to, in order to assist in 'making the case' for a population health approach. This book does not shy away from the 'tough questions' of politics and social policy. It's quite hard-hitting at times. That's a real positive."

—Victoria Barr, University of Victoria

"The book is very accessible to general/non-specialist audiences. My students commended the book for its accessibility and coherence. This volume is straightforward, easy to read, accessible to undergraduate students. Canadian content is also hugely important."

—Alan Davidson, University of British Columbia

SOCIAL DETERMINANTS OF HEALTH

Social Determinants of Health

Canadian Perspectives

———⬤———

Second Edition

Edited by Dennis Raphael

Canadian Scholars' Press Inc.
Toronto

Social Determinants of Health: Canadian Perspectives
Second Edition
Edited by Dennis Raphael

Published by
Canadian Scholars' Press Inc.
425 Adelaide Street West, Suite 200
Toronto, Ontario
M5V 3C1

www.cspi.org

Canadian Scholars' Press Inc. gratefully acknowledges financial support for our publishing activities from the Government of Canada through the Book Publishing Industry Development Program (BPIDP).

Library and Archives Canada Cataloguing in Publication

　　Social determinants of health : Canadian perspectives / edited by Dennis Raphael. – 2nd ed.

Includes bibliographical references and index.
ISBN 978-1-55130-350-5

　　1. Public health—Social aspects—Canada. 2. Public health—Economic aspects—Canada. 3. Medical policy—Social aspects—Canada. I. Raphael, Dennis

RA418.S63 2008　　　　　362.10971　　　　　C2008-902795-7

Interior design and composition: Brad Horning & Stewart Moracen
Cover design: John Kicksee/KIX BY DESIGN
Cover art: Courtesy of Krisztián Hoffer, kepesvagyok.hu

Printed and bound in Canada.

Canada

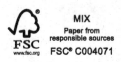

MIX
Paper from
responsible sources
FSC
www.fsc.org　FSC® C004071

For Alexander and Toba

TABLE OF CONTENTS

Part Three: Foundations of Lifelong Health: Education

Part Four: Foundations of Lifelong Health: Food and Shelter

Part Five: Social Exclusion

Part Six: Public Policy

FOREWORD
TO THE SECOND EDITION

When Tommy Douglas brought our first universal publicly funded health system to the province of Saskatchewan, he passionately argued that medicare must not only ensure that people get the health care they need when they need it, but it must implement public policies for keeping people well, not just patching them up once they get sick.

Unfortunately, since that time medicare has been pulled toward a commitment to the service contract of health care delivery. Thankfully, in Canada we have had Dennis Raphael sounding the alarm that just focusing on the "repair shop" is not only counter to our Canadian values of social justice, it will ultimately put the sustainability of our cherished health care system at risk. His scholarship and dogged advocacy on the need to address the broadest possible approach to social determinants of health has been a powerful antidote to the "tyranny of the acute."

It has been said that Canada led thinking on population health with the Lalonde Report of 1974, *New Perspectives on the Health of Canadians*. In 1986 the *Ottawa Charter* identified five action areas for health promotion, the fourth of which, "Building healthy public policy," called for "complementary approaches, including legislation, fiscal measures, taxation and organizational change. Health promotion policy requires the identification of obstacles to the adoption of healthy public policies in non-health sectors and the development of ways to remove them."

Since then, a tremendous amount of research has shown that health is influenced by a wide range of policies and interventions that go beyond health care. Interestingly, the Canadian Institute for Advanced Research estimates that only 25 percent of the health of the population is attributable to the health care system, while 15 percent is due to biology and genetic factors, 10 percent results from the physical environment, and 50 percent is attributable to the social and economic environments. Health can no longer be the sole responsibility of the ministers of health.

Throughout this volume there is a profound sense of frustration that despite the increasing discussions and evidence on the importance of dealing with the social determinants of health, Canadian public policy-makers have been embarrassingly resistant to these concepts.

I believe that as long as citizens think of the "sickness care system" whenever they hear the word "health," we are going to have real trouble in our efforts reorienting public policy to the social determinants of health. Surely the production of health through poverty elimination or workplace hazards reduction must fit side by side with a system mandated to operate emergency rooms and to reduce wait times for surgical services? Canadians must understand that upfront investment in the social determinants of health today will prevent larger amounts of money being spent on treatment and rehabilitation later on.

Dr. Halfan Mahler has said that "Health is politics," and that "If you want to move healthy public policies forward, you have to have political dynamite." SARS, Kashechewan, Hurricane Katrina, or the heat wave in France in 2004 that killed over 14,000 have been important teachable moments. I believe we have done a terrible job of explaining the "Pay now or pay a lot more later" economic arguments for investing in health of citizens. "A stitch in time saves nine," " penny-wise and pound foolish" are axioms we were all raised on. But the "tyranny of the acute" means that putting new drugs on the formulary and a new gamma knife for the world-class surgeon becomes the squeaky wheel and active measures on the social determinants of health take a back seat again and again. In Canada we have also suffered because the social determinants of health criss-cross many government departments and all jurisdictions. We have been unable to break through the gridlock of jurisdictional squabbles and vertical ministerial accountability for these complex challenges.

I think citizens do understand the social responsibility—health as a fundamental human need and therefore a basic human right and our moral obligation to do the right thing. But if they or a loved one are on a wait list, they expect their politicians to immediately respond and fix it. The medical model still rules.

There is no question that the political will to do the right thing dramatically improves with an educated public. Health literacy means that citizens can be pulling healthy public policy from their governments and politicians. I am a big believer in bottom-up solutions and the importance of improving the methodologies for true civic efficacy.

However, we have a formidable enemy in the sales department of modern media. Simple messages and simple solutions fit on a bumper sticker and in a seven-second sound bite. Every day I am reminded of the quote of H.L. Mencken: "For every complex human problem there is a neat simple solution, it's just that it's wrong." I believe that we must fiercely defend the complex solutions for the complex problems that are facing health and health care, but I believe we have to find simpler messages, plain language if we are going to have citizens onside.

The WHO Commission on Social Determinants of Health, which is headed by Sir Michael Marmot, is examining the "social determinants of health" and "health inequities," but he is now brilliantly talking about the causes and the "causes of the causes" that better explain the huge gaps in health outcomes.

Lately I have found that the following short health literacy quiz has been helpful in putting the public back into public health and replacing "health care" with "systems for health."

HEALTH 101
Do you think we should have
(a) strong fence at the top of the cliff or
(b) state-of-the-art fleet of ambulances and paramedics waiting at the bottom?

Would you prefer
(a) clean air or
(b) enough puffers and respirators for all?

Would you prefer that wait times be reduced by
(a) a falls program to reduce preventable hip fractures or
(b) private orthopaedic hospitals and more surgeons?

Should we invest in
(a) early learning, child care, literacy, the early identification of learning disabilities, and bullying programs or
(b) increase the budget for young offenders' incarceration?

Should we
(a) assume that the grey tsunami will bankrupt our health care system or
(b) include our aging population in the planning of strategies to keep them well?

Is the best approach to food security
(a) food banks and vouchers or
(b) income security, affordable housing, community gardens and community kitchens, and a national food policy?

Pick the one that is not correct:
Pandemic preparedness should focus on
• Tamiflu for all
• working with the vets to keep avian flu a disease of birds
• making sure people wash their hands, especially the doctors and nurses
• research on vaccines
• community care plans for our most vulnerable

Should governments boast about

(a) how much they spent on the sickness care system or

(b) the health of their citizens, leaving no one behind?

The profound structural change needed to secure investments in the social determinants of health in our complex federal system will occur only if we succeed in raising public awareness and developing political will. As you know, politicians tend to follow where the public goes, so helping the public understand the issues and demand change from governments will be crucial. For me, a major challenge in Canada is to make the public understand, believe, and take ownership that ill health, poverty, and social exclusion are unacceptable in one of the richest countries of the world. Progress toward a healthier world thus requires broad participation, sustained advocacy, and strong political action.

I firmly believe that this book provides an imperative for Canada to move from the description of the problem and the prescription of solutions to implementation of systematic and meaningful strategies and interventions to improve the health of our citizens and eliminate the inequity particularly among our First Peoples.

Population health is ultimately a question of what kind of society we wish to live in. The aim of population health is for human health to be seen as one of the most important overall objectives of public policy.

This is about advocacy, leadership, and action. It is about the civic literacy of putting health back into health care. Dennis Raphael has articulated a vision.

The other contributors have shown us that real solutions are out there in trenches. We need the political will to harvest those solutions into better public policy across government departments and across the squabbling jurisdictions.

I was there that Friday night in November 2002 at York University in Toronto for the opening of the conference "Social Determinants of Health across the Lifespan." I remember hearing John Frank and Dennis Raphael speaking so passionately about these things that seem so sensible and doable.

This book updates the progress to date in the scholarship and evidence of the interventions that can improve the overall health of the population and reduce health disparities, which will allow tens of thousands, and maybe even millions, of Canadians to lead longer lives in better health. This, in turn, will result in increased productivity because a healthy population is a major contributor to a vibrant economy, reduced expenditures on health and social problems, and overall social stability and well-being for Canadians. Perhaps even more importantly, a focus on interventions to deal with the social determinants of health will translate into a fairer and more equitable society.

Disraeli said that "The care of the public health is the first duty of a statesman." Unfortunately, in our present political system, statesmen, as defined by James Freeman Clarke, are rare: "A politician thinks of the next election, a statesman the next generation." If this book were compulsory reading for all elected officials and public servants, we could achieve not only a healthier, more equitable society but also the added dividend of more statesmen!

—Dr. Carolyn Bennett, MP, FCFP; assistant professor, Department of Family and Community Medicine, University of Toronto; Canada's first minister of state for public health, 2003–2006

FOREWORD
TO THE FIRST EDITION

One of the key points that I made in Building on Values: The Future of Health Care in Canada is that we have to set a national goal of making Canadians the healthiest people possible. One of the keys to achieving this goal is a greater emphasis on preventative health measures and improving population health outcomes.

Although I referenced this in my report, I will be the first to admit that even if all of my 47 recommendations are adopted, and even if they are implemented the way I would want them to be, it will only take us partway toward this goal.

A health care system—even the best health care system in the world—will be only one of the ingredients that determine whether your life will be long or short, healthy or sick, full of fulfillment, or empty with despair.

If we want Canadians to be the healthiest people in the world, we have to connect all of the dots that will take us there. To connect the dots, we have to know where they are. Those who have contributed to this volume have added valuable perspectives in this regard as they connect research and ideas on the social determinants of health to the health outcomes we seek as a nation.

Healthy lifestyle choices may be important and vital—and they are. A comprehensive, responsive, and accountable national health care system may be important and vital—and it is.

But the main factors—the main "determinants," as the experts call them—that will likely shape our health and lifespan are the ones that affect society as a whole. And if we want Canadians to be the healthiest people in the world, we have to deal with them at that level.

The editor of this text, Dr. Raphael, has gathered together some of Canada's important thinkers on the key determinants. This volume provides the latest research and ideas regarding income distribution; the importance of a healthy workplace; the critical role that early childhood education, and public education generally, plays in the life-cycle process; the importance of food and shelter; and the importance of belonging reinforced by various views of social inclusion.

I noted recently that our policy-making and program-developing mechanisms in Canada are suffering from what I call "hardening of the categories." Something useful is proffered by one government department with the intended gains stifled by something counterproductive in another department.

Our policy-making processes need to be integrated and integrating. We need to move from an illness model to a wellness paradigm that connects the dots of all of the factors that contribute to health for individuals and society at large.

Even if we make great strides to improve our systems of health care in Canada, our genuine gains in health will be hindered unless we pay serious attention to the other determinants of health. At present, there are too many children going to school and to bed hungry, too many people living on our urban streets, an increasing number of working poor, and too many people feeling like they are on the outside looking in when it comes to decision making in our communities.

How important is it that we think in new ways?

Historians and health experts tell us that we have had two great revolutions in the course of public health. The first was the control of infectious diseases, notwithstanding our current challenges. The second was the battle against non-communicable diseases.

The third great revolution is about moving from an illness model to all of those things that both prevent illness and promote a holistic sense of well-being.

In my view, the wellness model needs to be informed:

- by inspired leaders who genuinely share power with those less fortunate
- by a commitment to social inclusion and civil society that provides opportunities for all Canadians to participate in the things that count in our neighbourhoods across this great country

- by an understanding that hopelessness kills and hopefulness with opportunity is a prescription for good health

That's my kind of revolution. It's the kind that will ensure that Canadians are the healthiest people we can be. It's also the kind of revolution that understands that the exceptional health we seek, and how we achieve it, can provide a Canadian model for the world to emulate.

Social Determinants of Health provides a rich companion to our work on health care and a useful springboard for integrated healthy public policy.

—The Honourable Roy J. Romanow, PC
Saskatoon
February 2004

PREFACE

This volume updates and extends the analysis of the state of various social determinants of health in Canada contained in the 1st edition of *Social Determinants of Health: Canadian Perspectives.* This work represents a unique undertaking in the social determinants of health area as it brings together scholarship by those working in early childhood education and care, education and literacy, employment and working conditions, food security, gender, health services, housing, income and its distribution, social exclusion, the social safety net, and unemployment and job insecurity with work by those specifically focused on the health effects of these issues.

The 1st edition of *Social Determinants of Health: Canadian Perspectives* aimed to foster communication between those concerned with the current state of various social determinants of health and those knowledgeable about their health effects. Clearly the work contributed to this goal. The close to 8,000 copies of the work sold reached a wide range of sectors both inside and outside of academia. It contributed to the increasing diffusion of the social determinants of health concept into discussion of a wide range of issues. It is now common to find mention of the health-related effects of lack of child care, continuing income, housing, and food insecurity, inadequate social and health services, and other social determinants of health in a wide range of documents, reports, and related advocacy efforts.

The social determinants of health concept has been taken up by pioneering public health units across Canada striving to shift the discussion of health away from biomedical and behavioural risks toward emphasizing living conditions as the primary determinants of individual and population health. United Ways of Canada, Social Planning Councils, and numerous other agencies concerned with striving to improve the quality of life of

Canadians now draw upon the social determinants of health concept in their activities.

Yet for all of this increased discussion of the social determinants of health concept, there is precious little to show of its effects upon the development of public policy in Canada. There is little evidence that policy-makers draw upon these concepts and related research findings to create health-promoting public policy. Media coverage of health issues continues to be dominated by biomedical and behavioural approaches and, not surprisingly, public understandings of the determinants of health mirror these preoccupations. Clearly there is a continuing need to present the social determinants of health message.

The 2nd edition continues to raise these issues. There is greater attention paid to the ideological barriers to having these issues addressed by those working in the health field and the makers of public policy. In addition to the updating of the material presented in the chapter, new or newly authored chapters focus on:

- the pathways and mechanisms that explain how social determinants of health come to shape health
- early childhood and how a range of factors shape children's health
- the complexity of Aboriginal health and its determinants
- the health care system and how it serves as a social determinant of health
- public policy and the social safety net
- public policy and gender

As before, the aim of *Social Determinants of Health: Canadian Perspectives* is to promote more accurate public understandings and more mature public policy-making in the support of health. These have clearly proven to be difficult tasks to accomplish in Canada. This has not been the case in many other nations. It is reassuring, though frustrating, to note that the social determinants of health concept has taken root and been nurtured in many European nations such that public policy in the service of health is increasingly common. Hopefully, this volume will help to narrow the gap between Canadian action on the social determinants of health and those seen in other nations.

—Dennis Raphael
August 2008

A Note
from the Publisher

Thank you for selecting the 2nd edition of *Social Determinants of Health: Canadian Perspectives,* edited by Dennis Raphael. The editor, contributors, and publisher have devoted considerable time and careful development (including meticulous peer reviews) to this book. We appreciate your recognition of this effort and accomplishment.

This volume distinguishes itself on the market in many ways. One key feature is the book's well-written and comprehensive part openers, which help to make the chapter all the more accessible to both general readers and undergraduate students. The part openers add cohesion to the section and to the whole book. The themes of the book are very clearly presented in these section openers.

Each chapter contains the following structure: a formal introduction and conclusion, critical thinking questions, annotated recommended readings, annotated related Web sites, as well as references, which are consolidated at the back of the book.

Part One

Introducing the
Social Determinants of Health

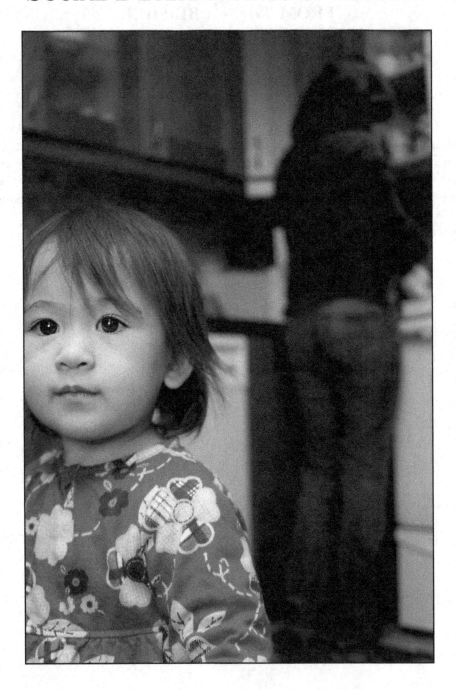

There is increasing recognition that the mainsprings of health are to be found in the manner in which societies are organized and resources distributed among the population. The concept of the social determinants of health is an illustration of how thinking is moving beyond a medical model and lifestyle approaches to understanding health and the means by which it can be maintained. In the medical model of health, the body is seen as a machine that is either running well or in need of repair. If the body is free of illness, the person is healthy. If it is either infected with pathogens or afflicted with system- or organ-malfunctioning disease, illness occurs. The remedy for such disease and illness is found in medical or curative care, which is located in the health care system and administered by doctors and nurses.

In the lifestyle model of health, the causes of disease are to be found in individuals' "unhealthy choices," such as diets lacking in fruits and vegetables, sedentary behaviours, or partaking of alcohol or tobacco. The remedy for these poor choices are health education, exhortations for individuals to change their behaviours, and even environmental adjustments (e.g., sin taxes, smoking and alcohol bans, etc.) to make the "healthy choice, the easy choice." Despite an extensive body of evidence that indicates that biomedical and behavioural indicators are rather poor indicators of health status as compared to the living conditions individuals experience, allocation of government spending to the health care system, research activities, and disease foundations reflect strong commitment to the medical and lifestyle approaches to health. The preoccupation of the public, the media, and governments with the medical and lifestyle approaches to health ensures that broader concerns with living conditions usually receive less attention.

In Chapter 1, **Dennis Raphael** defines and identifies the social determinants of health. He provides a brief history of the concept and an overview of Canadian evidence that indicates that living conditions—rather than biomedical and lifestyle indicators—related to the distribution of income, the provision of housing and food security, and the security of employment and quality of working conditions are the primary determinants of health. These social determinants of health help to explain how improvements in health status among Canadians over the past century came about, why there are important differences in health status among Canadians, and why Canadians are healthier than Americans, but less healthy than citizens of the nations of northern Europe. Raphael then identifies some key emerging themes that help inform the content of the chapters that follow.

In Chapter 2, **Dennis Raphael** discusses the latest research on how the social determinants of health come to be related to the health of individuals, communities, and entire jurisdictions. The chapter considers a variety of models of how living conditions come to "get under the skin" to shape health. These models include what are called materialist, psychosocial comparison, and neo-materialist approaches. How the social determinants of health influence health are also assessed by applying models of physiological and psychological processes that examine how the social determinants of health shape health. To understand how inequalities in the quality of the social determinants of healthy people experience come about and how these unequal experiences come to influence health, models of political economy are presented that identify the economic and political forces that shape these unequal distributions of social determinants.

Chapter 1

———————

SOCIAL DETERMINANTS OF HEALTH: AN OVERVIEW OF KEY ISSUES AND THEMES

Dennis Raphael

Introduction

Social determinants of health are the economic and social conditions that shape the health of individuals, communities, and jurisdictions as a whole. Social determinants of health are the primary determinants of whether individuals stay healthy or become ill (a narrow definition of health). Social determinants of health also determine the extent to which a person possesses the physical, social, and personal resources to identify and achieve personal aspirations, satisfy needs, and cope with the environment (a broader definition of health). Social determinants of health are about the quantity and quality of a variety of resources that a society makes available to its members.

These resources include, but are not limited to, conditions of childhood, income, availability and quality of education, food, housing, employment, working conditions, and health and social services. An emphasis upon societal conditions as determinants of health contrasts with the traditional health sciences and public health focus upon biomedical and behavioural risk factors such as cholesterol levels, body weight, physical activity, diet, and tobacco and alcohol use. Since a social determinants of health approach sees the mainsprings of health as being how a society organizes and distributes economic and social resources, it directs attention to economic and social policies as means of improving it. It also requires consideration of the political, economic, and social forces that shape policy decisions.

Concern with the social determinants of health is not new. It has been known since the mid-19th century that living conditions are the primary determinants of health (Engels, 1845/1987; Virchow, 1848/1985). And since then hundreds of studies have demonstrated that the material and social circumstances to which people in developed nations such as Canada are exposed to in their homes, workplaces, and communities are far more important to their health than so-called "lifestyle choices" such as using tobacco or alcohol, eating fruits and vegetables, or partaking in physical activity (Nettleton, 1997; Tesh, 1990). These findings have not been lost upon the writers of Canadian government and public health documents. Since the mid-1970s Canadian governmental and public health agencies have produced numerous statements and policy documents that have contributed to health promotion efforts worldwide. In large part, Canada's reputation as a "health-promotion powerhouse" comes from the high quality of the concepts and ideas contained within these documents (O'Neill, Pederson, Dupéré & Rootman, 2007).

Nevertheless, even a cursory examination of prevailing governmental and public health activities focused on actually promoting health—as opposed to documents talking about promoting health—sees little evidence that applications of these concepts have been made in practice (Raphael, 2007a). The profound gap between Canadian health promotion word and deed is documented (Canadian Population Health Initiative,

2002). Instead of efforts to improve Canadians' living conditions, individualized approaches focused on biomedical and behavioural risk factors—with some exceptions—dominate governmental, public health, disease association, and other health-promotion efforts (Raphael & Bryant, 2006b).

When living conditions are considered by these health authorities, it is usually to identify those Canadians whose living conditions are said to put them at risk for making "unhealthy lifestyle choices" rather than urging governmental authorities to improve their living circumstances. Rather than improving the primary determinants of health—the adverse living conditions people are subjected to—activities focus on targeting the victims of these adverse living conditions for behaviour change. This is the case even though health behaviours are known to be rather less important determinants of health. The effect of all this is to add insult—victim blaming—to injury—the experience of deprived living conditions (Raphael, 2002).

Not surprisingly, public understandings of the determinants of health mirror these activities (Canadian Population Health Initiative, 2004). Surveys show that Canadians have little awareness of the important role that living conditions play in determining health (Eyles et al., 2001; Paisley, Midgett, Brunetti & Tomasik, 2001). The mass media reinforces these understandings through its uncritical reporting of any and all studies of how a particular gene or behaviour (e.g., drinking coffee or white wine, eating peanuts, consuming tomatoes, sleeping more than or less than eight hours a night, watching too much TV, or playing computer games, etc.) either protects from, or predicts, some dire medical condition (Gasher et al., 2007; Hayes et al., 2007).

That these findings may be weak and contradictory to findings reported a week or two earlier does little to slow these reporting onslaughts (Davey Smith & Ebrahim, 2001). Therefore, this volume has two rather daunting tasks: (1) to counter the understandings Canadians hold concerning the determinants of health; and (2) to provide support for efforts to improve the quality of the social determinants of health through the development of health-promoting public policies.

In this chapter, I review the social determinants of health concept and present recent theoretical developments and empirical findings. I provide the rationale for selecting the social determinants of health included in the volume and explore a number of key themes in the field. Throughout this presentation the social determinants of health approach is contrasted with the traditional approach to disease prevention focused on biomedical and behavioural risk factors. I conclude by asking the reader to consider how Canadians' understandings concerning the determinants of health and current Canadian policy environments affect both the quality of these social determinants of Canadians' health and Canadian policy-makers' receptivity to the ideas contained within this volume.

An Historical Perspective on the Social Determinants of Health

During the mid-1800s political economist Friedrich Engels studied how poor housing, clothing, diet, and lack of sanitation led directly to the infections and diseases associated with early death among working people in England. Engels identified material living conditions, day-to-day stress, and the adoption of health-threatening behaviours as the primary contributors to social class differences in health (Engels, 1845/1987).

> All conceivable evils are heaped upon the poor.... They are given damp dwellings, cellar dens that are not waterproof from below or garrets that leak from above.... They are supplied bad, tattered, or rotten clothing, adulterated and indigestible food. They are exposed to the most exciting changes of mental condition, the most violent vibrations between hope and fear.... They are deprived of all enjoyments except sexual indulgence and drunkenness and are worked every day to the point of complete exhaustion of their mental and physical energies.... (Engels, 1845/1987, p. 129)

Around the same time, Rudolf Virchow (1848/1985) identified how health-threatening living conditions were rooted in public policy-making and emphasized the role that politics played in promoting health and preventing disease (see Box 1.1) These issues never completely disappeared from public health preoccupations, but over

---

Box 1.1: Rudolf Virchow and the social determinants of health

---

German physician Rudolf Virchow's (1821–1902) medical discoveries were so extensive that he is known as the "Father of Modern Pathology." But he was also a trailblazer in identifying how societal policies determine health. In 1848, Virchow was sent by the Berlin authorities to investigate the epidemic of typhus in Upper Silesia. His *Report on the Typhus epidemic prevailing in Upper Silesia* argued that lack of democracy, feudalism, and unfair tax policies in the province were the primary determinants of the inhabitants' poor living conditions, inadequate diet, and poor hygiene that fuelled the epidemic.

Virchow stated that *Disease is not something personal and special, but only a manifestation of life under modified (pathological) conditions.* Arguing *Medicine is a social science and politics is nothing else but medicine on a large scale,* Virchow drew the direct links between social conditions and health. He argued that improved health required recognition that: *If medicine is to fulfil her great task, then she must enter the political and social life. Do we not always find the diseases of the populace traceable to defects in society?* (Virchow, 1848/1985).

The authorities were not happy with the report and Virchow was relieved of his government position. But he continued his pathology research within university settings and went on to a parallel career as a member of Berlin City Council and the Prussian Diet, where he focused on public health issues consistent with his Upper Silesia report. Virchow also bitterly opposed Otto Von Bismarck's plans for national rearmament and was challenged to a duel by said gentleman. Virchow declined participation.

---

the past 30 years have received rather less emphases than biomedical and behavioural approaches to health promotion and disease prevention (Raphael, 2001a).

British Contributions

The 1980 publication of the Black Report and the 1992 publication of the *Health Divide* (Townsend et al., 1992) sparked interest in how social conditions shape health. These UK reports described how lowest employment-level groups showed a greater likelihood of suffering from a wide range of diseases and dying prematurely from illness or injury at every stage of the life cycle. Additionally, health differences occurred in a step-wise progression across the socio-economic range with professionals having the best health and manual labourers the worst. Skilled workers' health was midway between the extremes. These health differences emerged even though the UK had developed a universally accessible health care system at the end of the Second World War. These two reports—and the many that have followed up on these themes—stimulated the study of health inequalities, and the factors that determine these inequalities and directed attention to the role that public policy plays in either increasing or reducing health inequalities (Acheson, 1998; Benzeval, Judge

& Whitehead, 1995; Gordon, Shaw, Dorling & Davey Smith, 1999; Pantazis & Gordon, 2000).

Health inequalities and the social determinants of these inequalities continue as active areas of inquiry among British researchers (Benzeval et al., 1995; Gordon, 2000; Graham, 2004a; Shaw, Dorling, Gordon & Smith, 1999). These studies frequently focus on inequalities in health among members of different employment strata with recognition that membership in such groups is strongly correlated with income and education levels. British researchers also study the health effects of poverty and how indicators of disadvantage cluster together (Gordon & Townsend, 2000; Pantazis, Gordon & Levitas, 2006). Much of the available data on the links between social determinants of health and health status are British, as are some of the best theorizations of how these factors influence health across the lifespan. The UK is also the source of many ideas on how to apply these findings to promote health (Benzeval et al., 1995; Graham, 2004b).

Canadian Contributions

Canadians have actively theorized the relationship between economic and social conditions and health. In 1974 the federal government's *A New Perspective on the Health of Canadians* identified human biology, environment, lifestyle, and health care organization as determinants of health (Lalonde, 1974). The document was important in outlining determinants of health outside of the health care system.

Another Canadian government document, *Achieving Health for All: A Framework for Health Promotion*, outlined reducing inequities between income groups as an important goal of government policy (Epp, 1986). This would be accomplished by implementing policies in support of health in the areas of income security, employment, education, housing, business, agriculture, transportation, justice, and technology, among others. Health Canada's *Taking Action on Population Health: A Position Paper for Health Promotion and Programs Branch Staff* states that:

> There is strong evidence indicating that factors outside the health care system significantly affect health. These "determinants of health" include income and social status, social support networks, education, employment and working conditions, physical environments, social environments, biology and genetic endowment, personal health practices and coping skills, healthy child development, health services, gender and culture. (Health Canada, 1998, p. 1)

Canadian Public Health Association (CPHA) documents tell a similar story. In 1986, its *Action Statement for Health Promotion in Canada* identified advocating for healthy public policies as the single best strategy to affect the determinants of health (Canadian Public Health Association, 1996). Priority actions included reducing inequalities in income and wealth, and strengthening communities through local alliances to change unhealthy living conditions. In 2000, the CPHA endorsed an action plan that recognized poverty's profound influence upon health and identified means to reduce it (Canadian Public Health Association, 2000). Other CPHA reports document the health effects of unemployment, income insecurity, homelessness, and general economic conditions (Canadian Public Health Association, 2001).

The study of the social determinants of health therefore deals with two key problems:

1. What are the societal factors (e.g., income, education, employment conditions, etc.) that shape health and help explain health inequalities?
2. What are the societal forces (e.g., economic, social, and political) that shape the quality of these societal factors?

The next section presents various frameworks for considering the social determinants of health.

What Exactly Are the Social Determinants of Health?

The term "social determinants of health" appears to have grown out of researchers' attempts to identify the specific exposures by which members of different socio-economic groups come to experience varying levels of health status. While it was well documented that individuals in various socio-economic groups experienced differing health outcomes, the specific factors and means by which these factors led to illness remained to be identified.

The term "social determinants of health" made its debut in the 1996 volume *Health and Social Organization: Towards a Health Policy for the 21st Century* (Blane, Brunner & Wilkinson, 1996). In the chapter "Social Determinants of Health: The Sociobiological Translation," Tarlov took the environment health field from the Lalonde Report—the others being biology and genes, health care, and lifestyle—and fleshed out these environmental determinants of health (Tarlov, 1996). In his model, inequalities in the quality of social determinants of housing, education, social acceptance, employment, and income become translated into disease-related processes through individuals comparing themselves unfavourably to others. The World Health Organization followed this work up with its *Social Determinants of Health: The Solid Facts* document (Wilkinson & Marmot, 2003).

The relevance of the social determinants of health was also indicated by attempts to explain how nations come to differ in overall population health. As one illustration, the health of Americans compares poorly to the health of citizens in most other industrialized nations (Raphael, 2007b). This is the case for life expectancy, infant mortality, and death by childhood injury despite the US's overall greater wealth. In contrast, the population health of Sweden is generally superior to most other nations (Burstrom, Diderichsen, Ostlin & Ostergren, 2002). Could the same social determinants of health that explain health differences *within* national populations explain health differences seen *among* national populations? And why would nations differ so much in terms of the quality of the social determinants of health experienced by their citizens?

Current Concepts of the Social Determinants of Health

There are a variety of contemporary approaches to social determinants of health. The commonalities among these are particularly illuminative.

The *Ottawa Charter for Health Promotion* identifies the "prerequisites for health" as peace, shelter, education, food, income, a stable ecosystem, sustainable resources, social justice, and equity (World Health Organization, 1986). These prerequisites of health are concerned with structural aspects of society and the organization and distribution of economic and social resources. In 1992, Dahlgren and Whitehead formulated their rainbow model of health determinants, in which the "living and working conditions" arch identified agriculture and food production, education, work environment, unemployment, water and sanitation, health care services, and housing as contributors to health (Dahlgren & Whitehead, 1992).

Health Canada outlines various determinants of health—many of which are social determinants—of income and social status, social support networks, education, employment and working conditions, physical and social environments, biology and genetic endowment, personal health practices and coping skills, healthy child development, health services, gender, and culture (Health Canada, 1998). These determinants were adapted from work done by the Canadian Institute for Advanced Research (Evans, Barer & Marmor, 1994). Within this framework, the specific concepts of physical and social environments can be criticized for lacking grounding in concrete experiences of people's lives and lacking policy relevance—i.e., there usually is no Ministry of Physical Environments or Ministry of Social Environments. There is also evidence that these terms have little meaning for Canadians and for policy-makers (Bryant et al., 2004).

A British working group charged with specifying the social determinants of health identified the social [class health] gradient, stress, early life, social exclusion, work, unemployment, social support, addiction, food, and transport (Wilkinson & Marmot, 2003). This listing is more grounded in the everyday experience of people's lives and policy-making structures and avoids the potential problem of policy irrelevance. Indeed, the stimulus for this work was the European Office of the World Health Organization aiming to raise these issues among policy-makers and the public. Finally, the US Centers for Disease Control and Prevention highlights social determinants of health of socio-economic status, transportation, housing, access to services, discrimination by social grouping (e.g., race, gender, or class), and social or environmental stressors (Centers for Disease Control and Prevention, 2006).

Origins of the Canadian Social Determinants of Health Conference and This Volume

As I became more familiar with the social determinants of health field, my surprise grew at Canada's shortcomings in researching and addressing these important issues. As noted, numerous studies indicated that various social determinants of health have far greater influence on health and the incidence of illness than traditional biomedical and behavioural risk factors. Additionally, scholarship on the state and quality of various social determinants of health in Canada had been finding their quality to be deteriorating (Federation of Canadian Municipalities, 1999, 2001, 2003, 2004a, 2004b). Yet for the most part, policy-makers, the media, and the general public remained badly informed concerning these issues. Indeed, it appears at times—especially during the retrenchments in public policy that began during the late 1980s—that much of the public policy agenda seems designed to threaten rather than support the health of Canadians by weakening the quality of many social determinants of health (Raphael, 2001d; Raphael & Bryant, 2006a).

These concerns about the neglect of the social determinants of health led to my applying (through York University's School of Health Policy and Management) to Health Canada's Policy Research Program for funding to organize a national conference entitled "Social Determinants of Health across the Lifespan: A Current Accounting and Policy Implications." The purpose of the conference was to: (1) consider the state of several key social determinants of health across Canada; (2) explore the implications of these conditions for the health of Canadians; and (3) outline policy directions to strengthen these social determinants of health. The York University "Social Determinants of Health across the Lifespan" conference was organized around a synthesis that identified 12 key social determinants of health especially relevant to Canadians (see Box 1.2). Four criteria were used to identify these social determinants of health.

The first criterion was that the social determinant be consistent with most existing formulations of the social determinants of health and associated with an existing empirical literature as to its relevance to health. *All these social determinants of health are important to the health of Canadians.*

The second criterion was that the social determinant of health be consistent with lay/public understandings of the factors that influence health and well-being. This was ascertained through assessment of available empirical work on Canadians' understandings of what aspects of Canadian life contribute to health and well-being. *All these social determinants of health are understandable to Canadians.*

The third criterion was that the social determinant of health be clearly aligned with existing governmental structures and policy frameworks (e.g., ministries of education, housing, labour, Native affairs, women's issues, etc.). *All these social determinants of health have clear policy relevance to Canadian decision makers and citizens.*

The fourth criterion was that the social determinant of health be an area of either active governmental policy activity (e.g., health care services, education) or policy inactivity that have provoked sustained criticism (e.g., food security, housing, social safety net, etc.). *All these social determinants of health are especially timely and relevant.*

The inclusion of health services, the social safety net, and Aboriginal status as social determinants of health is not common to most conceptualizations. Health services are included in the belief that a well-organized and rationalized health care system could be an important

social determinant of health—if this is not currently the case. The social safety net is increasingly recognized as an important determinant of the health of populations, but to date has not been explicitly included in most formulations. Aboriginal status is another social determinant of health that is not explicitly explored in most conceptualizations of the social determinants of health. It represents the interaction of culture, public policy, and the mechanisms by which systematic exclusion from participation in Canadian life profoundly affects health. Gender and how its meaning is constructed within Canadian society is an important social determinant of health. It interacts with all other social determinants of health to influence the health and well-being of Canadians.

As a result of that conference, the profile of the social determinants of health was raised across Canada. One outcome was the 1st edition of *Social Determinants of Health: Canadian Perspectives* (Raphael, 2004). The second was the drafting and ratification of the *Toronto Charter on the Social Determinants of Health* (Raphael, Bryant & Curry-Stevens, 2004). The third was the establishment of a "Social Determinants of Health" listserv based at York University in Canada. Five years have passed since the 1st edition appeared and new insights have arisen concerning the social determinants of health and the barriers to their influencing public policy

---

Box 1.2: The social determinants of health framework

The 12 social determinants of health identified by the organizers of the York University conference form the basis for the content of this volume. These are:

- Aboriginal status
- early life
- education
- employment and working conditions
- food security
- gender
- health care services
- housing
- income and its distribution
- social safety net
- social exclusion
- unemployment and employment security

in the service of health. This volume updates and expands upon the findings presented in that volume and provides some of these insights.

Current Themes in the Social Determinants of Health Field

Five themes inform the presentation and understanding of the material in this volume: (1) empirical evidence concerning the social determinants of health; (2) mechanisms and pathways by which social determinants of health influence health; (3) the importance of a life-course perspective; (4) the role that policy environments play in determining the quality of the social determinants of health within jurisdictions; and (5) the role that political ideology plays in shaping state and societal receptivity to social determinants of health concepts. Each is considered in turn.

Theme 1: Empirical Evidence of the Importance of the Social Determinants of Health

Much of this volume is concerned with presenting the empirical evidence of how social determinants of health shape health. From an overall perspective, the quality of various social determinants of health to which citizens are exposed provides explanations for: (1) improvement in health status among Canadians over the past 100 years; (2) persistent differences in health status among Canadians; and (3) differences in overall health status among Canada and other developed nations.

The Social Determinants of Improved Health among Canadians Since 1900

Profound improvements in health status have occurred in industrialized nations such as Canada since 1900. It has been hypothesized that access to improved medical care is responsible for these differences, but best estimates are that only 10–15 percent of increased longevity since 1900 is due to improved health care (McKinlay & McKinlay, 1987). As one illustration, the advent of vaccines and medical treatments are usually held responsible for the profound declines in mortality from infectious diseases in Canada since 1900. But by the time vaccines for diseases such as measles, influenza, and polio and treatments for scarlet fever, typhoid, and diphtheria appeared, dramatic declines in mortality had already occurred.

Improvements in behaviour (e.g., reductions in tobacco use, changes in diet, etc.) have also been hypothesized as responsible for improved longevity, but most analysts conclude that improvements in health are due to the improving material conditions of everyday life experienced by Canadians since 1900 (McKeown, 1976; McKeown & Record, 1975). These improvements occurred in the areas of early childhood, education, food processing and availability, health and social services, housing, employment security and working conditions, and every other social determinant of health. Much of the current volume is concerned with the present state of these social determinants of health and how they shape the health status of Canadians. Particularly important is the question of how recent policy decisions are either improving or weakening the quality of these social determinants of health.

The Social Determinants of Health Inequalities among Canadians

Despite dramatic improvements in health in general, significant inequalities in health among Canadians persist (Health Canada, 1999; Wilkins, Berthelot & Ng, 2002). Access to essential medical procedures is guaranteed by medicare in Canada. Nevertheless, access issues are common and this is particularly the case with regard to required prescription medicines where income is a strong determinant of such access (Raphael, 2007d). It is believed, however, that health care issues account for a relatively small proportion of health status differences among Canadians (Siddiqi & Hertzman, 2007). As for differences in health behaviours (e.g., tobacco and alcohol use, diet, and physical activity), studies from as early as the mid-1970s—reinforced by many more studies since then—find their impact upon health to be less important than social determinants of health such as income and others examined in this volume (Raphael, 2007a).

Evidence indicates that health differences among Canadians result primarily from experiences of qualitatively different environments associated with the social determinants of health. As just one example, an overview of the magnitude of differences in health that are related to the social determinant of health of income is provided. Income is especially important as it serves as a marker of different experiences with many social determinants of health (Raphael, Macdonald et al., 2004).

Income is a determinant of health in itself, but it is also a determinant of the quality of early life, education, employment and working conditions, and food security. Income also is a determinant of the quality of housing, need for a social safety net, the experience of social exclusion, and the experience of unemployment and employment insecurity across the lifespan. Also, a key aspect of Aboriginal life and the experience of women in Canada is their greater likelihood of living under conditions of low income (Raphael, 2007e).

Income is a prime determinant of Canadians' premature years of life lost and premature mortality from a range of diseases (see Box 1.3). Numerous studies indicate that income levels during early childhood, adolescence, and adulthood are all independent predictors of who develops and eventually succumbs to disease (Davey Smith, 2003).

This is also the case in Canada. Income is an exceedingly good predictor of incidence and mortality from a variety of diseases. About 23 percent of excess premature years of life lost can be attributed to income differences among Canadians (see Figure 1.1). The figure of 23 percent in Figure 1.1 is calculated by using the mortality rates in the wealthiest quintile

---

Box 1.3: Statistics Canada study of income-related premature mortality

In Canada, data on individuals' income and social status are not routinely collected at death, so national examination of the relationship between income and mortality from various diseases uses census tract of residence to estimate individuals' income. There is potential for error in these analyses that relate income to death based on residential area, since some low income people live in well-off neighbourhoods and vice versa. Essentially, these analyses are conservative estimates of the relationship between income level and death rates. The most recent available data shows that in 1996, Canadians living within the poorest 20% of urban neighbourhoods were more likely to die from cardiovascular disease, cancer, diabetes, and respiratory diseases—among other diseases—than other Canadians (Wilkins et al., 2002).

Figure 1.1 shows the percentage of premature years of life lost in urban Canada than can be attributed to various diseases and to income differences. Cancers are the leading cause of premature years of life lost accounting for 31% of these. Injuries and circulatory diseases (heart disease and stroke) are also leading causes of premature years of life lost. However, the percentage of premature years of life lost that can be attributed to income differences among Canadians is also very high at 23%, a magnitude that is greater than all years lost to either injuries or circulatory disease and approaching the level of cancers.

Figure 1.1: Percentage of premature years of life lost (0–74 years) to Canadians in urban Canada due to various causes, 1996

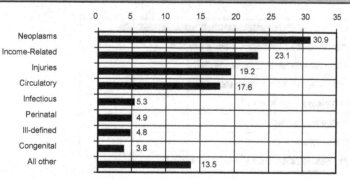

Source: "Percentage of premature years of life lost (0–74 yrs) to Canadians in urban Canada due to various causes, 1996," adapted from the Statistics Canada publication "Health reports—supplement," Catalogue 82-003, Volume 13, *2002 Annual Report*, Chart 9, p. 54.

of neighbourhoods as a baseline and considering all deaths above that rate to be "excess" related to income differences. Therefore, 23 percent of all of the premature years of life lost to Canadians can be accounted for by differences among wealthy, middle- and low-income Canadians (Wilkins et al., 2002).

What are the diseases that differentially kill people of varying income levels? Income-related premature years of life lost are focused upon specific diseases. As shown in Figure 1.2, the diseases most related to income differences in mortality among Canadians are heart disease and stroke. Importantly, premature death by injuries, cancers, infectious disease, and others are all strongly related to income differences among Canadians.

In 2002, Statistics Canada examined the predictors of life expectancy, disability-free life expectancy, and the presence of fair or poor health among residents of 136 regions across Canada (Shields & Tremblay, 2002). The predictors employed included socio-demographic factors (the proportion of Aboriginal population, the proportion of visible minority population, the unemployment rate, population size, percentage of population aged 65 or over, average income, and average number of years of schooling). Also considered in the analysis were the daily smoking rate, obesity rate, infrequent exercise rate, heavy drinking rate, high stress rate, and depression rate. Table 1.1 shows the proportion of variation (the total is

100 percent) in health outcomes explained by each of these predictors. Consistent with most other research, behavioural risk factors are rather weak predictors of health status as compared to socio-economic and demographic measures of which income is a major component (Diez-Roux, Link & Northridge, 2000; Lantz et al., 1998; Roux, Merkin & Arnett, 2001).

These differences in premature mortality are mirrored in the greater incidence of just about every affliction that Canadians experience. This is especially the case for chronic diseases such as heart disease and stroke, diabetes, cancers, as well as injuries and infectious diseases (Wilkins et al., 2002). Indeed, the incidence of, and mortality from, heart disease and stroke, and adult-onset of type 2 diabetes are especially good examples of the importance of the social determinants of health (Raphael, Anstice & Raine, 2003; Raphael & Farrell, 2002). While governments, medical researchers, and public health workers emphasize traditional adult risk factors (e.g., cholesterol levels, diet, physical inactivity, and tobacco and alcohol use), it is well established that these are relatively poor predictors of heart disease, stroke, and type 2 diabetes rates among populations. The factors making a difference are living under conditions of material deprivation as children and adults, stress associated with such conditions, and the adoption of health-threatening behaviours as means of coping with these difficult circumstances. In fact, difficult

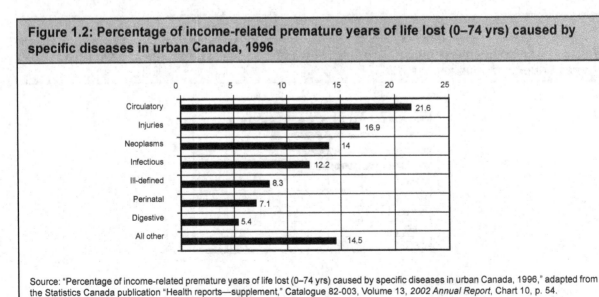

Figure 1.2: Percentage of income-related premature years of life lost (0–74 yrs) caused by specific diseases in urban Canada, 1996

Disease	Percentage
Circulatory	21.6
Injuries	16.9
Neoplasms	14
Infectious	12.2
Ill-defined	8.3
Perinatal	7.1
Digestive	5.4
All other	14.5

Source: "Percentage of income-related premature years of life lost (0–74 yrs) caused by specific diseases in urban Canada, 1996," adapted from the Statistics Canada publication "Health reports—supplement," Catalogue 82-003, Volume 13, *2002 Annual Report*, Chart 10, p. 54.

Table 1.1: Proportion of variation in life expectancy, disability-free life expectancy, and proportion of citizens reporting fair or poor health explained by different factors at the health region level in Canada (total variation for each outcome measure = 100%)

Predictors	Life expectancy	Disability-free life expectancy	Fair or poor health
Socio-demographic factors only	56%	32%	25%
Additional variation predicted by:			
Daily smoking rate	8%	6%	4%
Obesity rate	1%	5%	10%
Infrequent exercise rate	0%	3%	0%
Heavy drinking rate	1%	3%	1%
High stress rate	0%	0%	1%
Depression rate	0%	8%	9%

Source: Shields, M. and Tremblay, S. (2002), "The health of Canada's communities," *Health reports—supplement* 13 (July), p. 13.

living circumstances during childhood are especially good predictors of these diseases (Barker, Osmond & Simmonds, 1989; Davey Smith & Hart, 2002; Eriksson et al., 1999).

In addition to predicting adult incidence and death from disease, income differences—and the other social determinants of health related to income—are also related to the health of Canadian children and youth. Canadian children living in low-income families are more likely to experience greater incidence of a variety of illnesses, hospital stays, accidental injuries, mental health problems, lower school achievement and early dropout, family violence and child abuse, among others (Canadian Institute on Children's Health, 2000). In fact, low-income children show higher incidences of just about any health-, social-, or education-related problem however defined. These differences in problem incidence occur across the income range, but are most concentrated among low-income children (Ross & Roberts, 1999; Ross, Roberts & Scott, 2000).

The Social Determinants of Health Differences between Nations

Profound differences in overall health status exist between developed and developing nations. Much of this has to do with the lack of the basic necessities of life (food, water, sanitation, primary health care, etc.) common to developing nations. Yet among developed nations such as Canada, less profound but still highly significant differences in health status indicators such as life expectancy, infant mortality, incidence of disease, and death from injuries exist. An excellent example is comparison of health status differences and the hypothesized social determinants of these health status differences among Canada, the United States, and Sweden.

Table 1.2 shows how Canada, the US, and Sweden fare on a number of social determinants of health and indicators of population health. Scholarship has noted that the US takes an especially *laissez-faire* approach to providing various forms of security (employment, food, income, and housing) and health and social services, while Sweden's welfare state makes extraordinary efforts to provide security and services (Burstrom et al., 2002; Raphael & Bryant, 2006b). The sources of these differences in public policy appear to be in differing commitments to citizen support informed by the political ideologies of governing parties within each nation (Bambra, 2004; Navarro & Shi, 2002).

Emerging scholarship is specifically focused on how national approaches to security provision to citizens

Table 1.2: USA, Canada, and Sweden rankings on selected social determinants of health and indicators of population health in comparison to other industrialized nations (2000–2002)

	(Ranking, 1 is best)		
Measure	USA	Canada	Sweden
% in child poverty	22 of 23	17	1
Income inequality	18 of 21	13	3
% in low-paid employment	24 of 24	20	1
Public social expenditure	24 of 28	23	1
Public share health spending	28 of 29	23	1
Life expectancy	20 of 26	5	4
Infant mortality	24 of 30	16	1
Child injury mortality	23 of 26	18	1

Source: Raphael, D. (2003). "A society in decline: the social, economic, and political determinants of health inequalities in the USA," in Hofrichter, R. (Ed.), *Health and social justice: A reader on politics, ideology, and inequity in the distribution of disease.* San Francisco: Jossey Bass/Wiley, 59–88.

influence health by shaping the quality of numerous social determinants of health. Nations such as Sweden, whose policies reduce unemployment, minimize income and wealth inequality, and address numerous social determinants of health, show evidence of improved population health using indicators such as infant mortality and life expectancy (Diderichsen, Whitehead, Burstrom & Aberg, 2001). At the other end, nations with minimal commitments to such efforts such as the United States show rather worse indicators of population health (Raphael, 2000).

Theme 2: Mechanisms and Pathways by Which Social Determinants of Health Influence Health

To secure the policy relevance of the social determinants of health and build support for their strengthening, it is important to understand how social determinants of health come to influence health and cause disease. Recent theoretical thinking considers how social determinants of health "get under the skin" to influence health. The Black and the *Health Divide* Reports considered two primary mechanisms for understanding health inequalities: cultural/behavioural and materialist/structuralist (Townsend, Davidson & Whitehead, 1992).

The cultural/behavioural explanation was that individuals' behavioural choices (e.g., tobacco and alcohol use, diet, physical inactivity, etc.) were responsible for their developing and dying from a variety of diseases. Both the Black and the *Health Divide* Reports, however, showed that behavioural choices are heavily structured by one's material conditions of life. And—consistent with mounting evidence—these behavioural risk factors account for a relatively small proportion of variation in the incidence and death from various diseases. The materialist/structuralist explanation emphasizes the material conditions under which people live. These conditions include the availability of resources to access the amenities of life, working conditions, and the quality of available food and housing, among others.

The author of the *Health Divide* Report concluded: "The weight of evidence continues to point to explanations which suggest that socio-economic circumstances play the major part in subsequent health differences." Despite this conclusion and increasing evidence in favour of this view, much of the Canadian public discourse on health and disease remains focused on "lifestyle" approaches to disease prevention. The *Traditional Ten Tips for Better Health* reflects this lifestyle orientation while the *Social*

Box 1.4: Which tips for better health are consistent with research evidence?

The messages given to the public by governments, health associations, and health workers are heavily influenced by the ways in which health issues are understood. Contrast the two sets of messages provided below. The first set is individually-oriented and assumes individuals can control the factors that determine their health. The second set is societally oriented and assumes the most important determinants of health are beyond the control of most individuals. Which set of tips is most consistent with the available evidence on the determinants of health?

The traditional ten tips for better health

1. Don't smoke. If you can, stop. If you can't, cut down.
2. Follow a balanced diet with plenty of fruit and vegetables.
3. Keep physically active.
4. Manage stress by, for example, talking things through and making time to relax.
5. If you drink alcohol, do so in moderation.
6. Cover up in the sun, and protect children from sunburn.
7. Practice safer sex.
8. Take up cancer screening opportunities.
9. Be safe on the roads: follow the Highway Code.
10. Learn the First Aid ABCs: airways, breathing, circulation. (Donaldson, 1999)

The social determinants ten tips for better health

1. Don't be poor. If you can, stop. If you can't, try not to be poor for long.
2. Don't have poor parents.
3. Own a car.
4. Don't work in a stressful, low paid manual job.
5. Don't live in damp, low quality housing.
6. Be able to afford to go on a foreign holiday and sunbathe.
7. Practice not losing your job and don't become unemployed.
8. Take up all benefits you are entitled to, if you are unemployed, retired or sick or disabled.
9. Don't live next to a busy major road or near a polluting factory.
10. Learn how to fill in the complex housing benefit/asylum application forms before you become homeless and destitute. (Gordon, 1999; personal communication)

Determinants of Health Ten Tips for Better Health is consistent with more advanced thinking (see Box 1.4).

These conceptualizations have been refined such that analysis is now focused upon three frameworks by which social determinants of health come to influence health (Bartley, 2003). These frameworks are: (1) materialist; (2) neo-materialist; and (3) psychosocial comparison. The materialist explanation is about how living conditions— and the social determinants of health that constitute these living conditions—shape health. The neo-materialist explanation extends the materialist analysis by asking how these living conditions come about. The psychosocial comparison explanation considers whether we compare ourselves to others and how these comparisons affect our health and well-being.

To anticipate these analyses, evidence strongly supports materialist and neo-materialist explanations for understanding how the social determinants of health come to influence health status. Chapter 2 is devoted to these and other frameworks that identify mechanisms and pathways by which the social determinants of health shape health status.

Theme 3: The Importance of a Life-Course Perspective

Traditional approaches to health and disease prevention have a distinctly non-historical emphasis. Usually adults and, increasingly, adolescents and youth are urged to adopt "healthy lifestyles" as a means of preventing the development of chronic diseases such as heart disease and diabetes, among others (Chronic Disease Prevention Alliance of Canada, 2003; Health Canada, 2003). In contrast to these approaches, life-course approaches emphasize the accumulated effects of experience across the lifespan in understanding the maintenance of health and the onset of disease. It has been argued that:

> The prevailing aetiological model for adult disease which emphasizes adult risk factors, particularly aspects of adult life style, has been challenged in recent years by research that has shown that poor growth and development and adverse early environmental conditions are associated with an increased risk of adult chronic disease. (Kuh & Ben-Shilmo, 1997, p. 3)

More specifically, it is apparent that the economic and social conditions—the social determinants of health—under which individuals live their lives have a cumulative effect upon the probability of developing any number of diseases. This has been repeatedly demonstrated in longitudinal studies—the US National Longitudinal Survey, the West of Scotland Collaborative Study, Norwegian and Finnish linked data—that follow individuals across their lives (Blane, 1999). This has been most clearly demonstrated in the case of heart disease and stroke (Raphael & Farrell, 2002). And most recently, studies into the childhood and adulthood antecedents of adult-onset diabetes show how adverse economic and social conditions across the lifespan predispose individuals to this disorder (Raphael et al., 2003).

A recent volume brings together some of the important work concerning the importance of a life-course perspective for understanding the importance of social determinants (Davey Smith, 2003). Adopting a life-course perspective directs attention to how social determinants of health operate at every level of development—early childhood, childhood, adolescence, and adulthood—to both immediately influence health as well as provide the basis for health or illness during later stages of life. These issues are considered further in Chapter 2.

Theme 4: The Role of Public Policy and Policy Environments

Much social determinants of health research simply focuses on determining the relationship between a social determinant of health and health status, so a researcher may document that lower income is associated with adverse health outcomes among parents and their children. Or a researcher may demonstrate that food insecurity is related to poor health status among parents and children, as is living in crowded housing, and so on. This is termed a depoliticized approach as it says little about how these poor-quality social determinants of health come about (Raphael & Bryant, 2002).

Social determinants of health do not exist in a vacuum. Their quality and availability to the population are usually a result of public policy decisions made by governing authorities. As one example, consider the social determinant of health of early life. Early life is shaped by availability of sufficient material resources that assure adequate educational opportunities, food, and housing among others. Much of this has to do with the employment security and the quality of working conditions and wages. The availability of quality, regulated child care is an especially important policy option in support of early life (Esping-Andersen, 2002). These are not issues that usually come under individual control. A policy-oriented approach places such findings within a broader policy context.

Yet it is not uncommon to see governmental and other authorities individualize these issues. Governments may choose to understand early life as being primarily about parents' behaviours toward their children. They then focus upon promoting better parenting, assist in having parents read to their children, or urge schools to foster exercise among children rather than raising the amount of financial or housing resources available to families. Indeed, for every social determinant of health, an individualized manifestation of each is available. There is little evidence to suggest the efficacy of such approaches in improving the health status of those most vulnerable to illness in the absence of efforts to modify their adverse living conditions (Raphael, 2001c).

An important purpose of this volume, therefore, is to place the social determinants of health within a public policy perspective and to outline policy options for strengthening these social determinants of health. Since evidence indicates that strengthening these social determinants of health would improve the health status of Canadians, it would be expected that governments would be responsive to these ideas. This may not be the case.

> In fact, Canada has fallen behind countries such as the United Kingdom and Sweden and even some jurisdictions in the United States in applying the population health knowledge base that has been largely developed in Canada (Canadian Population Health Initiative, 2002, p. 1).

Canada's performance in implementing social determinants-relevant policy reflects a weakening commitment to supporting its citizenry. Canadian political economist Gary Teeple argues that a strong national Canadian identity and a willingness to reduce class conflict at the end of the Second World War led to the development of a strong Canadian welfare state (Teeple, 2000). The strengthened Canadian welfare state became associated with more equitable distribution of income and wealth through social, economic, and political reforms. These reforms included progressive tax structures, social programs, and governmental structures that supported health. These are the mainsprings of strong social determinants of health.

Yet, since the early 1970s—and coincident with increasing economic globalization—a fundamental change has occurred in national and global economies. In Canada, governments have weakened the structures associated with the welfare state. Federal program spending as a percentage of GDP is close to 1950s levels, and government policies have increased income and wealth inequalities, created crises in housing and food security, and increased the precariousness of employment (Raphael, 2001b). This has not been the case in all developed nations. What role does politics and political ideology play in these developments?

Theme 5: Politics, Political Ideology, and the Social Determinants of Health

Considering the evidence of the importance of the social determinants of health, how can we explain why certain nations take up this information and apply it in the formulation of public policy while others do not? Another way of considering this issue is inquire as to why there is such a gap between knowledge and action on the social determinants of health in Canada.

One way to think about this is to consider the idea of the welfare state and the political ideologies that shape its form in Canada and elsewhere. The concept of the welfare state is about the extent to which governments or the state use their power to provide citizens with the means to live secure and satisfying lives. Every developed nation has some form of the welfare state. Important questions are: (1) How developed is this welfare state? and (2) What are the implications of the welfare state for the social determinants of health?

Two literatures inform this analysis. The first concerns the three forms of the modern welfare state. Esping-Andersen identifies three distinct clusters of welfare regimes among wealthy developed nations: Social democratic (e.g., Sweden, Norway, Denmark, and Finland), liberal (the US, the UK, Canada, and Ireland), and conservative (France, Germany, Netherlands, and Belgium, among others) (Esping-Andersen, 1990, 1999). There is high government intervention and strong welfare systems in the social democratic countries and rather less in the liberal. Conservative nations fall midway between these others in service provision and citizen supports.

Social democratic nations have very well-developed welfare states that provide a wide range of universal and generous benefits. They expend more of national wealth for supports and services. They are proactive in developing labour, family-friendly, and gender equity-supporting policies. Liberal nations spend rather less on supports and services. They offer modest universal transfers and modest social-insurance plans. Benefits are provided primarily through means-tested assistance whereby these benefits are provided only to the least well-off. How do these forms of the welfare state come about? How do they shape the social determinants of health?

Navarro and colleagues provide empirical support for the hypotheses that the social determinants of health and health status outcomes are of higher quality in the social democratic rather than the liberal nations (Navarro, 2004; Navarro et al., 2004). Some of these indicators are spending on supports and services, equitable distribution of income, and wealth and availability of services in support of families and individuals. Health indicators include life expectancy and infant mortality.

Could this general approach to welfare provision shape Canadian receptivity to the concepts developed in this volume? And, if so, what can be done to improve receptivity to and implementation of these concepts? The final chapter of this volume revisits these issues.

Developments Since the 1st Edition of This Volume

There have been some notable developments in the social determinants of health field since the appearance of the 1st edition of this volume in 2004. Internationally, the World Health Organization's establishment of an International Commission on the Social Determinants of Health has stimulated discussion (World Health Organization, 2004). To date the commission has produced excellent background papers on the social determinants of health and has begun to produce numerous final reports dealing with a range of important issues (Irwin & Scali, 2007). Two of the commission's knowledge networks (Globalization and Health and Early Childhood Development) are centred in Canada, and another (Workplace Health) has significant Canadian representation. The concept has enjoyed increased mention in the international academic literature and reviews are available (Graham, 2004a, 2004b; Raphael, 2006). The Canadian Senate's Subcommittee on Population Health has undertaken a review of the social determinants of health (Canadian Senate, 2007).

Within Canada, a few Canadian health units have distinguished themselves by their work in raising the importance of the social determinants of health (Raphael, 2007d). And there is clear evidence that those working in specific social determinants of health concept areas such as employment security and working conditions, early childhood education and care, housing, income, and food security, health and social services, and poverty reduction are more aware of how their issues impact health. Non-

governmental agencies such as the United Ways across Canada and the United Nations Association of Canada have drawn upon the social determinants of health concept to advance their work (United Way of Greater Toronto & Canadian Council on Social Development, 2002; United Way of Ottawa, 2003; United Way of Winnipeg, 2003).

While it is clear that the social determinants of health concept has attained a greater visibility among these varied sectors, there is little evidence that the concept has significantly contributed to any Canadian public policy advances in the service of health. When governments have produced health-enhancing public policies such as new housing programs or enhanced early childhood education programs, it is difficult to discern if health considerations have been considered in their decisions. There has not been the case elsewhere where social determinants of health concepts have been actively incorporated into the making of public policy (Mackenbach & Bakker, 2002).

For the most part, the social determinants of health concept within the Canadian public health scene has been limited to the production of even more policy documents declaring its importance with rather little to show for the effort. This may be a result of governing parties' political ideologies shaping policy-makers' receptiveness to the social determinants of health concept (Raphael & Bryant, 2006a). Government policy-makers will hesitate to advocate public policies that are seen as inconsistent with the views of the elected representatives who effectively serve as their employer. Identifying how these barriers may be overcome constitutes an important goal of this volume.

Conclusion

As noted, a social determinants of health approach is not a wholly new development, but has its roots in critical examination of the causes of illness and disease that date from the mid-19th century. The modern resurgence of interest into how living conditions shape health dates from the 1970s. British researchers investigated the sources of health inequalities and contributed much to our conceptual and empirical understanding of these issues. At the same time, and continuing to the present,

Canadians developed health promotion and population health concepts that directed attention to various social determinants of health. But, unlike the British and others, Canada has lagged well behind other jurisdictions in applying this knowledge to developing economic and social policies in support of health.

The pages to follow contain assessments of the current state of 12 key social determinants of health in Canada and analyses of how these conditions affect the health of Canadians. As you read each chapter, reflect upon your own life situation and the others around you in relation to the specific social determinant of health. Are you and others experiencing a higher quality of this social determinant of health or a lower quality of it? Do you see the situation improving or declining?

Consider how the quality of these social determinants of health is influenced by decisions made by Canadian policy-makers in Ottawa, your province, and your local municipality. As you read the policy options that are provided for improving both the state of these determinants and the health of Canadians, keep in mind the importance of the broader political, economic, and social environments in which Canadians are now living. To what extent do these environments influence the quality of the social determinants of health and policy-makers' receptivity to these ideas on promoting the health of Canadians? What can be done to put these ideas into practice? How can these ideas be implemented to improve the quality of the social determinants of health and improve the overall health of Canadians?

Critical Thinking Questions

1. Reflect upon the degree of familiarity you had with the idea of living conditions as primary determinants of health prior to reading the chapter. When you thought of health and its determinants, what did you think of?
2. Were living conditions and the public policies that shape them considered as health issues in your previous studies?
3. What do your answers say about how health issues are framed in Canada in general and by governments, public health agencies, and the media?
4. What does it say about your previous studies in the health sciences or related fields?
5. Look at a few days' worth of health-related stories in *The Globe and Mail* or your local newspaper. How often is there a social determinants of health angle on a health story?
6. Why do you think the social determinants of health appear to be so low on just about everybody's agenda?

Recommended Readings

Bartley, M. (2003). *Health inequality: An introduction to concepts, theories, and methods.* Cambridge: Polity Press.

Large differences in life expectancy exist between the most privileged and the most disadvantaged social groups in industrial societies. This book assists in understanding the four most widely accepted theories of what lies behind inequalities in health: behavioural, psychosocial, material, and life-course approaches.

Davey Smith, G. (2003). *Health inequalities: Life-course approaches.* Bristol: Policy Press.

The life-course perspective on adult health and health inequalities is an important development in epidemiology and public health. This volume presents innovative, empirical research that shows how social disadvantage throughout the life course leads to inequalities in life expectancy, death rates, and health status in adulthood.

Graham, H. (2004). "Social determinants of health and their unequal distribution: Clarifying policy understandings." *Milbank Quarterly, 82,* 101–124.

This article outlines some of the emerging issues in the social determinants of health field and details how their consideration influences the framing of problems and their potential solutions.

Hofrichter, R. (Ed.). (2003). *Health and social justice: Politics, ideology, and inequity in the distribution of disease.* San Francisco: Jossey-Bass.

This volume offers a comprehensive collection of articles written by expert contributors representing the fields of sociology, epidemiology, public health, ecology, politics, organizing, and advocacy. Each article explores a particular aspect of health inequalities and demonstrates how these are rooted in injustices associated with racism, sex discrimination, and social class.

Raphael, D. (2007). *Poverty and policy in Canada: Implications for health and quality of life.* Toronto: Canadian Scholars' Press Inc.

This book focuses on how the social determinants of health cluster to create the most disadvantageous life circumstance: Poverty. It includes information on the lived experience of poverty, how public policy shapes its incidence, and how poverty shapes health and the quality of life.

Raphael, D., Bryant, M., & Rioux, M. (2006). *Staying alive: Critical perspectives on health, illness, and health care.* Toronto: Canadian Scholars' Press Inc.

This book provides a range of approaches for understanding health issues. In addition to traditional health sciences and sociological approaches, this new book also provides the human rights and political economy perspectives on health. It focuses on these issues in Canada and the United States, but provides an international context for these analyses.

Related Web Sites

Canadian Centre for Policy Alternatives (CCPA)—www.policyalternatives.ca

The centre monitors developments and promotes research on economic and social issues facing Canada. It provides alternatives to the views of business research institutes and many government agencies by publishing research reports, sponsoring conferences, organizing briefings, and providing informed comment on the issues of the day from a non-partisan perspective.

Canadian Senate Sub-Committee on Population Health—tinyurl.com/ypwhhq

This Senate committee has undertaken to examine and report on the impact of the multiple factors and conditions that contribute to the health of Canada's population, known collectively as the social determinants of health. The Web site contains transcripts of witnesses' presentations and will eventually produce a report on the issue.

Centre for Social Justice (CSJ)—www.socialjustice.org

The CSJ's work is focused on narrowing the gap between rich and poor, challenging corporate domination of Canadian politics, and pressing for policy changes that promote economic and social justice. It provides information, statistics, and reports on the gap between the rich and the poor, housing, and other issues related to social determinants of health.

National Council of Welfare (NCW)—www.ncwcnbes.net

The NCW advises the Canadian government on matters related to social welfare and the needs of low-income Canadians. NCW publishes several reports each year on poverty and social policy issues, presents submissions to parliamentary committees and Royal Commissions, and provides information on poverty and social policy.

World Health Organization Commission on the Social Determinants of Health (CSDH)—www.who.int/social_determinants/en/

The CSDH supports countries and global health partners to address the social factors leading to ill health and inequities. It draws the attention of society to the social determinants of health that are known to be among the most important causes of poor health and inequalities among and within countries.

Chapter 2

Social Structure, Living Conditions, and Health

Dennis Raphael

Introduction

As you work your way through this volume, it will become increasingly clear that there is little dispute that the social determinants of health, or living conditions, are the primary factors implicated in the incidence of disease and illness. Study after study finds that these conditions are the best predictors of health outcomes, and their effects swamp the influence of behavioural risk factors such as diet, physical activity, and even tobacco use. In this chapter, frameworks that explain how the experience of the social determinants of health leads to health outcomes are presented. There are very narrow health frameworks that limit attention to behavioural risk factors such as physical activity, diet, and tobacco and alcohol use and how these come to influence health. These approaches simply view the social determinants of health concept as identifying those individuals whose health-threatening behaviours are worthy of behavioural health promoters' attention. These approaches usually say nothing about how the social determinants of health directly affect these individuals' health and shape their adoption of these health-threatening behaviours. These narrow models certainly do not emphasize actions to improve the quality of the social determinants of health that Canadians may experience.

Of much greater value are broader frameworks that consider how the social determinants of health directly and indirectly influence health. These frameworks identify the immediate and more distant societal structures that shape the quality of the social determinants of health people experience and how these lead to health problems. More detailed biological and psychological frameworks are also available that consider how these experiences influence bodily systems and set the stage for present and future disease. These biological and psychological approaches consider how people's bodies respond to the experience of the social determinants of health thereby specifying how aspects of living conditions "get under the skin" to determine health.

There are also frameworks that examine how political and economic forces that shape the distribution of economic and social resources influence the quality of the social determinants of health people experience. These frameworks show that the quality of these social determinants of health reflect societal approaches to societal organization and resource provision. These frameworks also include the role that economic globalization can play in determining the quality of the social determinants of health people experience. Included within these broader frameworks are analyses of the pathways and mechanisms by which gender, race, and status are related to the quality of the social determinants of health people experience. Despite these advances in knowledge, however, there is still an inordinate amount of attention paid by researchers, health workers, and the media to individualistic approaches, i.e., those focused on individual risk behaviours. Numerous reasons are advanced in this chapter as to why this might be the case.

Individual Approaches

An individual perspective limits analysis of health risks to individual biomedical and behavioural risk factors for disease (Raphael et al., 2005). For biomedical indicators, this is associated with screening for physiological and medical risk factors such as hypertension, excess weight, cholesterol, and high blood glucose levels, among others (Labonte, 1993). The appropriate responses to these threats are some form of mandated behavioural regime or treatment with drugs. In the case of behavioural risk factors such as lack of physical activity, type of diet, and the use of alcohol and tobacco, the usual approach is to exhort the individual to carry out a series of changes in his or her behaviour.

These individual perspectives carry the assumption that these factors are the primary contributors to various health conditions (Nettleton, 1997). While these biomedical and behavioural risk factors may contribute to disease, there is little evidence to assign these risk factors a primary role in explaining how disease and illness comes about. Indeed, evidence has accumulated that biomedical and behavioural factors play a relatively minor role—as compared to the social determinants of health—in predicting life expectancy, cardiovascular disease and stroke, type 2 diabetes, respiratory disease, and stomach cancer, among other afflictions (Davey Smith & Gordon, 2000; Johnson et al., 2003; Lawlor, Ebrahim & Davey Smith, 2002). Additionally, there is an assumption that these risk factors can be modified—with resultant improvements in health—either by medical interventions or by the person at risk making "healthy choices" (Fitzpatrick, 2001).

There is also little evidence in support of the assumption that those most at risk can change their behaviours by making healthy choices. Biomedical and behavioural risk factors are heavily structured by the social determinants of health that people experience (Jarvis & Wardle, 1999; Shaw, Dorling, Gordon & Davey Smith, 1999). And there is little evidence of success for behavioural interventions applied to especially vulnerable populations (O'Loughlin, Paradis, Gray-Donald & Renaud, 1999). Finally, the focus on biomedical and behavioural risk factors puts forth a particular ideological view concerning the sources of health and disease in general and the especially problematic living situations and health status of populations that are marginalized by lack of material and social resources. Travers (1996) argues that:

> Individualism assumes that the current social system provides sufficient and equal opportunity for individuals to move within the social system according to their abilities. Within this ideological construct, poverty results from the individual's failure to seize the opportunity or to work sufficiently hard within the current social structure; it is not a reflection of inadequacies and inequities within that social order. (p. 551)

Despite their clear inadequacy for explaining the means by which various social determinants of health shape health, individualist approaches dominate public understandings, health care and public health discourses and messaging, and governmental policy to health promotion and population health (Canadian Population Health Initiative, 2004; Raphael, 2000). Why this is the case is considered following presentation of more relevant and useful frameworks that explain the pathways and mechanisms by which the social determinants of health come to be so strongly related to health.

Social Determinants of Health and Living Conditions

Social determinants of health can best be understood as specifying the material and social living conditions that people experience. The quality of these social determinants of health is a reflection of the organization of society and how a society distributes economic and social resources. Brunner and Marmot (2006) provide a broad descriptive model that outlines how the organization of society shapes various social determinants of health and health itself. Their model is presented as Figure 2.1.

In this model, social structure is provided as a catch-all for the organization of society and how it distributes access to actual material and social resources. The specifics of how societal decisions on the distribution

Figure 2.1: Social determinants of health

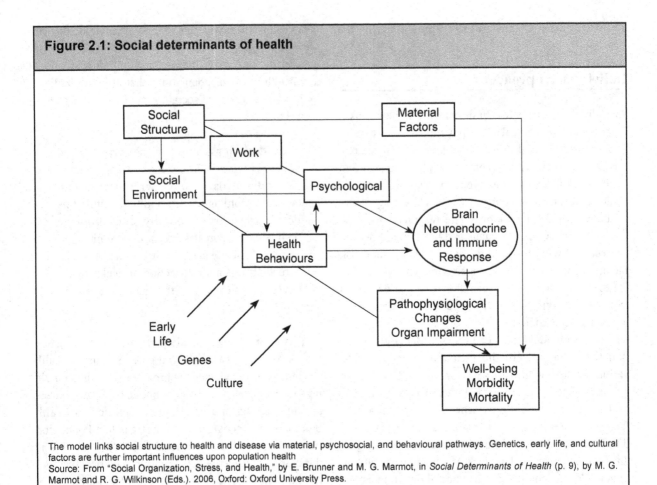

The model links social structure to health and disease via material, psychosocial, and behavioural pathways. Genetics, early life, and cultural factors are further important influences upon population health
Source: From "Social Organization, Stress, and Health," by E. Brunner and M. G. Marmot, in *Social Determinants of Health* (p. 9), by M. G. Marmot and R. G. Wilkinson (Eds.). 2006, Oxford: Oxford University Press.

of resources shape the social determinants of health and health status constitute the content of this volume. Suffice at this point to point out that Brunner and Marmot's model is depoliticized in that it makes little mention of the political, economic, and social forces that shape how a society's social structure comes about. Models presented later in this chapter begin to flesh out these dynamics.

The model shows three primary pathways that link social structure with health status (i.e., well-being, morbidity, and mortality). The first is a direct link between social structure, material factors (e.g., living conditions), and health status. Material factors are the concrete living conditions that include both positive exposures to health-enhancing events or situations as well as exposures to negative health-threatening events or situations.

In the second pathway, social structure shapes social and work environments to create psychological and behavioural responses that—operating through brain mechanisms—determine health status. The third primary pathway is one that sees these same environments creating behavioural responses that directly impair bodily organs thereby determining health. Early life, genes, and culture contribute to processes at all levels of the model. Though not elucidated in this model, social structure has a direct influence upon early life, which has effects that carry across the lifespan.

Like many linear models, this diagram does not take into account the complexity of the relationships among health determinants themselves and the relationships of these determinants with health outcomes. All of these factors are iterative in that each has both forward and feed-back effects. For example, conditions of work and the social environment both result from, as well as influence, the social structure. Social structure shapes conditions of work and quality of social environments. However, the conditions of work and wages that people are exposed to then feed back to influence their degree of power and ability to determine aspects of the social structure such as the degree of political influence, the responsiveness of governments to needs and aspirations, and societal attitudes toward the group to which they belong. Low-waged workers, for instance, will have less political influence, and governments will be less responsive to their needs because of the workers' lower standings in the social class hierarchy.

Similarly, neighbourhoods—usually low-income ones—experiencing health problems that result from the organization of social structure and its distribution of resources may develop adverse reputations that limit their ability to influence societal and governmental responsiveness and attitudes toward their community. Such feedback may further marginalize and stigmatize the community in question. And all of these specific environments have direct effects upon health through material factor pathways.

Similarly, psychological factors and health behaviours feed back to affect the quality of work and social environments as well as the social structure itself. Stress-producing circumstances associated with experiencing poor-quality social determinants of health may create unpleasant work and social environments that make coping and managing even more difficult. One way to think about this is to consider that all the factors in Figure 2.1 are interrelated as described in Table 2.1.

In the following sections, four models that fill in some of the underlying processes outlined in Figure 2.1 are presented: the materialist, neo-materialist, life-course, and social comparison models. Within these four broad models, more specific accounts of pathways mediating the social determinants of health and health status relationship are also presented.

Materialist Explanations for the Social Determinants of Health and Health Status Relationship

The materialist framework sees objective living conditions as explaining how social determinants of health shape health status (Bartley, 2003). Within a materialist view,

Benzeval and colleagues argue that there are three key mechanisms that link social determinants to health: (1) experience of material living conditions; (2) experience of psychosocial stress; and (3) adoption of health-supporting or health-threatening behaviours (Benzeval, Judge & Whitehead, 1995). All of these mechanisms reflect experience with concrete living conditions. The first part of the materialist argument is that individuals living within a society experience differing exposures to positive and negative living conditions throughout their lives. These different exposures accumulate to produce adult health outcomes (Shaw, Dorling, Gordon & Davey Smith, 1999).

Socio-economic position in a society such as Canada is a powerful predictor of health as it is an indicator of material advantage or disadvantage over the lifespan (Lynch & Kaplan, 2000). These material conditions of life include childhood advantage or deprivation related to quality of nourishment and housing, and adult issues of employment or unemployment, occupational quality and hazards, and access to resources such as health and social services, among others (Shaw, Dorling, Gordon & Davey Smith, 1999). Material conditions of life determine health by influencing the quality of individual development, family life and interaction, and community environments (Brooks-Gunn, Duncan & Britto, 1998).

And the quality of material life conditions—in a finely stepped pattern from poverty through to tremendous wealth—are associated with the likelihood of physical problems (infections, malnutrition, chronic disease, and injuries), developmental problems (delayed or impaired cognitive, personality, and social development), educational problems (learning disabilities, poor learning, early school leaving), and social problems (socialization, preparation for work, and family life) (Davey Smith & Gordon, 2000; Hertzman, 1999a; Roberts, Smith & Nason, 2001; Ross & Roberts, 1999).

As mentioned, these are graded effects whereby poor people do worse than lower middle-class people, who do worse than middle-class people, who in turn do worse than upper-middle class people, and so on (Benzeval, Dilnot, Judge & Taylor, 2001; Graham, 2001). Some have argued that this evidence of a graded effect suggests that psychological conditions—people's perception of their position in the social hierarchy—rather than material living conditions shape feelings of worth and health outcomes (Marmot, 2004; Wilkinson, 2001). However,

Table 2.1: How various social determinants of health are related to each other	
Health determinant	**Role played in the SDOH and health relationship**
Social Structure	Determines the availability of material and social resources available to the population and the organization and the quality of work and social environments. Illness results from a failure of the social structure to provide individuals with the resources necessary to avoid material and social deprivation, thereby leading to health and other problems.
Work Environment	Shapes work dimensions that promote health and well-being. Also determines the amount of money that results from work, the quality of benefits, and the degree of security. Work environments also shape a variety of psychological and behavioural responses that contribute to health. Primary effects concern the ability of workplaces to provide resources to meet material and social needs.
Social Environment	Degree of social support and quality of social interactions are influenced by availability of material resources and conditions of everyday life. Lack of these supports weakens the quality of the immediate social environments and are associated with a clustering of disadvantage among individuals living within specific spatial areas.
Psychological	Experience of control, reward, and status result from differing family, social, and work environments. Experience of stress related to the ability to meet basic needs and the experience of stigma and exclusion shapes the adoption of coping mechanisms. Distribution of societal resources shapes the presence of adverse experiences and these experiences, in turn, shape health.
Health Behaviours	Represent means of coping with effects of material and social deprivation associated with poor-quality environments. When chosen as a response to the experience of poor-quality social determinants of health, these have the potential to further threaten health, making receipt of additional material and social resources less likely.
Brain	Stress and autoimmune systems are weakened by accumulated adverse experiences associated with material and social deprivation, lack of control and adequate rewards, and chronic experience of fight-or-flight reaction. Adverse health outcomes feedback to weaken the quality of work, social, and material environments.
Pathophysiological Changes	Organ impairment results from adverse experiences associated with poor-quality social determinants of health. Degree of economic resources interacts with the availability of health and social services to further contribute to degree of health impairment and health status.
Health Status	Onset of disease and illness interacts with economic and societal supports available to shape the progression of illness as well as social, work, and other environments. Objective living conditions associated with the onset of illness deteriorate, making positive health outcomes even less likely.

materialists counter by arguing that findings of stepped differences among social classes and income groups occur because:

The social structure is characterized by a finely graded scale of advantage and disadvantage, with individuals differing in terms of the length and level of their exposure to a particular factor and in terms of the number of factors to which they are exposed. (Shaw, Dorling, Gordon & Davey Smith, 1999, p. 102)

Benzeval and colleagues (2001) also develop the concepts of income potential and health capital to explicate some of the means by which social determinants of health shape health:

> *Income potential* is the accumulation of abilities, skills and educational experiences in childhood that are important determinants of adult employability and income capacity. Education is seen as the key mediator in this association, being strongly influenced by family circumstances in childhood and a central determinant of an individual's income in adulthood.
>
> *Health capital* is the accumulation of health resources, both physical and psychosocial, inherited and acquired during the early stages of life which determine current health and future health potential. (p. 97)

In their model, childhood circumstances are a result of their parents' characteristics, their objective living conditions, and other aspects of their social environments.

These all contribute to their immediate health status and their potential to acquire income in adulthood. As adults, both the experiences of childhood and adult situations then go on to influence health as adults (see Figure 2.2).

A more detailed rendering of the influence of material factors upon health is provided by van de Mheen, Stronks, and Mackenbach (1998). In their model, childhood socio-economic circumstances: (1) are explicitly related to childhood health; (2) set a trajectory that, if left unchanged, will continue to accumulate socio-economic advantage or disadvantage over time; and (3) have both direct influence upon adult health and an indirect effect upon adult health through mediating processes of personality and health behaviours. These mediating processes include the psychological sense of personal control and efficacy, and the adoption of health-threatening behaviours such as tobacco use, diet, and alcohol use.

There are also selection processes by which unhealthy adults fall into a spiral of lowering socio-economic conditions. This model certainly seems plausible for Canada. The results from van de Mheen's and colleagues' study of Dutch citizens (1998) and many other similar studies support the usefulness for understanding the role that material and social resources, manifested in a variety of social determinants of health, plays in explaining health outcomes.

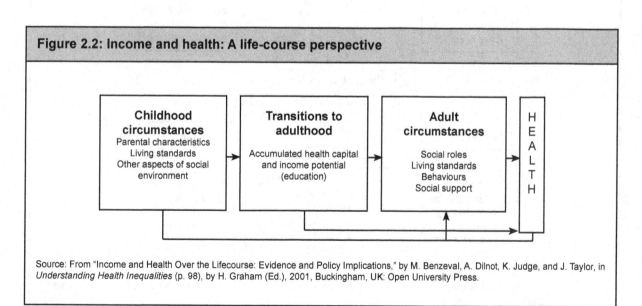

Figure 2.2: Income and health: A life-course perspective

Source: From "Income and Health Over the Lifecourse: Evidence and Policy Implications," by M. Benzeval, A. Dilnot, K. Judge, and J. Taylor, in *Understanding Health Inequalities* (p. 98), by H. Graham (Ed.), 2001, Buckingham, UK: Open University Press.

The second component of the materialist model is that living conditions determine the presence or absence of health-threatening stress. The fight-or-flight reaction evolved as a means of dealing with sudden and dangerous threats in the environment (Brunner & Marmot, 2006). The body is activated to respond to these immediate threats by either fighting or fleeing. Such activation involves a variety of bodily systems: the sympathetic and parasympathetic nervous systems, the neuroendocrine system, and the metabolic system. If, however, the reaction is elicited in a chronic way as a response to continuing threats associated with poor quality social determinants of health such as low income, insecure employment, and housing and food insecurity, among others, it takes a toll on health.

Chronic elicitation of the fight-or-flight reaction can weaken the immune system and disrupt the neuroendocrine and metabolic systems (Brunner & Marmot, 2006; Lupien, King, Meaney & McEwan,

2001). And evidence from surveys and explorations of the lived experience of low income, insecure employment, and housing and food insecurity indicate that these experiences make such stress especially likely (Allison, Adlaf, Ialomiteanu & Rehm, 1999; Avison, 1997; Cohen, Kaplan & Salonen, 1999; Davey Smith, Ben-Shlomo & Lynch, 2002; Stewart et al., 1996). Indeed, there is accumulating evidence that individuals who experience difficult living circumstances associated with poor-quality social determinants of health come to have maladaptive responses to stress, weakened immunity to infections and disease, and a greater likelihood of metabolic disorders (Davey Smith et al., 2002; Lupien et al., 2001; Sapolsky, 1992; Wamala, Lynch & Horsten, 1999) (see Figure 2.3).

A specific model of how chronic elicitation of the fight-or-flight reaction can come to shape two key chronic diseases—cardiovascular disease and type 2 or insulin-resistant diabetes—is provided by Brunner and Marmot

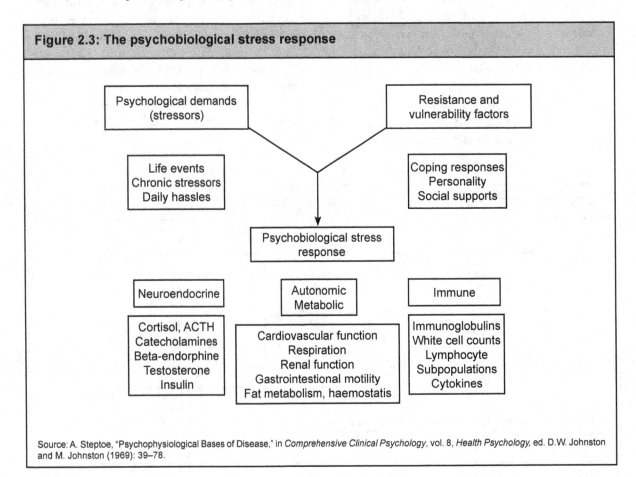

Figure 2.3: The psychobiological stress response

Source: A. Steptoe, "Psychophysiological Bases of Disease," in *Comprehensive Clinical Psychology*, vol. 8, *Health Psychology*, ed. D.W. Johnston and M. Johnston (1969): 39–78.

(2006). They clearly specify how the social environment can have a direct stress-related effect upon the circulatory and metabolic systems leading to cardiovascular disease and type 2 diabetes. Brunner and Marmot also specify how stress relations can promote the adoption of health-threatening behaviours such as tobacco use, lack of physical activity, and increased fat and sugar uptake, all of which further contribute to the incidence of these two diseases. Nevertheless, approaches to cardiovascular disease and type 2 or insulin-resistant diabetes are dominated by lifestyle approaches to risk and prevention despite the accumulating evidence in support of a broader, social determinants-oriented approach (Raphael, Anstice & Raine, 2003; Raphael & Farrell, 2002).

The third component of the materialist model is that experience of varying quality social determinants of health and the levels of stress associated with these experiences lead to the adoption of health-supporting or health-threatening behaviours. In the latter case, these behaviours can be seen as coping responses. Numerous Canadian studies show that people living under conditions of income, employment, housing, and food insecurity are more likely to take up risk-related behaviours such as smoking, excessive alcohol consumption, and lack of physical activity (Health Canada, 1999; Pomerleau, Pederson, Østbye, Speechley & Speechley, 1997; Potvin, Richard & Edwards, 2000; Williamson, 2000).

The materialist explanation, however, views these behaviours as reflecting life circumstances (Bartley, 2003; Shaw, Dorling & Davey Smith, 2006; Shaw, Dorling, Gordon & Davey Smith, 1999) rather than making unwise choices. Similarly, adoption of carbohydrate-dense diets and weight gain are also seen as means of coping with difficult circumstances (Wilkinson, 1996). As summarized by Shaw et al. (1999):

> We also see that some of the factors which contribute to health inequalities—such as smoking and inadequate diet—are themselves strongly influenced by the unequal distribution of income, wealth and life chances in general. These factors do not simply reflect the lack of knowledge or fecklessness of the poorer members of society. If we are to tackle inequalities in health we need an approach which deals with the fundamental causes of such inequalities, not one which focuses mainly on those processes which mediate between social disadvantage and poor health. (p. 105)

Life-Course Perspectives on the Social Determinants of Health and Health Status Relationship

It is important to consider how the material and social conditions associated with varying quality social determinants of health influence health across the lifespan (Davey Smith, 2003). Two such life-course models were provided earlier to illustrate the materialist approach to understanding how social determinants shape health status. While it is common to research contemporaneous living situations as contributors to health, it is important to not neglect the accumulated effects upon health of the social determinants of health across the lifespan. Life-course perspectives are concerned with how exposures to varying economic and social conditions have a cumulative effect upon health (Bartley, 2003). In Canada, the lack of longitudinal studies of health that can show these effects can reinforce this here-and-now emphasis, which focuses on the immediate health effects of various social determinants of health (Raphael et al., 2005). However, research from elsewhere provides evidence of the importance of these cumulative effects (Davey Smith et al., 2002; Davey Smith & Gordon, 2000; Davey Smith, Hart, Blane, Gillis & Hawthorne, 1997; Lynch, Kaplan & Salonen, 1997; Power, Bartley, Davey Smith & Blane, 1996).

Hertzman (2000a) outlines three types of health effects that have relevance for a life-course perspective: latent, pathway, and cumulative. *Latent effects* are biological or developmental early life experiences that influence health later in life. These biological or developmental factors, which impact at sensitive periods in human development, have a lifelong effect regardless of later circumstances. Some of these effects may occur prior to birth and are related to the quality of nutrients received, the incidence of infection, and the use of tobacco, all of which affect availability of oxygen to organs. These latent effects may come to affect blood clotting and cholesterol metabolism, leading to coronary heart disease and type 2 diabetes in later life.

During infancy, latent effects upon health may result from malnutrition and infection. Malnutrition may affect health, cognitive development, and educational attainment during childhood and later life. Infection can provide long-term developmental risk and increase problems with airway and respiratory function.

All of these latent effects are a result of exposures to varying quality social determinants of health. The incidence of low birth weight, which is a reliable predictor of incidence of cardiovascular disease and adult-onset diabetes in later life, is one such effect (Barker, Forsen, Uutela, Osmond & Eriksson, 2001; Bartley, Power, Blane, Davey Smith & Shipley, 1994; Davey Smith et al., 2002; Forssas, Gissler, Sihvonen & Hemminki, 1999). Exposures to varying quality social determinants of health can lead to differing likelihood of respiratory problems as an adult. Experience of varying nutritional intakes during childhood has a variety of lasting health effects (Forsen, Eriksson, Tuomilehto, Osmond & Barker, 1999; James, Nelson, Ralph & Leather, 1997; Sarlio-Lahteenkorva & Lahelma, 2001).

Pathway effects are experiences that set individuals onto trajectories that influence health, well-being, and competence over the life course. Living conditions shape children's vocabulary upon entering school (Willms, 1997, 2002). This then sets them upon a path that leads to differing educational expectations and achievement, varying employment prospects, greater or lesser accumulation of financial resources, and differing likelihood of illness and disease across the lifespan (Ronson & Rootman, this volume). Material and social conditions associated with varying-quality neighbourhoods, schools, and housing also set children on differing paths that either support or threaten health across the lifespan (Hertzman, 1998, 2000b).

The experience of varying quality social determinants of health therefore sets individuals upon life trajectories that affect health, well-being, and competence over time. Early life may be a particularly important period in itself (a critical or sensitive period) or it may be a marker for a path for which a person is headed. In either event, early life sets most people out on a pathway that leads to the accumulation of exposures that lead to varying health outcomes.

Cumulative effects represent the accumulation of these advantages or disadvantages over time (Hertzman, 1999a, 1999b). These involve the combination of latent and pathways effects. Children experience these advantages

or disadvantages, and over time these accumulate. If children escape disadvantage, the accumulation of disadvantage stops, but the previously accumulated health disadvantage continues with them into adulthood.

The effects of the accumulation of advantage or disadvantage over time are multifaceted and involve individual, family, and community factors. This is especially the case for diseases such as cardiovascular disease, type 2 diabetes, respiratory disease, and some cancers. Adopting a life-course perspective directs attention to how early experience of varying social determinants of health influences health at every level of development—early childhood, childhood, adolescence, and adulthood—to both immediately influence health and provide the basis for health or illness later in life. As noted, much of the specific evidence for life-course effects come from studies from outside Canada, but increasing availability of data from Canadian studies that follow people over time should confirm the robust findings of accumulative health advantage and disadvantage over time (Dooley & Curtis, 1998; Ross, Roberts & Scott, 1998).

Neo-materialist Explanations for the Social Determinants of Health and Health Status Relationship

The neo-materialist argument shares a concern with materialist approaches with how health outcomes come to be associated with exposures to varying quality social determinants of health over the lifespan, but extends the analysis to explicitly consider how these health advantaging or threatening living conditions come about (Bartley, 2003; Lynch, Davey Smith, Kaplan & House, 2000). In this analysis, the focus is upon how a society allocates economic and social resources among the population. Generally, nations that distribute income and wealth more equitably are also greater spenders on various aspects of social infrastructure that are associated with the social determinants of health. These include spending on—and quality of—health care and social services; education and libraries; employment and training opportunities; and supports for the unemployed, those with disabilities, and other forms of potential disadvantage. Not surprisingly, these jurisdictions with greater equity in distribution of resources and greater investment in social infrastructure frequently show superior population health profiles.

Canada has a less skewed distribution of income and wealth among the population and spends somewhat more than the US on social infrastructure in some key areas (Ross et al., 2000). And, not surprisingly, Canadians generally enjoy better health than Americans as measured by infant mortality rates, life expectancy, and incidence of, and mortality from, a range of diseases as well as childhood injuries (Innocenti Research Centre, 2000, 2001; Jackson, 2002; Organisation for Economic Co-operation and Development, 2005a, 2005b). But Canada does not do as well as many European nations where distribution of resources is more equitable, low-income rates are lower, and where health indicators are better. In essence, the quality of various social determinants of health in Canada lags behind many other developed nations.

The neo-materialist view, therefore, directs attention to both the effects of experiencing varying quality social determinants of health (materialist view) and identifying the societal forces that determine the quality and distribution of these living conditions (neo-materialist). How a society decides to distribute resources among citizens is an especially important theme that runs through much of the content of this volume.

Social Comparison Explanations for the Social Determinants of Health and Health Status Relationship

In the social determinants of health literature, the social comparison approach is usually presented as a competing explanation to the materialist framework (Bartley, 2003). In this model, material and social conditions of life are downplayed in favour of the view that individual placement in the social hierarchy and social distance explain differences in health status (Raphael, 2003). Rather than focus on material and social living conditions associated with varying quality social determinants of health, the argument here is that the health status of people in developed nations is largely shaped by citizens' interpretations of their standings in the social hierarchy (Kawachi & Kennedy, 2002). There are two mechanisms by which this occurs.

At the individual level, the perception and experience of personal status in unequal societies lead to stress and poor health. Comparing their status, possessions,

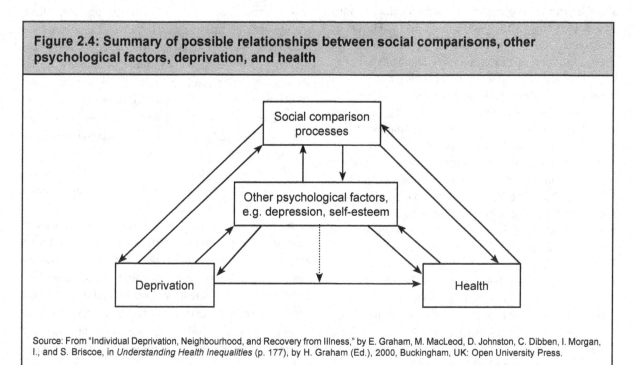

Figure 2.4: Summary of possible relationships between social comparisons, other psychological factors, deprivation, and health

Source: From "Individual Deprivation, Neighbourhood, and Recovery from Illness," by E. Graham, M. MacLeod, D. Johnston, C. Dibben, I. Morgan, I., and S. Briscoe, in *Understanding Health Inequalities* (p. 177), by H. Graham (Ed.), 2000, Buckingham, UK: Open University Press.

and other life circumstances to others, individuals experience feelings of shame, worthlessness, and envy that have psychobiological effects upon health. These comparisons lead to attempts to alleviate such feelings through overspending, taking on additional employment that threatens health, and adopting health-threatening coping behaviours such as overeating and use of alcohol and tobacco (Kawachi & Kennedy, 2002). Figure 2.4 illustrates this process.

At the communal level, widening and strengthening of hierarchy weakens social cohesion. Individuals become more distrusting and suspicious of others, thereby weakening support for communal structures such as public education, health, and social programs. The public's exaggerated desire for tax reductions weakens public infrastructure. This model can be criticized on various grounds. The first is that it neglects the profound and concrete effects of differences in material and social living conditions on health. This neglect is especially problematic when considering the material and social deprivation of people living in the most adverse conditions, i.e., in poverty (Lynch et al., 2000). Second, it depoliticizes issues of societal organization and distribution of economic and other resources among the population, obscuring the sources of varying quality social determinants of health and the political, economic, and social forces that maintain these differences (Muntaner, 2004). Third, it has the potential to reduce the health effects of varying social determinants of health to psychological processes of poor people's maladaptive coping (Shaw, Dorling, Gordon & Davey Smith, 1999).

This is not to suggest that some of the processes described by the model do not help explain how living under varying quality social determinants of health contributes to health status. Comparing oneself to others and seeing oneself come up short can clearly contribute to poor health. But the source of these comparisons lies not with individual interpretations of these shortcomings, but rather in the societal structures and processes that create such inequalities. In addition, the perception of coming up short may not originate with individuals who lack such resources, but rather with the attitudes and views of societal members who possess more of these resources. And these attitudes and views may be shaped by the same societal processes that create and maintain differing quality of a variety of social determinants of health, serving to justify their existence.

Tarlov (1996) attempted an integration of the materialist and social comparison approaches. In this model, the experience of differences in the material and social conditions of life contribute to health. People lacking quality social determinants of health experience inequity, limited opportunity, employment instability, and social segregation. These observations of inequality produce stress that reflects the dissonance between expectations and realities. These stress reactions lead to a variety of health-threatening biological reactions related to lipid disorders and the creation of atherosclerotic plaque formation in the circulatory system.

Social comparison processes appear relevant to the experiences of varying quality social determinants of health, but the sources of these interpretations must be seen as embedded in the material and social conditions of life that differ among individuals.

Societal Structures, the Experience of Material and Social Deprivation, and Psychosocial Stress

There are still some missing pieces to the materialist and neo-materialist models and how they explain how the social determinants of health operate. These are the specific mechanisms by which the experience of varying quality social determinants of health are shaped by immediate and more distant features of the environment. Raphael and colleagues use the term "horizontal structures" to refer to the more immediate social determinants of health with which people interact (Raphael et al., 2005). More distant societal structures that influence the quality of the social determinants of health are called "vertical structures" (Raphael et al., 2005). They then consider how these interactions come to produce health effects.

Some horizontal structures—and the associated social determinants of health—with which people interact are the health and social services within a community, availability and quality of housing, the educational, employment and recreational opportunities available, and other material and social resources found within a community. The following chapters detail how the organization of these horizontal structures shapes health.

Vertical structures shape the quality of these more immediate structures and represent the political, economic, and social forces that determine the quality of various social determinants of health that people experience. A focus on governmental support for opportunities for employment and training, distribution of income and social benefits, and social welfare and tax policies within a jurisdiction constitutes such an analysis (Raphael, 2004). Jurisdictions make decisions that shape the quality of virtually all the social determinants of health. To consider the immediate effects of the social determinants of health without considering the forces that shape these determinants would be derelict.

Gender, Race, and Disability-Related Pathways That Mediate the Poverty and Health Relationship

In addition to the materialist, life-course, neo-materialist, and social comparison approaches to understanding how social determinants of health shape health status, specific pathways and mechanisms related to gender, race, and disability have been outlined. The following sections provide an overview of these pathways and mechanisms. These themes run through the entire content of this volume.

Gender

Gender is an important pathway mediating the social determinants of health and health status relationship. Men and women experience differing quality social determinants of health. Much of this has to do with women being considered responsible for raising children and caring for the health needs of families (Armstrong, 2004). How this plays out is that women are less likely to be working full-time and are less likely to be eligible for unemployment benefits, an argument developed by Tremblay and Jackson in this volume.

Women are more likely to be employed in lower-paying occupations and experience discrimination in the workplace. In addition, just about every public policy decision that weakens the provision of social determinants of health associated with economic and social security—such as the failure to raise minimum wages or social assistance benefits, reducing access to public health services, limiting the availability of affordable housing or government-supported quality child care and introducing restrictive workfare requirements—disproportionately affects women more than men (Armstrong, 1996). These issues are considered by Armstrong and others in this volume.

Race

Race is becoming an important pathway mediating the social determinants of health and health status relationship. The social determinants of health situation of Aboriginal Canadians is problematic and is developed in Smylie's chapter. Other people of colour in Canada earn less income, are more likely to be unemployed, and experience more precarious employment than other Canadians, issues considered by Galabuzi. The social determinants of health situation of recent immigrants to Canada of colour is especially problematic.

Disability

People with disabilities are profoundly disadvantaged in a variety of social determinants of health areas (Fawcett, 2000; Lee, 2000). These include employment opportunities, wages, and receipt of benefits. Canadian public policy toward people with disabilities is under-developed in relation to other nations, a topic considered by Raphael (2007).

Political and Economic Pathways

Political and economic pathways are analyses specifically concerned with how political decisions shape the quality of the social determinants of health within a jurisdiction. This area is becoming increasingly important with growing economic globalization and its impact upon the distribution of economic and social resources and political decision making. This is a very underdeveloped area in the Canadian health sciences literature. A recent review found increasing attention being directed to this area by a few Canadian researchers (Raphael et al., 2005). Particularly important are two papers by Coburn and a response by Lynch (Coburn, 2000, 2004; Lynch, 2000).

In a 2000 paper, Coburn argued that neo-liberalism as a governing ideology was a useful explanatory device for explaining growing income, wealth, and health inequalities in nations such as Canada, the US, and the UK. He suggested that emphasis upon the marketplace as the arbiter of distribution of resources would be associated with deteriorating quality of any number of social determinants of health such as income and wealth distribution and quality of social infrastructure.

Lynch (2000) responded to Coburn's article and provided a model that outlines some of these key issues (see Figure 2.5).

In Lynch's model, income inequality—a key social determinant of health—represents the result of a series of processes. Income inequality reflects societies' decisions to allocate resources inequitably. This process results in poverty for many as a direct result of providing low wages and limited benefits to those in need: *individual income for those at the bottom of the social hierarchy*. At the same time, there is limited investment in community infrastructure. These limited commitments affect the health of the entire population, but especially those at the bottom of the hierarchy who lack the financial resources

to purchase these assets. The important addition of the Lynch model is noticing the degree to which income inequality and lack of investment in various social determinants of health result from adoption of neo-liberal ideology and public policy approaches to resource organization and distribution.

Neo-liberalism is the belief that the marketplace should be the arbiter of how economic and other resources are organized and distributed. It suggests a limited role for government in a wide range of areas. Neo-liberal-oriented governments are less likely to take action to strengthen the overall quality of various social determinants of health.

For Lynch (2000), whether a nation chooses to strengthen the social determinants of health is related to a number of factors such as history, traditions, institutions, and organization of civic society and culture. Political and economic traditions are probably key to

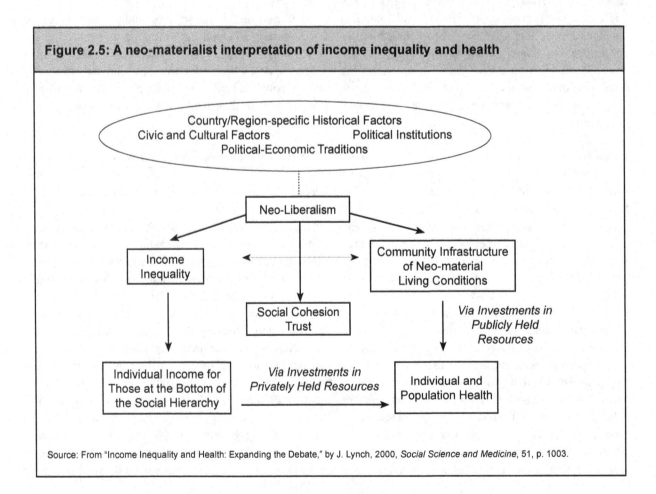

Figure 2.5: A neo-materialist interpretation of income inequality and health

Source: From "Income Inequality and Health: Expanding the Debate," by J. Lynch, 2000, *Social Science and Medicine*, 51, p. 1003.

understanding these processes. These traditions and the other components near the top of Lynch's model probably also influence how a nation's government responds to another important factor in health: economic globalization.

A more explicitly political model of these processes with relevance to Canada is provided by Coburn (2004) (see Figure 2.6). In this model, Coburn outlines how economic globalization is associated with both neo-liberalism and the power of capital (investment monies) to shape public policy in support of the social determinants of health (A). These forces interact with a nation's form of the welfare state and the market (B) to shape how these forces play out in a variety of indicators (C). The end result of these public policy approaches is quality of health status and well-being as well as a nation's overall economic wealth (D). In light of the situation in Canada, Coburn's analysis would suggest that increasing influence of the corporate elite in Canada has been driving a withdrawal from traditional Canadian support of the social determinants of health.

This withdrawal has been associated with increasing income inequality, consistently high levels of poverty, and stagnating or declining governmental expenditures on various social determinants of health such as education, income, employment, housing, and food security, and health and social services. As seen in later chapters, there is some evidence to suggest that this may indeed be happening in Canada.

Conclusion

Materialist explanations for understanding how the social determinants of health shape health status are concerned with the effects of differing material and social living conditions. These include the degree of exposures to conditions of advantage and deprivation. Neo-materialist explanations focus on the extent to which societies provide resources to the population, thereby strengthening the social determinants of health. Social comparison theories state that individuals compare their living situations to others, and if they find themselves

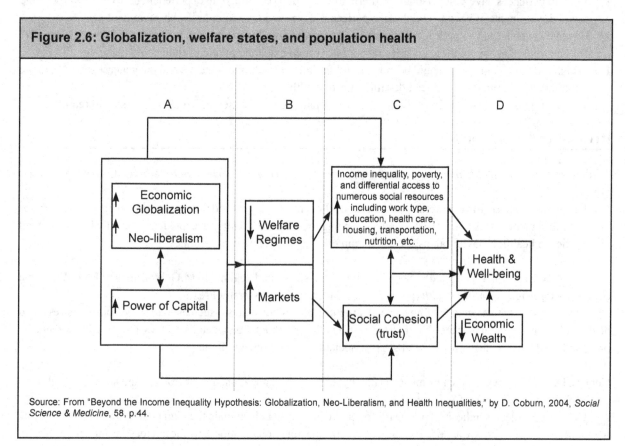

Figure 2.6: Globalization, welfare states, and population health

Source: From "Beyond the Income Inequality Hypothesis: Globalization, Neo-Liberalism, and Health Inequalities," by D. Coburn, 2004, *Social Science & Medicine*, 58, p.44.

lacking, experience feelings of stress, envy, and jealousy that threaten health. These latter approaches have the potential to downplay the importance of material and social living conditions associated with varying quality social determinants of health.

There are also other models that concern themselves with the specific features of immediate and distant environments that shape health status. Gender, race, and disability status interact with environments to shape health status. Finally, there are political and economic models that attempt to place public policy-making on the social determinants of health within broader frameworks of resource distribution that are influenced by globalization and other forces associated with the power of capital or wealth. These latter models suggest the importance of understanding the broad nature of policy-making in each nation and how this nature shapes the quality of the social determinants of health.

Explicit in some of these frameworks and implicit in others is that the social determinants of health are shaped by approaches to public policy. The implications of these frameworks are that governments should do whatever they can to strengthen the social determinants of health. What some of these approaches would be constitutes much of the content of this volume.

Critical Thinking Questions

1. Which of the models do you think may be most useful for explaining how the social determinants of health shape health status? On what grounds do you say this?

2. What experiences have you personally experienced or observed of people experiencing varying quality of the social determinants of health? Did these experiences have obvious health or health-related effects?

3. Have you ever had any experiences in which you compared your living situation to others and felt bad as a result? Do you think that having these negative responses over an extended period of time could make you ill?

4. Which models do you think would be most useful for influencing policy-makers and the general public as to the importance of improving the social determinants of health?

5. Why do you think these models are rarely, if ever, mentioned in the media? What can be done to rectify this?

Recommended Readings

Bartley, M. (2003). *Health inequality: An introduction to concepts, theories, and methods.* Cambridge: Polity Press.

Large differences in life expectancy exist between the most privileged and the most disadvantaged social groups in industrial societies. This book assists in understanding the four most widely accepted theories of what lies behind inequalities in health: behavioural, psychosocial, material, and life-course approaches.

Brunner, E. & Marmot, M.G. (2006). "Social organization, stress, and health." In M.G. Marmot and R.G. Wilkinson (Eds.), *Social determinants of health* (pp. 6–30). Oxford: Oxford University Press.

This chapter contains details of how social structure and its correlates—such as material resources, stress, and health behaviours—get under the skin to determine health. The chapter also details how various bodily systems are profoundly affected by the experience of stress associated with living conditions.

Coburn, D. (2004). "Beyond the income inequality hypothesis: Globalization, neo-liberalism, and health inequalities." *Social Science & Medicine, 58,* 41–56.

Coburn provides a synthesis of political-economy concepts to help explain the high poverty rates and increasing inequality seen in today's Canada. He outlines a key role for globalization and the increasing influence of neo-liberalism as a governing ideology in shaping the experiences of Canadians in general and people living in poverty in Canada in particular.

Graham, H. (2007). *Unequal lives: Health and socioeconomic inequalities.* Buckingham: Open University Press.

    Unequal Lives is an introduction to social and health inequalities that brings together research from a variety of fields to guide understanding of why people's lives and health remain unequal. Social determinants of health are seen as the mediating mechanisms by which public policy shapes health.

Keating, D.P. & Hertzman, C. (Eds.) (1999). *Developmental health and the wealth of nations.* New York: Guilford Press.

    This book provides contributions that explore the psychological and developmental processes by which health inequalities come about. Running throughout the volume is a concern about economic inequality and poverty as a source of health and other outcomes.

Raphael, D., Colman, R., Labonte, R., MacDonald, J., Torgeson, R. & Hayward, K. (2003). *Income, health, and disease in Canada: Current state of knowledge, information gaps, and areas of needed inquiry.* Toronto: York University. Online at tinyurl.com/2x2h63.

    This report provides a systematic overview of how income is conceptualized as a variable in health research in Canada. It contains detailed descriptions of various approaches to conceptualizing income and other social determinants of health, and how these studies measure their effects upon health. It also provides a critique of gaps in research.

Shaw, M., Dorling, D., Gordon, D. & Davey Smith, G. (1999). *The widening gap: Health inequalities and policy in Britain.* Bristol: The Policy Press.

    In this excellent volume, the authors identified the 15 "worst health" and 13 "best health" constituencies in Britain and examine area differences on a wide range of health and socio-economic indicators. Their analysis takes place within a lifespan perspective whereby health differences are seen as resulting from an accumulation of material disadvantages that reflect widely differing economic and social life circumstances.

Related Web Sites

Canadian Population Health Initiative (CPHI)—www.secure.cihi.ca/cihiweb/dispPage.jsp?cw_page=cphi_e

    The CPHI's role is to expand the public's knowledge of population health. It works with partners across the country to: (1) generate new knowledge about the factors affecting the health of different groups of Canadians; (2) analyze evidence about the effectiveness of policy initiatives and provide a range of policy options based on best evidence; and (3) bring researchers, policy-makers, and health practitioners together to move the most current population research findings into policy and practice.

Canadian Public Health Association Policy Statements—www.cpha.ca/english/policy/pstatem/polstate.htm

    This Web site contains numerous CPHA statements about income, housing, employment, and other social determinants of health.

Policy Press UK—www.policypress.org.uk/

    The Policy Press is the specialist publisher in the UK of social and public policy books, reports, journals, and guides. As a not-for-profit organization aiming to improve social conditions, it is committed to publishing titles that will have an impact on research, teaching, policy, and practice. Many of its volumes are concerned with income and wealth inequalities, poverty, and other social determinants of health.

Prairie Women's Health Centre of Excellence—www.pwhce.ca/research.htm

The Prairie Women's Health Centre of Excellence works with the community to conduct new research specific to women in Manitoba and Saskatchewan, and with others across the country. Its current focus areas are: Aboriginal women's health issues; women, poverty, and health; health of women living in rural, remote, and northern communities; and gender in health planning.

Research from the National Longitudinal Survey of Children and Youth (NLSCY)—www.statcan.ca/english/rdc/rdcprojectsnlscy.htm

This Web site provides details concerning the many studies and reports being carried out within this project.

Part Two

INCOME SECURITY AND EMPLOYMENT IN CANADA

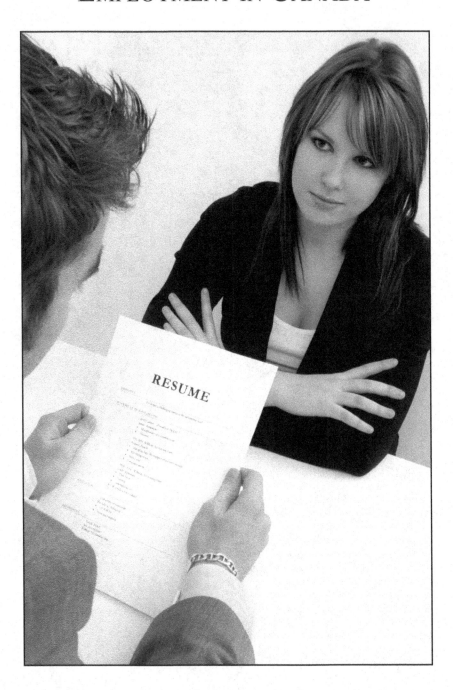

Income and its distribution, the availability and security of employment, and conditions of employment are prime social determinants of health. The availability of income, much of this a result of employment, is a determinant of other social determinants of health. Without adequate income, access to food, housing, and other basic prerequisites of health is increasingly difficult. Without adequate income, the likelihood of social exclusion increases as more and more Canadians are unable to participate in commonly assumed economic, social, cultural, and political activities. And even when employment is available, deteriorating working conditions, wages, and benefits, and increasing employment insecurity threaten health. Employment insecurity is a result of increasing economic globalization and the power of corporations and other employers. The contributions in this section document how Canadians are experiencing clear threats to health through the weakening of these social determinants of health. The sources of the deterioration of these social determinants of health are governments' political, economic, and social policy decisions. The contributors probe the origins of these decisions and present alternative policy futures to address these concerns.

Ann Curry-Stevens provides an overview of the meaning and importance of income and wealth inequality as well as the latest Canadian statistics. Despite long-standing beliefs about the equalitarian nature of Canadian society, not only is inequality increasing, but it is Canadians at the very bottom who are losing ground while those at the very top benefit. And non-White and new Canadians are especially likely to be losing ground. This skewing of Canadian society results from having governments leaving issues of income distribution to the marketplace and abrogating their responsibilities to meet the basic needs of many Canadians.

Nathalie Auger and Carolyne Alix provide an overview of what is known about the relationship between income and health. They provide different ways of measuring income and how these measures can be related to health. Their review provides conclusive evidence that income is a key social determinant of health. Detailed findings from recent studies on the relationship between income and health in Quebec drive home these points. The authors conclude that little will be accomplished in terms of improving Canadians'

health without focusing on issues of income distribution, poverty reduction, and providing Canadians with the basic prerequisites of health.

Dianne-Gabrielle Tremblay discusses how recent economic and demographic transformations are influencing the current Canadian employment market. Various definitions of employment insecurity are presented. Increases in "boundaryless careers"—in contrast to those jobs where some degree of security and upward progression could be expected—leads to increasing precariousness of employment. This is especially the case among Canadian women. The sources of these changes are a combination of economic and social forces, but their effects are strongly mediated by policy responses within nations. US and Canadian approaches are contrasted with those seen among Scandinavian nations where full employment and job retraining efforts are more valued.

Emile Tompa, Michael Polanyi, and Janice Foley focus on the productivity and health effects of increased labour market flexibility. While it is believed that such approaches increase productivity and efficiency, the evidence concerning this is mixed. What is clearer is that such approaches increase worker insecurity and threaten health and well-being. These negative effects are more likely to accrue to women, Canadians of colour, and those at the lower end of the economic ladder. The authors provide a range of ways by which economic competitiveness and employee health needs can be balanced. These include policy changes to balance power between employers and employees, research and education, and cultural and institutional changes to support health and well-being.

Andrew Jackson explains how a good job involves security, adequate conditions including pace and stress, opportunities for self-expression, and individual development at work, participation, and work-life balance. Evidence is systematically provided that indicates that there is significant deterioration in many of these workplace characteristics in Canada. He looks closely at injury rates in the workplace and teases out the factors contributing to their incidence. One factor strongly related to working conditions is degree of unionization whereby unionization is associated with improved conditions, security, and benefits. The Canadian scene is contrasted to that of European nations that direct resources to improving employment and employment training. Improvement will occur when governments help equalize bargaining power between workers and employers.

Peter Smith and Michael Polanyi provide recent findings concerning major work dimensions and their influence upon health. They focus on availability, adequacy of income, appropriateness of work arrangements with respect to non-work responsibilities and needs, and appreciation or involvement of workers as active workplace participants and contributors to society. Concepts such as "flexisecurity" and provision of a basic income are potential means of improving workplace conditions and improving health. They also suggest means by which available evidence can be translated into action involving democratizing policy-making processes and providing citizens with opportunities for meaningful engagement in democratic deliberation.

Chapter 3

WHEN ECONOMIC GROWTH DOESN'T TRICKLE DOWN: THE WAGE DIMENSIONS OF INCOME POLARIZATION

Ann Curry-Stevens

Introduction

Income inequality (also generically called the "growing gap") has generated significant attention over the last 10 years, with a substantial body of research profiling various elements of the gap. This chapter will walk the reader through an array of measures of inequality and unearth the learnings from such research. It is hoped that, simultaneously, the readers will become critical consumers of such statistical information, building skills to evaluate the adequacy of future data to which they are exposed. New research has also been done for this chapter—research that exposes the changing class structure of Canada, moulding us increasingly toward the poignant image of a rotten apple, eroding the middle class and increasing the rich and the poor.

We then place this research in the broader social and political context of the turn of the century, with a generation under our belts of the erosion of the social safety net and greater reliance on the market for meeting our economic needs. In conclusion, we profile the various forms of solutions, including policy solutions, campaign solutions, and vision-based solutions.

A note about the data: Most of the data in this chapter use income measures on families in which 85 percent of us reside. The reported data from the Centre for Social Justice refer to families (with one or two parents) raising dependent children.

Misleading "Average" Income Reports

When incomes are said to be growing, the data typically refers to a single measure of incomes, the mean (or average) for the entire population. One accentuated example reveals the inadequacy of this measure:

> If there are five people making $20,000/year and one person making $200,000/year, then the mean income level for those six people is $50,000/year. But to what degree does this measure reflect the real experience of those six people? Very little, for any of those involved.

In real life, Canadian families had an average market income of $70,300 in 2005, up from $69,500 in 2004. This is an increase, in one year, of 1.15 percent beyond the rise in inflation (since the figures are already adjusted to inflation, allowing for dollars to be constant across years). This continues a trend of rising annual growth in average incomes. At first glance, it would appear as though the economy is serving us well, in that our incomes were still rising despite stagnant economic growth. But remembering the illustration used above, the average income might be misleading as it might be unduly high if the incomes at the top are skewing the average to higher values. This is exactly what is happening.

Measures of Income Distribution: Market Incomes

Market incomes are the topic of discussion for the next few sections of this chapter as we focus on how well the market serves our income needs across the income spectrum. In later sections, we will examine other measures of income, including income measures that include the effects of transfers (such as unemployment insurance, child tax benefits, pensions, and social assistance) and taxes (provincial and federal income tax). Wealth measures (the total value of assets minus debts) are covered at the close of the review of income measures.

a. Median Incomes

The median income indicates the actual income of the middle-income earner in the population. In the scenario above, the median income would be that of the midpoint between the 3rd and 4th income earner. The middle-income earner is making $20,000/year, a picture that illustrates the actual environment for the majority, but does not provide any evidence of the incomes for anyone else. In reality, the difference between the average (also called the mean) and median incomes of all Canadians is substantial. The average family income in 2005 was $70,300 while the median income was $12,600 less at $57,700 (custom tabulation from Statistics Canada data, CANSIM table 202-0201). It is interesting to note that the difference between the median and the mean has been rising dramatically over the last 25 years from $4,000 to the high of $12,600 in 2005. This trend is due to the dramatic rise in mean incomes as they are swayed by the preponderance of very high incomes.

The problems with both the average and the median income measures is that they tell us very little about the incomes of those outside of the middle range—and the average actually tells us nothing about income earners at all, as our hypothetical example shows us. For those of us wanting to uncover the lived reality for Canadians, we have to turn to other income measures that explore various income groups; how they change in relationship over time; and uncover the trends during various time periods, such as the last generation, the last decade, and different cycles of booms and busts.

b. Quintiles

Analyses of Statistics Canada data reveals how the changes in income from 1980–2005 are spread across different slices of the population, namely quintiles (or 20 percent segments) of the population.

From this analysis, we can establish that, in fact, the reported gains in income for Canadian families over time are misleading. It is unequally borne by different sections of the population (see Figure 3.1).

One might claim that this is not really very much of a difference. In reality, the loss at the bottom was minimal (at $900). So maybe we are just making a fuss over relatively inconsequential issues. The value of these dollars for low-income earners is, however, significant as $900 can represent the purchase of winter clothing for one's children and being able to sustain telephone service. One important observation is that the loss for middle-income Canadian families is most dramatic of the quintiles, a fact we will return to later in this chapter.

To examine if these findings are typical or atypical, we need to turn to both longer term analysis and more detailed analysis, for the quintile investigation likely smoothes over variations within these groups.

c. Deciles and Ratios

The Centre for Social Justice, in 1998, published an explosive report on the growing gap in Canada, an attempt to understand the nature of inequality in Canada and how it had changed over time. This study turned away from the traditional evaluation of quintiles in favour of deciles and allowed for exploration of greater nuances of life at both margins—the top 10 percent of income earners and the bottom 10 percent of income earners. The preferred statistic in this situation was the ratio of the top and bottom 10 percent, and an assessment of how they had varied over time. The study in 1998 was repeated in 1999, with the cumulative findings presented in Table 3.1.

These findings revealed burgeoning inequality (as the ratio exploded from double to triple digits) yet showed some good news in its narrowing from 1993–1997. This good news appeared to stem from an eventual improvement of low income four years into an unprecedented economic boom. Yalnizyan (2007) has since extended this decile analysis to 2004 and revealed that the ratio has dropped below 1:100 in recent years, but that it remains in the high double digits. But please

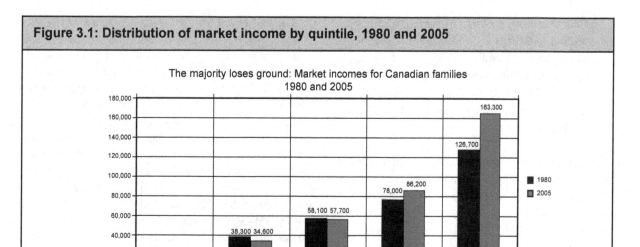

Figure 3.1: Distribution of market income by quintile, 1980 and 2005

The majority loses ground: Market incomes for Canadian families 1980 and 2005

Market income is income earned through employment (waged and self-employment), plus the value of gains on investments cashed in during the year.

Source: Statistics Canada. (2008). Survey of Labour and Income Dynamics and Survey on Consumer Finances. Ottawa: Statistics Canada.

Table 3.1: Distribution of market income by decile

Market income earnings	1981	1984	1989	1993	1997
Poorest 10%	4,866	1,938	3,741	511	1,255
Richest 10%	122,964	125,056	144,699	131,412	136,394
Ratio	25.27	64.53	36.68	257.17	108.68

Data Source: Statistics Canada, Survey of Consumer Finances.

Source: Yalnizyan, A. (1998). *The growing gap: A report on growing inequality between the rich and poor in Canada.* Toronto: Centre for Social Justice; Yalnizyan, A. (2000). *Canada's great divide: The politics of the growing gap between rich and poor in the 1990s.* Toronto: Centre for Social Justice.

do not assume that a 100-fold discrepancy is anywhere near acceptable in Canadian society.

d. Income Measures across Time: Boom and Bust Cycles

The next report from the Centre for Social Justice (Curry-Stevens, 2001) used a different measure of inequality. The measure used in the earlier reports was unduly influenced by relatively small increases in income, resulting in a shrinking of the gap during the economic boom cycle of the last 10 years. The calculations work as follows:

Let's say that the poorest Canadian families earned $1,000 in 1995 and the richest earned $100,000. Using the ratio measure, the gap ratio is 100; that is, the richest 10 percent earn 100 times more than the poorest 10 percent. Let's then say that in the next year, the poorest Canadians earn $2,000 and the richest earn $110,000. According to the ratio calculation, the measure of inequality drops to 55, and it appears that there is a drastic shrinking of inequality in the country. Yet, the distance between the two income-earning groups has increased since the poor got richer by only $1,000 while the richest earned an additional $10,000. It is the significance of the changes in incomes of the poorest that unduly influence this measure, and we know that their incomes are highly volatile.

Seeking to remedy this situation, the third report on the status of inequality in Canada from the Centre for Social Justice turned to periodic measures of inequality, that of measuring the performance of each decile over time and comparing the performance of different income groups. Additionally, the CSJ report analyzed the trends within economic cycles to see how incomes were affected by upturns and downturns in the economy. Those seeking to silence complaints about the market had increasingly voiced an argument akin to, "Well, we are likely entering a recession, so it is more important that we do *x*, *y*, or *z* than to put more money into income supports for poor people" (feel free to put whatever policy alternative you want in this sentence, such as tax breaks for the rich, reductions in environmental protections, or reduced labour legislation).

The CSJ report, entitled *When Markets Fail People*, was prepared with the intention of exploring the income performance of the deciles over the last two recessions (1981–1984 and 1989–1993) and the last three recovery periods (1973–1981, 1984–1989, and 1993–1998). The patterns of economic performance were dramatic (Table 3.2). For the bottom income earners, the last two recessions saw a drop in their incomes of 60 percent and then 86 percent, yet their income recovery performances during the boom years were actually negative in the first boom, and then somewhat significant during the next boom (up by $1,803) and then marginal in the third (up by $584). The companion data for the wealthiest Canadian families were that in the first recession they actually gained ground and had their incomes increase by 2 percent and the second saw their incomes drop by 9 percent. Yet during the recovery years, their incomes surged by $11,964, then by $19,643, and then by $17,158.

Turning our analysis to recovery periods, we find that all income groups eventually gain ground (with the sole exception of the poorest decile in the boom of the 1970s), but inequality widens dramatically as top incomes surge over the meagre improvements made at lower levels (Table 3.3). A supplemental calculation of "fair shares"

Table 3.2: Market incomes during recessions (1981–1984 and 1989–1993)

	1981	1984	1989	1993	1981 to 1984	% Change	1989 to 1993	% Change
Decile 1	4,866	1,938	3,741	511	-2,928	**60% drop**	-3,230	**86% drop**
Decile 2	21,296	14,853	19,000	10,392	-6,443	**30% drop**	-8,608	**45% drop**
Decile 3	31,747	26,250	30,614	22,306	-5,497	**17% drop**	-8,308	**21% drop**
Decile 4	39,395	35,117	39,879	32,314	-4,278	**11% drop**	-7,565	**16% drop**
Decile 5	46,498	42,911	47,813	40,946	-3,587	**8% drop**	-6,867	**14% drop**
Decile 6	53,187	50,073	55,508	49,611	-3,114	**6% drop**	-5,897	**11% drop**
Decile 7	60,886	57,708	63,945	59,216	-3,178	**5% drop**	-4,729	**7% drop**
Decile 8	69,739	66,739	74,681	70,012	-3,000	**4% drop**	-4,669	**6% drop**
Decile 9	83,169	80,433	89,707	84,782	-2,736	**3% drop**	-4,925	**5% drop**
Decile 10	122,964	125,056	144,699	131,412	+2,092	**2% increase**	-13,287	**9% drop**

Date source: Unpublished data from Statistics Canada, Survey of Consumer Finances. All figures are in constant 1997 dollars.

Source: Curry-Stevens, A. (2001). *When markets fail people: Exploring the widening gap between rich and poor in Canada.* Toronto: CSJ Foundation for Research and Education.

was done on the data—if the data distribution was to stay constant, each decile would receive 10 percent of the income gains. Our analysis revealed that every decile below 7—for every economic boom over the last 30 years—got less than their fair share. It is only the top three deciles that got more than their fair share. As consistent with our growing pessimism about the market, we find that the top decile takes the lion's share of all income improvements and that this share accelerated across the decades.

Noted is our failure to achieve fairness. This "fair share" approach would have sustained existing levels of inequality. We did not even consider whether remedial allocations of income could occur, whereby the poor would receive more income gains that the rich, which would have reduced the gap.

The comparisons of these two performances is dramatic—recessions cause the poor to lose far more earning power than any other group, yet after shouldering these huge losses, they fail to catch up, putting to rest the possibility that, when the full economic cycles are considered, these trends have a negligible effect on inequality. For decades, we have asked the working class to tighten their belts during recessions and have made promises that when the economy improves, more benefits

will be allocated. Recovery times endow the rich to accelerate their earnings with quite minor achievements resulting for the poor. This performance is pervasive over each economic cycle, and throughout the last generation (approximately 25 years), the trends have worsened with inequality being experienced more deeply across the population.

A final scan of the data posted above reveals a deeply troubling finding—that the market incomes of the bottom 30 percent of Canadian families are worse off in 1998 than they were in 1973. Troubling trends also exist for the middle class, who are basically treading water, gaining little ground, and have to cope with the rapid distancing of those richer than they. The social consequences of a deteriorating middle class have begun to be assessed (Curry-Stevens, 2008) as this broad income group holds the potential to exert greater political influence than those in at the lowest margins. When the promise of economic adequacy begins to ring hollow, pressure for political and economic change may be catalyzed.

Population Measures of Inequality

We now turn our attention to the shifting profile of the population and explore the numbers of people living at

Table 3.3: Market incomes during recoveries (1973–1981, 1984–1989, and 1994–1998)									
	1973	1981	1984	1989	1994	1998	1973–81	1984–89	1994–98
Decile 1	5,386	4,866	1,938	3,741	733	1,317	($520)	$1,803	$584
Decile 2	20,245	21,296	14,853	19,000	11,874	13,809	$1,051	$4,147	$1,935
Decile 3	29,189	31,747	26,250	30,614	24,715	26,093	$2,558	$4,364	$1,378
Decile 4	35,824	39,395	35,117	39,879	34,761	36,456	$3,571	$4,762	$1,695
Decile 5	41,752	46,498	42,911	47,813	43,510	46,073	$4,746	$4,902	$2,563
Decile 6	47,747	53,187	50,073	55,508	52,117	55,679	$5,440	$5,435	$3,562
Decile 7	54,239	60,886	57,708	63,945	61,091	65,562	$6,647	$6,237	$4,471
Decile 8	62,495	69,739	66,739	74,681	71,615	76,851	$7,244	$7,942	$5,236
Decile 9	74,113	83,169	80,433	89,707	87,225	94,122	$9,056	$9,274	$6,897
Decile 10	111,000	122,964	125,056	144,699	135,509	152,667	$11,964	$19,643	$17,158

Data source: Unpublished data from Statistics Canada, Survey of Labour and Income Dynamics, and Survey of Consumer Finances. All figures are in constant 1997 dollars.

Source: Curry-Stevens, A. (2001) *When markets fail people: Exploring the widening gap between rich and poor in Canada.* Toronto: CSJ Foundation for Research and Education.

these different income levels. Such investigation provides insights as to the changing nature of our class structure. First let's explore this theoretically. Prior to the rapid expansion of waged labour and the industrial revolution in the 19th century, the distribution of the population was pyramid-shaped, with the vast majority living in poverty. Through the 19th century and much of the 20th century, there is a massive expansion of the middle class as many move up the income ladder and, to a lesser degree, an expansion of the wealthy. These trends result in our becoming apple-shaped, and it was seen as a healthy sign of a flourishing democracy. A strong and stable middle class, with prognosis for upward mobility, seemed to mark the golden age of capitalism (1940s–1970s). We now investigate, statistically, the form that our population now takes.

Yalnizyan (1998) profiled the proportion of Canadian families in 1973 and in 1996 who were living at different income levels. Taking the decile distribution of 1973 and then measuring how much of the population was now based at those levels, she uncovered a grave hollowing out of the middle class (Figure 3.2). Where middle-income earners formerly composed 60 percent of the population,

this value slipped to just 44 percent by 1996. While the middle class shrank, the ranks of the very poor and the very rich rose significantly. This was the generational picture of the inequality from 1973–1996, but without the fuller picture of distribution for 1973, we do not know what form our class structure has, although we know it is more divided and polarized from that time on.

Subsequently, Curry-Stevens (2004) examined the shifting concentration along ranges of income, and provides a clearer picture of how the population is shaped at the start and the end of the last 20 years (Table 3.4).

From this study, we can see that the distribution of Canadian families is changing quite dramatically, especially if we examine how the recovery and recession times impact the population. The size of the middle class, relative to other income groups, decreased by 25 percent over the last 25 years. Surprisingly, losses are experienced in both the recovery (–5.6 percent) and recession (–5.0 percent) periods. This is counterintuitive. We would expect that the size of the middle class would increase as the economy would generate an increasing middle class as the ranks of the poor and struggling move up the ladder. After all, we were led to believe that a thriving

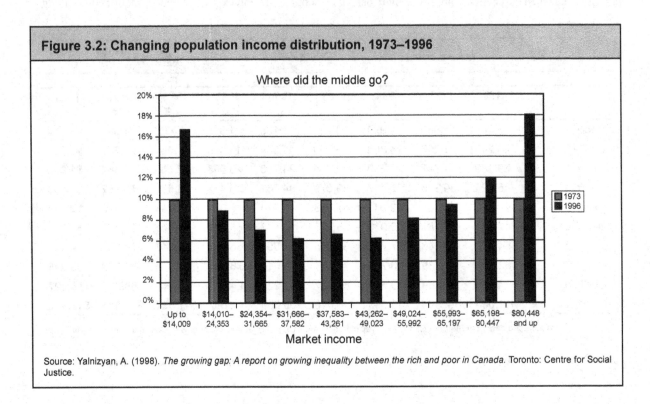

Figure 3.2: Changing population income distribution, 1973–1996

Where did the middle go?

Source: Yalnizyan, A. (1998). *The growing gap: A report on growing inequality between the rich and poor in Canada.* Toronto: Centre for Social Justice.

Table 3.4: Distribution of market incomes of Canadian families 1980 to 2000, highlighting most recent recession and recovery data, as well as data for last two decades.

	Poor < $5,000	Working poor $5,000–$19,999	Struggling $20,000–$29,999	Middle class $30,000–$59,999	Well off $60,000–$99,999	Rich $100,000–$149,999	Very rich >$150,000	TOTAL rounded to nearest 1%
1980	7.3%	10.1%	8.1%	34.7%	29.7%	8.0%	2.2%	100%
1989	7.7%	10.6%	8.5%	32.1%	28.1%	9.6%	2.9%	100%
1993	10.9%	12.9%	9.9%	30.5%	25.0%	8.4%	2.3%	100%
2000	7.3%	12.0%	8.7%	28.8%	27.9%	11.1%	4.3%	100%
Calculations								
Recovery	-33.0%	-7.0%	-12.1%	-5.6%	11.6%	32.1%	87.0%	
Recession	41.6%	21.7%	16.5%	-5.0%	-11.0%	-12.5%	-20.7%	
2 Decades	**0.0%**	**23.0%**	**6.9%**	**-17.0%**	**-6.1%**	**38.8%**	**95.5%**	

Source: Curry-Stevens, A. (2004). "Arrogant capitalism: Changing futures, changing lives," *Canadian review of social policy* 51(June), 137–142.

middle class is the foundation of a healthy democracy. Yet, the economy is not generating such results.

The chart also reveals another troubling dynamic. Note the pattern of those earning between $60,000 and $99,999 a year. This well-off group has shrunk by 6.1 percent over the last generation. The erosion of the size of this group creates a structural barrier to a more affluent Canada, whereby decreasing odds of moving up thwarts the middle class. The ranks of the economic elite are growing in strength, drawing in numbers from those well off, but not being replaced by mobility upwards from the middle class.

We now use the same data set to more fully examine the profile of our changing class structure over the last 25 years. For this study, we portray the data in graphic form, enabling us to compare the 1980 and 2005 patterns. Such investigation allows us to address the shifting structures and companion problems (Figure 3.3).

We can see that population measures of economic inequality reveal profound changes in our class structure, with the predominant features of the years 1980–2005 being an erosion of the middle class while increasing the ranks of the wealthy and the poor. This hollowing out begins our image of becoming more of a rotten apple than an apple. The data taking us to 2005 shows that Canadians are marginally less likely to be very destitute (making

less than $5,000), but are more likely to be working poor (earning less than $20,000), and struggling (making between $20,000–30,000). They are today much less likely to be in the middle class and in ranks of the well-off. In total, they are much less likely to earn incomes up to $100,000, except if they are at dismal income levels, and then they are more likely to be low income. Yet they are also more likely to be rich and very rich—meagre carrots given the rest of the scenario facing the majority of Canadians. The ranks of the rich and very rich today total 22.0 percent of Canadian families.

If we ask ourselves why this deteriorating situation for almost 80 percent of the Canadian population is tolerated across various classes, we need to more fully understanding patterns of taxes, transfers, consumption, and also of politics and rhetoric. We will return to this question at the close of the chapter, and also direct the reader to consider the materials in the Raphael and Curry-Stevens chapter at the end of this text.

Taxes and Transfers: Establishing Our Lived Experiences

We have just spent considerable time reviewing the status of market incomes in Canada for reasons that stem from

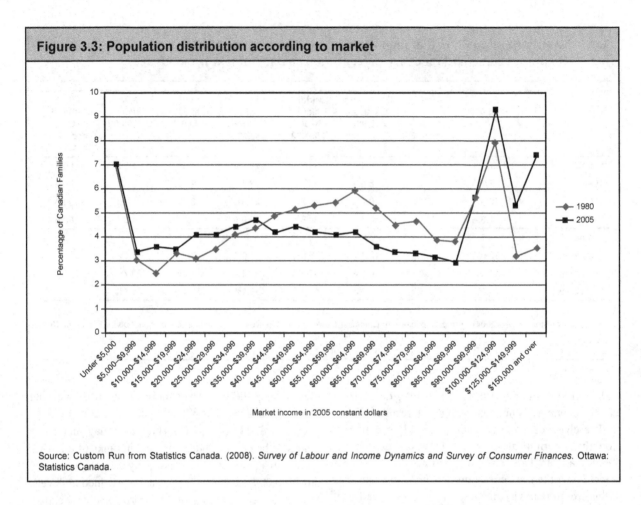

Figure 3.3: Population distribution according to market

Source: Custom Run from Statistics Canada. (2008). *Survey of Labour and Income Dynamics and Survey of Consumer Finances*. Ottawa: Statistics Canada.

its prime generative role in creating inequality. Turning to the role of transfers and taxes (the redistributive factors), we concurrently turn our focus to the incomes that people actually live on—government transfers provide them with additional income through pensions, welfare, and unemployment benefits (the largest transfers) and taxes reduce the incomes that people end up with as governments remove taxes in order to pay for essential services and the transfers noted earlier. Overall, these interventions have an equalizing effect as they raise the incomes of those at the bottom (through transfers) and lower the incomes at the top (through income taxes). Our key areas of concern are the trends in these taxes and transfers, issues that rest with the government and various politicians in power. It is government policy that sets the levels of the taxes and transfers, and thus creates the net redistributive effect on the income patterns established in the marketplace where we earn our income.

Overall, this redistributive effect dramatically reduces inequality. Before taxes and transfers, the inequality between rich and poor is in the triple digits, with the richest 10 percent earning 109 times the income of the poorest 10 percent. When taxes and transfers are added, the ratio drops (in 2004) to 9.9 (Yalnizyan, 2007). The cumulative effect is obviously significant and progressive. But the study of Yalnizyan was not a good news story, for while this ratio shows the moderating effect of government policy, it also showed that this effect is becoming less significant over the last generation. Her data reveals that the ratio has grown from a low of 7.5 in 1988 to its highest level of 9.9 in 2007 (Yalnizyan, 2007, p. 48).

Another way to understand this trend is that our governments have become increasingly tolerant of income inequality and are reducing the levers that promote income equality. Specifically, drops in income transfers (with employment insurance coverage being dramatically reduced at the federal level and social assistance reduced in many provinces) and decreased progressivity in our income tax system increase inequality. The significance of these levers must be appreciated, for as the attack on government spending occurred at the start of the 1980s, so too did the attack on the progressive tax system.

While the deteriorating situation of redistribution via government policies is distressing, remember that the causal factor for income inequality is wages and incomes, factors that are under the responsibility of employers and corporations. We must remember that wages paid by employers are the primary culprit for burgeoning inequality (Figure 3.4).

From the position of those concerned with equality, such moves by federal and provincial governments are indefensible, illustrating that they have led, at the bottom decile, to a reduction in net income during this most recent era of economic growth. Again, we witness the pulling away of the top income group in whose ranks we find our political and economic leaders. This trend generates considerable concern about the growing isolation and resulting social exclusion of the rich from the majority population below them.

Already in evidence is income growth at the uppermost income levels. Murphy, Roberts, and Wolfson (2007) analyzed incomes at various definitions of "high income" using both relative and absolute thresholds. Following the relative measure used in this chapter, we will look

at incomes at the top 5 percent, 1 percent, 0.1 percent, and 0.01 percent of the population (as we have already examined the top 10 percent). We will also continue to use family measures to maintain continuity.

From Figure 3.5, we can see that the richer one becomes, the more significant are one's income gains over the years. When looking at the values of these incomes and also drawing from Figure 3.1, we can see evidence that the economy greatly favours those at the top and is harmful to those in the middle and at the bottom of the income ladder. This should raise questions in our minds when we consider the impact of the economy on our social structures and the interventions advanced by governments to influence the economy and the quality of jobs available. Consider the ethics involved when the top 0.1 percent of Canadian families bring home an extra $1.35 million annually, and the top 0.01 percent bring home an extra $5 million annually! We have also learned that across the last generation, governments are doing a less adequate job in advancing equality—they are increasingly tolerating the ravages of inequality created by deeply unequal wages.

Wealth Measures

A final method through which to measure inequality is the measure of wealth. This is the total sum of the value of

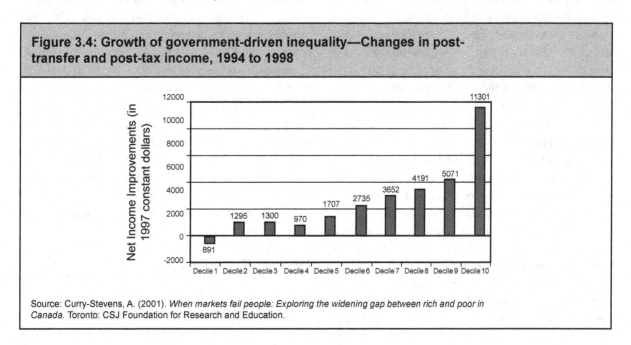

Figure 3.4: Growth of government-driven inequality—Changes in post-transfer and post-tax income, 1994 to 1998

Source: Curry-Stevens, A. (2001). *When markets fail people: Exploring the widening gap between rich and poor in Canada.* Toronto: CSJ Foundation for Research and Education.

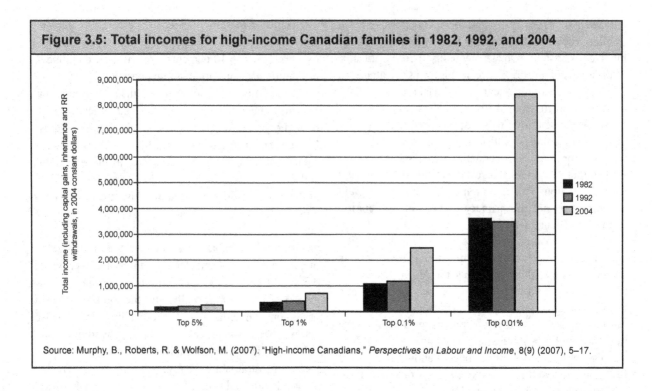

Figure 3.5: Total incomes for high-income Canadian families in 1982, 1992, and 2004

Source: Murphy, B., Roberts, R. & Wolfson, M. (2007). "High-income Canadians," *Perspectives on Labour and Income*, 8(9) (2007), 5–17.

all assets minus all debts owed, and allows us to review the cumulative impact of years of differential incomes on the net assets of various groups within the population. The years of available statistics are limited to 1984, 1999, and 2005, which still illuminate generational trends, but miss the nuance available through annual reviews. This problem is moderated somewhat by the more stable nature of wealth as opposed to income measures. The exception to this stability is the value of assets held in the stock market, volatile in general, but relatively stagnant in recent years, and substantially more significant for upper income groups and of rapidly shrinking significance as one moves down the prosperity ladder.

Again, the average wealth measure paints a rosy picture, with a 79 percent increase in mean wealth recorded for Canadian families over the last generation. The decile picture reveals an answer to the question "For whom is this true?" by showing the distribution of those effects (Figure 3.6). The poorest 40 percent of Canadian families actually lost ground over the last six years. The poorest decile lost the most ground, now owing $9,600 to their debtors. The richest 10 percent of families saw their wealth increase by a dramatic 123 percent, to a value of

$1,194,000. Figure 3.7 shows the uneven distribution of improvements in wealth over the last 21 years.

The net change in family wealth over the generation is illustrated showing how wealth inequality shows a rapid deterioration that cannot help but have wider social effects. In Morissette and Zhang's (2006) analysis of the cause, they attribute the primary causes to disparities in home equity, RRSPs, and LIRAs (totalling 60 percent of the growth in inequality); stocks, bonds, and mutual fund holdings (13 percent); and other real estate (21 percent). Inequality in inheritances between income groups also contributes to wealth inequalities, with the average inheritance for the bottom 20 percent found to be $13,200 and the top 20 percent to be $136,600 in 2005. Sharp increases in RRSP contributions occurred for high-income families between 1986 and 2003, mirroring the federal government's tax incentives for large contributions.

Hardest-Hit Populations

Within our patterns of income inequality are features that help put a face to inequality today. Increasingly, that

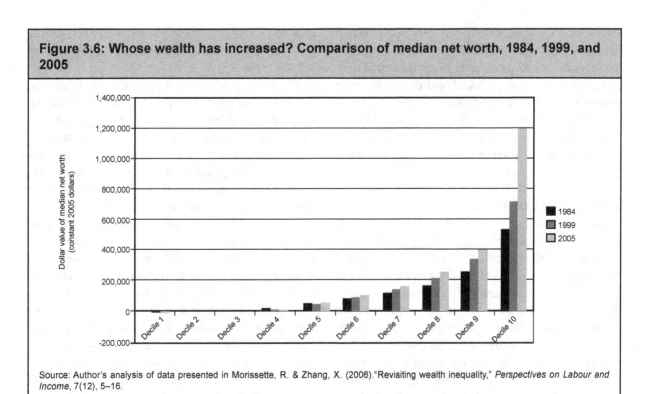

Figure 3.6: Whose wealth has increased? Comparison of median net worth, 1984, 1999, and 2005

Source: Author's analysis of data presented in Morissette, R. & Zhang, X. (2006)."Revisiting wealth inequality," *Perspectives on Labour and Income*, 7(12), 5–16.

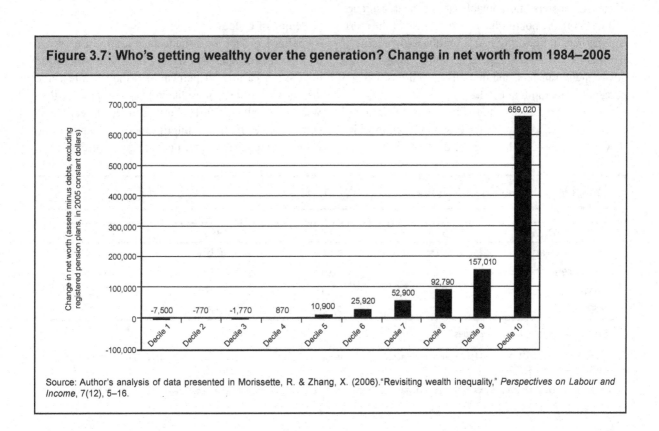

Figure 3.7: Who's getting wealthy over the generation? Change in net worth from 1984–2005

Source: Author's analysis of data presented in Morissette, R. & Zhang, X. (2006)."Revisiting wealth inequality," *Perspectives on Labour and Income*, 7(12), 5–16.

face is racialized, destitute, female, and young. This is not to say these dynamics are exclusive to these groups, but that market and government trends have been most damaging to these groups. As we consider the growth in income inequality, severe social consequences emerge from the ways in which this issue hits home in different communities. There are several faces to this impact, three of which are covered in this chapter: the poorest Canadians, people of colour, and women.

a. The Poorest Canadians

Those at the bottom of the income ladder, those in the poorest decile and quintile have already exhibited the worst form of market failure, for their market incomes are completely insufficient to sustain their families or even themselves. They lose by far the most in recessions (up to 86 percent of their incomes were lost in the last recession) and fail to gain much ground in recoveries (earning only another $584 in the last recovery). In fact, when surveying the total income for the bottom decile, Curry-Stevens (2001) revealed that 91 percent of their total income comes from government transfers. In an era of cuts to transfers (most notably employment insurance and welfare), the poorest income groups suffer the most. It is perhaps noteworthy that more than 40 percent of families derive at least 10 percent of their incomes from government transfers, and that this level drops below 5 percent for the top four deciles.

The poverty rates themselves have fluctuated according to the point within the economic cycle in which they are measured. While the incidence of poverty has gone down in this last economic boom (and this is truly good news), they remain higher than the levels reached in 1989 (Table 3.5).

Further calculations by Scott (2002) reveal that the news is not as good as originally assessed. While the levels of poverty have gone down, the depths of their poverty have increased. This poverty gap is the distance that the average income level for those in poverty live below the poverty line itself. All groups, except lone-parent families, are worse off than they were in 1989, living typically $1,000 deeper in poverty.

A profile of Canada's poor (meaning they fall below Statistics Canada's Low-Income Cut-off line) was conducted by the National Council of Welfare (2006) with alarming revelations. The depths of poverty and its persistence are worsening. More than 30 percent of Canadians were poor at some point between 1996 and 2001, although the annual poverty rate is at 15.5 percent. The depth of poverty is revealed in Figure 3.8. Please note that these figures include government transfers such as welfare, child tax credits, and pensions. Even with these programs, the level of destitution is profound.

b. People of Colour

Racialized groups in Canada face a strong earnings disadvantage compared to Whites. In 1998, the racialized population earned 30 percent less than Whites, and they were 2.3 times more likely to live in poverty than Whites (Galabuzi, 2001). Furthermore, the economic performance of recent immigrants is deteriorating, with real incomes falling, on average, 7 percent from

---

Table 3.5: Selected poverty rates

Rate of Poverty	1980	1989	1996	2005
All Canadians	16.0%	14.0%	20.6%	15.3%
Children	16.2%	15.1%	23.6%	16.8%
Working Age	13.3%	12.1%	19.5%	15.5%
Seniors	31.0%	22.6%	20.6%	14.5%

Based on before-tax low-income cut-offs

Source: Scott K. (2002). "A lost decade: Income inequality and the health of Canadians." Presentation to the "Social Determinants of Health across the Lifespan" conference, Toronto, November 2002.

Additional source: Author's analysis of Statistics Canada (2008). *Survey of Labour and Income Dynamics*. Ottawa: Statistics Canada.

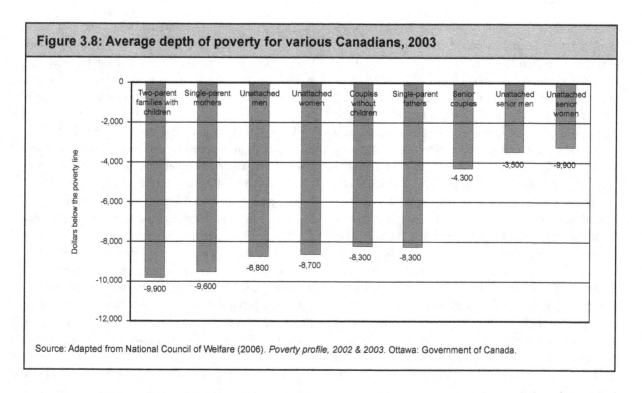

Figure 3.8: Average depth of poverty for various Canadians, 2003

Source: Adapted from National Council of Welfare (2006). *Poverty profile, 2002 & 2003*. Ottawa: Government of Canada.

1980–2000 despite general income growth of 7 percent for Canadian-born men (Frenette & Morisette, 2003).

Several hypotheses tend to surface to explain these differences, with each one debunked as they emerged:

1. Perhaps it is because they are immigrants? No. White immigrants earn an average of 22 percent more than immigrants of colour, thus showing that most of the difference is a function of skin colour and much less due to immigrant status (Galabuzi, 2001).

2. Perhaps it is because they are not as well educated? No. When we compare recent immigrants to the Canadian-born population, 44 percent of recent male immigrants have a university degree while only 19 percent of those Canadian-born are similarly accomplished. The pattern for women is similar but less pronounced. Even in the 1980s, the educational attainment of new immigrants was double that of the Canadian-born (Frenette & Morisette, 2003).

3. Perhaps it is because of their language skills? No. The Canadian government demands competency in one of the two official languages to be eligible for immigration. They may be strongly accented, but will have English language proficiency.

There is one other possible causative factor: The length of time in Canada affects the type of jobs available, so it would be unreasonable to expect that new entrants to the job market would have earnings parity with more seasoned workers. To answer this question, we turn to Frenette and Morisette (2003). Seeking to understand how earnings between immigrants and non-immigrants could achieve parity, they reviewed the economic performance of immigrants who arrived during different time periods with those who were Canadian-born. Immigrants who arrived within the last five years had dramatically lower incomes than the Canadian-born workers. In 2000, recent immigrant men earn 28 percent less than Canadian-born men. This is double the rate of 1980, indicating a worsening of the employment crisis for new immigrants. For women, the difference is even worse as they earn 31 percent less than their Canadian-born counterparts.

Their investigation of the longer-term impact of immigration status is also profoundly unsettling. Even

15 years after arrival, immigrants who arrived between 1985 and 1989 earned between 15 percent and 24 percent lower earnings than non-immigrants. Earlier immigrants fared better, with those arriving from 1975–1979 earning only 13 percent less. One troubling consequence is the "potential drop in immigrants' permanent income, and in the absence of offsetting changes in their savings rates, a potential decline in immigrants' wealth and precautionary savings.... Recent immigrants will be more likely to have difficulty making ends meets and will also be more vulnerable to shocks such as job loss or unexpected expenditures" (Frenette & Morisette, 2003, p. 15).

Immigrant workers can be expected to sustain this pattern over time unless there is "abnormally high earnings growth in the future" (Frenette & Morisette, 2003, p. 1). Such "abnormal" growth could be induced by an array of policy initiatives such as employment equity or acceptance at par of foreign credentials or foreign work experience, interventions that have been largely voluntary as opposed to mandatory (with the notable exception of the federal government's commitment to employment equity within the public service).

It seems we are skirting around the obvious—that instead of immigration status, education, or language skills, the problem is one of skin colour, and that racism (as it shows up in our institutions and individual behaviours) is the strongest component of the differential earnings level.

Is this a fair accusation to level at Canadian society, a country that prides itself in its racial diversity and its embrace of immigrants from all countries around the world? When one looks beyond this surface image, one finds a strong legacy of racism, land theft, colonization, occupational segregation, and even slavery. Few know it, but 200 years of slavery existed from the early 1600s to 1833, followed shortly thereafter by ongoing segregation in schools and other institutions. Racism was deemed legal by Canada's highest court (until 1939) and Ontario segregated Black students until 1964.

The enslavement of Native peoples that began in the 1600s continues today, with Aboriginal rights limited to reserves, severely curtailing the political and social rights of Aboriginals who live off-reserve. The federal government's continued failure to introduce Aboriginal self-government and to resolve outstanding land claims maintains the marginalization and exploitation of Aboriginals. The residential school system of 1879 to the mid-1980s forcibly removed children from their homes, denied them access to their families and culture, and forced British culture onto them. Aboriginal communities throughout the country continue to struggle with recovery.

What do we imagine the impact of this history to be? Current pronounced labour issues carry over from more clearly apparent exploitation. Modern-day servants exist in the form of those who clean our toilets, wash our dishes, package our foods, mow our lawns, care for our children, sew our clothes, drive us around, and harvest our foods. Such occupations are typically low-wage and rely heavily on the labour of racialized groups. We must ask ourselves how much our legacy of slavery and ongoing racism creates the employment conditions of these occupations. Is our ongoing failure to adequately pay those who service the needs of Whites a legacy of slavery and how Whites devalue those who perform such jobs?

We must face this history, and the companion evidence of reports that illustrate racism is embedded in various Canadian systems: criminal justice (Commission on Systemic Racism in the Ontario Criminal Justice System, 1994); education (Canadian Race Relations Foundation, 1999; Lewis, 1992); immigration (Canadian Council for Refugees, 2000); public service (Task Force on the Participation of Visible Minorities in the Federal Public Service, 2000); housing (Ornstein, 1994, 1999); and employment (Abella, 1984; Canada Employment and Immigration Advisory Council, 1992).

c. Women

Despite popular opinion that women have achieved equality with men, women's incomes remain a stubborn 62 percent lower than men ($24,400 instead of $39,300 for total income in 2003) (Lindsay & Almey, 2006, p. 133). At first glance, one might think that this is a function of choice and that women might work fewer hours to accumulate this income. But when we compare income levels of women who work full-time to those of men who work full-time, the earnings remain inequitable. While there is a significant improvement, female workers still earn only 71 percent of male earnings (Table 3.6).

Remember that the occupational and educational attainment data have been collected for full-time, full-

Table 3.6: Selected annual income data, 2003 for women and men in Canada

Employment and family status	Women	Men	Earnings ratio
Annual earnings	24,800	39,100	63%
Full-time, full-year earnings	36,500	51,400	71%
Family status for full-time, full-year workers			
Separated, divorced, or widowed	37,600	48,600	77%
Married	36,800	56,400	65%
Single, never married	34,600	37,000	94%
65 and over	24,400	39,300	62%
Lone-parent families	32,500	54,700	59%
Education level for full-time, full-year workers			
Secondary school graduate	30,500	43,000	71%
Certificate or diploma	34,200	49,800	69%
University degree	53,400	77,500	69%
Occupation for full-time, full-year workers			
Sales/service	24,100	43,300	56%
Trades/transportation	24,800	43,500	57%
Primary	19,200	31,500	61%
Manufacturing	26,200	45,100	58%
Professionals			
Business/finance	55,800	80,400	69%
Social sciences/religion	63,900	91,200	70%
Medicine/health	61,100	116,300	53%
Teaching	47,500	63,300	75%
Managerial	46,600	69,000	68%
Administrative	35,500	55,700	64%

Source: Adapted from Lindsay, C. & Almey, M. (2006). "Income and earnings." In *Women in Canada: A gender-based statistical report* (pp. 133–158). Ottawa: Statistics Canada.

year workers, thus eliminating the impact of part-time work. And still women make significantly less money than men.

If we think about this dynamic another way, we can consider that men receive a significant premium for their gender regardless of their education, age, and profession. The size of this premium will vary, but men are being financially rewarded for the simple fact that they are male. Given that this premium transverses all forms of family status, education, profession, and age, we can deduce that this premium is unearned and undeserved.

Patriarchy remains alive and well in the employment market.

Summary of Findings

Reviewing the data in this chapter, we uncover the following problems with the distribution of market income, total income, and wealth:

1. Inequality is growing throughout time, with the market's performance widening the economic

(and subsequently social) gap between the rich and the poor.

2. The severity of these problems is accelerating through the last generation as incomes at the top surge and those at the bottom falter.

3. There is much greater income volatility at the bottom of the income ladder and less further up the ladder, indicating that this form of insecurity (that of not knowing how poor people will become in a given year) necessitates assured incomes through social transfers.

4. The incomes at the bottom are completely inadequate to live on, with the bottom decile being destitute and the next decile earners living well below the poverty line. Even the third decile is below the poverty line. Despite improvements in the poverty levels, they are still higher than in 1989, leading us to understand that the market is unable to provide sufficient work or income for the most marginal Canadians.

5. The ratio of top earners to bottom earners moves from double digits in the 1970s and 1980s to triple-digit inequality in the 1990s. Different measures of this gap generate different results as to whether the gap is widening or narrowing. Earlier ratio measures have been discarded in favour of absolute measures.

6. Upward income mobility is harder today than 25 years ago. There is an erosion of upper (but not top) income groups in society, meaning that it is harder today to break out of middle incomes and into upper incomes.

7. Governments today are tolerating more inequality as the post-tax, post-transfer income measures reveal a trend toward greater inequality. The erosion of the progressive nature of income taxes and transfers is responsible for this change.

8. Greater reliance on markets for the overall financial well-being of its citizens is a dismal failure for both absolute and relative inequality, but most poignantly for relative inequality. Today we are a much more socially and economically divided nation, with lives increasingly proscribed by the fortunes and misfortunes of our birth.

9. Women's economic situation has stalled in its gains toward equity with men. Regardless of women's education, occupation, family status, and age, they continue to be curtailed in achieving equity with men. Men's patriarchal advantage continues in the payroll departments across the nation.

10. The particularly vulnerable position of people of colour reflects deep racial divisions within our society that are exacerbated by income inequality and occupational segregation.

Solutions

Let us distinguish the various forms of solutions that exist: policy solutions, campaign solutions, and vision-based solutions. All provide insights as to how to reduce income inequality. While more research questions may surface as one becomes familiar with the existing research, it is worthy to note that this author gives little priority to further research. The trends are established, durable, and largely resistant to minor tinkering. We have proven our case; it is time to move to solutions.

There are several sources for quite comprehensive "shopping lists" of various policy solutions. We direct the reader to those covered in each of the three Centre for Social Justice reports on the growing gap. Items covered include strategies to address jobs, wages, services, and supports and specifically include items such as a living wage, increased access to unionized jobs, employment equity, and reversing the trends toward free trade and corporate globalization.

Specific attractive policies include improved unionization access; the median income for non-unionized workers in 2006 is $15.00/hour while those who are unionized earn $21.42/hour, resulting in a union wage advantage of $6.42/hour (Statistics Canada CANSIM database from Labour Force Survey). Racialized workers also benefit as the union advantage for them dramatically decreases the earnings gap from approximately 30 percent to 8 percent, so their incomes much more closely match those of Whites when they are union members (Galabuzi, 2001).

These lists are a combination of returning to what worked in the past (more reliance on progressive taxation, higher overall tax revenues, and increased social spending on services and income supports) and innovative solutions that have worked in other countries (guaranteed annual incomes, living wages that take income earners above the poverty line, reduced work weeks that increase overall employment levels, and creating disincentives for excessive corporate incomes). While the progressive community is reluctant to return to the days of old (especially given the successful campaigns of the right that have undermined support for a healthy tax base), it was a system that provided base minimums of support to those who needed it. Ask anyone who has been denied employment insurance or who has suffered cuts to welfare cheques, and the days of old look pretty good.

The problem with such shopping lists is that they are just that—a list of possible interventions. When proposed, they offer no sense of strategic priorities or sense of agreement on which interventions would yield better results than others. That is the job of social movement organizations and coalitions that would select one or two specific initiatives for the base for a campaign. In order to shift from the shopping list to the campaign priorities, we need an assessment of the viability of various policy initiatives, which in turn requires assessments of the resources within social movements and which issues stand a chance of winning, entailing full consideration of the decision makers on the issues, whether broad public support can be activated, and whether political will can be generated for the initiative.

Vision-based solutions attempt to speak to a different vision for Canada, galvanizing citizens around particular objectives and directions. While most typically articulated by political parties (especially during political campaigns), the lack of such political visioning has given rise to non-governmental groups doing such work. One example is the dialogue process as conducted by the Canadian Policy Research Networks, in which they engaged 408 citizens in a dialogue on Canada's future (Michalski, 2001).

Occasionally, governments themselves pass motions that are visionary in orientation. The all-party motion passed in 1989 to end child poverty by the year 2000 was one such initiative that generated considerable public interest in ending child poverty, yet failed dismally in actually reducing it. Another is Quebec's anti-poverty law, which in 2002 made "poverty reduction an explicit and central policy priority" (Noël, 2002, p. 1), which has resulted in improvements to employment assistance, minimum wages, improved parental wage assistance, and expansion of affordable housing.

We close with a vision for the future of economic inequality that stems from the analysis conducted in this paper:

> We must proclaim that the market fails more and more of us at an accelerated pace, resulting in a growth of both absolute and relative inequality. The most significant of these trends is the growing social exclusion of the economic and political elite, who have pursued narrow economic interests in a self-serving and anti-democratic manner. Their isolation by gender, race, and class deepens the emerging crisis of mistrust in our political leadership. It is time for a redirection of our collective resources that ensures that the social identity of our birth does not dictate our life's achievements. It is time to educate ourselves as to the political dimensions of this economic and cultural reality and build a nation that ensures decency of jobs and wages for all working people and extends compassionate support to those who slip through our existing systems.

Conclusion

As we enter 2008, cracks in the armour of conservative pundits have widened. They have, through their faulty economic performance, induced their own political losses in several areas of Canada. The neo-liberal agenda of downsizing, privatization, and deregulation has destabilized quality of life and moved political sensibilities further to the left. Concurrently, movements for democratic reforms are moving to the forefront, for the problems of income inequality have strong ties to the activities of our political leadership (both elected officials and top bureaucrats). It is also a time for civil society to influence the economic and ideological debates in the nation. Controlling capitialism and its companion ideological doctrines must move to the forefront of our policy agenda.

Box 3.1: The Poor and Us

It is common, among the non-poor, to think of poverty as a sustainable condition—austere, perhaps, but they get by somehow, don't they? They are always "with us." What is harder for the non-poor to see is poverty as acute distress: The lunch that consists of Doritos or hot dog rolls, leading to faintness before the end of the shift. The "home" is also a car or a van. The illness or injury that must be "worked through" with gritted teeth because there's no sick pay and the loss of one day's pay will mean no groceries for the next. (Ehrenreich, 2001, p. 214)

Now that the overwhelming majority of the poor are out there toiling in Wal-Mart or Wendy's—well, what are we to think of them? Disapproval or condescension no longer apply, so what outlook makes sense? Guilt, you may be thinking warily. Isn't that what we're supposed to feel? But guilt doesn't go anywhere near far enough; the appropriate emotion is shame—shame at our own dependency, in this case, on the underpaid labour of others. When someone works for less pay than she can live on—when, for example, she goes hungry so that you can eat more cheaply and conveniently—then she has made a great sacrifice for you, she has made you a gift of some part of her abilities, her health and her life ... the working poor neglect their own children so that the children of others will be cared for; they live in substandard housing so that other homes will be shiny and perfect; they endure privation so that inflation will be low and stock prices high.... Some day, of course ... they are bound to tire of getting so little in return and demand to be paid what they're worth. There'll be lots of anger when that day comes, and strikes and disruption. But the sky will not fall and we will all be better off for it in the end. (Ehrenreich, 2001, p. 221)

It is imperative for us to loudly proclaim the market's failure to deliver enough decent jobs, especially for those at and close to the bottom of the income ladder. Incomes are insufficient, and the burdens placed on the tax and transfer system (via the government) to remedy this situation poise us for a worsening of the tax revolt movement as Canadians focus their blame on the taxes they must pay as opposed to their low and stagnating incomes levels. Blame squarely rests with the market and its inability to offer us a decent living.

So, what are we to do? The task is simultaneously pragmatic, tactical, and visionary. At its root, we must require our politicians to work in our best interests. They must be separated from the moneyed interests that undermine their capacity to work for the common good, and be held to standards that reflect deep understanding of their own privilege. It is time to engender boldness and courage in all of us to build a society with justice for all.

Critical Thinking Questions

1. What amount of inequality between rich and poor is tolerable? At what point do people become too rich or too poor? Should society be able to say, "That is just too much income?"
2. Increasing the government's involvement in controlling capitalism is not popular, and yet this is how initiatives such as medicare, rent control, minimum wage, labour standards, and social housing have emerged. What do you think it will take for popular opinion to extend into more direct control over the supply and the quality of jobs, including incomes?
3. What can you do to help advance civil society's control of capitalism? Who can you have these discussions with?
4. Capitalism is also an ideology. It includes ideas such as private property, private ownership of wealth, accumulation of wealth across generations, consumption on the ability to pay, and increasing consumption as

the signs of a "good life." All of these ideas reflect values and beliefs about life and people. What could you do to narrow your support for these cultural dimensions of capitalism?

5. Often social justice requires a redistribution of the benefits of our current economic situation. What are you willing to forego in order for others to have more?

Recommended Readings

Canadian Centre for Policy Alternatives. (2007). *The alternative federal budget 2007: Strength in numbers*. Ottawa: Canadian Centre for Policy Alternatives

This document provides an excellent assessment of government spending and income collection, and yields a balanced budget that favours the interests of middle- and lower-income Canadians. Anyone seriously interested in the alternatives to corporate domination and the levers that exist for governments to generate better incomes and services for the majority of Canadians should become familiar with the alternative budget process, conducted yearly by the CCPA.

Ehrenreich, Barbara. (2001). *Nickel and dimed: On (not) getting by in America*. New York: Owl Books.

This book is a profound narrative of the experiences of a journalist who goes undercover and works in several different low-wage jobs, attempting to make ends meet. She works as a waitress, hotel maid, house cleaner, nursing home aide, and Wal-Mart salesperson. This book is an easy and evocative read, leading readers to contemplate issues of their privilege and build considerable empathy and outrage for the low-wage workers of North America.

Hobgood, M. (2000). *Dismantling privilege: An ethics of accountability*. Cleveland: Pilgrim Press.

Written by a Christian ethicist, this text profiles the ethical dimensions of an increasingly isolated privileged class that exerts considerable political influence over the policy environment. Hobgood proposes that with social separation comes ignorance of the lived realities of those with less, and that over time this ignorance breeds an arrogance of presuming one understands the lives of those who struggle. It is about the ethical processes and duplicity of the elites and will inform the reader of the deep changes required to effect broader social change.

Lakoff, G. (2004). *Don't think of an elephant: Know your values and frame the debate*. White River Junction: Chelsea Green Publishing.

This is Lakoff's most clear and direct writing on the issue of framing debates. Lakoff writes in the US context, but his lessons are very important for social justice campaigns, suggesting that we emphasize the values base of specific campaigns and establish congruent messages that are likely to resonate broadly throughout the population. Excellent case studies are included in this text.

Yalnizyan, Armine. (1998). *The growing gap: A report on growing inequality between the rich and poor in Canada*. Toronto: Centre for Social Justice.

This is the most comprehensive profile of the growing gap in Canada. Covering the broad measures as well as population-specific issues (gender, youth, and seniors), this report provokes alarm and documents alternate policy options to narrow the gap. A must-read for beginning researchers on economic inequality in Canada.

Related Web Sites

Campaign 2000 and the Child Poverty Working Groups— www.campaign2000.ca

Their Web site is an excellent source of child-centred information on federal and provincial budgets, political debates, and demographic reports. The campaign began shortly after the all-party motion to end child poverty by 2000.

When it appeared that little progress was underway, a group of NGOs and associated researchers came together to influence public policy and to strengthen family life in Canada, with the goal of making sure that no Canadian child is raised in poverty. The deadline has come and gone, with one-sixth of Canadian children living in poverty.

Canadian Centre for Policy Alternatives—www.policyalternatives.ca

There is a significant but untold story (in this chapter) about taxes, progressivity, and hidden bias toward the wealthy as reflected in federal and provincial taxes. These resources provide a great introduction to the current and pressing tax issues that have dramatic effects on inequality.

Council of Canadians—www.canadians.org

Since 1985, the Council of Canadians has consistently supported campaigns on significant issues such as free trade, privatization of water, close integration with the US, health care, genetic engineering, and more. Their Web site is an excellent source of information on many topical issues. Individuals can join the council and become active at the local level.

———— ● ————

Chapter 4

INCOME, INCOME DISTRIBUTION, AND HEALTH IN CANADA

Nathalie Auger and Carolyne Alix

Introduction

Canadian social policies have for some time included poverty reduction as a goal. There has been a particular focus in eliminating poverty in groups at risk. Some policies have been successful, such as those focusing on poverty reduction among the elderly, and others unsuccessful, such as policies for reduction of childhood poverty (Barrett et al., 2003). Canada has also been a leader in generating income-related health research. In fact, many Canadian studies have shown a positive association between income and health (Wilkins et al., 2002).

At the provincial level, there is also a great interest in income issues by public health. For example, Quebec has for some time had provincial objectives for population health. These began with the 1992 Politique de la Santé et du Bien-Être, which outlined six strategies for reaching nineteen population health objectives (Ministère de la Santé et des Services Sociaux, 1992). The strategies focused on developing personal skills, creating supportive environments, building healthy public policy, working with high-risk groups, and improving life conditions. In the last strategy, one specific objective was poverty reduction in families with young children. The 1992 objectives evolved over time into the current National Public Health Program, which includes a multitude of health objectives in the domains of chronic disease, unintentional injury, infectious disease, environmental health, workplace health, and social health (Massé & Gilbert, 2003).

In this chapter, we will focus on Canadian studies assessing the relationship between income and health. There are two general types of studies looking at income and health: (1) those assessing the relationship between income and health, and (2) those assessing the relationship between income inequality and health. In Canada, most studies have been done using income per se. Consequently, this chapter focuses mainly on studies of income and health. Nevertheless, the relationship between income inequality and health remains important. Before turning to a discussion of these studies, a brief mention of their inherent characteristics and weaknesses is warranted.

Characteristics of Income-Health Studies

The problems found in studies assessing the relationship between income and health have been reviewed in detail elsewhere (Kawachi, 2000; Phipps, 2003). In this section, we will provide only a general overview in order to better understand the underlying concepts. Many of the critiques pertain to defining poverty. Others pertain to finding a suitable measure of poverty, which usually involves a measure of income. Unfortunately, income measures do not necessarily encompass factors such as social deprivation and social capital: the social aspects of poverty.

To further complicate matters, studies may use data in which the unit of measurement is at the macro (population) level rather than at the micro (individual) level. The former have been called ecologic studies. Macro-level analyses may also be subject to a bias called the ecologic fallacy, which occurs when macro-level data are used to make inferences at the individual level. There are also criticisms of individual-level study designs. For example, cross-sectional studies that assess the poverty-health relationship at one point in time do not allow one to determine whether poverty preceded poor health. In fact, it is feasible that poor health precedes poverty. This bias has been called reverse causation (Phipps, 2003).

We will first discuss the definition of poverty. There is no clear consensus on what is meant by poverty. Although all measures of poverty are essentially relative, one option is to conceptualize poverty as either absolute, relative, or subjective poverty (Phipps, 2003):

1. Absolute poverty usually refers to having less than an absolute minimum income level based on the cost of basic needs. One of the disadvantages of this definition is that it is difficult to objectively select a minimum set of necessities. Another disadvantage is that the cut-off changes over time. Although there is no official poverty line in Canada, the Statistics Canada low-income cut-off has traditionally been used (Phipps, 2003). Recently, the market basket measure has been introduced as another tool to measure poverty (Human Resources Development Canada, 2003).

2. Relative poverty usually refers to having less than the average standard in society. This form of poverty is often measured as the proportion of individuals below a certain percentage of the median income (Phipps, 2003).

3. Subjective poverty refers to individuals feeling that they do not have enough to meet their needs. Information on subjective poverty can be obtained from surveys. In industrialized countries, there is a general consensus that relative measures of poverty are more appropriate for studies on income and health (Phipps, 2003). In practice, however, studies tend to vary greatly on the type of indicator used to measure poverty.

Some of the indicators used to measure poverty in ecologic studies of income inequality include: (1) proportion of aggregate income earned by the poorest proportion of households; (2) the ratio of income shares earned by the upper 90th percentile to the 10th percentile of households; and (3) a multitude of other indices. These studies have been critiqued for arbitrarily choosing indicators or for using data-driven indicators (Kawachi, 2000). This critique has, however, been countered and it has been shown that income studies usually reach the same conclusion irrespective of the indicator used (Kawachi & Kennedy, 1997).

The indicators selected for study may have other drawbacks, some of which may have implications for identifying the income-health relationship (Phipps, 2003):

1. The indicator may not reflect annual disposable income. Ideally, income should be calculated after taxes and governmental transfers. Likewise, income should take into account the costs of public services. If services such as health care are not publicly financed, disposable income will be reduced since individuals who rely more heavily on these services will have to pay out of pocket.

2. In households composed of more than one person, the indicator may not take into account the advantage of shared resources. Researchers have proposed equivalence scales to calculate income per person; however, the choice of equivalence scale may not be objective. Also, equivalence scales may not adjust for unequal sharing of resources within families.

3. The indicator may not take into account volatility of income. Long-term measures of income may be more appropriate. Alternatively, it may be that acute changes in income are more important determinants of health.

4. Indicators do not take into account accumulated assets or debts.

5. Indicators do not account for time required to acquire income.

6. It may be that depth of poverty, or just how far income falls short of the poverty line, is more important.

7. Similarly, duration of poverty may be important.
8. The timing of poverty during the life cycle may play a role. Exposure to poverty during the early years of a child's life may have a greater effect on health (Phipps, 2003).
9. The study may not adequately adjust for other factors, known as confounders, which could account for the income-health relationship (Kawachi, 2000). Some studies use other measures of socio-economic status as a proxy for income (e.g., place of residence). This is because socio-economic data on ill or deceased individuals are not routinely collected in Canada.

These methodological constraints would lead one to question the validity of the income-health relationship. However, many researchers have countered these criticisms with credible arguments (Kawachi, 2000). Also, given that the number of studies finding positive associations between income and health continues to increase, the importance of income as a determinant of health becomes clear. We now turn to a discussion of some of the most recent studies performed in Canada.

Canadian Studies on Income and Health

Income Inequality and Health

We will begin by reviewing the evidence linking income inequality and health in Canada. Income inequality refers to the extent to which income is unequally distributed in a population. In an early study using Census data and vital statistics, Ross et al. (2000) found no relation between income inequality and mortality in Canada, but a strong relation in the United States. Income inequality was defined as percentage of total household income received by the poorest 50 percent of households. The authors speculate that the social policies widely present in Canada, but less so in the United States, could partly account for the differences in mortality (Ross et al., 2000). In a later study using survey data that accounted for neighbourhood income, Hou and Chen (2003) found that income inequality was associated with poor self-reported health in Toronto, but not with chronic conditions or distress. In their analyses, income inequality

was measured with the coefficient of variation for family income. Xi et al. (2005) also found that income inequality, measured as the Gini coefficient of Ontario public health units, was associated with poor self-reported health beyond individual and neighbourhood income.

Meanwhile, using Canadian survey data, McLeod et al. (2003) did not find a relation between self-reported health and income inequality (measured as the percentage of total income for the bottom 50 percent of the income distribution). Thus, depending on study methodology, differing results have been obtained. Consequently, the association between income inequality and health remains a subject of debate. Nevertheless, one of the implications of these studies is that policies that reduce income inequality may be favourable for public health.

Individual Income and Health

A large body of Canadian evidence, much of which was collected prior to the millennium, will not be discussed here since it has been reviewed elsewhere (Wilkins et al., 2002; Phipps, 2003). Suffice it to say that at least 17 Canadian studies of individual-level income data and 11 studies of small geographic area-based socio-economic data have found a link between income and health (Wilkins et al., 2002).

There is a large body of evidence linking individual income and health status in Canadian children (Phipps, 2003). The evidence has been summarized by the Canadian Institute of Child Health (Kidder et al., 2000). Briefly, income has been associated with low birth weight; injury-related mortality (including fire and homicide deaths); developmental problems such as hyperactivity, psychosocial problems, delinquent behaviour, and delayed vocabulary development, among others. For many of these analyses, data was taken from the "National Longitudinal Survey of Children and Youth" and the "National Population Health Survey" (Ross & Roberts, 1999). Data from the "Longitudinal Study of Child Development in Quebec" indicates that not only poverty, but duration of poverty as well, are associated with childhood health, even after taking into account socio-demographic characteristics (Séguin et al., 2005; Séguin et al., 2007). Other researchers have linked poverty to obesity, asthma, and health service utilization in children (Phipps et al., 2006; Lethbridge & Phipps, 2005; Kozyrskyj et al., 2004). The relation between income and childhood health remains a subject of study.

Few Canadian studies have looked at trends over time. This issue was addressed in a recent ecologic study by Wilkins et al. (2002). The investigators examined changes in mortality rates by income in small geographic areas of urban Canada from 1971–1996. They divided their population into quintiles based on the proportion of people in the neighbourhood below the low-income cut-off. They measured life expectancy at birth, infant mortality, potential years of life lost (PYLL), income-related excess PYLL before age 75, cause-specific mortality rates, and various other indicators of health. They found that for most causes of death, differences in mortality between rich and poor neighbourhoods had diminished over the study period. However, some causes of death changed little and some, such as suicide mortality among females, had increased. They also estimated that, in 1996, 24 percent of total PYLL were related to income differences. Using a similar methodology, but without examining trends over time, Lemstra et al. (2006) found that low neighbourhood income was associated with higher health care utilization in Saskatoon.

A recent study by the Institut de la statistique du Quebec looked at the association between income and health over time using individual level data (Ferland, 2003). All data was taken from the 1987 "Santé Québec" survey and the 1998 "Enquête sociale et de santé." In this study, individuals were classified into five groups based on gross income before taxes adjusted for household size. Health status for several outcomes (perceived health, mental health, long-term activity limitation, psychological stress, and functional gastrointestinal problems) was found to be negatively associated with gross annual income. Furthermore, the study concluded that there had been no weakening of the income-health relationship over time. In fact, for one health outcome, psychological stress, there appeared to be an increase in inequality of health outcomes between the richest and poorest individuals (Ferland, 2003).

Other studies performed in Quebec have linked higher income to favourable levels of general health, mental health, stress, and obesity (Bordeleau & Traoré, 2007; Aubin & Traoré, 2007). In an influential 1998 study (Lessard et al., 1998), poverty in Montreal was found to be associated with health at all stages of the life cycle, including infant mortality, lung cancer, fertility rates, psychological distress, and suicide. The study, which was widely circulated in Quebec, spurred greater interest in social inequality as a determinant of health in Montrealers. In a follow-up to the 1998 report, a more widespread study was conducted in 2002 on the urban health of Montrealers (Lessard et al., 2002). This second study demonstrated that neighbourhood poverty was associated with a variety of health indicators, such as infant mortality, life expectancy, and cause-specific mortality. It confirmed the findings of the 1998 study and demonstrated that the health gap between rich and poor continued to exist in Montreal. This report has been instrumental in pushing forward the poverty agenda in Quebec.

What Do Recent Quebec Data Show?

While previous research in Quebec has looked at the city of Montreal, this section gives an updated portrait of the income and health relationship at the provincial level. In order to better understand the data presented in this section, we will begin by going over the methods used to look at these associations. Box 4.1 outlines the methodological approach.

What follows is a bit of background to better understand the results (all data are based on the 2001 Census unless otherwise specified). Quebec is a province with 7.4 million residents. About 52 percent of the population resides in Montreal, Montérégie, and the provincial capital. Compared to Canada as a whole, Quebec has fewer immigrants (9.9 percent vs. 18.4 percent); a larger proportion of the population without a high school diploma (24.4 percent vs. 22.7 percent); a higher unemployment rate (8.0 percent vs. 6.3 percent, 2006 Census); and a lower personal disposable income per capita ($23,274 vs. $25,624, 2006 Census). Quebec is also the province with the highest proportion of the population living below the low-income cut-off (19.1 percent), with Newfoundland having the second highest proportion (18.8 percent), and Canada averaging at 16.2 percent (Figure 4.1). However, these data do not take into account the generally lower cost of living and more widespread social services in Quebec relative to other Canadian provinces (Institut National de Santé Publique du Quebec, 2006). These differences may in part

---

Box 4.1: Income and health in Quebec

The data were taken from provincial vital statistics registries, surveys, and the 2001 Census. Health data include outcomes such as mortality (infant mortality, life expectancy, all-cause and cause-specific mortality); morbidity (general health perception, obesity, birth outcomes such as pre-term birth and poor fetal growth); and behavioural risk factors (smoking, physical activity, nutrition, breastfeeding).

Different sources of income data were used. Personal income is usually collected and therefore available in surveys. Therefore, for survey data, individual income was used and rates for health outcomes were calculated for different income categories. Unfortunately, individual income is not available in sources such as vital statistics registries. For these types of data, we used proxy measures of income based on the income level of the neighbourhood of residence. Here, neighbourhoods were specified as dissemination areas, an area originally created by Statistics Canada for data-collection purposes of the 2001 Census. The dissemination area is the smallest area for which Statistics Canada provides population data, including socio-economic data. We used two indicators of neighbourhood income, both of which were linked to the health data sets via the postal code. Here is how the two indicators were calculated:

1. Like Wilkins et al. (2002), income levels of dissemination areas were calculated according to the proportion of individuals living below the low-income cut-off before taxes. Statistics Canada considers the low-income cut-off to be the income level where a family tends to spend a significantly higher proportion of its income on food, shelter, and clothing compared to the average family (Webber, 1998). It is based on family and community size.
2. Dissemination areas were also categorized according to level of deprivation. In Quebec, a material-deprivation index is available for dissemination areas. The deprivation index is a composite index calculated from 2001 Census data using data on education (proportion of residents with no high school diploma), employment (ratio of employment to population), and mean income (Pampalon & Raymond, 2000).

Dissemination areas were next stratified into five income groups (low, low average, average, high average, high) for both neighbourhood income and neighbourhood material deprivation. These data were linked to the health data sets using a program supplied by Statistics Canada (Wilkins, 2006). Last, we calculated rates for a spectrum of health indicators by neighbourhood quintile (for vital statistics data), or by personal income (for survey data).

---

explain why Quebec's rank tends to improve when other indicators of income are used (Institut de la Statistique du Quebec, 2006).

In terms of health status, Quebec varies markedly. Although life expectancy at birth in Quebec (men, 76.4; women, 82.1 years) is similar to that for Canada (men, 77.0 years; women, 82.0 years), the same cannot be said for the leading causes of mortality. Quebec has a higher cancer mortality than Canada (194 vs. 179 cancer deaths annually per 100,000 population, 2000–2002), and surpasses all provinces for colorectal and lung cancer mortality. Meanwhile, mortality from circulatory system diseases is lowest in Quebec compared to Canada (184 vs. 201 deaths annually per 100,000 population, 2000–2002) despite having less favourable nutrition (47.6 percent

consume at least five servings of fruits and vegetables per day vs. 56.4 percent for Canada) and more smokers (24.4 percent vs. 21.8 percent for Canada, data are for the population 12 years and over, 2005).

In terms of health perception, a lower proportion of Quebecers report good health (9.7 percent vs. 10.2 percent) and mental health (3.7 percent vs. 4.9 percent) compared to Canada. Quebec is also the only province with a higher proportion than Canada for reported life stress (26.1 percent vs. 23.3 percent). The suicide rate is highest in Quebec (16.5 per 100,000 population annually), with Alberta coming up second (14.1) (Figure 4.2).

The reasons for these differences are unclear. The aforementioned socio-economic conditions of life, which are clearly different across Canadian provinces, may

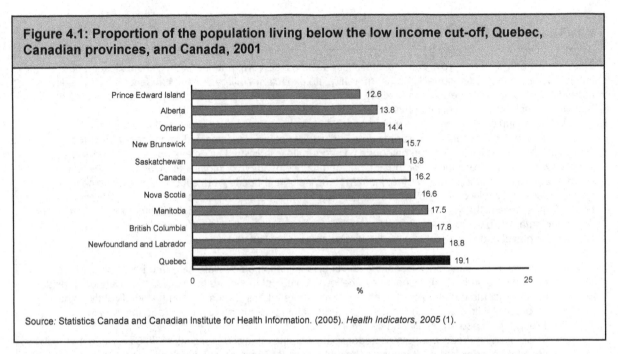

Figure 4.1: Proportion of the population living below the low income cut-off, Quebec, Canadian provinces, and Canada, 2001

Source: Statistics Canada and Canadian Institute for Health Information. (2005). *Health Indicators, 2005* (1).

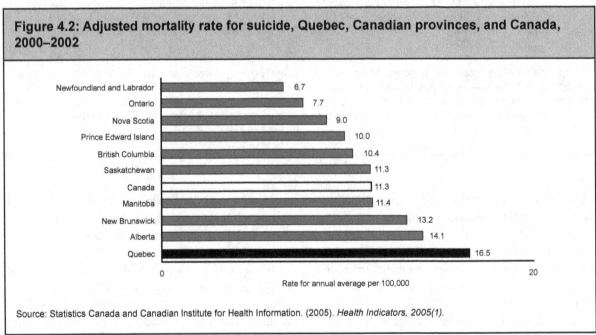

Figure 4.2: Adjusted mortality rate for suicide, Quebec, Canadian provinces, and Canada, 2000–2002

Source: Statistics Canada and Canadian Institute for Health Information. (2005). *Health Indicators, 2005(1)*.

partly account for the differences. We therefore turn to a look at health differentials across income in Quebec.

From the very beginning of life, income is linked to health. In fact, a relationship exists between income and most measures of infant health. Table 4.1 shows infant mortality, pre-term birth, and fetal growth according

to income over a 25-year span in Quebec. The lowest income quintile consistently has poorer outcomes. Keeping in mind that infant mortality is widely regarded as a general indicator of population health and adequacy of social services, this table illustrates the following three points:

1. Infant mortality fell in all income quintiles over the past two decades.
2. Despite this improvement, infant mortality continues to be highest in the low-income quintile.
3. The increase in infant mortality is relatively constant as we move from high- to low-income quintiles.

Table 4.1 also shows trends for pre-term birth and small-for-gestational-age birth. Pre-term birth has become more frequent in all income categories over time, despite a reduction in babies born small for gestational age. Another interesting point is that there is a linear increase in these adverse birth outcomes as we move from to high to low income, and that this linear trend is as present today as it was 20 years ago.

A similar trend is seen in gender and life expectancy. Figure 4.3 shows life expectancy at birth by sex and neighbourhood income. This figure illustrates the following:

1. Life expectancy is highest in high-income quintiles for both women and men.

2. Life expectancy decreases steadily for both genders as we move from high to low income.
3. This decrease is more pronounced in men than in women. In fact, men residing in the low-income neighbourhoods can expect to live 4.2 years less than men in high-income neighbourhoods, whereas the difference is only 2.1 years for women.

Figure 4.4 indicates that mortality rates for the leading causes of death differ depending on level of deprivation. Strikingly, the trend can be seen for all deaths and for four leading causes of death (cancer, circulatory system, respiratory tract, and accidental injury). This figure illustrates the following:

1. Mortality is highest in the most deprived neighbourhoods.
2. The increase in mortality is relatively constant as we move from low to high material deprivation.
3. The difference in mortality due to accidental injuries is particularly large between the most and least deprived neighbourhoods.

Table 4.1: Birth outcomes,* by neighbourhood income and period, Quebec, 1981–2004

	Year	Neighbourhood income				
		Low	Low-average	Average	High-average	High
Infant mortality rate (per 1,000 live births)	1981–1984	8.5	8.4	8.1	7.4	7.9
	1991–1994	7.1	6.2	5.3	4.5	5.0
	2001–2004	5.6	4.4	4.8	4.2	3.9
Pre-term birth (%)	1981–1984	6.1	6.0	5.8	5.7	5.5
	1991–1994	7.7	6.9	6.7	6.4	6.2
	2001–2004	8.4	7.9	7.6	7.2	7.1
Small for gestational age (%)	1981–1984	16.9	16.1	15.4	15.3	14.5
	1991–1994	13.0	11.7	10.6	9.9	9.3
	2001–2004	9.6	8.4	8.0	7.4	6.9

Source: Minister of Health and Social Services, birth and death registry, Quebec, 1981–2004.

*Infant mortality is the number of deaths among children less than 1 year of age in a given period divided by the number of live births in the same period; pre-term is defined as less than 37 completed weeks of gestation; small for gestational age is defined as birth weight below the 10th percentile for sex and gestational age.

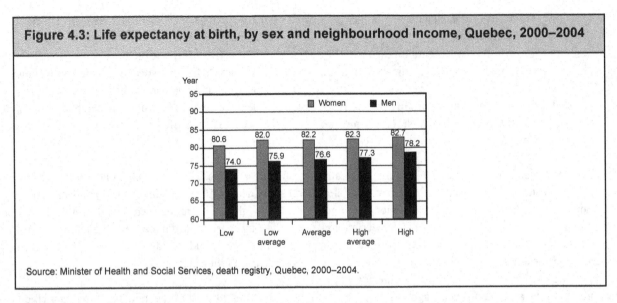

Figure 4.3: Life expectancy at birth, by sex and neighbourhood income, Quebec, 2000–2004

Source: Minister of Health and Social Services, death registry, Quebec, 2000–2004.

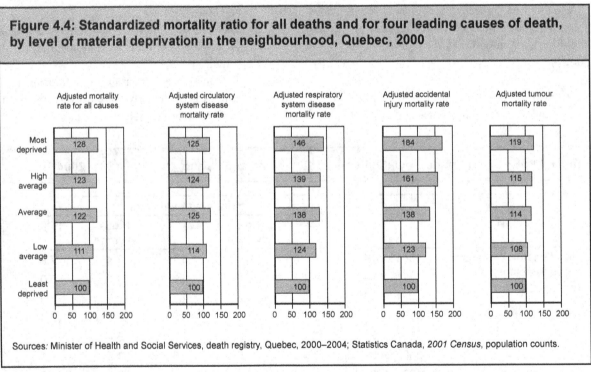

Figure 4.4: Standardized mortality ratio for all deaths and for four leading causes of death, by level of material deprivation in the neighbourhood, Quebec, 2000

Sources: Minister of Health and Social Services, death registry, Quebec, 2000–2004; Statistics Canada, *2001 Census*, population counts.

As mentioned earlier, suicide is a particularly important problem in Quebec. Figure 4.5 shows suicide mortality according to income quintile in Quebec. This figure shows that even suicide is linked to income. In fact, suicide mortality is almost twice as large in low-income neighbourhoods as compared to high-income neighbourhoods.

Personal income of individuals, like neighbourhood income, is also associated with health and its determinants in adults. Table 4.2 shows some examples of the discrepancy between extremes of income for some determinants of health (smoking, not consulting health professionals, job insecurity) and for health status (poor self-rated health, chronic health conditions, poor self-

Figure 4.5: Adjusted suicide mortality rate (per 100,000 population), by sex and neighbourhood income, Quebec, 2000–2004

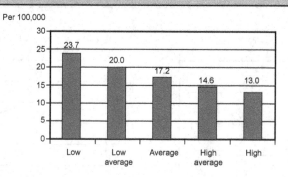

Source: Minister of Health and Social Services, death registry, Quebec, 2000–2004.

rated mental health, suicidal ideation). For both men and women, the frequency of all these outcomes and risk factors was higher in low-income groups (Table 4.2). Give the elevated suicide mortality in Quebec, one cannot help noticing the large difference in suicidal ideation between high- and low-income groups.

The association between personal income and health is also present for young people. Figure 4.6 shows various indicators of health for children and youth. This figure shows how the income of one's parents (i.e., family income) is also linked to health. Even from the earliest point in life, a mother in a low-income family is more

Table 4.2: Frequency of various determinants of health and health outcomes, by sex and personal income, Quebec, 2005

	Men		Women	
	High income	Low income	High income	Low income
Determinants of health				
Smoking	16.3	31.8	18.4	26.1
No consultation with health professionals past 12 months	4.8	11.2	1.1	4.7
Job insecurity	21.6	34.3	19.8	39.9
Health outcomes				
Poor or fair self-rated health	1.8	6.1	2.0	5.7
Has a chronic health condition	60.7	62.7	61.5	74.9
Poor or fair self-rated mental health	3.6	17.2	3.2	15.6
Seriously considered suicide past 12 months	14.2	21.8	10.0	22.1

Source: *Canadian Community Health Survey*, Cycle 3.1, 2005.

Acknowledgements: The authors wish to thank Geneviève Perreault for calculating the data in the table.

Figure 4.6: Health indicators for infants, children, and youth of Quebec according to household income

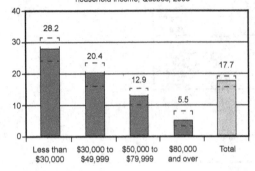

Proportion of mothers who smoked during pregnancy according to household income, Quebec, 2005

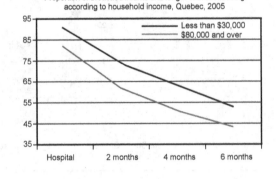

Proportion of breastfed infants and length of breastfeeding according to household income, Quebec, 2005

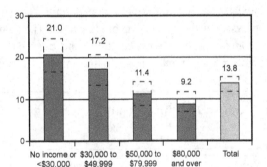

Proportion of youth aged 12–24 years who smoke, by household income, Quebec, 2005

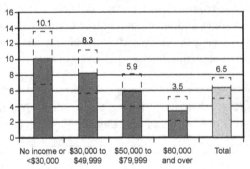

Proportion of youth aged 12–24 years who had an elevated psychological index of distress, by household income, Quebec, 2005

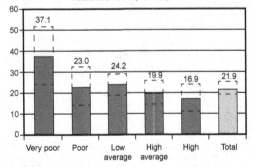

Proportion of 13-year-olds with low self-esteem according to relative household income, Quebec, 1999

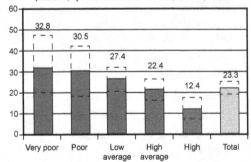

Proportion of 13-year-olds with a learning difficulty or behavioural problems, by relative household income, Quebec, 1999

Source: Minister of Health and Social Services, Quebec Public Health Institute (in press) 3e *Rapport national sur l'état de santé de la population du Quebec.*

likely to smoke and less likely to breastfeed. Furthermore, children and young adults in poor households are more likely to smoke, suffer from psychological distress, have low self-esteem, and have learning difficulties or behavioural problems, to name a few.

In summary, these data show that socio-economic conditions such as income and material deprivation are strongly associated with a large spectrum of health outcomes in Quebec. These associations are present throughout the life course.

Theories Explaining Income and Health

Having demonstrated the relationship between income and health indicators, it is pertinent to wonder why such a link exists. In fact, several theories have been proposed in the literature (Phipps, 2003). In general, these can be divided into two types, those pertaining to absolute income per se and those pertaining to relative inequality of income.

Briefly, the absolute income hypothesis proposes that there is a positive association between personal income and health, but that the association is non-linear. That is, even though the health of both rich and poor improves with income, the poor are much more responsive to income changes. The implication is that redistribution of income from rich to poor should cause average health to improve (Phipps, 2003). The absolute-deprivation hypothesis goes even further to say that income below a certain deprivation threshold is adverse for health, but once past this threshold, there are minimal gains in health to be made (Phipps, 2003).

There are at least three theories explaining how income inequality affects health (Kawachi, 2000):

1. Income inequality may result in underinvestment in human capital, manifested through lower social spending in sectors such as education. This may be because, in societies with rising inequalities, the rich have diverging interests from the poor and exert pressure to decrease public spending (Kawachi, 2000). A variant is the neo-materialist hypothesis, which states that income inequality is a manifestation of underlying historical, political, cultural, and economic processes (Lynch et al., 2000). These processes result in systematic underinvestment in public infrastructure, including education, health services, transportation, housing, occupational regulations, etc. The result is that not only do individuals have a lack of private resources, but there is also reduced access to material infrastructure necessary for health.

2. Income inequality leads to underinvestment in social capital by diminishing community solidarity confirming and social cohesion (Kawachi, 2000).

3. The third pathway occurs through psychosocially mediated effects, in which perceived widening of the income gap leads to frustration and biological processes that are harmful to health (Kawachi, 2000).

Some authors have argued that the link between income inequality and population health could be a statistical artifact. However, several authors have demonstrated that statistical issues cannot entirely account for the link between income and health (Phipps, 2003).

Conclusion

Data from Quebec and the rest of Canada contribute to the growing evidence confirming a link between poverty and health. Economic policies in Canada have not been entirely successful in reducing poverty, as evidenced by the increasing number of poor Canadians over time and the growing income inequality between the richest and poorest members of society (NAPO, 2006).

A decade ago, Canada was ranked first by the United Nations Development Programme (United Nations Human Development Report, 1999) for its performance on human development. The most recent data indicate that Canada now ranks 6th for human development and 8th for poverty among industrialized nations (United Nations Human Development Report, 2006). These global trends illustrate the growing importance of poverty in Canada.

Poverty has a significant impact on health, as emphasized by the director of the Montreal Public Health Department (Lessard et al., 1998, p. 60):

Having scanned the health and well-being of Montrealers from one end of the life cycle to the other, we note the important role played by poverty. Inequalities in health and well-being can be traced back to socio-economic inequalities, that is to the harsh living conditions that marginalize so many of our fellow citizens, not only limiting their access to essential goods, but depriving them as well of any meaningful role in social life.

Poverty weighs heavily on health in both its material and social dimensions: poor education, dependence, precarious jobs, inactivity. And the consequences of this are reflected in most of our social and health indicators: globally, in reduced life expectancy and, more particularly, in the higher proportion of diseases or psychosocial problems, in low-birth-weight babies, in developmental problems, in school dropout rates, in adolescent pregnancies, in psychosocial distress, etc.

If, as a society, we want to make significant gains on the health front, we must energetically pursue our efforts to improve living conditions. It is no exaggeration to say that poverty in Montreal constitutes a major health problem—a problem all the more worrisome seeing that it persists in a global context of unprecedented wealth and technological progress.

The advocacy of the Montreal Public Health Department has led to the development of the Observatoire Montréalais des Inégalités Sociales et de la Santé (OMISS), an organization aiming to reduce social and health inequalities by encouraging knowledge development and linking research to decision making. The newer Léa-Roback Centre for research on health inequalities also contributes to this process. Continuing efforts by organizations such as these could have a significant impact on policies for poverty reduction. In 2002, the government of Quebec unanimously passed Bill 112, a law to combat poverty and social exclusion (Bill 112, 2002). Bill 112 describes a provincial strategy to combat poverty and includes five key action areas: (1) prevention of poverty, with a focus on developing the potential of individuals; (2) strengthening social and economic safety nets; (3) promoting access to employment; (4) promoting the involvement of society as a whole; and (5) ensuring intervention at all levels. This law, while not perfect, is unique in North America and is a significant step in recognizing poverty as a priority for policy-making (Nöel, 2002, 2004).

Without fighting poverty, we have little hope of improving public health. Public health policies in Canada necessarily must address the upstream determinants of health, particularly that of poverty.

Notes

The authors are grateful for the advice of Robert Choinière and Marc Goneau on the tables and figures.

Critical Thinking Questions

1. What health conditions have been linked to income?
2. What is the difference between individual income versus income inequality, and which of these is most associated with health?
3. Why is it more difficult to study the relationship between income and health than it is to study other factors such as smoking and health?
4. What are the mechanisms that can explain how income manages to influence health?
5. Is it possible to significantly increase the level of health of Canadians by focusing on the medical system alone, or is it important to also consider social factors such as low income?

Recommended Readings

Marmot, M. & Wilkinson, R.G. (Eds.) (2006). *Social determinants of health*, 2nd ed. New York: Oxford University Press.

This textbook is a classic reference that addresses not only poverty and health, but also other social determinants in relation to health.

Nöel, A. (2002). *A law against poverty: Quebec's new approach to combating poverty and social exclusion.* Background Paper-Family Network, Canadian Policy Research Networks, December 2002. Online at www.cpds. umontreal.ca/fichier/cahiercpds03-01.pdf.

This paper was written as a backgrounder to the new Quebec anti-poverty law. Its purpose was to make the law better known and to open a discussion on the law.

Nöel, A. (2004). *A focus on income support: Implementing Quebec's law against poverty and social exclusion.* Canadian Policy Research Networks. Online at www.cprn.org/documents/29659_en.pdf

Subsequent to Quebec's anti-poverty law, which was passed in 2002, the government released its action plan against poverty and social exclusion in 2004. This paper is a critical appraisal of this action plan.

Phipps, Shelley. (2003). *The impact of poverty on health: A scan of research literature.* Canadian Institute for Health Information, June 2003. Online at secure.cihi.ca/cihiweb/dispPage.jsp?cw_ page=GR_323_E

This paper, prepared by the Canadian Population Health Initiative, is a summary of the state of knowledge between poverty and health.

Ross, N.A. (2004). *What have we learned studying income inequality and population health?* Canadian Institute for Health Information, December 2004. Online at secure.cihi.ca/cihiweb/splash.html

This paper, prepared by the Canadian Population Health Initiative, is a summary of the association between income inequality and health.

Related Web Sites

The five Web sites that follow contain extensive information on income and other social determinants of health at the local, national, and international levels. They also provide links to additional relevant Web sites.

Canadian Institute for Health Information—secure.cihi.ca/cihiweb/splash.html

The Canadian Institute for Health Information (CIHI) is an independent, not-for-profit organization that provides essential data and analysis on Canada's health system and the health of Canadians. CIHI tracks data in many areas, thanks to information supplied by hospitals, regional health authorities, medical practitioners, and governments.

Léa Roback Centre for research on the social inequalities of health (in French)—www.centrelearoback.ca

The Léa Roback Centre is funded by the Institute of Population and Public Health as part of a strategic initiative of Health Research Canada for the establishment of centres for research development.

National Anti-poverty Organization (NAPO)—www.napo-onap.ca

NAPO is a non-profit, non-partisan organization working for the eradication of poverty in Canada. It strives to: (1) ensure that the concerns of low-income people are reflected in government policy and decision making; (2) defend the human and economic rights of low-income people in Canada; and (3) assist local and regional organizations to include the voices of low-income people in Canada in decision-making and policy-making processes in their communities.

PovNet—www.povnet.org

PovNet is an online resource for advocates, people on welfare, and community groups and individuals involved in anti-poverty work. It provides up-to-date information about resources in British Columbia and the rest of Canada. PovNet links to current anti-poverty issues and also provides links to other anti-poverty organizations and resources in Canada and internationally.

Quebec Public Health Institute (INSPQ)—www.inspq.qc.ca/english/default.asp?A=7

The INSPQ is a government organization founded in 1998 to improve the coordination, development, and use of expertise in public health. Its creation involved uniting the province's principal public health laboratories and centres of expertise and transferring and assigning staff from a number of regional public health departments and from the Ministère de la Santé et des Services Sociaux.

Chapter 5

Precarious Work and the Labour Market

Diane-Gabrielle Tremblay

Introduction

This chapter deals with unemployment and transformations within the labour market. We are interested in those issues arising from the perspective of economic security and insecurity of individuals. I will first locate my position in the general context of economic transformation, the evolution toward a knowledge economy, and the effects this evolution may have for individuals, particularly from the perspective of the transformation of careers. The current context also translates into new modes of learning, which are more informal and less focused on internal labour markets, and which also have an effect on job security or insecurity. This raises issues about individuals' employment possibilities. The chapter will deal generally with seven questions and is therefore divided into the following sections:

1. What are the main labour market transformations and their effects?
2. What does job security mean today?
3. What is the definition of insecurity? What are its causes?
4. What are the connections between jobs and security/insecurity?
5. What effects do employment and social policies have on job security?
6. Is job security still important?
7. How can job security be ensured?

Transformation of the Labour Market

For a number of decades, certain regions of Canada have known relatively high levels of unemployment. While the situation has improved, especially in the central regions, a number of regions still experience problems, particularly those that depend on natural resources.

In the context of the knowledge economy, careers are increasingly fragmented, with individuals being involved in a growing number of jobs, projects, and businesses over the course of their working lives. This reinforces both the problems faced by some unskilled people and certain regions where there is a lower percentage of people with higher education.

The knowledge economy also translates into the development of "projects." In this context, the intelligence of a business is a function of the quality of the "skill network" it contains, not only of the skills of its individual employees (Tremblay, 2002b, 2003a, 2003c). Thus, both young people entering the labour market and those undergoing a career change must face new labour market realities, broadly determined by the development of the knowledge economy (Tremblay, 2003c).

Knowledge economy businesses, with their focus on projects, bring into question a number of the dominant principles and theories of labour economics, particularly with regard to the advantages of internal markets that allow individuals to develop skills and careers within an organization (Tremblay, 2003a).

The new boundaryless careers follow a different pattern than careers based on a vertical promotion ladder as are found in internal labour market models (Tremblay, 2004a). In the latter model, careers were lived out within a single company, and often within a single union. The new nomadic careers present new challenges for both individuals and organizations.

Boundaryless Careers

Careers have most often been analyzed in the context of an internal labour market, or within the context of large hierarchical companies, frequently unionized ones, where one moves up the hierarchy in one's career. Horizontal and other forms of mobility have received less attention, partly because these forms are traditionally seen as non-promotion and, therefore, non-career moves. This may also be because unions have strongly adopted the ladder or closed internal market model as the archetypal career (Tremblay & Rolland, 1998). However, in recent years, the concept of career has evolved (Cadin et al., 2000). Some career theorists have begun to show evidence of a different vision of careers. Some have even spoken of a new paradigm, which is counterposed to the dominant hierarchical ascending career model. We refer here to the concept of "boundaryless careers" (Arthur & Rousseau, 1996; Tremblay 2003a).

In a number of sectors, new forms of organization of work and collaboration are being developed, such as teamwork (Tremblay & Rolland, 2000), mobile work (Thomsin & Tremblay, 2006), networks, and virtual communities of practice (Tremblay, 2002b). However, while such developments may be positive for certain sectors, they entail precariousness, lack of stability, and the lack of a career for others. New types of employment often arise. As examples, we have the case of self-employment and "false" self-employment—that is, those who are dependent on one or more order-givers (Tremblay, Chevrier & Di Loreto, 2007).

In general, the context of new organizations entails more flexibility, often through development of multiskilling and enriched jobs, but just as frequently through the development of a greater range of tasks at one level. This includes rotation through a number of equivalent tasks, as well as the development of precarious conditions of work.

The following question thus arises: Where have all the industrial jobs, with employment security and a guaranteed salary, gone? In the past, the standard-bearer for job security was the male industrial worker, with a full-time, unionized job. He had protection; a stable, "permanent" job; and any interruptions in the continuity of his employment were covered by unemployment insurance, which protected the family income. Today, this type of worker is clearly on the decline.

We have entered the age of flexibility. This has meant a range of new employment statuses and periods of unemployment (Tremblay, 2003a, 2003b, 2003c, 2004a, 2007a). But it has also entailed variable intensity of employment, including part-time, casual, and contract work. The types of work and levels of income are variable and, according to labour market experts, are leading to a review of the traditional definitions of the various groups within the labour force (Standing, 1999; Tremblay, 2004a).

While the foregoing poses definite challenges for economic theory, it challenges income security as well! In fact, it leads us to wonder how unemployment and insecurity should be redefined in this new context, given that the unemployment rate no longer offers a correct measurement of the true labour supply or of insecurity. This situation is clearly seen in the case of self-employed workers (Tremblay, Chevrier & Di Loreto, 2006, 2007). The traditional categories within labour economics are no longer sufficient. The categories of employees, unemployed people, and inactive members of the labour force are too simplistic for an analysis of the reality of self-employment or the new diversity of employment status (casual, temporary, reduced-time, part-time, etc.).

Therefore, the concept of "active labour force" itself becomes questionable, given the diversity of forms of employment explained above. The various forms of work (third sector, social economy, non-governmental organizations, volunteers, and informal) are multiplying; some are more recognized than others. Homework, parenting, and caregiving are increasingly recognized as legitimate, which raises the issue of distinctions between work and non-work, and, accordingly, between the active and inactive labour force, with work-family or work-life balance issues taken into account (Tremblay, 2006; Tremblay, Paquet & Najem, 2006; Tremblay, Najem & Paquet, 2006).

In short, the concepts of unemployment, inactivity, and active participation are questioned, while a range of employment and unpaid work gain legitimacy. With all these challenges to forms of employment and what is considered "real work," the concept of job security is also in doubt. All this leads to a challenge to the notions of security and insecurity.

What Does Security Mean Today?

The need for security can be defined in different ways, according to the discipline's approach or specific area of interest.

Box 5.1: Definitions of security

According to Standing (1999, p. 37), security involves a sense of well-being or control, or mastery over one's activities and development, as well as the enjoyment of certain self-esteem. Conversely, insecurity involves anxiety and uncertainty.

Collective security can also be distinguished from other forms of security or insecurity. Again citing Standing (1999, p. 37), collective (or societal) security could be seen as the need to identify with or belong to a group, typically to exercise control over the behaviour of others or to limit their control. Security arises from multiple forms of identity, such as class, occupation, and community membership (Standing, 1999), to which we would add territorial belonging (Tremblay & Fontan, 1994; Fontan, Klein & Tremblay, 2005a, 2005b), which are also sources of social identity and, therefore, a certain level of security.

The company can also be considered a source of security, so it is therefore possible to refer to a certain amount of "company security," such as that found within the Japanese company, which generally ensured employees a long-term job (Tremblay & Rolland, 1998, 2000). There is also individual security: A person's curriculum vitae, skills, and union membership can provide a feeling of personal security (Standing, 1999, p. 37).

Given this, how can we define security? To return to Standing (1999, p. 84), security can be defined as a

system of defence against the development of a technical division of labour, often through measures that preserve some of the social division of labour or segmentation of the labour process. It is appropriate to wonder if the definition is applicable in the context of the international division of labour.

In the context of mass production and large organizations (Fordism), employees' stability was considered to be a desirable standard for industrial society. The development of trade unionism and the seniority standard contributed to making it expensive for a person to quit his or her job, which tended to favour employees' job stability and non-mobility. We might wonder why the regulation of the job market occurred. In fact, historically speaking, employment standards, unionization, and unemployment insurance came about as a result of workers' struggles, as a way to compensate for workers' weaker power, but also to ensure stable labour supply for companies who wanted to counter chronic labour instability among farm workers at the beginning of the industrial era.

Over the years, income security became associated with the welfare state. However, benefits were only for full-time workers, and women were frequently dependent on their spouses' family benefit coverage. We can now discuss the meaning of job insecurity.

What Does Job Insecurity Mean?

Despite the existence of male industrial workers with more or less stable jobs, and despite labour regulations favouring job stability, slow growth in the 1970s resulted in workforce rationalization and layoffs, long-term unemployment, and a reduction in the coverage of as well as the level of employment insurance benefits for jobless people. Today only about one of every two workers is eligible for employment insurance, and in the resource-dependent regions of the country, where unemployment is higher and long periods of unemployment are more frequent, many workers end up excluded from the employment insurance regime. Furthermore, available jobs are often precarious and poorly paid, which leads to lower benefits.

In the current economic environment, companies are in an endless search for improved competitiveness and productivity, which often results in demands for flexibility, diversified types of employment, changing work shifts, and, ultimately, insecurity. Globalization and the international division of labour have contributed to the displacement of investment and jobs toward developing countries, which leads to an increased feeling of job insecurity. As discussed above, job insecurity is largely subjective, something an individual feels given his or her job situation and the overall economic situation. Job insecurity can thus be considered a symptom of income insecurity and insecurity about the labour market in general.

This leads us to ask how workers' insecurity can be reduced. This reduction can be achieved in a variety of ways, both direct and indirect. To reduce insecurity directly, one can try to ensure either greater job security or greater coverage of costs (benefits) when unemployed. While the latter approach does not reduce insecurity at its source, increased benefit coverage does make insecurity easier to bear. Insecurity can also be reduced indirectly by attacking its causes (Standing, 1999, p. 183).

Another question arises: How can insecurity and security be measured? This is a particularly complex issue, which has been the subject of relatively little study.

However, Dasgupta (2001, p. 9) emphasizes that there are both objective and subjective measures, which brings us to the debate we discussed earlier about labour market indicators, and their validity or relevance. Objective measures are interesting but limited, as we saw earlier. We have already mentioned individual measures: unemployment rates, average length of period of employment vs. unemployment, fixed term contracts vs. indefinite employment, skill transferability, etc. These constitute individual measures of the likelihood that given individuals will maintain ongoing employment and stability and security. There are also contractual measures, such as the rate of non-standard jobs or job status, and institutional measures such as legal protection and collective agreements (Dasgupta, 2001, p. 9).

As well, there are subjective measures. These may relate to the feelings that one's permanence in employment is guaranteed by the company (as in Japan), or by society and public employment policy (such as in Sweden) (Tremblay & Rolland, 1998). In order to assess an individual's relative insecurity or security, the following measures would be of interest: the likelihood of losing one's job, the likelihood of finding another, the value of the current job, and the value of the future job or period of unemployment (Dasgupta, 2001, p. 9).

We may therefore conclude that insecurity is related to the perception of risk. In theory, manual or manufacturing jobs should be associated with greater perceived insecurity, but in fact, this feeling of insecurity rises in countries with higher levels of education. A number of studies on the perception of risk have shown this, in particular those carried out by the Organisation for Economic Co-operation and Development (OECD) (1996). The OECD found an overall increase in people's perceived job insecurity. Standing (1999) notes that perceived insecurity does not appear very differentiated by sex, possibly because women have lower expectations regarding security and stability. In fact, as women are more highly represented in part-time and otherwise precarious jobs than men (Tremblay, Chevrier & Di Loreto, 2006, 2007), this may affect their expectations of job stability.

Let us examine in greater detail the situation of the Canadian labour market in order to specify to what degree individuals may perceive or experience economic insecurity.

What Are the Connections between Jobs and Security/Insecurity?

Over the recent years, unemployment has decreased in many provinces, although there is a big difference in unemployment rates between Alberta's booming economy and the Maritime provinces or even Quebec, especially outside large cities. But the main evolution that sparks insecurity is the increase in non-standard work—that is, part-time, occasional, contract work, and the like.

Less than two-thirds of Canadian workers have a regular or permanent full-time job, which is considered a standard job (Kapsalis & Tourigny, 2004). While the majority of workers have a standard form of employment, the number of non-standard jobs has increased significantly in the last three decades as Figure 5.1 shows. Indeed, non-standard forms of employment such as self-employment, part-time, multiple job holders,

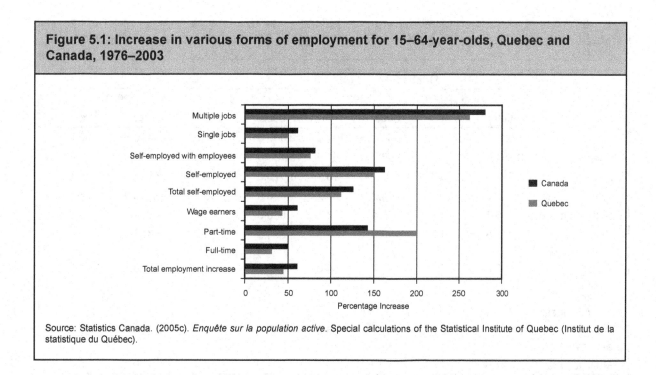

Figure 5.1: Increase in various forms of employment for 15–64-year-olds, Quebec and Canada, 1976–2003

Source: Statistics Canada. (2005c). *Enquête sur la population active.* Special calculations of the Statistical Institute of Quebec (Institut de la statistique du Québec).

and the like have increased more than full-time jobs, salaried employment, or single jobs.

As can be seen in Table 5.1, self-employment represents 14.4 percent of workers in Canada, 9 percent on their own, and 4.9 percent with employees. Multiple job holders are 5 percent and part-time workers are 18.4 percent. All these forms of employment can represent some form of job and revenue insecurity, although it is not always the case for the self-employed, especially for those self-employed with employees.

The increase in non-standard employment affects all age categories of both sexes. However, women and men are more concentrated in shorter hours and in non-standard employment (Figure 5.2, Table 5.2).

Young workers aged 15–24 are overrepresented in non-standard work—for example, in part-time and temporary work—and the percentage has increased over time (Statistics Canada, 2005a; Statistics Canada, 2005b).

Table 5.2 presents the evolution of part-time work and self-employment for men and women in Canada, from 1975 to 2000.

It is clear that, to varying degrees, those in precarious employment situations perceive a measure of job

---

Box 5.2: Precarious work in Canada

In Canada, excluding those who are unemployed, only about half of all Canadians have a single, full-time job that has lasted six months or more. The current Canadian labour force includes the following (some overlap is possible—for example, part-timers can also be temporary workers):

- 14 percent self-employed workers
- 10 percent temporary workers
- 18 percent part-time workers
- 6 percent employed in their current job for less than six months
- 5 percent are employed in more than one job

---

insecurity due to their employment status. However, we must interrogate the sources of this insecurity and of these diversified forms of employment. We can certainly observe such forms in the job market, but their development should not be seen as a "fact of nature." Thus, many question the contribution of employment policies on the diversification of types of employment.

Table 5.1: Forms of employment of workers 15–64 years, Quebec and Canada, 1976–2003

	Quebec				Canada			
	1976		2003		1976		2003	
	000s	%	000s	%	000s	%	000s	%
Total	2,513.1	100.0	3,604.2	100.0	9,608.5	100.0	15,478.9	100.0
Full-time	2,294.6	91.3	2,952.3	81.9	8,433.4	87.8	12,631.7	81.6
Part-time	218.5	8.7	652.0	18.1	1,175.0	12.2	2,847.1	18.4
Wage earners	2,265.0	90.1	3,144.2	87.2	8,476.9	88.2	13,213.3	85.4
Self-employed	216.7	8.6	453.4	12.6	1,000.3	10.4	2,232.3	14.4
Lone self-employed	118.5	4.7	288.5	8.0	574.3	6.0	1,469.0	9.5
Self-employed with employees	98.2	3.9	164.9	4.6	425.8	4.4	763.3	4.9
Single employment	2,475.5	98.5	3471.2	96.3	9,403.6	97.9	14,699.3	95.0
Multiple jobs	37.6	1.5	133.0	3.7	204.9	2.1	779.6	5.0

Source: Statistics Canada. (2005). *Enquête sur la population active.* Special calculations of the Statistical Institute of Quebec (Institut de la statistique du Québec), p. 129.

Figure 5.2: Percentage of women constituting those in various forms of employment

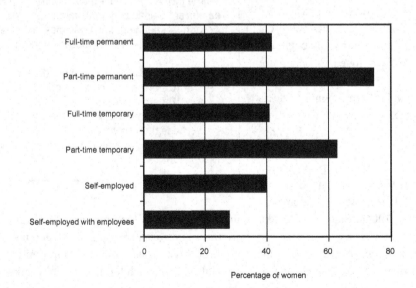

Source: Vosko, L., Zukewich, N. & Cranford, C. (2003). "Le travail précaire: Une nouvelle typologie de l'emploi." *L'emploi et le revenue en perspective* (Graph C, p. 23). Ottawa: Statistics Canada.

Table 5.2: Evolution of part-time workers and self-employed in Canada, 1975–2000

	Part-time workers		Self-employed	
	Women	Men	Women	Men
1975	13.6%	3.6%	3.4%	2.4%
1980	26.0%	6.9%	9.2%	14.9%
1985	28.4%	8.8%	10.6%	17.4%
1990	26.9%	9.2%	9.9%	17.4%
1995	28.6%	10.8%	11.7%	19.1%
2000	27.3%	10.3%	12.4%	19.4%

Source: Statistics Canada. (2001) *Femmes au Canada: Une mise à jour du chapitre sur le travail.* Publication no. 89F0133XIF. Ottawa: Statistics Canada, p. 21.

What Are the Effects of Employment and Social Policies on Insecurity?

This is a highly complex issue that requires an in-depth analysis. In this chapter, we can only provide an overview of the importance of policy on insecurity. We can use Esping-Andersen's well-known welfare state typology as a basis for analysis of the different types of social policy and welfare states. According to Esping-Andersen (1985), countries can be divided into three main categories. The first are liberal states based on *laissez-faire*. The US and Great Britain are the main representatives of this group. The second group includes conservative countries where there is some government intervention of a conservative nature, such as Germany, the Netherlands, and France. The third category includes social-democratic countries, principally the Scandinavian nations of Sweden, Norway, and Denmark. In such countries, the policies are based on revenue sharing at the national level to reduce income gaps between rich and poor. To varying degrees and at different points in their history, such countries have imposed controls on capital exportation and on foreign investment in national sectors, all in aid of full employment. This is what characterizes social and employment policies, although we have seen the typology applied equally well to family policies as well. Employment policies and social policies both impact on security and insecurity (Tremblay, 2006).

The contribution of employment entry, employability, social economy, and other programs to the de-standardization of forms of employment should be questioned. These programs have, in our view, played a major role in challenging the existing norm of full-time, full-year employment. In some cases, this translates into a simple perception of insecurity, while in others, the de-standardization and insecurity are objective: fixed-term contracts, part-time, reduced benefits, etc. (Tremblay, 2003c, 2004a, 2007a).

Nonetheless, there is also a subjective dimension associated with these job-market-entry or short-term employment programs. This dimension can be measured, although not easily. It is linked to various probabilities such as the likelihood of losing one's job or finding another (or, in fact, the perception of such likelihood). The likelihood of finding a job varies by program, but it is generally higher than before taking part in the program, although sometimes participation results in stigmatization of participants, which damages their job possibilities afterward.

Participation in such programs also can result in a reduction of expectations, especially among women. It appears that women lower their employment expectations more readily than men. The value of the current or future job is a further dimension of a subjective nature.

Comparisons between Scandinavia and North America

The evaluation of the effects of participation in a public job or a job-market-entry program also varies according to the place and philosophy reflected in the public policy of the country. Scandinavia provides active support for entry into regular employment. For many years, the nearly full-employment situation in the region made it easier to reintegrate people into jobs after participating in such programs. Job program participants are less undervalued than in other countries of Europe or the Americas, where such programs are less likely to lead to a steady, regular job. Scandinavia also supports integration into work through job-training programs, work-time adjustment measures, family-friendly policies, and longer family leaves (up to 18 months), including time reserved for the fathers—two months in Sweden and Finland, as well as three months in Iceland (Tremblay, 2007c, 2004b). All these policies influence the overall labour market, the chances of finding work, and, accordingly, the subjective assessment of the effects of taking part in a publicly funded job program.

In contrast, in North America, there is more emphasis on palliative and passive measures such as workfare. There are few alternate work-schedule arrangements and little support. In terms of family-supportive policies, there are virtually none in the US, and such policies are minimal in English-speaking Canada (although the federal government enacted a parental-leave policy), but slightly more developed in Quebec. There, parents have lower costs for state-funded child care and, since January 2006, a new parental leave, which offers higher benefits than the Canadian scheme, has three to five weeks reserved for fathers, and is more flexible (longer leave with lower benefits or shorter leave with higher benefits) (Tremblay, 2006). However, Quebec is still far from the Scandinavian standard, and some political parties (the ADQ, which came second in the 2007 election) propose policies that are quite conservative, such as "cash for care" of $100 a week for parents of children who are not in the daycare system, or a "baby bonus" of $5,000 for the third child. While this is apparently attractive to stay-at-home moms, it is very risky for those less educated to stay out of the labour market for many years since they lose their skills and often run more risks of being in poverty, especially if they end up as single mothers. In any case, Quebec's family policy appears to be somewhere in between the Scandinavian and the *laissez-faire* at the moment (Tremblay, 2006).

What Are the Effects of Social Policy on Insecurity?

From a social policy perspective, the differences in countries' places in the typology translate into major variations in the way unemployed people are considered. In the US, an unemployed person is considered to be responsible for his or her condition. Social assistance benefits are seen as a compensation for work. This is *laissez-faire* economics, in which the state sees no need to intervene since individuals are responsible for their lot and the market should allow them to overcome their unemployment if the market is working well. In the US there are the "deserving" poor (disabled people) and the undeserving poor (those who are considered responsible for their own condition).

In Scandinavia, on the other hand, the accent is on lifelong professional development, labour force integration, and the participation of civil society actors (associations, third sector, social economy) in the strategies of integration. In Sweden and Denmark, trade unions oversee the compensatory mechanisms, which is quite a different situation from that of the US.

In France, at least in theory, there is greater emphasis on integration and collective solidarity than on simple compensation benefits for unemployed workers. There is a shared view among a number of researchers that the true results of the minimum integration income (*revenu minimum d'insertion* in French or RMI), supposedly different from workfare, indicate only a qualified success (Paugam, 1998). There appears to be a gap between the objectives and philosophy and the reality. While the objectives were quite lofty at the beginning of the project, they became decidedly less so over the years. Those who gained the most from the program were those who needed it the least, while at the same time the program was unable to help those with less formal education or lower skill levels escape their dependence (Paugam, 1998; Chapon & Euzéby, 2002).

There is clearly a risk of downward convergence and homogenization in the context of the European Union, which many see as being constructed along the lines of the liberal model. The European social models are therefore facing a risk of downward adjustment. The same type of question arises with respect to integration in the Americas (NAFTA, FTAA). Will the liberal model (or US/British model) occupy the space of social policy? The question is not a trivial one, since such a development could lead to a significant increase in insecurity and relative risk of unemployment and underemployment.

From the perspective of women and their particular situation, social policy has important effects. A first class of policy would favour women's integration into the labour force, with work-family measures, including those that would promote a greater role for men in exercising parenting responsibilities. A second type would support women who choose to remain in the home with their children through social advantages given to men who support stay-at-home wives, or generous benefits for sole-support mothers.

If we attempt to classify countries by the type of policy they have, we see that the Scandinavian countries favour women's labour force participation and men's role in parenting, although with mixed results. Such politics are based on equality between men and women. They offer women the same insurance programs created for men, and while failing to be completely appropriate, they consider women as autonomous rather than as a husband's dependant.

Conservative welfare states such as Germany and the Netherlands support men whose wives remain at home (Germany), promote women's part-time work (Netherlands, France), and women's temporary withdrawal from the labour force for maternity leave (Tremblay, 2006, 2007c).

Finally, countries with a liberal or *laissez-faire* approach try to require women to integrate into the labour force (workfare) without providing measures to help work-family balance, nor do they provide for proper wages or working conditions.

There are two major social risks for women, namely, unemployment and family responsibilities. When there are problems with dependants (children or aging or ill parents), women tend to reinvest in the family. Very often, there is some reinforcement of women's traditional role between the private sphere and the labour force, which some call the "gender trap." In fact, since they have not invested themselves enough in the sphere of work, and are often denied their individual rights or benefits due to their limited participation in the labour force, women may become trapped and forced into a return to the home sphere.

Two options appear open. We may argue for the importance of labour force participation as a source of benefits and income security, or argue for citizen's income and other measures of this type (a point to which we will return). However, in the current context, it is in the labour market where rights take shape in most countries. It is, therefore, certainly preferable for women to participate in this market. Failure to participate leads women into the "gender trap," which often translates into poverty.

Is Job Security Still Important?

In light of the reservations set out in the foregoing paragraph about the importance of the labour market as the source of rights, insurance, and income, certain questions arise, such as whether job security is still important today and, if so, why, for whom, and how.

From employers' point of view, job security is a constraint on efficiency and flexibility in adjusting production. The OECD's publications have shown an inverse relationship between job flexibility and job security. We have observed that in Canada, the various forms of precarious conditions have a tendency to cluster (Tremblay, 2004a, 2007a). That is, people working part-time are more likely to be employed in fixed-term and contract positions that do not have benefits. Further, a recent study of several European countries showed that the economic slowdown Europe recently experienced has relaunched the debate about labour flexibility, including precarious forms of employment and wage reductions (Freyssinet, 2003). Some raise the notion that workers should adapt to having less security. In fact, insecurity or weak job security is becoming the norm in those countries where precarious or non-standard jobs are beginning to outstrip traditional forms of employment.

In support of job security, some defend the idea of job security as the main source of income security, and thus criticize the restrictions imposed on the employment insurance regime several years ago in Canada. Job security is considered important for the well-being of workers and their families, as well as being seen as favouring macroeconomic stability. Furthermore, it appears that flexibility and wage reductions do not always favour job creation (Freyssinet, 2003).

Also, recent work on business issues indicates that job security is a source of loyalty, commitment, and increased motivation. Furthermore, job security is seen as essential to the interest of both employees and employers in training and skill development. Job security can therefore be seen as positive for business as it favours productivity and innovation (Tremblay, 2007d).

There are certainly other avenues, and some theorists defend the concept of a guaranteed or citizen's income, mentioned above. While flexibility is necessary, and some consider that job protection works against flexibility, other forms of security can be provided: citizen's income, minimum guaranteed income, etc. Some writers believe that this would simultaneously ensure social justice and efficiency (Standing, 1999, p. 184).

However, this position is highly contested. It overlooks the non-financial advantages of work, including participation in social life, self-esteem, and personal development. Other critics hold that the cost of providing such a citizen's income at an appropriate level would be extremely high, and that a true minimum income is more realistic. Finally, it is argued that the stigma attached to social assistance would not necessarily disappear by just changing the name of the program, even though some believe that a "citizenship" income, considered the right of every citizen, might change people's perspective (Standing, 1999).

Feminist economists fear a marginalization of women and their return to the home since a formula providing a minimum integration or citizen's income would compete with the low wages many women earn, and would tend to encourage women to leave the labour force (Tremblay, 2007b).

Ultimately, security is important for both sides of this debate. On one side, income security is seen as the most important rather than job security, and providing a decent income for all would solve the problem. In this view, it would be possible to ensure a decent income for many without affecting low-income earners' interest in continuing to work. On the other side, the expectations of the majority are more along the lines of ensuring a job for everyone since working is highly valued both socially and as a source of income. We share this position. In our view, it would be impossible to ensure a citizenship income or guaranteed minimum income for more than a small minority of people without levies or taxes that would be totally unacceptable to working people. The debate has

been around for quite a few years, but the dominance of the liberal perspective reduces the likelihood of movement toward this option unless it were to occur in the context of extremely limited programs (both in philosophy and scope) as was the case with the minimum-integration income (*revenu minimum d'insertion*, RMI) introduced in France (Paugam, 1998).

How Can Job Security Be Assured?

This remains the fundamental question. How can we ensure the security of individuals, which we believe must involve job security? In our view, an existence income or citizen's income cannot be a viable solution to ensure income security for all, and such a guarantee would not ensure job security. On the contrary, it might make it less important in the labour market.

Social security is recognized as a favoured instrument for redistribution of time and money, but it also possesses a symbolic power in the construction of family roles. Social security might therefore be used as a source of redistribution, not just of income, but of societal roles, as is the case with parental leave, when time is reserved for fathers (as is now the case in Quebec) (Tremblay, 2006). It could give every person the chance to participate in both spheres, both the workplace and the family, both men and women (Tremblay, 2004b; Tremblay, Paquet & Najem, 2006).

How can this be done? Women's participation in the labour force must be encouraged through proper measures to help balance work and parenting roles (Tremblay, 2003a, 2002c), as well as through high-quality jobs and pay-equity measures. This can be seen as going beyond social policy toward essential workplace measures, while social policy can be only a safety net at best. Without such measures, however, women remain trapped within the family and continue to be their husbands' dependants.

Fathers' participation in parenting and family responsibilities (including caring for aging or ill parents) must be encouraged. This can be achieved through incentive measures such as those implemented in Sweden or Iceland, e.g., offering respectively a two- or three-month parenting leave only for fathers (Tremblay, 2004b, 2007c). The extension of parental leave in Canada and the opportunity to share such leave between spouses is not enough to increase the participation of fathers, especially given that women earn, on average, 70 percent of what men make. The time reserved for fathers in the new Quebec regime of parental leave—that is, three or five weeks, depending on the regime chosen—has translated into a participation rate of 36 percent in 2006 (first year of application), an increase over the average of 11 percent for Canadian fathers in general from 2001–2005, with the Canadian parental leave (which has no time reserved for fathers, although they can, in principle, share the time with mothers) (Tremblay, 2006).

There will always be a role for social security. More should be done to counteract material or financial insecurity and family instability. The latter is not within the scope of the state's responsibility, although the government can reduce the costs of such instability to women by ensuring women's autonomous rights. Social security measures should, in fact, be provided to the dependent person to ensure continuity and a degree of autonomy in decision making. Provision should be made to cover all forms of risks, including the risk of withdrawal from the labour force, loss of a job, illness, and unemployment. There also needs to be more adaptation to the diversity of employment status as applied to self-employed, part-time, and contract employees. Finally, there should be a broad definition of "close dependants" to ensure coverage of all social risks. Otherwise, there is a risk that women will withdraw from the labour force in order to care for close family without formal recognition of this responsibility. On the contrary, currently such withdrawal puts the rest of their working lives in peril, and some find themselves permanently excluded from the paid labour force or end up living in poverty.

Therefore, the key is to ensure income and job security at the same time for both men and women and, above all, to avoid trapping women in the private sphere and relegating them to dependence on a spouse. Furthermore, men must not be trapped in the public sphere or labour market, or saddled with the obligation to earn a "family wage" through overtime work that deprives them of essential parenting activities. They should be encouraged to increase their participation in family life and parenting. Financial autonomy of people with a disability or who are otherwise dependent is also to be ensured.

Conclusion

It is no surprise that we are putting forward a model similar to the Scandinavian model as one that allows for individuals' economic security, and that we see a strong association between economic security and job security. In the US and the Anglo-Saxon world, we are seeing the opposite. The model is based instead on liberal ideology, which considers that markets work well and can assume the regulatory role they have been given, and that the free movement of goods around the world is a source of growth and, ultimately, of economic security. Unfortunately, while the model achieves a certain level of economic security, it does not apply to everyone, and certainly does not apply to American women excluded from the labour market or those who earn low wages. However, over the years, the American model has been applied more and more despite some resistance and opposition. This model appears to be imposed despite our view that it endangers the very objective of economic security, especially for women, which is currently threatened, given the prevailing standards and conditions (unequal wages, discrimination, family responsibilities imposed on women, sole-support parents, etc.).

In recent years, the liberal vision has certainly spread, ignoring a number of basic aspects of "economic life." Dominant economic theories are also headed in this direction, which properly gives rise to concern for the economic security of people in the future. This is not the place to expand on the opposite views found within a range of proponents of economic thought (Tremblay, 2002a). Clearly, orthodox theories stemming from the American model or, more generally, Anglo-Saxon models, are based on quantitative and positivist methods, and contribute to the spread of the dominant Anglo-Saxon model. They do not favour the social-democratic visions linked to an alternative role for the state and social policy.

There are three main concerns that should be considered in our search for economic security. First, it is important to contest the dominant economic model in favour of institutionalist theories that are more respectful of the historic, social, and political reality of societies, and more likely to support social democratic policies that provide for true economic security for all. Furthermore, economic security needs to be better defined in the current context. The various types of risk described above must be taken into account, as well as different types of security (food, physical, etc.). Third and finally, the full range of types of work and social situations should be considered; we have progressed beyond the era of full-time work for men and women being assigned to the home. This should be taken into account in any reflection about economic security for men and women.

Critical Thinking Questions

1. Reflect upon your knowledge of the issue of job security and insecurity before you read this chapter. What is the main difference in what you thought then and what you think now?
2. What did you think about the issue of job security as a component of employment or job quality and what do you think now?
3. Was job security and insecurity considered as a health issue in your mind and in your previous research or work?
4. Are public policies concerning job security important to you as a health issue?
5. How do you consider Canadian public policies act upon job security?
6. How do you think governments, public agencies, and the media frame public policies regarding job security and employment? Is it an important public policy in Canada?
7. Do you think job security has a place in employment and health policies in Canada? Should this issue have more prominence in these policies?
8. Look at articles in *The Globe and Mail* or other Canadian papers (*Le Devoir*, *La Presse*, chronicles on work) or your local newspaper. How frequently do they deal with employment issues, job security, and income security?
9. Why do you think employment and job security appear to be rather invisible in the public debate and in the public policy agenda?

Recommended Readings

Tremblay, D.-G. (2003). *The new division of labour and women's jobs: Results from a study conducted in Canada from a gendered perspective.* Research Note no. 2004-10A of the Canada Research Chair on the Knowledge Economy. Online at www.teluq.uquebec.ca/chaireecosavoir/pdf/NRC04-10A.pdf.

   This paper contains the results of a Canadian study on the division of labour and women's jobs from a gendered perspective.

Tremblay, D.-G. (2003). *New types of careers in the knowledge economy: Networks and boundaryless jobs as a career strategy in the ICT and multimedia sector.* Research Note no. 2003-12A of the Canada Research Chair on the Knowledge Economy. Online at www.teluq.uquebec.ca/chaireecosavoir/pdf/NRC03-12A.pdf.

   This paper examines career transformations related to the new, knowledge-based economy, particularly in terms of occupational training, mobility, and career development. Learning and training are emphasized.

Tremblay, D.-G. (2004). *Labour issues and the labour market as a social construction: An institutionalist perspective.* Research Note no. 2004-9 of the Canada Research Chair on the Socio-organizational Challenges of the Knowledge Economy. Online at www.teluq.uquebec.ca/chaireecosavoir/pdf/NRC04-09A.pdf.

   This paper presents a theoretical analysis of labour issues and the labour market from an institutionalist perspective.

Tremblay, D.-G. (2006). *Networking, clusters, and human capital development.* Research Note no. 2007-4 of the Canada Research Chair on the Socio-organizational Challenges of the Knowledge Economy. Online at www.teluq. uquebec.ca/chaireecosavoir/pdf/NRC06-08A.pdf.

This paper presents the various concepts related to clusters and the role of information circulation in innovation, knowledge development, and employment.

Tremblay, D.-G., Davel, E. & Rolland, D. (2003). *New management forms for the knowledge economy: HRM in the context of teamwork and participation.* Research Note no. 2003-14A of the Canada Research Chair on the Knowledge Economy. Online at www.teluq.uquebec.ca/chaireecosavoir/pdf/NRC03-14A.pdf.

In this paper, the authors present a number of theoretical and contextual elements on the introduction of teamwork and participation in organizations.

Tremblay, D.-G., Paquet, R. & Najem, E. (2006). *Work, family and aging; Towards a new articulation of social times over the lifetime?* Research Note no. 2007-4 of the Bell Canada Research Chair on Technology and Work Organization. Online at www.teluq.uqam.ca/chairebell/pdf/NR_CB_2007_04.pdf.

This paper presents data from Statistics Canada's workplace employment survey on working-time situations and aspirations, as well as work-life balance issues. It also presents the challenge of aging in Canada and presents working-time arrangements as a possible solution.

Related Web Sites

Bell Canada Chair on Technology and Work Organization—www.teluq.uqam.ca/chairebell

Specifically created in order to promote and coordinate scientific research within partnerships between industries and the academic world which it represents, the Network for Computing and Mathematical Modeling (ncm2) signed a partnership agreement with Bell Canada in 1998, thereby creating the Bell University Laboratories. Technology and Work Organization is one of the research chairs of Bell University Laboratories.

Canada Research Chair on the Knowledge Economy—www.teluq.uqam.ca/chaireecosavoir

The chair's objective is to re-examine the various theories of firm, in particular the evolutionary theory according to which knowledge of an organization is, above all, the function of its members' individual knowledge.

Human Resources and Social Development Canada—www.hrsdc.gc.ca/en/home.shtml

A division of the federal government of Canada, Human Resources and Social Development Canada investigates social development, human resources, labour, and homelessness.

Interventions Économiques—www.teluq.uquebec.ca/interventionseconomiques

Interventions Économiques is a journal that is interested in critical theoretical debates relating to the political economy and the socio-economic transformation of society. It is a journal devoted to economic interventions and social change. It examines key social issues such as reconciling the family/home life with work, changing work and workplace trends, etc.

Statistics Canada—www.statcan.ca

From publications to electronic data, Census to survey information, www.statcan.ca is *the* official source for Canadian social and economic statistics and products.

Chapter 6

———◆———

LABOUR MARKET FLEXIBILITY
AND WORKER INSECURITY

Emile Tompa, Michael Polanyi, and Janice Foley

Introduction

Over the past 20 years, the arrangement, content, and organization of work in industrialized countries have been changing. In an effort to remain competitive in the global economy, many firms have adopted flexible production strategies aimed at responding quickly to market signals in order to increase productivity and decrease costs.

While autonomy and quality of work may have improved for some workers, particularly in the high-end service sector, there is evidence that flexible strategies are intensifying work demands, increasing levels of labour-market insecurity, and exacerbating the polarization of wages and working conditions along lines of class, gender, and race.

This chapter outlines some of the direct and indirect health consequences of labour-market restructuring arising from the widespread adoption of flexible production strategies, in particular high-performance work organization and cost-cutting tactics. Based on a consideration of the health consequences of current work practices, we propose rethinking labour-market regulations in Canada, and outline a set of policy initiatives to promote healthy and productive practices.

Flexible Production in the New Economy

Technological change, deregulation, intensified international competition, and declining productivity gains have combined to stimulate fundamental changes in work systems, employment relations, firm structures, and the labour-market experiences of workers in Canada, the United States, and other industrialized countries (Tompa et al., 2007).

The liberalization of trade and finance has resulted in significant growth in the trade of goods and services and the flow of money across international borders. Meanwhile, technological advancements in computers, telecommunications, and transportation have increased the mobility of physical and financial capital as well as goods and services. Improvements in technology have allowed firms to produce goods more quickly and cheaply, leading to the saturation of domestic markets and exacerbating competition for markets. Technological advancements have also reduced the time it takes to develop new generations of products, thus reducing the shelf life of goods and forcing firms to constantly innovate. Furthermore, technological advancements have allowed consumers fuller access to information about products and the capacity to change brands more readily, again pressuring firms to innovate or reduce prices in order to maintain customers.

Labour-market norms and structures have also changed. For example, layoffs are no longer used solely in response to a downturn in the economy; they are also used to rationalize operations in thriving markets. The level of unionization has decreased in many developed countries, as has the extent of labour-market regulation.

Social safety net programs, such as employment insurance, have also been eroded in many cases.

In this highly competitive environment, many firms have adopted flexible strategies of production. Two primary forms adopted by firms have emerged: "task flexibility" (or "functional flexibility") and "numerical flexibility" (Smith, 1997).

Functional flexibility aims to increase productivity and improve profitability and service. It includes practices intended to elicit greater employee commitment and effort by enriching jobs and streamlining production processes.

The economic impacts of such strategies may not be as uniformly beneficial as is sometimes assumed. Re-engineering, or redesigning business practices with a focus on outcomes (Hammer & Champy, 1993), can yield performance improvements, but is often unsuccessful (Carter, 1999; Elmuti & Kathawala, 2000). "Lean production," which utilizes problem-solving teams and just-in-time production techniques, has had positive impacts on productivity, quality, and costs, but only by making employees work longer and harder (Fairris & Tohyama, 2002; Yates et al., 2001). Efforts to increase employee commitment—such as employee participation in decision making, self-directed work teams, and training—can result in improved bottom lines, service, and product innovation (Appelbaum et al., 2000; Varma et al., 1999). However, results have been mixed in terms of productivity, job satisfaction, organizational commitment, absenteeism, and turnover (Farias & Varma, 1998), and are dependent on employee and organizational and intervention characteristics (Belanger, 2000; Morissette & Rosa, 2003; Ramsay et al., 2000; Wood, 1999).

Numerical, or staffing, flexibility is focused on cost reduction. Numerical flexibility is often achieved by reducing labour costs through downsizing, and shifting to short-term contracting and part-time work (see Figure 6.1). It can also be achieved by using overtime as a buffer for fluctuations in demand. The upward drift in part-time employment as a main job over the last 25 years is particularly noteworthy for the youngest and oldest age groups of the working population (see figures 6.2 and 6.3). Predictably, involuntary part-time employment has also increased substantially over this time period (Tompa et al., 2005).

The impact of these practices on the bottom line has also been mixed (Wagar, 1998), beneficial only in the short-term (Appelbaum et al., 1999), and more successful at improving profit than productivity (CFO Forum, 1995). The growing evidence that downsizing

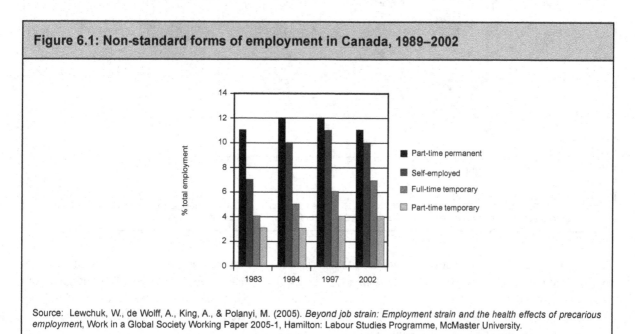

Figure 6.1: Non-standard forms of employment in Canada, 1989–2002

Source: Lewchuk, W., de Wolff, A., King, A., & Polanyi, M. (2005). *Beyond job strain: Employment strain and the health effects of precarious employment*, Work in a Global Society Working Paper 2005-1, Hamilton: Labour Studies Programme, McMaster University.

Figure 6.2: Part-time work as a main job among men in Canada as a proportion of all employed men, 1976–2002 (excludes full-time students)

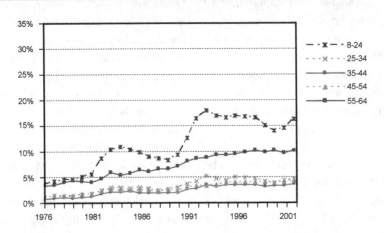

Source: Tompa, E., Dolinschi, R., Trevithick, S., Scott-Marshall, H., & Bhattacharyya, S. (2005). *Work-related precariousness: Canadian trends and policy implications*. Institute for Work & Health Working Paper no. 218. Toronto: Institute for Work & Health.

Figure 6.3: Part-time work as a main job among women in Canada as a proportion of all employed women, 1976–2002 (excludes full-time students)

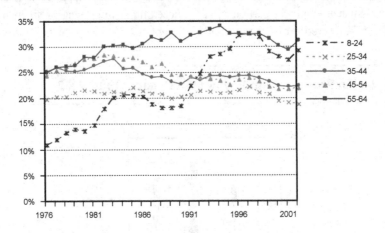

Source: Tompa, E., Dolinschi, R., Trevithick, S., Scott-Marshall, H., & Bhattacharyya, S. (2005). *Work-related precariousness: Canadian trends and policy implications*. Institute for Work & Health Working Paper no. 218. Toronto: Institute for Work & Health.

does not always achieve its objectives has not halted the trend toward laying off workers in an effort to improve financial performance.

Despite the increased use of contingent workers, there has been little examination of the economic impacts associated with their use. Indeed, costs associated with their use—such as reduced quality of services, reduced employee commitment, increased turnover and training costs—are frequently ignored (Davis-Blake et al., 2003).

In sum, the economic impacts of downsizing, re-engineering, and high-performance practices have been mixed. The health impacts, however, are of significant concern.

Flexible Organizational Strategies and the Experience of Work

Flexible production strategies have direct and indirect implications for the health and well-being of labour-force participants. While it may be that the increased flexibility of labour markets and workplaces has increased autonomy, motivation, and quality of work experiences for some high-skilled workers (Appelbaum et al., 2000), this appears not to be the case for those who are already disadvantaged in the workplace: low-skilled workers, women, and people of colour (Betcherman & Chaykowski, 1996). While there is some evidence of increases in employee control for standard workers in the United States and Europe (Landsbergis, 2003), there is also evidence in countries such as the United Kingdom of declining employee control (Green, 2002).

In general, studies indicate that work is intensifying, insecurity is growing, and market incomes are stagnating and polarizing.

Intensification of Work
The intensification of work—or increased effort expended by employees—has been identified as "one of the most significant trends of recent years" (European Foundation for the Improvement of Work and Living Conditions, 2002). Data from the United States (Landsbergis, 2003) and Europe (Burchell et al., 2002; European Foundation for the Improvement of Work and Living Conditions, 2002) show that, since the 1980s, workers increasingly report working at high speed, with high effort and tight deadlines. Data from Europe suggest that the increase in work intensity during the 1990s has been greater for women than for men, closing the gap that had previously existed (Fagan & Burchell, 2002).

Working hours for many employees have also increased. The proportion of Canadian men and women working more than 40 hours a week increased significantly between 1980 and 1995 (Shields, 1999). Similar increases have occurred in the United States (Schor, 2002), and about one in five men and one in 10 women work more

than 48 hours per week in Europe (Fagan, 2003). A recent study by the International Labour Organization (2007), reports that one in five workers around the world are working excessive hours, defined as working more than 48 hours per week. Among developed countries, the United Kingdom, Israel, Australia, Switzerland, and the United States have the highest incidence of long working hours in 2004–2005 (ranging from 19.2 percent to 25.7 percent of workers). The study notes that shorter hours benefits the health of workers and their families, reduces workplace accidents, and increases productivity and equality.

Not surprisingly, given the rise in work hours, one in three Canadian workers experiences conflict between work and family (Duxbury & Higgins, 2001), with evidence of similar conflict in the United States (Ferber & O'Farrell, 1991), the United Kingdom (Franks, 1999), and Europe (Fagan, 2003).

Increased Insecurity
A second trend related to widespread workplace and societal changes is an expanding and deepening sense of insecurity. Job insecurity has become widespread in Canada and other industrialized countries (Betcherman & Lowe, 1997; Burchell et al., 2002).

Workers are not only more uncertain about the likelihood that they will be retained in their current job, they are also uncertain about whether they will be able to find another job that meets their needs (Burke & Shields, 1999; Heery & Salmon, 2000). Finally, there is a broader sense of income insecurity as evidenced in Canada by workers' low level of confidence in the adequacy of the social safety net (Burke & Shields, 1999). Its inadequacy is corroborated by a rise in the percentage of Canadians living in poverty, and the average depth of poverty, from the 1980s to 1990s (Heisz et al., 2002).

Insecurity is not randomly distributed: Women's work in particular has become more precarious in Canada (Cranford et al., 2003), and women are twice as likely as men to work in low-paid jobs (Maxwell, 2002) (see Box 6.1).

Stagnation and Polarization of Incomes
The third key labour-market trend is that average incomes have stagnated and compensation for work has become more polarized, particularly among male workers

(Beach et al., 2002). Formerly well-paid, unionized, manufacturing-sector employees have been forced to seek employment in the expanding service sector, where full-time jobs are scarce, few employees have benefits or earn living wages, hours are irregular, and many employees hold multiple jobs in an effort to survive (Broad, 2000). One in six Canadians receive an inadequate wage of less than $10 per hour (Maxwell, 2002). While women continue to be paid at lower rates than men at all levels of the hierarchy, and continue to be concentrated in low-end jobs in industrialized countries, the income gap between men and women has lessened somewhat in Canada, as women, on average, experienced better income growth than men during the 1990s (Heisz et al., 2002). Although family disposable income equality remained steady from the 1970s to the mid-1990s due to government transfers and supports, there is some evidence that inequality had risen by the late 1990s (Heisz et al., 2002). In summary, significant changes to the work landscape are taking place, and these have significant health implications, which we explore below.

Box 6.1: Precarious jobs: A new typology of employment

- Between 1989 and 1994, the share of the workforce aged 15 and over engaged in part-time work, temporary work, own-account self-employment, or multiple jobholding grew from 28% to 34%. Since then, it has hovered around this level.
- The rise in non-standard employment in the early 1990s was fuelled by increases in own-account self-employment and full-time temporary paid work. Although employees with full-time permanent jobs still accounted for the majority of employment, this kind of work became less common, dropping from 67% in 1989 to 64% in 1994 and 63% in 2002.
- In 2002, women accounted for over 6 in 10 of those with part-time temporary jobs or part-time self-employment (own-account or employers) and for nearly three-quarters of part-time permanent employees.

Source: www.statcan.ca/english/indepth/75-001/online/01003/hi-fs_200310_02_a.html

---

Employer Flexibility and Employee Ill Health

Recent economic and workplace transformations have been accompanied by mixed changes in workers' health. The number of work fatalities (Marshall, 1996) and work-related injury and illness claims (Mustard et al., 2001) has decreased substantially over recent decades in Canada and other developed countries.

However, Canada still has the highest work-related mortality rate of Organisation for Economic Co-operation and Development (OECD) countries, and is the fourth highest in workplace injuries (Osberg & Sharpe, 2003). While this may be attributable in part to different classification criteria and the resource-based nature of the Canadian economy, Canada also performs poorly on within-country trend data. Canada has had little success in reducing its fatality rate over a 21-year period (only 6.6 percent compared to Italy's 60 percent decrease) and only modest success in reducing work-related injuries; six other countries had higher decreases (Osberg & Sharpe, 2003). Most recently, workplace fatalities have increased in Canada, from 758 in 1993 to 958 in 2004, and to 1,097 in 2005 (Sharpe & Hardt, 2006).

While causal connections between changing work conditions and health are difficult to establish, there is reason to believe that both the intensification of work and rising levels of job, employment, and income insecurity are having ill-health effects. There are at least four potential pathways through which these adverse labour-market experiences may influence health: (1) stress-induced physiological changes such as increased cholesterol and changes in the nervous, immune, and endocrine systems (Bosma et al., 1998; Kasl et al., 1998; Mattiasson et al., 1990); (2) increased risky health behaviour, such as a decrease in physical activity and an increase in smoking, drinking, and unhealthy dietary habits (Duxbury & Higgins, 2003; Morris et al., 1992); (3) loss of social support (Ali & Avison, 1997; Aneshensel, 1992; Gore, 1978); and (4) inadequacy of income that results in material deprivation (Bjarnason & Sigurdardottir, 2003; Bobak et al., 2000; Borrell et al., 2004). Below we discuss the evidence of negative health implications of intensification of work; non-standard work arrangements; and rising levels of job, employment, and income insecurity.

Intensification of Work and Its Health Consequences

Reports of work intensification and job stress have increased dramatically in the last decade, posing a significant threat to workers' physical and mental health (Benach et al., 2002; Duxbury and Higgins, 2003). Intensification may arise due to the underbidding of contracts by their employers, or workers being called upon to fill in only during peak demands. European data shows that individuals working continuously at high speeds report roughly twice the rates of stress, injuries, and back, neck, and shoulder pain as individuals who never work at high speeds (European Foundation for the Improvement of Working and Living Conditions, 2002). Other unique health conditions arising from work intensification have also been identified. A Dutch study found that "leisure sickness" on weekends and holidays, characterized by headaches, sore muscles, fatigue, and nausea, is common among employees who are perfectionists, carry large workloads, and feel very responsible for their work (Burrell, 2001).

Non-standard Work Hours and Health

The trend toward longer hours for core employees and people in managerial and professional ranks has been well established over the past decade. Long hours of work have been directly linked to negative physiological and psychological health symptoms, as well as to family relationship difficulties (Sparks et al., 1997; Landsbergis, 2003). Disturbed relaxation ability, correlated with elevated blood pressure and coronary heart disease, is related to working more than 50 hours per week (Ertel et al., 2000).

Non-standard hours of work (e.g., rotating shifts, compressed work weeks, and irregular hours) have also been linked with ill health (Martens et al., 1999). However, in general there has been conflicting evidence on the health impacts of non-standard or flexible work hours (Sparks et al., 2001). What seems to be key is whether employees are able to choose and are satisfied with their hours and schedules (Ala-Mursula et al., 2002; Sparks et al., 2001). Long hours at work may be more detrimental to the health of those workers (most often women) with heavy domestic workloads. The inability to balance work and family, which is exacerbated by long or unpredictable work hours, has also been directly linked

with increased stress and negative health symptoms (Duxbury et al., 1994; Ertel et al., 2000; Frone et al., 1997).

Precarious Work Arrangements and Health

Studies show that temporary and contract workers tend to have poorer working conditions, are more stressed, and are less healthy overall than the rest of the working population (European Foundation for the Improvement of Living and Working Conditions, 2002). Quinlan, Mayhew, and Bohle's (2001) review of 93 studies of contingent work and occupational health in various countries found that a substantial majority of studies showed a negative association between precarious employment and health.

The reasons why precariously employed workers experience poorer health are complex. Such workers may face more difficult working conditions, experience higher levels of job insecurity, have lower levels of control over their working conditions and arrangements, experience poorer quality social interactions, or be exposed to particular demands associated with their employment arrangements (Lewchuk et al., 2003).

Job Insecurity and Health

In general, studies have found an association between job insecurity and various disease and sickness outcomes (Sverke et al., 2002). A recent review by Ferrie (2001) found a consistent impact of perceived job insecurity on psychological morbidity, and emerging evidence of a relationship between job insecurity and self-reported morbidity. Job-level insecurity—or downsizing—has been associated with increased sickness absence (Kivimaki et al., 2000). Downsizing has been linked to increased workplace fatalities, workplace accidents, musculoskeletal injuries, and psychiatric disorders (Landsbergis, 2003; Probst & Brubaker, 2001). Perceived job insecurity also has negative effects on workers' marital relationships, parenting effectiveness, and their children's behaviour (Nolan, 2002).

Turnover and absenteeism rates, as well as stress-related disorders, increase after downsizing (Appelbaum et al., 1999), and Cohen (1997) found that employees who became disabled after experiencing downsizing took substantially longer to recover. If the downsizing trend continues, the costs associated with employee stress, which is estimated at $200 billion in the US annually (Carter, 1999), will only worsen.

Employment Insecurity and Health

The health effects of job insecurity appear to be moderated by the prevailing level of labour-market opportunities (Mohr, 2000; Turner, 1995). In other words, job insecurity can be less harmful when there are other employment opportunities available to workers. There is considerable literature exploring the mental and physical ill-health impacts of unemployment (Jahoda, 1982; Warr, 1987). Emerging research suggests that there are also negative health impacts of underemployment (Dooley, 2003). In Canada, certain vulnerable groups tend to have a higher exposure to underemployment, specifically visible minorities and younger individuals, and negative health impacts from such exposures are unevenly distributed across different age and gender groups (Scott-Marshall et al., 2007).

Income Insecurity and Health

The health impacts of employment insecurity and inadequacy are, in turn, affected by the perceived adequacy and security of income. Price and colleagues (2002) found that financial strain explains a significant portion of the relationship between employment status and subsequent depression. In general, income inadequacy, or poverty, has been clearly established as a predictor of ill health (Raphael, 2001).

Income insecurity and ill health are not equally distributed. Women and people of colour are more likely to work in low-income jobs, less likely to have benefits, and more likely to live in poverty (e.g., Maxwell, 2002). Saunders (2006) notes that one in six full-time workers in Canada earn less than $10 per hour in 2000, and this fraction has not changed since 1980. This is largely due to firms shifting risk to workers in the face of pressures from globalization, leaving large segments of society struggling to make ends meet. There is evidence that the degree of income inequality at the local and national levels is predictive of poorer health outcomes of groups across the income spectrum (Wilkinson, 1996). The polarization of incomes associated with flexible labour markets is hence a health concern.

In summary, there is reason to believe that stress and strain in today's flexible economy is related not just to the worker's job, but to the worker's broader experience of the organization and arrangements of employment (see Table 6.1 for one depiction of employment strain). While further quantitative and qualitative research is needed on the health impacts of cost-cutting and high productivity strategies, there is now enough evidence to justify action to reduce the negative health effects of neo-liberal, flexible employment strategies, and to promote the adoption of healthier and more authentically productive workplace practices and labour-market conditions.

Conclusion: Toward Healthy and Productive Work

While many firms focus on short-term profits and flexibility at a cost to employee health and well-being, there are opportunities for firms to adopt a wider array of employee-friendly organizational practices that better balance the dual aims of health and productivity.

Research and Education

Research and education are needed to promote a fuller recognition of the health- and productivity-related impacts of cost-cutting and high-performance strategies. There is a need to raise awareness of the magnitude of the problems, as well as educate employers and governments about how it wastes human capital. There is a particular need to dispel the assumption that cost-cutting and flexible staffing necessarily lead to economic competitiveness. New forms of knowledge transfer and education are needed. It has become increasingly clear that in order for research to be understood and used, stakeholders must be involved in the research process.

Culture Change

There is need for a culture change within and beyond organizations. This requires the same kind of sea change of thinking about work that has taken place on issues of drinking and driving, and smoking, both of which were driven by coordinated legal, policy, and community action. Workers, employers, government officials, researchers, and others need to come together to develop a shared vision of healthy and productive work. Developing this shared vision of "good" or "decent" work is the first step toward developing the kind of multilevel strategy that is needed to prevent, hinder, and stigmatize unhealthy workplace practices.

Table 6.1: Employment strain		
Components	**Control /demand/effort**	**Measures**
1. Employment relationship uncertainty	Control over access to work, where work is performed, the work schedule, setting terms and conditions of work	Employment uncertainty Earnings uncertainty Scheduling uncertainty
2. Employment relationship workload	Effort required to find work, balance demands associated with multiple workplaces and employers, keep work	Effort getting work Effort associated with multiple jobs Effort keeping work
3. Employment relationship support	Availability of help with a job, assistance if worker is stressed, presence of union and level of support provided by it	Same factors as the ISO-strain (Johnson, 1991)
4. Household Insecurity	Adequacy of household earnings and benefits	Individual and household earnings Household benefit coverage Presence of children under 18

Source: Lewchuk, W., de Wolff, A., King, A. & Polanyi, M. (2006). "The hidden costs of precarious employment: Health and the employment relationship." In L.F. Vosko (Ed.), *Precarious employment: Understanding labour market insecurity in Canada.* Montreal: McGill-Queen's University Press.

To encourage increased social accountability of employer practices, freer and fuller flows of information will be needed. This might include more systematic sharing of good or best organizational practices that have buy-in from both workers and management, as well as the provision of more complete information about the nature of production practices.

Institutional Change

Countries need to ensure that competitive pressures encourage high-road rather than low-road innovation. One possibility is through international trade and investment agreements that incorporate minimum labour standards. Taxation measures may also be used to deter non-productive and destabilizing investments (e.g., financial transfer taxes). It requires moving from a framework of free trade to one of "fair trade" (Mehmet et al., 1999). At the firm level, this requires rethinking corporate governance so that those interested in short-term profit alone (i.e., employers or shareholders) do not dictate decisions that impact on workers, families, and communities (Ackerman & Alstott, 1999).

Policy and Legislation

Individual countries and even individual firms have it within their power to react to global economic pressures in a variety of ways, thus suggesting the possibility that policy can be instituted at the national and provincial levels. The challenge is to find ways to redistribute risk between governments, workers, and employers so that social and health inequalities are reduced without jeopardizing competitiveness. This can be achieved through a mix of levers such as macroeconomic policy, education and training policy, regulation of workplace practices and benefits, and policies supportive of various forms of worker empowerment through organization and representation.

Particular attention needs to be given to low-paid employment and to non-standard forms of work. Minimum wage and income supplements need to be increased so that full-time workers can afford the basic costs of living. There could be requirements of prorating retirement, sick leave, holiday, and health care benefits for temporary and part-time workers. Regulation could also extend to training and advancement opportunities, and the requirement that temporary agencies hire staff on a permanent basis after a specific tenure of service. Legislation could also be designed to facilitate collective bargaining for non-standard forms of work through the expansion or reinterpretation of craft-like guilds and unions that cut across several employers. More generally, multifirm labour and management groups could provide support for workers throughout their careers with services such as career counselling and job-referral systems.

Low-paying work systems should be a specific target of public policy since workers in these systems are particularly vulnerable. Labour-force participants need to be aware of the types of skills demanded by the labour market, and have access to financing, appropriate training opportunities, and assistance with job search (e.g., access to job banks and career counselling). On the demand side, policy needs to provide a stimulus for firms operating in low-wage systems to raise productivity levels and, in turn, place more value on their human resources. Other policy concerns associated with these work systems are the predictability and length of work hours and autonomy, and control issues related to the pace and intensity of work.

Attention should be paid to enhancing job, employment, and income security of all workers. Job and income security can be promoted by requiring temporary agencies to hire employees after a certain time frame on a full-time permanent basis. Employment insurance premiums can be experience-rated to provide incentives for industries and employers who depend heavily on seasonal, part-time, and short-tenure work to consider a more complete set of costs that arise from these employment practices. Employment security can be promoted through increasing access to training, and by providing further options for reduced (and hence redistributed) work hours. Income security can be promoted by expanding access to employment insurance and pensions (Townson, 2003). Broader income security also requires the protection of public services such as health care, education, and recreation.

Finally, the design of workers' compensation and occupational health and safety regulation need to be revisited. Public policies and programs need to create incentives for firms to safeguard worker health and well-being rather than focus simply on reducing injuries and illnesses. Innovative regulatory practices directed at empowering workplace parties and encouraging firm-level solutions, such as providing employers, particularly smaller ones, with customized training and incentive programs would be helpful since firms often do not have the knowledge or resources to evaluate the direct and indirect costs of illness and injury and the benefits of investing in preventative measures.

Power and Equity

The growing power imbalance between employees and employers needs to be redressed. In part, this will depend on traditional and new forms of employee representation. In part, it will depend on creating a context of greater employment and income security so that workers are not forced to choose between poverty and workplace-induced illness.

Inequalities across various labour-force subgroups (along with characteristics such as gender, age, cultural background, and education level) need to be reduced. Indeed, it appears that economically marginalized groups such as women, youth, recent immigrants, low-wage, and non-White workers are being disproportionately harmed by flexible workplace strategies. There is a need, therefore, for stronger legislation governing equal opportunity in hiring, pay, training, and career advancement. Consistent with the notion of reducing inequalities, the requirement of certain accommodations for health conditions would allow freer labour-force participation for older individuals and individuals with functional deficits.

This chapter has described labour-market and workplace changes that have been shown to impact health. While some work-related health outcomes (like lost-time work accidents) have shown improvement, other outcomes (like stress and non-acute conditions) seem to be on the rise. Moreover, the outlook in terms of key work-related determinants of health, such as job demands, job control, job security, and income equality, is ominous. Stakeholders concerned about work and health need to better understand the health implications of today's workplace and labour-market conditions, and come together to establish a shared vision of, and agenda to create, healthy work for all in the very near future.

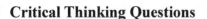

Critical Thinking Questions

1. Given the multiple and complex ways in which labour-market experiences can have adverse health consequences, how do policy-makers prioritize options to address them?
2. How do societies approach critical health issues when there is a trade-off between efficiencies of the market mechanism and the need for legislation, policies, and practices to protect and promote the health of workers?
3. How can developed countries address health and productivity issues related to labour-market experiences, given that markets transcend national boundaries and many multinational firms seek to operate in the lowest-cost markets?

Recommended Readings

Broad, D. (2000). *Hollow work, hollow society? Globalization and the casual labour problem in Canada.* Halifax: Fernwood.

Explains the contemporary casualization of work as integral to global economic restructuring, and explores the human impact of these trends.

Burchell, B., Ladipo, D. & Wilkinson, F. (2002). *Job insecurity and work intensification.* London: Routledge.

Reviews current research on flexibility, job insecurity, and work intensification and examines the impact of these developments on individuals, their families, the workplace, and the long-term health of the British economy.

European Foundation for the Improvement of Living and Working Conditions. (2002). *Quality of work and employment in Europe: Issues and challenges* (Foundation Paper). Dublin: EFILWC. Online at www.eurofound. eu.int/publications/files/EF0212EN.pdf.

Reviews challenges and opportunities associated with changes in work, based on a multicountry survey of European workers.

Landsbergis, P.A. (2003). "The changing organization of work and the safety and health of working people: A commentary." *Journal of Occupational and Environmental Medicine 45*(1), 61–72.

Reviews an important new US report on the current state of knowledge on work organization and health.

Vosko, L.F. (2006). *Precarious employment: Understanding labour market insecurity in Canada.* Montreal: McGill-Queen's University Press.

Contributions from multiple authors give treatment to the issue of precarious employment from a social, statistical, legal, political, and economic perspective.

Related Web Sites

Canadian Policy Research Network—www.cprn.com

This is the Web site of a non-profit policy think tank that undertakes research to guide decision makers as they craft social and economic policy.

Centre for the Study of Living Standards—www.csls.ca

This is the Web site of a non-profit organization that undertakes research to better understand trends in the determinants of productivity, living standards, and economic and social well-being.

European Foundation for the Improvement of Work and Living—www.eurofound.ie

This is an important and voluminous source of free reports on the changing nature of work and health.

International Labour Organization—www.ilo.org

This is the source of leading-edge thinking about the promotion of an international agenda for decent work.

Winning Workplaces—www.winningworkplaces.org

This has a range of information, success stories, and research on small and mid-size organizations' workplace practices.

Chapter 7

—————◆—————

THE UNHEALTHY
CANADIAN WORKPLACE

Andrew Jackson

Introduction

The purpose of this chapter is to provide a broad overview
of the impact of employment, working conditions, and
the work environment on health. The focus is on the
quality of work as opposed to wider conditions in the
labour market.

Health researchers have demonstrated a clear link
between income and socio-economic status and health
outcomes, such that longevity and state of health rise with
position on the income scale (Raphael, 2004). Very little
of this relationship is explained by important lifestyle
differences among income groups, or by differential
access to health care in countries like Canada that provide
universal health care. The fact that higher-income people
are in better health and live longer than middle-income
people suggests that the health gradient is linked to
relative position on the income scale rather than to
absolute deprivation or poverty.

Given the simple fact that the experience of work
dominates the lives of most working-age people, it
seems plausible that the close link between socio-
economic status and health runs, in significant part,
through different workplace experiences. Those at the
lower end of the income spectrum are most likely to
experience stress from job insecurity and from stress in
the workplace itself, and they are also most likely to face
workplace hazards to physical health.

Research has established strong links between
unemployment/precarious employment and poor health

outcomes, and between poor working conditions and
poor physical and mental health. Poor employment
conditions include: dirty and dangerous jobs, including
exposure to harmful substances that pose risks to physical
health in terms of injuries and occupational disease;
jobs that are stressful by virtue of the pace, demands,
or repetitive content of the labour process; jobs that are
stressful because of the exercise of arbitrary power in the
workplace and the lack of social supports; jobs that are
stressful because they do not meet human developmental
needs; and jobs that are stressful because they are a source
of conflict with the lives of workers in the home and in
the community.

Work and Health

In recent years, health researchers have increasingly
emphasized the links between work stress and physical
and mental health. Stress can arise from many sources,
including job insecurity, the physical demands of
work, the extent of support from supervisors and co-
workers, work-life conflict, and job strain (Wilkins &
Beaudet, 1998). High job strain—a combination of high
psychological demands at work combined with a low
degree of control over the work process—has been linked
to an increased risk of physical injuries at work, high
blood pressure, cardiovascular disease, depression and
other mental health conditions, and increased lifestyle
risks to health.

Work poses physical risks, and is clearly a major source of psychosocial stress, which has been identified as one major cause of increased morbidity and mortality. As the leading population health researcher Richard Wilkinson puts it, "to feel depressed, bitter, cheated, vulnerable, frightened about debts or job or housing insecurity; to feel devalued, useless, helpless, uncared for, hopeless, isolated, anxious. These feelings can dominate people's whole experience of life, colouring their experience of everything else. It is the chronic stress arising from feelings like these which does the damage" (cited in Dunn, 2002, p. 26).

It is ironic, not to say tragic, that the shift to a post-industrial society with an increasingly well-educated and skilled workforce is associated with rising levels of stress rather than increased well-being at work. Research has shown some negative consequences for health to date, but the full impact of current conditions is likely to be slow to appear. Many of today's older workers and retirees were workers in the golden age of postwar capitalism when working conditions were more closely regulated, and conditions were improving. The health impacts of 21st-century work may just be appearing.

This chapter provides a general overview of current conditions and the overall direction of change to look at some important cleavages among workers in terms of access to good jobs, and to place the situation in Canada in a comparative context. Comparisons are made with the European Union because better working conditions in the EU along some dimensions do suggest that improvement of the quality of the Canadian work environment is not incompatible with having a highly productive economy.

What Is a Good Job?

An appropriate starting point is to consider what constitutes a good job from the perspective of workers. For all of the emphasis that is (rightly) placed on the fundamental importance of waged employment as the critical source of income, other dimensions of employment are at least as important to workers. On the economic front, non-wage benefits, job security, and opportunities for advancement are as important as wages. The content of work and the nature of the labour process are less tangible and measurable, but count for

a lot as well. The EKOS/CPRN survey of changing employment relationships (which is a key part of the set of indicators of job quality in Canada to be found at www.jobquality.ca) confirmed that a large majority of workers place a high value on having interesting and personally rewarding work, enjoying some autonomy on the job, and having the ability to exercise and develop their skills and capacities. Lowe (2007, p. 56) finds that the most important criterion of job quality, cited by 72 percent of workers as being "very important," is being in a healthy and safe workplace, followed closely by work-life balance, which 63 percent see as "very important." Jencks et al. (1988) found that there is much more unequal distribution of quality jobs along valued dimensions other than pay, indicating that even large pay differences are an imperfect proxy for large class differences in the quality of employment.

The statement that quality of employment involves much more than pay will come as a surprise only to economists who have been trained to view work as a "disutility" endured in order to gain income. Work is better seen as a potential sphere for the development of individual human capacities and potentials. Production is also a social process. Good workplaces are those in which there are valued relationships with co-workers and some degree of active participation and democratic control of the work process. Bad workplaces, by contrast, are alienating and authoritarian.

For the purposes of this chapter, seven key dimensions of employment with relevance to well-being and health are considered:

- Job and employment security
- Physical conditions of work
- Work pace and stress
- Working time
- Opportunities for self-expression and individual development at work
- Participation at work
- Work-life balance

Before these dimensions are considered in detail, it is useful to briefly summarize some of the wider economic and social forces impacting upon Canadian workplaces.

Forces Shaping Workplace Change in Canada

The terms of employment—wages and benefits, hours, and working conditions—reflect the relative bargaining power of workers and employers, and the related willingness of governments to establish minimum rights and standards. Over the 1980s and 1990s, the context was one of high unemployment and underemployment, increased employer ability to shift production and new investments to lower-cost regions and countries, and an ideologically driven retreat from state intervention on behalf of workers.

There has been a pervasive and ongoing restructuring of employment relationships intended to promote productivity and competitiveness, as opposed to promotion of a worker-centred agenda of good jobs (Lowe, 2000). The basic direction of change is best understood as employers' simultaneous intensification and casualization of work. The most common forms of organizational change have been downsizing, contracting out of non-core functions, and securing greater flexibility of time worked through a combination of increased overtime and increased part-time and contract work.

The restructuring of work has been driven by employers. Governments have been mainly, at best, passive bystanders. But countervailing forces do continue to exist in workplaces in the form of unions and regulation of some working conditions.

Dimensions of Job Quality

Job Security

In considering the linkages from labour market conditions to health, researchers have studied both the availability of work and the nature of work. It is well established from studies of laid-off workers in the high unemployment decades of the 1980s and 1990s that the state of unemployment is bad for health for both material and psychological reasons. However, the relatively well-studied transition from stable employment to long-term unemployment, which followed rapid deindustrialization and major layoffs in response to shocks like the Canada–US Free Trade Agreement in the late 1980s and early 1990s, is less frequent today than alternation between short-term unemployment and precarious employment.

Frequent short-term unemployment is a source of stress and anxiety due to lack of income, uncertain prospects for the future, and its potential to undermine social support networks (World Health Organization, 1999). Workers who must often move between short-term jobs are also likely to derive less satisfaction and meaning from their paid work.

Most Canadians are familiar with the national unemployment rate, which is reported monthly and stood at about 6 percent in 2007. Taken at face value, this number considerably understates the true extent of employment insecurity. To be counted as employed, one need only have worked for a few hours in a week, so employment includes temporary employees, part-time workers who want more hours, and people working in low-wage survival jobs while looking for regular jobs matching their skills. To be counted as unemployed, a person has to have been unable to find any work at all, and to have been actively seeking work even if he or she knew that no suitable jobs were available. Moreover, there is continual turnover in the ranks of those who are counted as unemployed over a year. While well down from levels in the early 1990s, a 6 percent average monthly unemployment rate, combined with an average unemployment spell of about 20 weeks, still means that up to 15 percent of the workforce were unemployed at some point in 2007.

Long-term unemployment in Canada is much lower than in other advanced industrial countries. In 2005, just 17 percent of unemployed workers had been out of work for more than six months compared to a 47 percent average in Organisation for Economic Co-operation and Development (OECD) countries, and 64 percent in the European Union (OECD Employment Outlook, 2006, Table G). The Canadian job market is marked less by chronic long-term unemployment than by frequent transitions for many workers (especially women, recent immigrants, and racialized minorities) between low-paid, precarious jobs and relatively short periods of unemployment. Precariously employed workers also tend to be trapped in low-wage jobs. Layoffs from relatively good jobs also began to rise from 2005 because of large manufacturing job losses in Ontario and Quebec.

Precarious work in Canada is not only widespread, it is much more precarious than in many other countries. In the European Union, there are often job-security laws and

Box 7.1: Fear of job loss

As one would expect from the unemployment data, many working Canadians worry about losing their jobs. The Personal Security Index (PSI) of the Canadian Council on Social Development (CCSD) is used to track the proportion of people who think there is a good chance they could lose their job over the next two years. This stood at 37 percent in 1998, but fell to just 21 percent in 2006, based on data from an identical question in a major EKOS survey. Fear of job loss is slightly higher among men than women, and much higher in lower-income households. The PSI also tracked the proportion of workers who are confident they could find an equivalent job within six months if they lost their current job. Thirty-three percent were not confident in 2006, according to the EKOS survey, down much less dramatically from 38 percent in 1998. This suggests that while risk of job loss has been falling, many workers still fear they would be unable to find as good a job as the one they have if they were to be laid off.

regulations that limit employers' power to lay off long-tenure workers. A binding policy directive establishes that there should be limits on renewals of temporary contracts. Minimum-pay laws and widespread collective bargaining provide a wage-and-benefit floor to the job market. As a result, there are far larger pay gaps between precarious and core workers in Canada than in most EU countries.

Job insecurity in the precarious labour market is heightened by lack of supports and services to promote access to better employment. The dominant ethos is that heavy sticks are needed to drive the unemployed into available low-wage jobs. Our minimal and deeply punitive social welfare system is designed to make even poverty-line wages look attractive, and qualifying hours requirements for employment insurance (as high as 700 hours or 20 weeks of full-time work) effectively cut off many precariously employed workers who need income support between jobs the most. Employment insurance rules effectively disqualify many who survive by patching together sequences of paid employment with self-employment.

Canadian analysts of linkages from work to ill health have developed the concept of "employment strain" (Lewchuk et al., 2006). They argue that, in addition to stress arising from specific job characteristics (such as high job demands, fast speed of work, and low degree of control), stress with adverse implications for health arises from the precarious nature of many employment relationships in today's job market. Precarious work, such as temporary and contract work, is stressful in its own right, and also carries a high risk of exclusion from the protections and support networks to be found in more secure and stable jobs in larger workplaces. Studies have found a higher risk of injury and illness; greater workload and greater exposure to dangerous substances among the self-employed and those who work for small contractors; and a higher risk of self-reported ill health and a greater incidence of working in pain among precarious workers compared to workers in similar jobs who are in more secure forms of employment.

Another key difference between relatively secure and more precarious employment with direct implications for health is access to employer-sponsored health benefits. The most important benefit for the working-age population is prescription drug coverage. Drug benefits are typically provided by governments only to seniors, social assistance recipients, and sometimes people leaving welfare for work. Having a low-wage job with no health benefits can mean an inability to buy medically necessary prescription drugs, as well as needed dental and other health services not provided by physicians and hospitals whose costs are covered by medicare. In 2000, just 50 percent of employees had extended medical, dental, and life/disability coverage, usually provided as a package. While 70 percent of union members were covered, only 40 percent of non-union members were so fortunate, and coverage was very low in small firms with less than 20 employees (27 percent), part-time jobs (14 percent), and temporary jobs (17 percent) (Marshall, 2003, Table 2). Lowe (2007, p. 26) considers the best data to show that health benefits coverage has been falling. Moreover, the rising cost of employer health plans, especially drug costs, has led to reduced coverage for many workers, imposing heavier co-pays and more limitations on allowable prescriptions. In a better world, all citizens would be covered by a comprehensive public health care plan, but the large gaps in our current system mean that there is a tight link between having a good job and having good health-related benefits, and between having a more unhealthy job and having no or very limited benefits. There are also large gaps between secure and more precarious workers in terms of access to paid sick leave, though here there is at least entitlement to a modest floor through the Employment Insurance program. Many precariously employed workers thus face directly higher risks to health because of the quality of their employment.

Lack of employer-sponsored pension coverage for many precarious workers, combined with a relatively ungenerous public pension system, implies longer working lifetimes. Many low-wage older workers are significantly better off after they retire at 65 and qualify for the combined Old Age Security pension and Guaranteed Income Supplement, which at least provide an income close to the poverty line.

To summarize, a large minority of workers experience continuing precarious employment and a significant risk of periodic unemployment. The risks to health of precarious employment caused by stress and anxiety are compounded by lack of access to benefits.

Physical Conditions of Work

One might have thought that dirty and dangerous work was a thing of the past, banished along with the dark satanic mills of the Industrial Revolution. But deaths, occupational diseases, and injuries rooted in the physical conditions of work are still very much a feature of the contemporary workplace.

Unlike workplace fatalities, the incidence of work-related accidents and injuries appears to be falling. Reported injuries are those that are made known to provincial workers compensation boards since they involve time lost from work and payment while off the job. In British Columbia, reported lost-time claims fell from 8.8 to 5.4 per 100 full-time equivalent male workers between 1990 and 2001, and fell from 6.1 to

---

Box 7.2: Five deaths a day: Workplace fatalities in Canada

According to data collected by the Association of Workers' Compensation Boards of Canada, 1,097 workplace fatalities were recorded in Canada in 2005, up 45 percent from 758 in 1993, and up 8 percent from 958 in 2004. As Canadians work on average 230 days per year, this means that there were nearly five work-related deaths per working day.

The chances of a worker dying from a workplace-related accident or disease in Canada vary greatly by industry, occupation, gender, and age group. The most dangerous industry in which to work over the 1996–2005 period was mining, quarrying, and oil wells (49.9 deaths per 100,000 workers or one out of 2,000), followed by logging and forestry (42.9 per 100,000 workers or one out of 2,300), fishing and trapping (35.6 fatalities per 100,000 workers or one out of every 2,800 workers), agriculture (28.1 fatalities per 100,000 workers or one out of every 3,600 workers), and construction (20.6 per 100,000 workers or one out of 4,900). Finance and insurance was the least dangerous industry, with only 0.2 fatalities per 100,000 workers or one death for every 500,000 workers.

Men are much more likely than women to die on the job. In 2005, the incidence of workplace death was 30 times higher among men than women: 12.4 deaths per 100,000 workers versus 0.4 deaths.

Workplace fatalities arise from both accidents and occupational diseases. In 2005, out of the 1,097 workplace fatalities, 491 (44.8 percent) were from accidents and 557 (50.8 percent) from occupational diseases. Asbestos-related deaths alone accounted for about 340 deaths in 2005.

The ILO Workplace Fatality database shows that, in 2003, Canada had the 5th highest incidence of workplace fatalities out of 29 OECD countries. Only Korea, Mexico, Portugal, and Turkey had higher workplace fatality rates and all four countries are at a much lower level of development than Canada. Unfortunately, definitions of workplace fatalities differ from country to country and the ILO makes no attempt to standardize the data. Nevertheless, even if one fully adjusted for definitional differences, it is very unlikely that Canada would emerge as a low workplace fatality country relative to its peers.

Source: This is an abbreviated version of the Executive Summary of a report by Sharpe, Andrew & Hardt, Jill. (2006). *Five deaths a day: Workplace fatalities in Canada*. Centre for the Study of Living Standards Research Paper 2006-06. Online at www.csls.ca/reports/csls2006-04.pdf).

2.8 reported workplace injuries per 100 male workers in Ontario. Lost-time claim rates are much lower among women, but have fallen more modestly. For example, claims for women in Ontario fell from 3.3 to 2.0 per 100 workers over the same time period (Breslin et al., 2006). As one might expect, workplace injuries, like work-time fatalities, are heavily concentrated among men in blue-collar industrial jobs. These kinds of jobs shrank over much of the 1990s, but have recently grown as a result of the resource boom in Western Canada and a strong housing construction market.

The release of the CSLS report on growing workplace fatalities in 2006 (see Box 7.2) sparked a major public debate on the real trend in workplace injuries. It is generally recognized that workplace fatalities are at the tip of an iceberg, standing above workplace injuries and "near misses," so a decline in injuries combined with an increase in fatalities is curious. The CBC Radio program "The Current" ran a program on this issue as part of a series on health and safety in the workplace (www.cbc.ca/thecurrent/2007/200701/20070108.html). Focusing on the situation in Alberta, some argued that workplace accidents are seriously underreported. Troy Ophus, whose hand was crushed against an I-beam by a falling trolley, said that "a lot of injuries don't get reported" because workers feel they will be fired or treated as troublemakers. Dr. Louis Francescutti, an Alberta emergency room physician and university teacher, said that there is "not a shortage of injuries; it's just not being reported."

Part of the problem is that provincial workers' compensation systems have shifted toward experience-rating the premiums paid by employers, so that higher accident rates result in higher costs to them (Lippel, 2006). The laudable aim has been to increase employers' incentive to take workplace health and safety seriously, but, at the same time, it also now makes sense for employers to contract out the most dangerous jobs, and to persuade their own workers not to report injuries. Some employers provide awards for days worked without injuries, increasing peer pressure on workers not to report an injury.

Workplace health and safety issues are usually taken most seriously in larger workplaces, which are often unionized, where formal procedures and rules are in place, where safety training is most frequently provided, and where government inspections of health and safety conditions in response to worker or union complaints are most likely to take place. The shift of jobs to smaller, usually non-union workplaces and the growth of more precarious forms of employment, such as self-employment and employment with small subcontractors, has thus worked to undermine physical safety on the job. Self-employed workers are generally not covered by government health and safety legislation or by workers' compensation legislation and programs even though they may be working for large employers, so work-related accidents among them will not be reported (Lippel, 2006). Contract employees, who are covered in theory, may not know that they are protected by legislation and workers' compensation programs. These kinds of arm's-length employment are quite common in some high-risk industries, such as construction. Also, some quite dangerous jobs, such as farm jobs, are often not covered by health and safety legislation at all. Seasonal agricultural workers who come to Canada from other countries under special, temporary work permits are especially vulnerable.

The nature of workplace injuries and conditions is also changing. There has been a disturbing upward trend in repetitive strain and other soft-tissue injuries associated with highly repetitive machine and keyboard work. These account for an upward trend in the proportion of workplace injuries reported by women. As one would expect, physical injuries—sprains and strains to backs and hands, cuts, punctures, lacerations, fractures, and contusions—are associated with physically demanding jobs. Manufacturing and construction account for 20 percent of employment but about 40 percent of injuries, explaining the gap between injury rates among men and women. But injury rates are also high in sectors such as retail trade, and health and social services, which involve repetitive physical work.

Sullivan (2000) argues that workers' compensation practices, which were designed to address physical trauma in a world of manual, blue-collar, male work, have not changed to sufficiently recognize the growing reality of less visible physical injuries, which develop over a period of time. Soft-tissue injuries, such as repetitive strain injuries affecting women clerical and service workers, are underreported and undercompensated.

Musculoskeletal pain and chronic back pain are on the increase, especially with an aging workforce in physically demanding jobs, and are a major cause of work absence and disability (Shainblum et al., 2000). Many of these conditions have no specific causal event, are slow in onset, and develop progressively over time, and it is hard to separate out the specific job-related factors that may be involved. There is a clear link to the poor ergonomic conditions of work in specific kinds of jobs involving heavy work and repetitive tasks, but few workers are able to make successful worker-compensation claims. Often, workers will have moved between jobs and even occupations while a condition has been developing, so a condition cannot be attributed to a specific work experience with a specific employer. Similarly, Canada is experiencing a rapidly rising rate of chronic stress-related disability, which often has workplace roots, but cannot be identified as solely work-related or solely attributable to a specific job and employer. Many critics of the current workers' compensation system feel that it is inadequate in terms of measuring, let alone compensating for, work-related risks to health in a post-industrial environment.

Occupational diseases are, of course, also related to workplace risks and exposures. Lung diseases and cancers are linked to physical risks, including inhalation of toxic fumes, handling of hazardous chemicals, and exposure to carcinogens. In a very limited number of cases, there is a very clear causal linkage from occupational exposure to disease onset, which has been recognized by workers' compensation boards. For example, boards recognize that occupational exposure causes asbestosis among asbestos mine workers and a range of lung diseases among other miners. A handful of highly specific cancers have been demonstrably linked to exposure to specific carcinogens at work, but the overall incidence of occupational disease compared to workplace injuries is extremely low if we go by the official data.

The workers' compensation system demands high standards of scientific proof of cause and effect in order to keep down costs, but many carcinogens are present in the general environment as well as in the workplace. Experts estimate that anywhere from 10–40 percent of cancers may be caused primarily by workplace exposures, but only a tiny proportion of cancer victims qualify for workers' compensation. Similarly, workplace stress and heavy physical exertion are associated with heart conditions, but only a tiny proportion of heart attack victims (e.g., firemen) qualify. The key point is that occupational diseases due to the physical hazards of work are prevalent, but are largely unrecognized. Somewhat ironically, employers end up bearing a large share of the costs anyway through employer-funded, long-term disability plans.

An official European Union institution, the European Foundation for the Improvement of Living and Working Conditions regularly conducts surveys on European working conditions. The third survey for 2000 followed surveys for 1990 and 1995. It found that "[e]xposure to physical hazards at the workplace and conditions such as musculoskeletal disorders and fatigue caused by intensification of work and flexible employment practices are on the increase" (European Foundation for the Improvement of Living and Working Conditions, 2000, p. 10).

In 2000—defining significant exposure as exposure at least one-quarter of the time—29 percent of European workers were exposed to noise; 22 percent to inhalation of vapours, fumes, and dust; 37 percent reported having to move or carry heavy loads; and no less than 47 percent reported having to work in painful or tiring positions. In each case, a little under half of those reporting the hazard were exposed all of the time. Fortunately, given increasing rather than declining exposure to all of these risks (except inhalation exposure), 76 percent of European workers reported that they had been well informed of hazards. As one would expect, exposure is greatest in occupations such as machine operators, but the EU data also indicate quite widespread exposure to physical hazards.

The European survey also provides data on the incidence of repetitive work, for which no general Canadian information is available. In the EU, 31 percent of workers report continuous, repetitive, hand/arm movements, and 23 percent report working at short, repetitive tasks with cycle times of less than one minute. One in four (24 percent) workers report continuously working at high speed, with the level being highest among machine operators (35 percent), but still is high among clerical workers (20 percent) and service workers (23 percent). The incidence of high-speed work due to tight deadlines has been modestly increasing, though there is variation between countries and between different categories of workers. The survey found that those working at high speed were much more likely to report negative health effects, such as muscular pain, stress, and anxiety.

The 2005 survey found that intensity of work in the European Union has continued to increase, with a steadily rising proportion of workers expected to work at very high speed and/or working to tight deadlines. Between 1991 and 2005, those working at very high speed at least three-quarters of the time rose from just over one in five to about one-third, and the proportion working to tight deadlines at least three-quarters of the time rose from about one-quarter to more than one-third. There has also been a modest decrease in the proportion of employees who can exercise autonomy at work, though a majority still report an ability to change the order of tasks, the speed of work, and methods of work. Reported job satisfaction has been declining, with 22.8 percent of workers reporting being not very or not at all satisfied with working conditions in 2005, up from 15.2 percent in 1991. These trends are rather disturbing given that the European Union has given priority to measuring, monitoring, and improving working conditions. On a more positive note, however, only about one in four EU workers feel that their health and safety are threatened at work, down from about one in three in 1991, and there has been some increase in working-time flexibility and a decline in very long working hours (European Foundation for the Improvement of Living and Working Conditions, 2007).

Comparable data on the physical demands of work are simply unavailable for Canada, though one recent Canadian survey suggests that the incidence of high-speed work in Canada and the US is well above the average of all advanced industrial countries (Brisbois, 2003). There is little reason to believe that the situation here is any better than in the EU.

To summarize, despite the transition to a post-industrial society, the risks of occupational injury and disease are still high. One-third of Canadian workers (31.3 percent) feel that their employment puts their health and safety at risk, a bit above the average for advanced industrial countries (Brisbois, 2003). Regrettably, little hard data are available on the physical hazards of work in Canada. One aspect of work reorganization likely has been the intensification of physical demands on

some groups of workers. Highly repetitive work with short cycle times is likely just as prevalent as in the EU, explaining the sharply rising incidence of repetitive strain injuries among clerical and industrial workers.

Workplace Control and Stress

Sources of stress at work include the pace and demands of work, and the degree of control that workers have over the labour process. Karasek and Theorell (1990) and others have stressed that jobs are particularly stressful if high demands on workers are combined with a low level of decision latitude with respect to the use of skills and discretion on how to do the job. Stress from high-strain jobs (high demands, low control) is greater among women than men, primarily because of lower levels of job control (Wilkins & Beaudet, 1998). A Statistics Canada indicator judges that 28 percent of women had high-strain jobs in 2002 compared to 20 percent of men. High-strain jobs are most prevalent among lower-income sales and services workers (Park, 2007).

High-stress jobs have been found to be a significant contributing factor to high blood pressure, cardiovascular diseases, mental illness, and long-onset disability. Workers in high-strain jobs are about twice as likely to experience depression as other workers of the same age and socio-economic status with the same social supports (Shields, 2006). There is a link between low levels of control over working conditions to stress as well as to higher rates of work injuries. Even where work is physically demanding, there is less risk of injury if workers can vary the pace of work, take breaks when needed, and have some say in the design of workstations.

While there have been case studies pointing to high levels of stressful work in many Canadian workplaces (Lewchuk & Robertson, 1996), general data are again limited. Statistics Canada's *General Social Survey* provides some information. In 2000, 35 percent of workers reported experiencing stress at work from "too many demands or too many hours," up slightly from 33 percent in 1994, and up from 27.5 percent in 1991. Stress from this source is highest among professionals and managers, at 49 percent and 48 percent respectively, but is still high among blue-collar workers (28 percent) and sales and service workers (29 percent). By industry, the incidence of stress from "too many demands or hours" is highest in education, health, and social services at over 40 percent (see data at www.jobquality.ca). As one would expect, there is a strong relationship between working long hours and working in jobs that impose high demands. A 2005 survey with a somewhat different question found that one in three workers (32.4 percent) find most days "quite a bit or extremely stressful," with self-reported work stress being well above average in finance and insurance, and in health care (Lowe, 2007, p. 47).

Women are more likely than men to report high levels of stress from "too many hours or too many demands"—37 percent compared to 32 percent. This partly reflects work-life balance issues considered below, but it also reflects the high proportion of women working in the high-stress educational, health, and social services sectors, as well as in clerical positions that involve highly routinized, fast-paced work.

With respect to job control, data from the *General Social Survey* indicate that, in 1994, just 40 percent of Canadian workers reported that they had "a lot of freedom over how to work," down sharply from 54 percent in 1989. Data from a 2002 survey suggest there was a very slight increase in decision latitude in jobs between 1994–1995 and 2002 (Lowe, 2007, p. 49). It should, however, be taken into account that the education level of the workforce increased significantly over this period. Men generally exercise more control than women (43 percent compared to 38 percent in 1994). Professionals and managers predictably report that they exercise much more control than skilled workers who, in turn, have more freedom than unskilled workers (51 percent vs. 35 percent vs. 31 percent, respectively). The same survey indicates that about half of all working Canadians believe that their jobs involve a high degree of skill, with self-reported levels of exercising a high level of skill being a bit higher among women than men.

Data from the *National Population Health Survey* for 1994–1995 have been used to construct a measure of decision latitude based on responses to two questions: "I have a lot to say about what happens in my job" and "My job allows me the freedom to decide how I do my job." This response is now being used as an official population health indicator. In 1994–1995, 48.8 percent of all respondents, 52.3 percent of men and 44.5 percent of women, reported high decision latitude, while 36.6–30.7

percent of men and a full 44 percent of women reported low or medium decision latitude (Statistics Canada, 2001).

To summarize, while we lack detailed information on changes in the overall incidence of work involving high demands and low worker control, high-stress work is common and likely on the increase.

Opportunities for Self-Development

As noted, a valued characteristic of work is the opportunity it provides for the exercise and development of skills and capacities. Most of us welcome the chance to work in interesting, challenging jobs, and the opportunity to learn new things. The data presented above suggest that skilled workers, particularly professionals, are usually able to utilize their skills on the job, and enjoy a fair degree of control over the labour process. Educational credentials are increasingly the major requirement to obtain these kinds of good jobs. Access to training on the job is also an important determinant of well-being over the course of a working lifetime, since it provides opportunities for further skills development and for advancement to more challenging and rewarding work. However, there are major barriers to training for those who lack time, resources, and employer support.

There is abundant evidence that many jobs are structured to minimize the need for skills rather than to further develop the capacities of workers, and that overqualification is a serious problem (Livingstone, 2002). More than one in four Canadian men and women—and 40 percent of young people under 25— feel overqualified for their current job according to a survey by Canadian Policy Research Networks (www. jobquality.ca). Employers routinely overlook the skills and credentials of many new immigrants with the result that they are sidelined into low-paid, dead-end jobs.

Working Time

A historic goal of the organized labour movement has been to expand free time. Important breakthroughs were the 10- and then the eight-hour working day, the five-day working week and the advent of the weekend, the negotiation of paid days off, and pensioned retirement at progressively earlier ages. By the 1950s, the healthy norm of the standard, five-day, 40-hour week with paid annual vacation and retirement with a decent pension was firmly entrenched.

While progress was made through the 1970s and into the 1980s in terms of reducing weekly hours, annual hours, and the length of a working lifetime, the 1990s saw an increase in daily, weekly, and annual hours for many core workers in full-time jobs. Long hours are most prevalent among salaried professional and managerial workers, and among skilled blue-collar workers, who frequently work paid overtime. From an employer's perspective, overtime helps adjust production to changing market demand, and provides a particularly high cost-saving if the extra hours are not paid for. Even overtime pay premiums are often cheaper than the costs of hiring, training, and providing non-wage benefits to additional workers. Unpaid overtime is increasingly required not just of managers and professionals, but also of public and social services workers attempting to cope with increased workloads. Self-employed workers also tend to work very long hours.

While some workers want to work overtime for higher pay or out of commitment to the job or a career, most have limited ability to refuse demands for longer hours under employment standards legislation and under collective agreements. In most provinces, overtime well in excess of 40 hours can be required up to varying maximum levels of up to 50 hours or so, sometimes provided an overtime premium is paid. Only 25 percent of unionized workers have some right (usually conditional) to refuse overtime. Today, about one in four workers work overtime in any given week, averaging 8.5 hours or the equivalent of an extra day's work. About half of this overtime, usually that worked by salaried managers and professionals, is unpaid, suggesting that a large share is the result of too many demands compared to a normal work week (Lowe, 2007, p. 56).

The *Workplace and Employee Survey* found that 9 percent of all workers and 12 percent of workers in firms of more than 500 in 1999 would have preferred to work fewer hours for less pay. This can be considered an underestimate of involuntary long hours to the extent that many other workers would choose to take part of a compensation increase in the form of reduced hours. Reduced work time has recently been emphasized by several major industrial unions. For example, the

Communications, Energy, and Paperworkers' Union (CEP) have limited overtime in pulp and paper mills, and the CAW have increased paid days off in the auto assembly sector.[1]

There was a strong trend to long (and short) working hours for both men and women in the 1980s and 1990s at the expense of the 40-hour work week norm.[2] The proportion of so-called core-age men aged 25–54 working more than 50 hours per week in their main job rose steadily from 15 percent in the early 1980s to about 20 percent in 1994, and has continued at that level through 2006. Over the same period, the proportion of core-age women working more than 50 hours per week rose from 5 percent to about 7 percent.[3] About one in three core-age men and one in eight core-age women in paid jobs—those most likely to face work-family time conflicts—now work more than 41 hours per week. Moreover, work is increasingly taken home, especially with the rise of laptops and the BlackBerry, which make electronic work easily portable. About one in five workers now work from home in addition to their normal work hours, with this being most prevalent among professionals in both the public sector and working for large private-sector employers (Lowe, 2007, p. 19). So-called "good" jobs today make major demands on unpaid time outside of the workplace.

As noted above, working long hours is closely associated with working in high-demand jobs. While these jobs may be interesting and challenging and give rise to opportunities for advancement, long hours and high demands can be harmful to both physical and mental health. Studies suggest that very long hours are linked to high blood pressure and cardiovascular disease. Statistics Canada has found that moving to longer working hours has some negative impacts on health risks, such as smoking, drinking, and poor diet.[4] Long hours also create a high risk of stress in terms of balancing work with domestic and community life.

The shift of core workers to long daily and weekly hours of work is much more characteristic of the US and Canada than the more regulated job markets of continental Europe. The usual weekly hours of full-time paid workers in the EU are below 40, and falling (European Industrial Relations Observatory, 2006). Some countries, notably France, the Netherlands, and Germany, are now close to a 35-hour norm. The proportion of men working weekly hours much in excess of 40 hours is generally very low.

Weekend working appears to be increasing rapidly. The incidence has gone from 11 percent in 1991 to 15 percent in 1995, to 25 percent in 2000, and to 27 percent in 2003.[5] Women are more likely to work on weekends than men (28 percent compared to 21 percent), reflecting high employment rates in retail and health services. More than one in three production workers work on weekends, reflecting the rising incidence of continuous industrial production.

As noted, regular hours are shorter and jobs are less precarious in most European countries. These countries also provide much more generous paid time off work. In Canada, the minimum vacation entitlement under provincial employment standards is two weeks after a minimum length of service of about one year. (As of 2007, only Saskatchewan provided a minimum of three weeks.) Most provinces—but not Ontario as of 2007—provide for three weeks for workers with a lot of seniority, between five and 15 years. In collective agreements, the norm is three weeks of paid vacation, rising to four weeks after 10 years. (Seventy percent of unionized workers qualify for four weeks after 10 years, and 28 percent qualify after five years.) By contrast, in the EU, the minimum statutory entitlement to paid vacation leave is 20 days or four weeks, and the average provided in collective agreements is 25.7 days, or more than five weeks. German, Danish, and Dutch workers get six weeks of paid vacation per year (European Industrial Relations Observatory, 2006). Statutory paid holidays on top of paid vacation entitlements are comparable between Canada and European countries.

The average age of retirement in Canada has been steadily falling, but there is generally very limited provision for a phased-in retirement process that would allow older workers to voluntarily reduce their hours of work. Indeed, most defined pension plans create an incentive to maximize earnings (and, therefore, hours) just before retirement. By contrast, most European countries rely more heavily on public than on private pensions, and the tendency in many continental European countries has been to provide more flexible options for older workers.

To summarize, there is a strong trend to longer hours for core workers, as well as to more unsocial hours and more variable hours. Vacation entitlements and phased-in retirement provisions in Canada are quite limited compared to many European countries. These conditions all have direct implications for stress and for physical and mental health.

Work-Life Balance

Longer and more unpredictable hours, combined with high and rising job demands, are particularly likely to cause stress and anxiety in families where both partners work, and for single-parent families. In both cases, women bear the brunt of the burden (Duxbury & Higgins, 2002).

Increased family working time has been a critical factor in maintaining real incomes in a labour market marked by more precarious employment and stagnating wages. Family work hours obviously determine both income and the time potentially available to spend with family, children, and in the community. While long hours may result in higher incomes, work-family time conflict may affect the physical and mental health of parents and also influence the well-being of children. Much of the burden of caring for elderly parents as well as children is borne by working families. These pressures to balance work and family are greater than in many other countries

---

Box 7.3: Working families

There has been a very large increase in the total working hours of two-person families with children since the mid-1970s. This has come through increased work hours for many men, the increased entry of women into the workforce, and the shift of women into full-time jobs. About three in four (73 percent) of two-person families with children have two earners today compared to one in three in 1975, and three in four (73 percent) working women in two-parent families are full-time. Thus, the majority of women in two-person families with children now work full-time. Six in 10 women single parents (63 percent) with children work, 77 percent of whom work full-time. Full-time employment rates for women are only slightly lower for those with preschool children, reflecting maternity and parental leaves taken after the birth of a child.[6]

because of the relative underdevelopment of publicly financed and delivered early childhood, elder care, and home-care programs.

Time pressures are steadily increasing. Between 1992 and 1998, 25- to 44-year-old parents employed full-time put in an average of two hours more per week in paid-work activities. In 1998, fathers averaged 48.3 hours and mothers averaged 38.5 hours per week of paid work and related activities, up 5 percent for fathers and 4 percent for mothers from 1992. Lone-parent mothers increased their time in paid work even more than married mothers.

Work-family conflicts arise not just from longer and longer hours, but also from the frequent incompatibility of work schedules with the schedules and needs of children. While a minority of employers do offer flextime arrangements that are responsive to the needs of employees, the great majority of part-time jobs do not offer comparable pay, benefits, and career opportunities.

Levels of time stress and work-family stress among parents with children are extremely high. More than one-third of 25- to 44-year-old women who work full-time and have children at home report that they are severely time-stressed, and the same is true for about one in four men. Twenty-six percent of married fathers, 38 percent of married mothers, and 38 percent of single mothers report severe time stress, with levels of severe stress rising by about one-fifth between 1992 and 1998. About two-thirds of full-time employed parents with children also report that they are dissatisfied with the balance between their job and home life. Fathers and mothers alike blamed their dissatisfaction on not having enough time for family, which tends to lose out in the event of conflict.[7] Work-family conflict is driven by mounting demands from work, the still largely unchanged division of domestic labour between men and women, and the governments' failure to provide child care and elder care on a sufficient scale.

A major 2004 report for Health Canada explored the links between work-life conflict and Canada's health care system (Higgins, Duxbury & Johnson, 2004). Their premise was that an employee's ability or inability to balance work and life demands would be associated with key outcomes such as absenteeism, job satisfaction, job stress, family life satisfaction, level of overall stress in

life, and that these outcomes would be in turn linked to mental and physical health outcomes. The majority (58 percent) of workers in their sample of employees of medium to large organizations experienced high levels of "role overload," or having too much to do in a given amount of time. They found that, compared to their counterparts with low levels of role overload, employees with high role overload were almost 2.9 times more likely to say their health was just fair or poor, 2.6 times more likely to have sought care from a mental health professional, and about twice as likely to have made frequent visits to a physician. As a result, work-life stress results in high public and private health care costs, which could be avoided through better work organization, more family-friendly workplaces, and more supports for working families. The authors concluded that current workloads are not sustainable over the long term. Indeed, in a subsequent study, they find that lack of serious progress toward creating more family-friendly workplaces has been a key reason why today's younger workers are putting off having children for many years, if at all. Those who get ahead today are those who put work first.

Social Relations and Participation at Work

Work is a social process, and the social relations of production are an important aspect of the quality of jobs and of working life, but little hard information is available on this relatively intangible dimension. In 2000, 15 percent of workers reported stress in the workplace from "poor interpersonal relations," down slightly from 18.5 percent in 1994, but up from 13 percent in 1991.[8] Women report higher levels of stress from this cause than do men. Less than one-half of employees feel that they have much influence on their jobs. A survey by Canadian Policy Research Networks found that only 10 percent of workers feel that they can strongly influence employer decisions that affect their job, and 45 percent feel that they have no influence at all. There are few significant differences by age or gender.[9]

Unionized workers do have some influence through the process of collective bargaining. About one in three paid workers in Canada are covered by the provisions of a collective agreement. Coverage is highest by far in the public sector and in large private sector firms, particularly in primary industries, manufacturing, transportation, and utilities. By definition, collective agreements give access to a formal statement of conditions of employment, such as hours and working conditions, and access to a formal grievance and arbitration process. A formal grievance system militates against the exercise of arbitrary managerial authority, and against harassment by co-workers. Collective agreements also often provide for joint processes to govern working conditions over the life of a contract, such as labour-management, training, and health and safety committees. While the great majority of agreements contain a management rights clause clarifying management's power to assign and direct work, the majority also provide for some advance notification of, and consultation over, technological and organizational change. Many collective agreements also feature detailed job descriptions, meaning that changes in tasks are subject to joint agreement.

Most Canadian unions have adopted formal policies relating to workplace health and safety, work-family balance, work reorganization, and access to training, and have paid some attention to all of these qualities of work-life issues in bargaining. Improvement of the work environment has been on the agenda, and some unions have made gains. However, there are continuous pressures to increase productivity to maintain employment and wages, which tend to militate against an agenda of humanizing work and creating more healthy workplaces.

While some non-union workers also enjoy access to formalized (if non-binding) processes of dispute resolution and collective consultation, worker "voice" in the Canadian workplace is much weaker than in countries where unionization rates are much higher. Moreover, many European countries have legislation providing for joint works councils with powers to at least discuss working conditions. The EU survey shows that 78 percent of workers believe they have the possibility to discuss working conditions and 71 percent the possibility to discuss organizational change, most frequently on a formal basis.

John O'Grady (Sullivan, 2000) shows that effective workplace health and safety committees effectively reduce rates of injuries and disability, but are largely absent from the precarious labour market.

To summarize, institutions of collective representation are relatively weakly implanted in Canadian workplaces,

undercutting the ability of workers to shape working conditions.

Conclusion

This overview suggests many grounds for concern over the potential health impacts of trends in Canadian workplaces. Workplace threats to physical health in the form of fatalities, injuries, and occupational disease remain significant for many workers. Pervasive job insecurity is a source of stress. In core workplaces, the pace and intensity of work are on the rise, and many are working very long hours in very demanding jobs. The incidence of high-strain jobs that combine high demands and limited control is quite high, particularly among women. The best available evidence suggests that the quality of work along most dimensions valued by workers is deteriorating. Summarizing the most recent trends, Lowe (2007, p. vii) concludes that "economic prosperity has not brought commensurate gains to workers in terms of job quality since the millennium." These negative trends exist across the skills and income spectrum, with well-paid professionals enduring high levels of stress from overwork, while the less skilled and less well paid endure stress from unstable work, physical risks, poor working conditions, and high job demands combined with low levels of control.

We need more information about the level and trends of workplace determinants of health. We lack systematic evidence of the kind collected in Europe. This could be remedied if Statistics Canada conducted regular surveys on the quality of the work environment and working conditions. The now discontinued *Workplace and Employee Survey* (WES) provided only very limited information in this area, and the *National Population Health Survey* provides only very limited information on working conditions.

Governments must intervene to help shape and improve workplace conditions. A wide range of relevant recommendations have been made over the years, most recently in the 1990s by two major Human Resources Development Canada-initiated consultations. These were the Donner Task Force (the *Report of the Advisory Group on Working Time and Redistribution of Work*) and the *Report of the Collective Reflection on the Changing Workplace*. The thrust of the first was to regulate working time by limiting long hours and by making precarious work more secure. The thrust of the second, which included a very wide range of options, was to propose changes to employment standards and forms of collective representation. A more recent milestone report was the report of a federal task force on employment standards, *Fairness at Work: Federal Labour Standards for the 21st Century*. Commissioner Arthurs in 2006 again called for limits on long working-time and arbitrary work schedules, more paid time off the job, and measures to secure respect

for human rights in the workplace. He set out a "decency principle," which stated in part that "no worker should be subject to coercion, discrimination, indignity or unwarranted danger in the workplace, or be required to work so many hours that he or she is effectively denied a personal life" (Government of Canada, 2006). At the end of the day, it is unlikely that there will be significant positive changes in the workplace if everything is left to employers, and if governments do not help equalize bargaining power between workers and employers.

Notes

1. On working time issues, see *Report of the Advisory Group on Working Time and Distribution of Work, Human Resources Development Canada* (1994).
2. "The Changing Work Week: Trends in Weekly Hours of Work," Statistics Canada, *Canadian Economic Observer*, September 1996.
3. Labour Force Survey data, available at www.jobquality.ca.
4. "Longer working hours and health," *The Daily*, November 16, 1999.
5. 1991 and 1995 data from the *Survey of Work Arrangements*. 2000 data from the *Workplace and Employee Survey* (WES).
6. Statistics Canada, Cat. 71-535 MPB #8, Work Arrangements in the 1990s, tables 3.1, 3.2.
7. Statistics Canada, *The Daily*, November 9, 1999.
8. *General Social Survey*, 2003.
9. www.jobquality.ca.

Critical Thinking Questions

1. How important are work and working conditions as a determinant of physical and mental health in a post-industrial society?
2. How would you set out to clearly establish links between work and health?
3. High-stress jobs are often defined as those with high demands but low levels of control. What kinds of jobs are most stressful by this definition?
4. Does it seem plausible to you that work is generally becoming more and more stressful and demanding?
5. What are some of the different ways in which work-related stress and conflicts affect women and men?

Recommended Readings

Duxbury, Linda & Higgins, Chris. (2002). *The 2001 National Work-Life Conflict Study*. Health Canada. Online at www.hc-sc.gc.ca.
    Duxbury and Higgins have conducted several major studies of conflicts between work, family, and community life over the past several years, sparking increased interest in work-related stress as a key determinant of health.

European Foundation for the Improvement of Living and Working Conditions. (2008). "Report on the European Survey on Working Conditions." Online at www.eurofound.ie.

   Reports based on this regular European Union-wide survey provide a much more detailed picture of working conditions than is available for Canada.

Government of Canada. (2006). "Fairness at work." *Federal Labour Standards for the 21st Century*.

   Written by a noted labour lawyer and academic, Harry Arthurs, this sets out a detailed account of what is wrong in Canadian workplaces, and how governments should intervene to promote positive change.

Karasek, Robert & Theorell, Tores. (1990). *Healthy work: Stress, productivity, and the reconstruction of working life*. New York: Basic Books.

   The classic study of the impacts of workplace stress on health. Stress is seen as the result of high job demands combined with low levels of control.

Sullivan, Terrence (Ed.). (2000). *Injury and the new world of work*. Vancouver & Toronto: University of British Columbia Press.

   Contains recent studies of trends in workplace injuries, showing how soft-tissue injuries attributable to fast-paced work have grown compared to traditional workplace accidents.

Related Web Sites

Canadian Labour Congress—canadianlabour.ca

   This is the Web site of the Canadian Labour Congress, which represents more than 3 million union members and speaks out on issues of interest to working people. There are a number of research and other documents related to work and health on the sub-sites of the social and economic policy department and the health and safety department, as well as links to national and international union Web sites.

Canadian Policy Research Networks—www.jobquality.ca

   Maintained by the Canadian Policy Research Networks (CPRN), this site contains a wealth of data on job quality in Canada, including the results of CPRN surveys.

European Foundation for the Improvement of Living and Working Conditions—www.eurofound.europa.eu

   This is the Web site of the European Foundation for the Improvement of Living and Working Conditions, a European Union institution that closely monitors and reports on changing conditions of work and their implications for physical and mental well-being.

Health Canada—www.hc-sc.gc.ca/ewh-semt/occup-travail/index_e.html

   This is the sub-site of the Health Canada Web site, which is devoted to occupational health and safety issues and provides access to a number of recent research studies. Provincial governments maintain similar sites.

Programme on Safety and Health at Work and the Environment—www.ilo.org/public/english/protection/safework/whpwb/index.htm

   This is the Web site of the Programme on Safety and Health at Work and the Environment (SafeWork) of the International Labour Organization, the United Nations organization that specializes in labour and work issues. This site provides access to numerous ILO studies and databases, and looks at working conditions in a truly global context.

Chapter 8

———————●———————

Understanding and Improving the Health of Work

Peter Smith and Michael Polanyi

Introduction

The chapters in this book demonstrate that social and economic conditions strongly influence health. This is something that health-promotion researchers and practitioners have long recognized. Despite this recognition, we have had only limited success in stimulating action to improve these health-affecting conditions. In this chapter we discuss four steps to addressing key workplace determinants of health: (1) gathering research evidence; (2) undertaking critical reflection and analysis; (3) envisioning a desirable future; and (4) advocating for action. These steps are all important if we are to turn our knowledge of the social determinants of health into actual improvements in health for all (see Figure 8.1).

The relationship between working conditions and health outcomes is an important public health concern. For example, work injuries account for almost 30 percent of the total injury burden in the United States (Smith, Wellman, Sorock, Warner, Courtney, Pransky & Fingerhut, 2005) and working conditions are as least as important as health behaviours in the development of long-term conditions such as cardiovascular disease (Marmot, Bosma, Hemingway, Brunner & Stansfeld, 1997) and deterioration in health status (Borg & Kristensen, 2000). However, the relationship between working conditions and health is complex, with research into work and health occurring in multiple disciplines and

at numerous levels (e.g., the individual, the workplace, and the economy).

This complexity is one reason for the limited success that work and health research has had in creating change. Even as we try to understand the linkages between working conditions and health, social and economic conditions are being transformed. There is also a lack of agreement among policy-makers, health practitioners, and researchers themselves on what should (or could) be done to improve work and social conditions, which inevitably leads to inaction until more (or better) evidence is generated (Baum, 2007; MacIntyre, 2003). In addition, our *approaches* to research have not always been conducive to stimulating public understanding and action. Conventional scientific research is unlikely to lead to shared understandings of today's complex social problems. New forms of collective inquiry and dialogue between researchers and non-researchers are needed to stimulate understanding and action (Israel, Schurman & House, 1989; Mergler, 1987). For example, workers possess valuable knowledge about their work conditions and the informal practices within their workplace. As such, they may be able to provide insights that researchers, positioned outside of the workplace, may not be aware of (Cornwall & Jewkes, 1995). Literature on "knowledge transfer" and "transdisciplinarity" recognizes that researchers need to find ways to involve community members and policy-makers in joint processes of inquiry throughout the research process as a way of creating

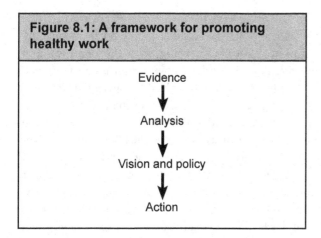

Figure 8.1: A framework for promoting healthy work

Evidence

↓

Analysis

↓

Vision and policy

↓

Action

research solutions that are feasible, socially acceptable, appropriate, effective, and sustainable. However, these approaches are not without challenges, which have been described in more detail elsewhere (Polanyi & Cole, 2003; Smith, 2007).

Evidence

There is a growing body of research showing that the content, organization, and arrangements of work are centrally linked to health outcomes (Polanyi, Frank, Shannon, Sullivan & Lavis, 2000). While it is beyond the scope of this chapter to fully review research on such linkages, it is worth highlighting, using guidelines originally proposed by Bradford-Hill (Hill, 1965), some of the key aspects of this research that support the assertion that certain working conditions *cause* poor health.

Longitudinal studies examining the effects of the psychosocial work environment[1] on health have consistently shown proper temporality between psychosocial working conditions and health outcomes. In other words, the work environment exposure precedes the change in, or onset of, the health outcome (Belkic, Landsbergis, Schnall & Baker, 2004; de Lange, Taris, Kompier, Houtman & Bongers, 2003; Schnall, Landsbergis & Baker, 1994). There is also strong evidence that the proposed pathway between working conditions and health is biologically plausible (Brunner, 1997; McEwen, 1998; Steptoe & Marmot, 2002). That is, there are logical and believable pathways through which

the work environment might worsen health status. The first is through a neuroendocrinological response to the stressful working conditions—referred to as allostatic load (McEwen, 1998)—and another is through changes in health behaviour patterns, possibly as a mechanism of coping.

The associations between dimensions of work (such as psychosocial working conditions) and poor health have been found across numerous working populations in a variety of countries (Belkic et al., 2004; de Lange et al., 2003; Malinauskiene, Theorell, Grazuleviciene, Azaraviciene, Obelenis & Azelis, 2005; Schnall et al., 1994) providing evidence that the relationship between working conditions and health is not a chance finding in one population group. That said, there has also been some inconsistency in the associations between psychosocial working conditions and health, in particular related to coronary heart disease risk, across gender (Eaker, Sullivan, Kelly-Hayes, D'Agostino & Benjamin, 2004; Lee, Colditz, Berkman & Kawachi, 2003; Niedhammer & Chea, 2003; Riese, Van Doornen, Houtman & De Geus, 2004), age (Hammar, Alfredsson & Johnson, 1998; Kuper & Marmot, 2003) and socio-economic groups (Landsbergis, Schnall, Warren, Pickering & Schwartz, 1999; Macleod, Davey Smith, Heslop, Metcalfe, Carroll & Hart, 2001), with weaker (or, in some cases, non-existent) associations found among women, older age groups, and higher socio-economic status groups. Finally, higher levels of (or greater exposure to) a psychosocial work environment exposure (e.g., lack of job control) at one point in time are associated with a larger current and future risk of poor health. That is, there is a dose-response relationship between the level of the psychosocial work exposure and the risk of poor health (biological gradient). However, the evidence has been less consistent about the cumulative exposure (measured at multiple time points) to different psychosocial working conditions on health, with the available research producing mixed results. (Amick, McDonough, Chang, Rogers, Pieper & Duncan, 2002; Johnson, Stewart, Hall, Fredlund & Theorell, 1996; Landsbergis, Schnall, Pickering, Warren & Schwartz, 2003). In addition, research is only just starting to examine the effects that changes in psychosocial working conditions (e.g., moving from having low job control to having high job control) have on health outcomes (Head, Kivimaki, Martikainen, Vahtera, Ferrie & Marmot, 2006;

Kivimaki, Elovainio, Vahtera & Ferrie, 2004; Vahtera, Kivimaki, Pentti & Theorell, 2000).

Key dimensions of the working environment that have been linked to health status are job strain, (Karasek & Theorell, 1990), effort-reward imbalance (ERI) (Siegrist, 1996; Siegrist & Peter, 1996), and, more recently, the level of organizational justice (De Vogli, Ferrie, Chandola, Kivimaki & Marmot, 2007; Ferrie, Head, Shipley, Vahtera, Marmot & Kivimaki, 2006; Kivimaki, Elovainio, Vahtera & Ferrie, 2003). Additional important aspects of work include long working hours (Shields, 1999; Spurgeon, Harrington & Cooper, 1997), work-life conflict (Duxbury & Higgins, 2001; Duxbury, Higgins & Johnson, 1999), job insecurity and precarious employment (Scott, 2004; Sverke, Hellgren & Naswall, 2002; Tompa, Scott-Marshall, Dolinschi, Trevithick & Bhattacharyya, 2007), and status inconsistency (being overqualified for your job) (Crompton, 2002; Peter, Gassler & Geyer, 2007; Smith & Frank, 2005). These measures are briefly described in Table 8.1.

In summary, there is compelling evidence that the social organization of work matters profoundly to health. Given the changing nature of work, more research is needed to develop a better understanding of the specific dimensions of healthy and unhealthy jobs in order to build support for particular interventions to improve working conditions. Research is also needed to better demonstrate the costs of unhealthy working conditions, and the benefits that changing working environments might make to companies and to societies in general since productivity, not health, is the ultimate aim of economic enterprises in capitalist society.

Analysis

Despite growing evidence of the negative health impacts of working conditions, so-called high-quality employment practices have been adopted only by a minority of companies in Canada (Duxbury & Higgins, 1998; Lowe, 2000). Clearly, information and evidence alone do not determine which workplace practices will be implemented and which will not. Instead, organizational practices and policies—for better and for worse—are influenced by an array of factors, including technology change, deregulation, declining unionization, and international competition and associated pressures to innovate, improve quality, and increase productivity.

As Eakin suggests, the health interests of workers will seldom prevail if they conflict with corporate profitability (Eakin, 2000). Grappling with the complex and conflicting relationship between firm productivity and workplace health is key to the development of strategies to improve the quality of working conditions.

One can identify three current analyses of the relationship between workplace health and competitiveness. The first assumes that companies need the flexibility to respond freely and rapidly to changes in consumer preference and demands and thus compete effectively. The policy prescription, therefore, is for governments to pull back from the regulation of business employment practices, and to allow a further "flexibilization" of employment contracts. While it is recognized that this may increase job insecurity in the short term, the benefits of economic growth and job creation outweigh this cost, and the emphasis should be on employability rather than job security.

The problem with this view is that it supports the development of work systems that compromise the health-determining conditions discussed above (e.g., jobs with reasonable demands, job control, work-life balance, and job security) (Landsbergis, 2003). It also allows firms to externalize these social costs of production, and provides little incentive for firms to improve working conditions. Moreover, this view rests on the now largely discredited assumption that the benefits of rising profits and economic growth will trickle down to all, a claim proved false during the past decade of rising inequality in Canada and the United States (Saunders, 2005). A recent review by Graham Lowe clearly demonstrating that economic prosperity in Canada through the last decade has not led to concurrent gains in job quality for Canadian workers (Lowe, 2007).

The second perspective is to suggest that the problem is just the opposite: an *excess* of employer flexibility. This, the traditional left view, is that a shift in the balance of power from workers to management (due in part to declining unionization rates, greater employer ability to relocate to other jurisdictions, and reduced government regulation) has undermined working conditions in general, and job security in particular. The prescription is for a re-regulation of employers and collective action among employees, in order to limit an employer's ability to engage in flexible employment practices.

Table 8.1: Key dimensions of the working environment that are related to health		
Work dimension	**Description**	**Key references and reviews**
Job strain	Job strain exists when people's autonomy over their work and their ability to use their skills are low, while the psychological demands placed upon them are high.	(Belkic et al., 2004; de Lange et al., 2003; Karasek, 1979; Karasek & Theorell, 1990)
Effort-reward imbalance	The "effort–reward imbalance" model (ERI) underlines the health importance of rewards (monetary, esteem, respect from supervisors and colleagues) being in line with the demands (time pressures, interruptions, responsibility, pressure to work overtime). When efforts are perceived to be higher than rewards, this leads to emotional distress.	(Siegrist, 1996; van Vegchel, de Jonge, Bosma & Schaufeli, 2005)
Organizational justice	Organizational justice reflects the extent to which people believe that their supervisor considers their viewpoints, shares information concerning decision making, and treats individuals fairly.	(De Vogli et al., 2007; Ferrie et al., 2006; Kivimaki et al., 2003)
Work hours	Work hours are measured as the number of hours usually worked, although questions can also incorporate preferences (e.g., Would you like to work less hours, more hours, or the same?). More research is needed to examine the relationship between working hours on health as it is likely that too many, and too few, are both related to health problems.	(Spurgeon et al., 1997)
Work-life conflict	Work-life conflict can occur when individuals have to perform multiple roles at the same time—as worker, spouse, parent, caregiver, or volunteer. The cumulative demands of multiple roles can result in two types of role strain: overload (having too much to do with too little time to do it) and interference (facing conflicting demands from different roles, such as having to be in two places at the same time).	(Duxbury & Higgins, 2001; Duxbury et al., 1999)
Precarious work	Precarious employment describes work experiences that are associated with instability, lack of protection, insecurity across various dimensions of work, and social and economic vulnerability.	(Scott, 2004; Sverke et al., 2002; Tompa et al., 2007)
Status inconsistency	Status inconsistency refers to a situation where an individual's level of education is higher than the skills he or she requires for the occupation. This situation has also been termed "goal-striving stress."	(Benoit-Smullyan, 1944; Dressler, 1988)

The strength of this view is that it recognizes the serious human problems that may result from rising employer flexibility and power. Its limitation is that it fails to acknowledge the legitimacy of employers' need for flexibility in today's global economy, nor the fact that some workers prefer to engage in part-time, flex-time, short-term, and other non-standard working arrangements (Marshall, 2001). In other words, there are positive dimensions to flexibility—*if* it is not simply flexibility for employers at the cost of employees, which has too often been the case.

The third view falls in the middle of the previous two. It suggests that there are potential benefits for all to be found in the emerging flexible organization of work (European Commission, 1997). It acknowledges both businesses' need for flexibility *and* employees' (and citizens') need for security. It recognizes that job security, in the form of full-time, permanent employment, is not something that can be retrieved in the new economy. However, it does not hold that *economic* insecurity is either a morally acceptable or an economically positive phenomenon. Instead it aims to forge a new framework of "flexicurity" by accepting the emergence of employment flexibility and short-term jobs, while providing generous social welfare and unemployment benefits along with active training support for the unemployed (see Box 8.1).

In sum, quite different analyses of the health-productivity dynamic exist. While it is important to be clear about the assumptions that we bring to this complex issue, it is unlikely that a shared analysis can be easily forged. Rather, focusing discussion on developing a shared vision for the future of healthy work may be more likely to stimulate change (Cooperrider & Srivastva, 1987; Weisbord & Janoff, 1995). Hence, while recognizing the importance of delineating and analyzing the roots of the negative impacts of work on health, it is also important that researchers work to support the development of a shared vision of work and policy options to achieve it.

Vision and Policy

Given the central focus on work in contemporary capitalist societies, it is astounding how little attention has been paid to the development of broadly shared policy goals with respect to work. In Canada, government committees and commissions have periodically considered aspects of

---

Box 8.1: Flexicurity

Over the past decade, Denmark has experienced a dramatic decline in unemployment. Denmark seems to have created a unique combination of stable economic growth and social welfare since the mid-1990s. The term flexicurity is used to characterize this successful combination of adaptability to a changing international environment and a solidaristic welfare system, which protects the citizens from the more brutal consequences of structural change. The recent success of the Danish model of flexicurity thus points to a third way between the flexibility often ascribed to a liberal market economy and the social safety nets of the traditional Scandinavian welfare state.... The Danish "miracle" is not just a trivial mixture of demand-driven growth and the hiding of a large share of the population in various welfare programmes. The relative success of the Danish model in recent years has stimulated ideas about the occurrence of a new employment system model in the form of the so-called "golden triangle," where people are enabled to move between different positions within work, welfare, and active labour market programmes. For instance large numbers of workers are affected by unemployment every year, but most of them return to employment after a short spell of unemployment. Active labour market programmes assist those who do not quickly go back into employment before re-entering a job.... Due to a non-restrictive employment protection legislation, which allows employers to hire and fire workers with short notice, the Danish system has a level of flexibility. At the same time, through its social security system and active labour market programmes, Denmark resembles the other Nordic welfare states in providing a tightly knit safety net for its citizens. The Danish model of "flexicurity" ... could serve as a source of inspiration for new ideas about alternative configurations of flexible labour markets and economic security for the individual rather than as a simple scheme that is ready for immediate export.

Source: European Foundation for the Improvement of Living and Working Conditions. (2002). *Quality of work and employment in Europe: Issues and challenges* (Foundation Paper). Dublin: EFILWC.

work (Advisory Committee on the Changing Workplace, 1997; Arthurs, 2006), but there has been no broad-based public visioning process on what elements might be part of "a good job" in Canada.

There is reason to believe that such a shared vision may be achievable. There is some consistency in terms of what employees as a group want from work: jobs that are interesting (something they like to do), jobs that provide opportunities to develop one's abilities, and jobs that allow for freedom to decide how one's job is done (Lowe, 2000; Polanyi & Tompa, 2002). In short, people want jobs that "enable them to live the lives they have reason to value" (Marmot, 2006).

Research on worker experiences and policy directions suggests four interrelated dimensions of healthy and productive work: *availability* of work; *adequacy* of income from work; *appropriateness* of work arrangements with respect to non-work responsibilities and needs; and *appreciation* or involvement of workers as active workplace participants and valued contributors to society (see Figure 8.2).

Available Work

Work is central to human existence and fulfillment and well-being. It provides us with an income, a sense of worth, and access to social networks. It is not surprising, therefore, that unemployment and job creation are central public concerns, and important agenda items for politicians and various organizations.

What *kind* of jobs should be promoted? Should we promote only highly paid full-time permanent jobs as unions often suggest? Or should there be an acceptance that the provision of highly paid, full-time jobs to all is

neither possible nor desirable, and that a range of work arrangements need to be promoted? Or, more radically, should we accept that there may no longer be enough paid work for all of us, and instead focus on creating conditions of income security, increasing the viability of a range of citizenship roles (e.g., parenting, caregiving, volunteering as well as paid work)?

It may be right to emphasize waged employment. However, there has been some rethinking of the relative importance of paid work, versus unpaid work, in recent years. This is partly because of the coexistence of chronic unemployment on one hand, and social and community needs going unaddressed on the other. Some question whether it is right that paid work should be highly rewarded while unpaid family, community, and civic contributions go largely unrewarded (Brown & Lauder, 2001). The growing importance of early childhood development and social and citizen participation to population health, as explored elsewhere in this book, also suggest a need to rethink the relative importance and rewards given to waged employment as opposed to broader social and civic participation.

Indeed, renewed attention has been directed toward the idea of a basic income policy over the last decade in Canada (Lerner, Clark & Needham, 1999), the United States (Aronowitz, Esposito, DiFazio & Yard, 1998) and Europe (Brown & Lauder, 2001; Gortz, 1999). While there are difficulties with this approach, including its economic feasibility, it does merit consideration by those concerned about population health (see www.basicincome.org for more details).

Increasing income security would prevent workers from being forced to take jobs that are unsafe and

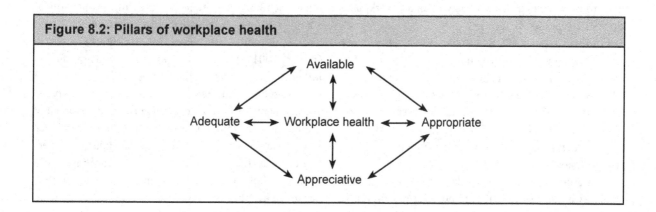

Figure 8.2: Pillars of workplace health

underpaid. It would also afford workers greater choice and control over their work content, work conditions, and work arrangements. At the same time, firms would gain a greater degree of flexibility as workers and their representatives would be less economically dependent on long-term job security and more open to a range of different work arrangements.

Providing a greater degree of income security will not necessarily change the fact that bad jobs continue to be disproportionately allocated to women, people of colour, and people with less education and of a lower socio-economic class. Indeed, socio-economic conditions before working life (childhood and adolescence) and outside of work (social networks, education, employability, and financial independence) shape the way that workplace experiences impact on health. Hence a key consideration in all these dimensions of work is to reduce inequalities in the distribution of quality work, by gender (Reskin & Padavic, 1994), class (Johnson, 2005; Johnson & Hall, 1995), and race (Cheung, 2005; Palameta, 2004).

Adequate Work

Most would agree that those who work should earn an adequate income to meet their needs. However, minimum wages have stagnated in Canada and the United States. Canadian data, adjusted for changes in the cost of living, suggest the wage rates for low-paid workers (full-time employees earning less then $10 per hour, in year 2000 dollars) did not improve between 1980 and 2000, and may have actually decreased (Chung, 2004; Morissette & Picot, 2005). Over the same time period wages for the people in the highest occupational groups more than doubled. In addition, wage rates for women within similar occupational skill groups are substantially less than men, even after adjustment for a variety of other workplace factors (Drolet, 2002).

Findings from the US on changes in wage rates describe a similar story of inequality in the benefits across different levels of the labour market over time. Information from the US Congressional Budget Office shows that over the 18-year period between 1979 and 1997, after-tax incomes of the bottom 40 percent of workers stagnated, while incomes for those in the top 20 percent soared (Johnson, 2005).

Numerous authors in Canada and the US call for increases in and, better still, an indexing of, minimum wages for both social and economic reasons (Bluestone & Harrison, 1999; Murray & Mackenzie, 2007). Wage levels are a "health" issue: Maxwell (Maxwell, 2002) indicates that wage supplements, the living wage, and individual development account strategies in both Canada and the US "can have significant positive effects on the well-being of beneficiaries" (p. 11).

There is also a widespread view that there is a need to extend and enforce adequate wages, benefits, and rights to non-full-time workers. Books and reports from both the US (e.g., Herzenberg, Alic & Wial, 1998; Skocpol, 2000) and Canada (Advisory Committee on the Changing Workplace, 1997; Lowe, 2007; Saunders, 2006) recommend the extension of pro-rated benefits, pensions, and health insurance to part-time workers. Others suggest that temporary workers should be treated more like permanent workers with their placement agencies (European Foundation for the Improvement of Living and Working Conditions, 2002), with agencies being obliged to provide benefits (King, McPherson & Long, 2000).

Requiring employers to provide pro-rated benefits to part-time workers would help to address the further problem of fixed costs and perverse incentives that deter the hiring of additional employees and instead encourage firms to ask or demand overtime work, which is often unpaid (Advisory Committee on the Changing Workplace, 1997). Finally, it should be made easier for workers to transfer their pensions from employer to employer (so-called "portable pensions") (Advisory Committee on the Changing Workplace, 1997; Herzenberg et al., 1998).

Appropriate Work

Contemporary work and family (or home) lives are highly interdependent as workers—a growing proportion of whom are now women—are increasingly combining paid work with family and home responsibilities (Jacobs & Gerson, 2001). Movement away from goods-producing industries to service-related industries has resulted in the need for different measures of productivity by management. Some researchers suggest the assessment of productivity in white-collar industries is the use of "face time" (Maume Jr. & Houston, 2001). That is, workers demonstrate their productivity and commitment to a firm by being the first to arrive in the morning and the last to leave in the evening (Fried, 1998). Research from

Australia suggests that more than one in five mothers are back at work by the time their child is six months old (Australian Institute of Family Studies, 2005). The impact these changes in working hours will have on family environments, and its subsequent impact on childhood health measures such as childhood self-esteem and obesity levels, is yet to be fully explored. However, it is of fundamental importance that workers can control their time—how much they work, when, and where.

Appreciative Work

Finally, new efforts are needed to ensure that workers are appreciated as actively contributing members of workplaces. As discussed earlier in this chapter, workers' ability to have input into decision-making processes, and their perceptions of justice and fairness at work have important health consequences (De Vogli et al., 2007; Kivimaki et al., 2003). Proposals for improving democratic voice in companies include elected single- or multi-employer worker committees established on a voluntary basis; mandated employee-participation councils; and greater worker, consumer, and community representation on company boards (Herzenberg et al., 1998; Vail, Wheelock & Hill, 1999). Appreciative work also means providing work that is linked to workers' interests, is meaningful to workers, and that encourages learning and growth (Polanyi & Tompa, 2002). Here again, the importance of increasing worker choice over the content of their work is central.

In summary, a range of policy directions seem to offer the possibility of creating social and economic conditions conducive to improved population health. However, it is important to recognize that different workers in fact want different kinds of jobs, working conditions, and arrangements, depending on their interests, life situations and responsibilities, skills, values, personalities, and so on (Polanyi & Tompa, 2002). Workers may be more or less able to deal with difficult working conditions, depending on the level of social support, financial independence, employability, and education outside of work. This is not to excuse poor working conditions for people who have minimal skills or awareness of other opportunities. Rather, it is to say that workers need the opportunity to choose and engage in work that fits with their desires, interests, and needs.

Work is complex and people are diverse, so researchers should not expect, on their own, to be able to identify the desirable dimensions of work. The specific policies at this point are less important than underlining the need to generate a broad-based dialogue on policy options conducive to healthy and productive work. There is a need for all stakeholders to collectively develop, in dialogue, a shared vision of the future of work and a program to achieve it.

Policies are also influenced by and reflective of the power distribution among various interest groups. Given that labour-market changes have reduced the power of workers and unions in many places, we need to focus on strategies to rebalance the distribution of power in workplaces. This could be done by expanding opportunities for representation among high-skilled and autonomous workers, and developing new forms of representation such as sector-based representation systems and multi-employer bargaining systems for smaller service sector firms (Advisory Committee on the Changing Workplace, 1997; Herzenberg et al., 1998).

In part, changing power relations requires changing the structures of decision making and the opportunities that are provided to influence decisions in various institutions. We have already spoken of the importance of creating increased opportunities for worker participation at the workplace level. However, there is also a need to create opportunities for broader democratic participation in social and political institutions (government, media, schools, community-based organizations). There is reason to believe that enhancing democratic participation will lead to more equitable decisions, build social cohesion, increase social support, and develop a greater sense of power and capacity among citizens, all of which are key to health.

Conclusion: Advocating for Action

There is a need to strengthen evidence of the links between work and health, to better grapple with the complex relationship between worker health and firm competitiveness, and to articulate a shared vision for work and set of policy options conducive to healthy work. The above issues are important, but if they do not lead to action, they will have failed.

In our pursuit of action, those of us who are concerned about population health can learn from the successes and failures of health promotion. One of the great successes of health promotion has been to make a strong argument for broadening the participation of communities, professionals, and policy-makers in processes of social and political change. Specifically, the case has been made that those whose health is affected by research and policy have a right to participate in these endeavours; that involving those affected by issues will lead to better understanding of health issues; and that involving those whose health is at stake is more likely to bring sustainable and practical solutions for change. Today, there is still a need to open up the research and policy process to meaningful involvement of these players.

We also need to learn from the failure of health promotion to shift attention and resources from health care to the social determinants of health. "Failure" may be too strong a word, for this is a monumental task when the vested interests of professional groups and other political and institutional barriers to change are taken into account. Yet it does suggest that new kinds of efforts are needed to place the social determinants onto the political landscape.

Some modest proposals are worth mentioning. First, population health researchers and professionals need to pay more attention to the constraints under which policy-makers function if we are to expect action on the so-called determinants of health. Government structures militate against the kind of future-oriented, cross-sectoral policy analysis and development that action on social determinants of health requires, and policy-makers' time is often consumed by fighting today's fire, protecting the programs and services they currently run, and wresting money from the finance department.

This means ceasing to lament oversimplistically that policy-makers and bureaucrats are "too political" and pay insufficient attention to population health research evidence. It means starting to provide clear and manageable policy options that resonate with specific policy-makers. It means shifting from "research transfer" and "knowledge dissemination" to processes of interactive policy development.

Of course, research evidence is only one part (and only sometimes a part) in the policy-making process. Not only do policy-makers get input from multiple sources, but policy decisions are also based on what is politically acceptable and what is practical (Nutbeam, 2003). Hence, those concerned with population health need to build a constituency supportive of action. To do so, we can work through existing national health-*care* coalitions (e.g., Canadian Healthcare Association, The Health Action Lobby, and the Canadian Health Coalition), encouraging them to go beyond their focus on health care into upstream social and political determinants of health. However, many of the determinants of health lie outside of the formal health sector. As such, we also need to work with numerous national, regional, and local social policy and community organizations concerned outside of the health sector, learning from their social policy analysis and experience in advocating for improvements to social and economic conditions. Finally, now may be the time to develop our own national network to put the social determinants of health on the political landscape. Such a network or coalition could articulate a vision for population health and a set of principles and specific policy options for its achievement. We could identify the core social determinants of health, and raise a strong population health-based voice for income, employment, labour, child care, housing, and welfare policies conducive to meeting these core determinants of health.

Above all, we should build on the revived interest in democratizing policy-making processes and providing citizens with opportunities for meaningful engagement in "democratic deliberation." People often have a better sense than we acknowledge of what makes them and their communities healthy or sick. Pushing for meaningful citizen involvement in the development and implementation of social, economic, and political policies and practices that impact on their well-being may be the best thing we can do to improve population health. It is through this pressure for change from community groups, combined with top-down political commitment—which Baum (2007) refers to as a "nutcracker" effect—that we hope might lead to healthier workplaces and societies.

Acknowledgements

Thanks are given to Tom McIntosh and an anonymous reviewer for helpful comments on an earlier draft of this paper, and to Ann Bishop for editorial assistance.

Note

1. The psychosocial work environment is defined as "the range of opportunities given to an individual to meet his or her need of well-being, productivity and positive self-experience" (Siegrist & Marmot, 2004).

Critical Thinking Questions

1. What do you personally think are some of the key dimensions of the working environment? Are these dimensions of work covered by current research on working conditions and health?
2. Think about the apparent trade-off between healthy working conditions and the need for business competitiveness. Are they necessarily antagonistic? Where do you think the balance should be? Why?
3. What do you think are some of the reasons that research on working conditions and health is not widely discussed and acted on? What can be done to change this?

Recommended Readings

Dunham, J. (Ed.). (2001). *Stress in the workplace: Past, present, future.* London: WHURR Publishers.
    Collection of writings by key authors offering various perspectives on the relationship between working conditions and health.

Karasek, R. & Theorell, T. (1990). *Healthy work: Stress, productivity, and the reconstruction of working life.* New York: Basic Books.
    Classic book on psychosocial demands at work and health that outlines the theory and evidence of the job-strain model.

Lowe, G.S. (2007). *21st-century job quality: Achieving what Canadians want.* Research Report W37. Ottawa: Canadian Policy Research Networks.
    A nice up-to-date summary of measures related to the quality of work in Canada.

Marmot, M. & Siegrist, J. (Eds.) (2004). "Health inequalities and the psychosocial environment." *Social Science & Medicine 58*(8), 1461–1574.
    A special issue of *Social Science & Medicine*, guest edited by Michael Marmot and Johannes Siegrist, covers a number of original research contributions on health inequalities and the psychosocial work environment.

Related Web Sites

Institute for Work and Health—www.iwh.on.ca
    Canadian research organization focused on preventing and treating work-related injuries and illness.

The Job Stress Network—www.workhealth.org

A Web site run through the Center for Social Epidemiology in California, which brings together information about psychosocial working conditions, in particular job strain, and facilitates communication among researchers and the public interested in the relationship between the work environment, the individual, and health.

National Institute for Occupational Safety and Health—www.cdc.gov/niosh/homepage.html

US federal agency responsible for conducting research and making recommendations for the prevention of work-related injury and illness.

Part Three

FOUNDATIONS OF LIFELONG HEALTH: EDUCATION

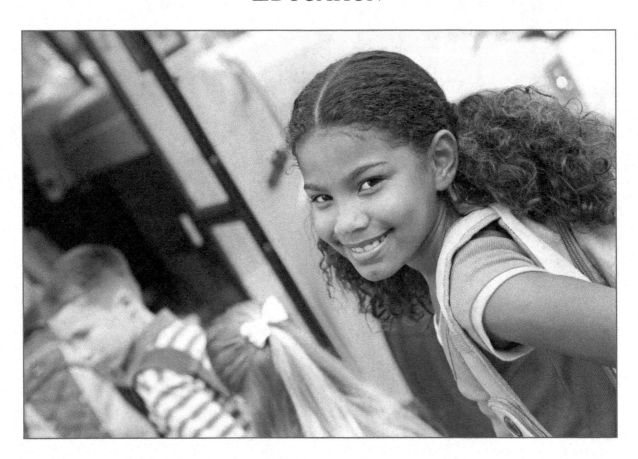

A consistent theme in the social determinants of health literature is the importance of early experience. Hertzman outlines three health effects that have their origins in early childhood. *Latent effects* are biological or developmental early life experiences that produce health effects later in life. Low birth weight, for instance, is a reliable predictor of incidence of cardiovascular disease and adult-onset diabetes in later life. *Pathway effects* are experiences that set individuals onto trajectories that influence health, well-being, and competence over the life course. For example, children who enter school with delayed vocabulary are set upon a path that leads to lower educational expectations, poor employment prospects, and greater likelihood of illness and disease across the lifespan. *Cumulative effects* represent the accumulation of advantage or disadvantage over time that manifests itself in incidence of a range of indicators of poor health. These involve the combination of latent and pathway effects. Education and literacy are important not only for providing children with key experiences that may have lifelong effects but for setting individuals on a life-course trajectory for either health or illness. In this section, the authors outline the importance for health of early childhood education and care and education and literacy.

Martha Friendly makes the argument for early childhood education and care (ECEC) as a crucial determinant of health for Canadians in general and children in particular. She provides an overview of what is known about what constitutes quality ECEC and its health effects upon both children and their families and for society as a whole. She then describes the current state of ECEC in Canada and compares this to developments in other nations. Canada's ECEC policies are woefully inadequate for the needs of Canadian families. Despite numerous governmental commitments to ECEC, only a small minority of Canadian families have access to quality regulated child care. Numerous policy lessons are provided and an analysis of recent developments in Canada is given.

Brenda Smith-Chant examines the rationale behind and available evidence concerning the effects of early childhood education and learning interventions. She outlines what is known about early childhood development and relates these findings to the effects of early interventions. She suggests that such interventions— in the face of many children's experience of material and social deprivation—must be intensive and ongoing. Dr. Smith-Chant outlines some of the barriers to developing these kinds of interventions. Finally, two means of promoting early development are presented. One of these represents more traditional approaches of supporting family interaction. The second proposes developing more responsive social services where the provision of child care and early education while parents work promotes early childhood development.

Charles Ungerleider, Tracey Burns, and Fernando Cartwright review the state of public education in Canada. The importance of education to Canadian society is argued. After providing a snapshot of some of the factors that determine educational success, they show how changing Canadian values are influencing the perceptions of the Canadian educational system. They look closely at issues related to Aboriginal students and their school performance. The authors argue that public education is doing well by Canadians as our children perform very well in international comparisons of achievement. But commitment to shared communal institutions such as public education is wavering, threatening public education and our futures.

Barbara Ronson and Irving Rootman detail the pivotal importance of literacy for health across the lifespan. Literacy has direct and indirect effects upon health. The mechanisms by which this occurs are presented. Factors that support or hinder literacy—such as income and its distribution, culture, and gender—and the interaction among these and other social determinants of health are considered. Since governmental policies are crucial influences upon literacy attainment, these are reviewed and policy directions to improve literacy and current research needs are provided. They conclude with an analysis of the purposes and effects of literacy testing, which is becoming increasingly common in Canada.

Chapter 9

———————

EARLY CHILDHOOD EDUCATION AND CARE AS A SOCIAL DETERMINANT OF HEALTH

Martha Friendly

The Child is father of the Man.
——William Wordsworth

Introduction

That early childhood experiences shape adult physical and mental health has been well documented and is today quite widely accepted. As the 1996 *Report on the Health of Canadians* (Federal/Provincial Territorial Advisory Committee on Population Health, 1996) observed: "There is strong evidence that early childhood experiences influence coping skills, resistance to health problems and overall health and well-being for the rest of one's life." There are two aspects to this: first, that development in early childhood has direct effects on health and, second, that early childhood development provides a platform for adult health through such factors as education, income, status, employment, and lifestyle, which are, in turn, linked to adult health.

Early childhood education and child care (ECEC) outside the family is only one factor known to have an impact on children during the early years. A sufficient income, adequate food and good nutrition, a healthy environment, parenting, housing, and educational early childhood programs all have an effect on young children's well-being, development, and health, then on the young school-aged child, and on into the child's development into an adult. Some of these, such as a non-toxic environment and good nutrition, affect children directly; some, such as an adequate income, have their main impact more indirectly through their effect on the child's first and primary environment, the family.

While all these factors are important, this chapter will concentrate on early childhood education and care programs. There is strong evidence that ECEC programs are a central—even a determining—factor that can affect children directly as well as indirectly through their impact on their parents.

What Is Early Childhood Education and Care?

More than 30 years ago, a landmark report from the Royal Commission on the Status of Women first recommended that Canada develop a national "daycare" program to support women's equality. Since then, the labour force participation rate of mothers has risen to 75 percent. Canada has become one of the most diverse countries in the world and as child development research has demonstrated that high-quality ECEC has positive benefits for children, a variety of objectives in addition to mothers' employment have come to drive what was once "the daycare debate." Today what was customarily called "daycare" in the 1970s, then "child care" in the 1980s and 1990s, is commonly called "early learning and child care" or "early childhood education and care." The term "early childhood education and care," or ECEC, is used internationally to describe inclusive and integrated services that play multiple roles for children and families. The Organisation for Economic Co-operation and Development (OECD) uses the term "ECEC" to:

> Reflect the growing consensus in OECD countries that "care" and "education" are inseparable concepts ... this term describes an integrated and coherent approach to policy and provision which is inclusive of *all* children and *all* parents regardless of employment or socioeconomic status. This approach recognizes that such arrangements may fulfill a wide range of objectives including care, learning, and social support. (OECD, 2001)

In Canada, the term "early childhood education and care" is used to encompass child-care centres and other care services like family child care in private homes whose primary aim is to allow mothers to participate in the paid labour force. It also includes kindergartens and nursery/preschools whose primary purpose is early childhood education. However, while well-designed ECEC programs enhance child development and simultaneously support parents in a variety of ways in and out of the paid workforce, Canada has barely even begun to develop policy and programs that meet the OECD's holistic approach.

The first part of this chapter reviews how ECEC is linked to a number of social domains that play a role in determining health over the life course. Its second part examines Canada's ECEC situation using a policy framework for effective ECEC systems based on a cross-national comparative policy analysis carried out by the OECD. The first edition of this chapter examined Canada using 2001 data and the first evidence from a decade-long ECEC study conducted by the OECD. This edition uses 2006 data and draws on the OECD's full comparative analysis, as well as its review of Canada, using the same policy framework as the first edition.

The previous edition concluded that "meeting the goal of high quality early childhood education and care for all ... will require mustering vision, commitment, and political will." As part of the context, this edition describes the shifting vision, commitment, and political will that have shaped how Canada has approached ECEC issues since the previous edition.

Early Childhood Education and Care as a Social Determinant of Health

That child development is complex is more than an overworked cliché. Research identifies many factors that contribute to whether children develop into healthy, competent adults—innate or genetic characteristics, prenatal conditions, the physical environment, nutrition, family attributes and interaction, peers, the community, schools, civil society, and the larger social-economic environment. Many of these have an impact on one another, combining in intricate ways to produce children who are successful, confident, content, competent, and resilient, or, conversely, who lack these attributes. Among these factors, there is considerable research that supports the idea that ECEC programs can be a key factor in child development and well-being and, ultimately, in life as a successful, healthy adult. As we shall see, ECEC programs are an especially good social determinant of health because if they are well designed, at one and the same time they can fulfill a multiplicity of goals that have effects on health.

Policy Goals for Early Childhood Education and Care

Over the past two decades, shifting Canadian rationales for ECEC have included early learning, lifelong learning, school readiness (or "readiness to learn"), child development, parents' employability, women's equality, balancing work and family, anti-poverty, alleviating at-risk status, and social integration.[1] Some of these (well-being, early learning, school readiness, lifelong learning) are focused on children. Others—women's equality and labour force participation, alleviating poverty and unemployment—are more focused on families or parents. Others are associated with the community or the larger society. These rationales fall into four policy goals, which are explored below.

Goal 1: Enhancing Children's Well-being, Healthy Development, and Lifelong Learning

That ECEC programs play an important role in child development is well supported by research. High-quality ECEC programs provide intellectual and social stimulation that promotes cognitive development and social competence. These effects persist into the school years to establish a foundation for later success. Although poor children may derive more benefit, the benefits of ECEC programs pertain regardless of social class and whether or not the mother is in the workforce.

There is overwhelming evidence that the positive effects of ECEC programs occur only if they are high quality and that, indeed, poor-quality programs may have a negative effect, especially for children from low-resourced families. Thus, it is the *quality* of ECEC programs that is critical in determining how developmentally effective they are, not merely whether children participate in them (Shonkoff & Phillips, 2000).

While there is no single universal definition of quality ECEC, there are some values so critical to the well-being of children that they are widely perceived to be the foundation of any definition of quality (see Friendly, Beach & Doherty, 2005, for a fuller discussion of quality issues in ECEC).

Moss, Penn, and Mestres point out that:

> ... while there is a range of culturally- and time-linked ways of defining quality in ELCC programs, more generally there is a consensus in much of the current child development literature that children need to feel loved, respected and listened to; that they are sociable and enjoy the company of other children and adults besides their immediate family; and that through affection, through social intercourse and with a stimulating environment, they mature, learn and develop a remarkably wide range of skills and competencies in the first five or six years. (Moss, Penn & Mestres, 2004, p. A19)

Generally in Canada, the term "quality" is used as shorthand for characteristics of ECEC programs that go beyond basic health and safety requirements to those that support children's development, learning, and well-being. From this perspective, studies show that high-quality ECEC programs:

- employ staff who are well educated for their work and have decent working conditions and wages
- organize children into groups of manageable size with adequate numbers of adults

- provide challenging, non-didactic, play-based, creative, enjoyable activities
- ensure consistent adult and peer groups in well-designed physical environments

High-quality ECEC services are also responsive to diverse populations of children and parents, include children with disabilities in a meaningful way, have connections to the community, and involve parents as partners by supporting them both in employment and in the parenting role.

The evidence shows that the positive effects of high-quality ECEC persist into later life. This is especially, but not exclusively, true for low-income children. A longitudinal study of very low-income American children who attended high-quality child care in infancy found that participants had lower juvenile crime and school dropout rates and much higher earnings as adults (the earnings of their mothers became much higher than those of a control group as well) (Masse & Barnett, 2002). This study of full-day infant child care reinforces research on ECEC's long-term benefits for low-income American children in part-day programs that began between two and three years of age (Schweinhart & Weikart, 1993).

At the same time, research shows that high-quality ECEC has a lasting impact on all children, not only those who are disadvantaged. A study of children in Sweden's universal high-quality child-care centres found that entry sometime around the first birthday meant that children performed better in school at eight years and 13 years regardless of family income and received more positive socio-emotional teacher ratings than children who began child care later or who were in family daycare or were not in child care outside the family at all (Andersson, 1992).

There is good evidence, then, that high-quality ECEC contributes to a platform of healthy child development that can have effects over the lifespan. In this way, ECEC programs can be conceptualized not only as reducing risks or deficits, but also as playing a positive role in ensuring that opportunities are not missed.

Goal 2: Supporting Parents in Education, Training, and Employment

In Canada, labour force participation of mothers of young children has risen steadily so that by 2005, 76 percent of mothers with a youngest child three to five years old worked outside the home, up from 73.4 percent in 2001 and 68 percent in 1995 (Friendly et al., 2007). As financial pressures on families began to mount in the 1980s, it became the norm for affluent and middle-class as well as poor families to have both parents (if there are two parents) in the labour force. At the same time, paid employment and careers have become appropriate and desirable roles for women. A third motivation for employment, especially for lone mothers, is associated with Canada's diminished social safety net, including the introduction of mandatory workfare programs in the 1990s.

Whatever the motivation, dependable alternative care for children is essential if mothers who would have been expected to provide it two generations ago are to participate in the workforce, training, or education. Without access to child care, women may be compelled to remain out of the labour force, work at poorly paid part-time or precarious employment, or may be forced to rely on social assistance. While a low-paid insecure job is not necessarily a route out of poverty, without child care, poor women and their families lack even the possibility of escaping poverty.

ECEC, as it supports parental employment and training, is linked to social determinants of health such as family income and poverty, which are both directly experienced by the child and mediated through the family. Thus, children benefit in the short and longer term if child care to help sustain their families economically is accessible. However, as described in the previous section, if the quality of child care upon which parents rely so they can go to work or training is not high enough to support healthy development, children may not benefit.

Goal 3: Strong Communities

The third goal—strengthening communities through social solidarity and social cohesion—is especially pertinent in diverse societies like Canada. Early childhood is a critical period for learning about difference and diversity and establishing a basis for tolerance; research shows that children recognize racial differences and hold opinions about race by the age of three. Consequently, inclusive childhood education programs can enhance respect for diversity through their impact on children as future adults. But ECEC programs have the capacity to have a significant impact on adults, too, and, in turn, on their children. Community-based programs that are holistic and welcoming can support neighbourhood, community, and interpersonal co-operation and social solidarity in the sense that they can be "forums located in civil society" through which parents can participate

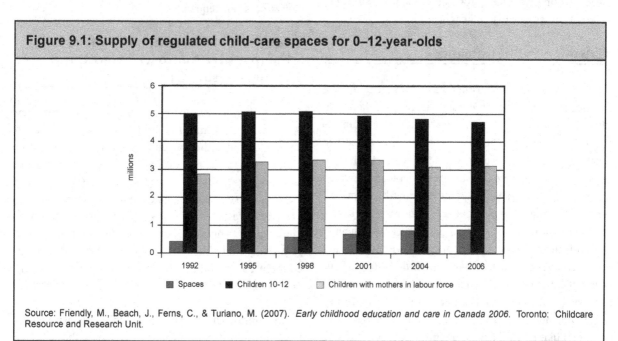

Figure 9.1: Supply of regulated child-care spaces for 0–12-year-olds

Source: Friendly, M., Beach, J., Ferns, C., & Turiano, M. (2007). *Early childhood education and care in Canada 2006.* Toronto: Childcare Resource and Research Unit.

in common activities related to the well-being of their children. In this way, ECEC programs that include parents are connected with community resources, and that demonstrate respect for diversity can promote solidarity and equity among classes, racial and ethnic groups, and generations.

Goal 4: Providing Equity

ECEC contributes to equity for multiple groups in society, but for two groups in particular—children with disabilities and women—access to ECEC is a particularly important equity and social justice issue. Ensuring the rights of children with disabilities is a matter of basic social justice. For children with disabilities and their parents, the opportunity to participate in early childhood programs with typical children is critical for child development, for supporting parents as parents and as workers, and for normalizing their lives. From a feminist perspective, that universal child care is critical for women's equality is certainly not new. As an equity issue, this goes beyond pragmatic considerations of access to employment and training as discussed in a previous section. That ECEC is a basic citizenship right for women is associated with the idea that social rights constitute a key element of citizenship and go way beyond training or employment. Putting it simply, equality for women cannot be a reality without full access to child care.

Canadian Political Realities

Canada's ECEC programs have developed as a hodgepodge of separate programs and policies that mean that no region of Canada has adequate ECEC opportunities for children and parents. This situation has, at least in part, been shaped by two key Canadian realities. The first is linked to the nature of Canadian federalism in which responsibility for social programs is primarily provincial/territorial. Within this political reality, the respective roles and responsibilities of the two orders of government—federal and provincial/territorial—have shifted and changed over the years. Compared to the 1960s–1970s when the modern social safety net was created, Canada underwent a deconstructing trend in the 1990s. In this environment, developing a national approach to a social program like ECEC is not straightforward. This has had

profound implications for the way ECEC has developed in the modern era (see Friendly, 2000).

A second political reality is that Canada is a liberal democracy with a relatively weak welfare state. As Meyers and Gornick, in their comparative application to child care of Esping-Andersen's typology of welfare regimes point out, Canada's ECEC provision relies on "market-based solutions and means testing, mak[ing] only limited public investments in ECEC" (2000, p. 23). In this analysis, the liberal-democratic (Canada, the US, and the UK) regimes are distinguished by their reliance on the marketplace for child care in several ways: high use of informal care; reliance on parent fees with subsidies for those who can qualify; and private, sometimes for-profit provision, compared to the considerably stronger role for the state that characterizes ECEC in continental Europe. Perhaps the clearest symbol of Canadian child care's private nature is that almost all responsibility for developing and managing it (even finding capital funds) is assumed by the private sector—parent groups, voluntary organizations, or entrepreneurs.

It is interesting to note that while Canadian responsibility for child care is primarily private, kindergarten under public education is a public responsibility. This is consistent with Meyers and Gornick's description of the liberal regimes' relatively strong commitment to public education as an "equalizer."

What We Can Learn about Canada Using a Comparative Approach? How Does Canada Measure Up?

Through the absence of comprehensive public policy development, Canadian ECEC has developed so unevenly that although each province/territory has multiple programs, only a small minority of children and families have access to needed services. ECEC services are either in short supply, inaccessible for many because user fees are too high, of mediocre quality, or—like kindergarten—not sensitive to the labour force needs of parents. And although a majority of young Canadian children have mothers in the labour force, most rely on unregulated arrangements privately arranged by parents.

In contrast, almost all continental European nations have developed publicly funded systems that provide good-quality early childhood programs with reasonable sensitivity to parents' labour force needs. Although different countries have different approaches to program delivery, generally, publicly funded ECEC programs become widely available to children by age three years, and a number of countries have relatively broad coverage for infants and toddlers as well.[2] Comparisons with other countries are valuable because they show that, although no country is entirely "perfect," ECEC programs can be organized to be relatively seamless and universal.

Thus far, this chapter has discussed how ECEC is linked to four social goals—healthy child development, family income, strong communities, and equity—that contribute to health in the broad sense. But these links are in place only if certain characteristics of public policy and service delivery are present. In recent years, a consensus has emerged from policy analysis in the ECEC field that specific conditions are essential at the system level to ensure access and quality at the program level. Thus, it is a high-quality early learning and child care *system* that is key to ensuring that high-quality programs are the rule rather than the exception; strong public policy is the basis for a high-quality early learning and child-care system (Friendly, Beach & Doherty, 2005).

An international policy study conducted by the OECD between 1998 and 2006 provides a good basis for examining the enabling conditions for ECEC programs and their implications for public policy. The OECD's Thematic Review of ECEC was launched as a result of a 1996 meeting of OECD education ministers about strengthening the foundations of lifelong learning. In 2001, *Starting Strong,* the project's first major report, observed that:

> Policy makers have recognized that equitable access to quality early childhood education and care can strengthen the foundations of lifelong learning for all children and support the broad educational and social needs of families. (Organisation for Economic Co-operation and Development, 2001, p. 7)

All OECD member countries were invited to participate in the study, and by the study's end, 20 countries were part of the project. A common framework and process were established and, following preparation of a background report that provided information about context and provision of Early Learning and Childcare (ELCC), each country was visited by an international expert team for several weeks. This group met with officials and community groups, visited ELCC programs, and prepared a *Country Note* presenting an analysis of the country's ELCC issues. (The two Canada reports were published in 2004.) The OECD also commissioned research on key topics (curricula and pedagogies; financing; children from low-income families; data).

The 50 reports that make up the OECD's Thematic Review of Early Childhood Education and Care comprise the largest body of comparative policy research to date in the field. This eight-year study provides an opportunity not only to compare how well Canada is doing using common international criteria, but also offers a unique opportunity to draw conclusions about what is known about best practices in ELCC policy and practice.

Analysis of the comparative data from 20 nations compiled for the Thematic Review's summary report shows that Canada is:

- a wealthy country (fourth highest GDP per capita among countries included)
- a country with a high child poverty rate (seventh highest of 20)
- a low spender on social programs, with only four countries lower (as a proportion of GDP)
- a country with a fairly high rate of mothers of young children working outside the home (seventh highest for mothers with children under three; eighth highest with children under six)
- a low spender on all child and family programs with only three countries lower (as a proportion of GDP)
- a not-generous provider of paid maternity and parental leave (in the lower third on "effective" parental leave, with duration and payment included)
- a country where costs to parents for ELCC programs are high with only three where they're higher
- a country where most children don't attend an ELCC program until age five, compared to six countries in which most (in some, almost all), attend by age three, and another five countries where most attend by age four

- the very lowest spender on ELCC programs of the 14 countries for which data were available. (Organisation for Economic Co-operation and Development, 2006; Friendly, 2006)

One of the OECD study's most valuable findings is that eight interrelated aspects of policy and program are the "key elements ... that are likely to promote equitable access to quality ECEC" (Organisation for Economic Co-operation and Development, 2001, p. 125). These eight policy lessons form a useful framework for examining Canadian ECEC.

Policy Lesson 1

Policy lesson 1 stresses the value of a systematic and integrated approach to policy development and implementation, including a coordinated policy framework and a lead ministry. That Canada does not have a systematic approach to policy and services was discussed previously. Canada has neither a national approach to ECEC nor is the approach in most of the provinces/territories (the level of government with the jurisdictional responsibility) coherent or integrated. The absence of coherent policy at the two senior levels of government not only has negative implications for accessibility and quality, but also means that public financing and other resources are used ineffectively.

At the service-delivery level, each province/territory has a program of regulated child care and separate kindergarten for five-year-olds; in each, there are child-care centres, kindergartens, nursery schools/preschools, regulated family child care, parenting programs, and an array of funding arrangements. However, at a practical level, although each province/territory has a tangle of programs, only a minority of children and families have services that provide the reliable care that parents need or the early childhood education programs that benefit child development.

The absence of a systematic approach to ECEC in Canada can be directly linked to poor accessibility and inadequate quality. Fragmentation of services engenders inconsistency, so is a poor fit with knowledge about the kinds of environments that enhance child development. In a more societal sense, Canadian families and children have to fit into narrow eligibility categories, segregated into class, income, racial, and lifestyle "silos" to qualify for different ECEC programs. This not only means that programs are irregularly available, but it weakens solidarity and undermines the potential that ECEC services have to serve as focal points for social cohesion.

In the *Canada Country Note*, OECD expert team recommended that "governments, policy makers, researchers and other stakeholders involved in ECEC in Canada [as first task] sit down together to conceptualize a coherent, long-term vision for each province and the country as a while, based on the best available evidence and prioritized into defined steps and time frames" (2004, p. 147).

Policy Lesson 2

Policy lesson 2 is that a strong and equal partnership with the education system is a valuable basis for a workable and equitable ECEC system. It suggests a lifelong-learning approach to recognize ECEC as a foundation of the education process and encourage smooth transitions for children.

Although there is now some recognition in Canada that care and early childhood education are inevitably tied together (as the term "early learning and child care" connotes), in practice Canadian ECEC rarely blends these two functions at either program or policy levels. Kindergarten as part of the education system is regarded as a foundation for lifelong learning and treated as a public good. With regard to child care, while provinces/territories regulate elements of child-care services such as staff training and ratios that are linked in research to child development, there is little infrastructure in place to go beyond basic regulation. Child-care programs are of such uneven quality that it is questionable as to whether they are "educational."

The OECD review's *Canada Country Note* said that:

> The aim is to conceptualize and deliver care and education as one seamless program to young children.... In the view of the OECD review team, greater intgegration of kindergarten and child care would bring real advantages in the Canadian context. (2004, p. 158)

Although Quebec took positive steps beginning in 1998 to reinforce the partnership between education and child care by publicly funding child care for all 0 to four-year-olds (not just for those whose mothers are in the labour force), the overall partnership between child care and the education system in Canada is divided and limited, not "strong and equal."

Policy Lesson 3

Policy lesson 3 calls for a universal approach to access to high-quality ECEC regardless of family income, parental employment status, special educational needs, or ethnic/ language background with particular attention to children in need of special support. To be accessible, ECEC must be available, affordable, and appropriate. This requires an adequate supply of services, affordable parent fees (either free, very low cost, or geared to income) and services that fit the needs and characteristics of the family and the child (for example, they must be responsive to parents' work schedules).

In 2006, few Canadian children under the age of five (when most go to part-day kindergarten) have a chance to participate in high-quality ECEC programs that benefit their development, and only a minority of parents can rely on the care they need to go to work or school. Access to regulated child care has improved little in the past decade

with limited impact on the sizable gap between need and provision. Canada-wide coverage—the proportion of children for whom there was a space in regulated child care—improved only from 7.5 percent to 17.2 percent in the 14 years between 1992 and 2006, lacklustre improvement for that period of time.

While there is now provision in every province/ territory in kindergarten for just about all five-year-olds, this is primarily only part-day (generally 2.5 hours), and only Ontario has introduced widespread kindergarten for four-year-olds. In contrast, close to 100 percent of three-year-olds are in publicly funded ECEC programs in Italy, France, and Belgium, and in most of the other European OECD countries, coverage of three-year-olds is 50 percent or better. Indeed, most European countries provide all children with at least two years of free, publicly funded ECEC provision before they begin primary school (Organisation for Economic Co-operation and Development, 2006).

The way Canadian ECEC is financed also plays a key role in making it inaccessible to many families. Parent user fees in child-care programs create barriers to access for poor, most modest, and many middle-income families. While fee subsidies targeted to low-income families are available in all regions (outside Quebec), modest and middle-income families are usually not eligible for

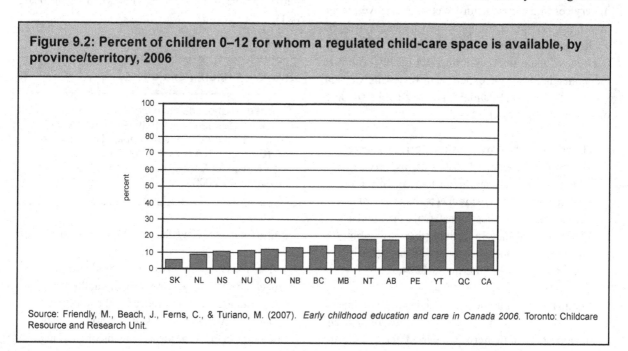

Figure 9.2: Percent of children 0–12 for whom a regulated child-care space is available, by province/territory, 2006

Source: Friendly, M., Beach, J., Ferns, C., & Turiano, M. (2007). *Early childhood education and care in Canada 2006*. Toronto: Childcare Resource and Research Unit.

them and underfunding may mean that subsidies are not available even to families who qualify.[3]

In the *Canada Country Note*, the OECD's expert international team noted a "market-determined fee structure (except Manitoba and Quebec), resulting in high parental contributions to child care costs, ranging from 34% to 82% of costs. The average across the country, excluding Quebec, is just under 50% of costs compared to a maximum 15% parental contribution in Finland or approximately 25% across Europe," and "an inefficient subsidy system with widely varying and complex eligibility criteria, accessed by only 22% of lone parents and around 5% of married mothers from low-income families" (2006, p. 301).

In general, Canadian child care is characterized by eligibility based on narrow categories, scarcity, children in need of special support being left unserved, and targeting to selected populations. It cannot be said that we are moving toward "a universal approach to access with particular attention to children in need of special support." Indeed, with the exception of public kindergarten and Quebec's evolving child-care program, Canada has not defined universality as an objective.

Policy Lesson 4

Policy lesson 4 calls for substantial public investment in services and infrastructure. Substantial government investment is required to support a sustainable system of quality, accessible services. In ECEC programs, financing is directly linked to accessibility and quality. The first recommendation of the expert team reviewing Canada was that Canada "substantially increase public funding of services for young children," noting that:

> Even in those provinces/territories that are keen to develop their ECEC systems, services are under funded, and neither the quality nor the quantity of provision meets the aspirations of parents and professionals. Only the regular funding that state investment brings is able to guarantee access and quality on a fairly equitable basis for all groups. (2004, p. 73)

Public funding must be substantial enough to finance capital costs; to cover all or most of the cost of program operation so that if there are parent fees, they are affordable by families across the income spectrum; and to ensure adequate infrastructure and training at all levels. According to the OECD, "Only the regular funding that state investment brings is able to guarantee access and quality on a fairly equitable basis for all groups" (2004, p. 73). The final report of the Thematic Review identified Canada as the lowest spender on ECEC programs among 14 OECD countries; according to their calculations, Canada spent only .25 percent of GDP (2006).

However, in financing ECEC programs, not only the amount but *how* public funds are delivered is important. The best practice is direct funding of programs, not vouchers, allowances, or parent subsidies. The OECD notes that supply-side (direct program) funding provides greater stability for programs with, in return, greater government control over planning, size, and location of services, quality levels, and evaluation and data collection (2006). Arguments made for demand-side mechanisms are primarily associated with parent choice and the idea that ECEC is a commodity in the marketplace. This supposition presumes not only that a choice is available, but that parents can accurately judge ECEC quality. Neither experience nor research suggests that this is so; American research has documented that in actuality, parents often overestimate the quality of their child care relative to objective measures (Helburn, 1995; Mocan, 2001).

Box 9.1: Funding and quality

"The debate about demand-side and supply side funding is often really a debate over what kind of quality will be provided and what kind of standards set" (Cleveland & Krashinky, 2003, quoted in Organisation for Economic Co-operation and Development, 2006).

In the Canada review, the OECD recommended:

> ... a move away from personal subsidy mechanisms toward operational funding and an entitlement for children, as in the traditional education model. Earmarked operational grant funding seems to be a surer means of ensuring

more highly qualified personnel and enriched learning environments in the centres—both of which are strong indicators of quality and learning. (2004, p. 8)

Policy Lesson 5

Policy lesson 5 suggests that both pedagogical frameworks focusing on children's holistic development and strategies for ongoing quality improvement are key, and also recommends that all forms of ECEC be regulated and monitored. As described earlier, the characteristics of ECEC services that determine whether they are likely to meet not only basic health and safety requirements but also provide environments that ensure development and learning have been well documented in research.

Two structural elements have been shown to be key in determining a baseline for quality in ECEC programs. The first of these—financing—was discussed in the previous section. While the second—regulation—has been shown to be linked to quality through the form and content of programs, especially staffing (Gallagher et al., 1999), regulation per se does not guarantee quality. Indeed, several Canadian studies have identified concerns about quality in regulated child-care services. *You Bet I Care!* (YBIC!), a cross-Canada study of process quality (that is, derived from structured observations of multiple program activities and elements) in child care, found that:

> Fewer than half of the preschool rooms (44.3%) and slightly more than a quarter of the infant/toddler rooms (28.7%) are providing activities and materials that encourage children's development. Instead, the majority of the centres in Canada are providing care that is of minimal or mediocre quality. The children's physical and emotional health and safety are protected but few opportunities for learning are provided. (Goelman et al., 2000)

Two more recent Quebec-wide studies showed similar results in regulated child care in Quebec (Japel, Tremblay & Côté, 2005; Fournier & Drouin, 2004), with both studies also showing much poorer quality in for-profit programs.

At the same time, the unregulated child care (unregulated family or in-own-home child care) that provides care for most Canadian preschool-age children while mothers work is outside systems of quality assurance altogether. While research on the precise details of these arrangements is sparse, enough is known to suggest that the majority of preschool-age children

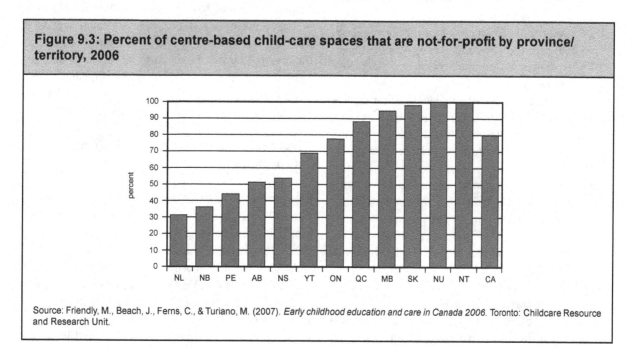

Figure 9.3: Percent of centre-based child-care spaces that are not-for-profit by province/ territory, 2006

Source: Friendly, M., Beach, J., Ferns, C., & Turiano, M. (2007). *Early childhood education and care in Canada 2006.* Toronto: Childcare Resource and Research Unit.

whose mothers work outside the home spend a good deal of time in child-care arrangements that lack early childhood-enhancing environments.

Policy Lesson 6

Policy lesson 6 suggests that appropriate training and working conditions for staff in all forms of provision is a foundation for quality ECEC services, which depend on strong staffing and fair working conditions. Strategies for recruiting and retaining a qualified, diverse, mixed-gender workforce, and for ensuring that a career in ECEC is satisfying, respected, and financially viable, are essential. As human interaction makes up the substance of a child's ECEC experiences, staff are the essence of ECEC programs. Research shows that adequate training and fair working conditions—wages and benefits, working environments, turnover, training, and morale—are all strongly and directly associated with the quality of a child's experience and development (Goelman et al., 2000; Whitebook et al., 1990).

Data from 2006 pertinent to human resources in Canadian child-care programs show that in 2006:

- No province/territory requires all child-care staff to have post-secondary education in early childhood, a key indicator of quality. In a number of them, ECE training is required only for a minority of staff
- Required ECE training for staff in regulated child-care centres and nursery schools ranges from none to a community college diploma (one to three years)
- While a number of provinces/territories now require ECE training of at least one year for a centre director, management or other supervisory training is required for centre directors in only one province
- Since 1992 there has been a steadily improving trend in ECE training requirements. Since 2004, however, improvements have been quite limited
- Only two provinces require regular in-service training

There are no current comparable data on staff wages, a key indicator of child-care quality. Statistics Canada data show that for women working full-time, full-year,

ECEs and assistants earn about 60 percent of the average and about 57 percent of the average for those with a post-secondary credential (Beach & Flanagan, 2006).

Policy Lesson 7

Policy lesson 7 calls for systematic monitoring and data collection with coherent procedures on the status of young children, ECEC provision, and the early childhood workforce. An analysis of Canadian ECEC data needs concluded that Canada essentially has no reliable, consistent, comparable data on various aspects of ECEC that can inform policy or improvements to service provision, or assess changes and effects on children and families over time (Cleveland et al., 2003). However, provisions and funds to develop strategies for "data and monitoring" that were part of the 2005 "national early learning and child care program" were cancelled in 2006 with the rest of the program.

Policy Lesson 8

Policy lesson 8 suggests that a stable framework and long-term agenda for research and evaluation requires sustained investment to support research on key policy goals and is a necessary part of a process of continuous improvement. While some research and evaluation studies, mostly conducted through a series of federal funding programs, have yielded valuable information, there has not been a *stable framework and long-term agenda*. The systematic data collection discussed in the previous section is linked to this research agenda; basic data to provide public accountability should be a complement to a research and evaluation agenda that can help provide answers to more complex questions.

First Steps, Next Steps, and Shifting Landscapes

One concern about ECEC in Canada has been that while other OECD countries have spent the past 15 years establishing and building their ECEC systems, in Canada, the process of establishing a coherent, sustained system of ECEC has not even begun. Nationally, several abrupt shifts in ECEC policy have occurred in a very short space of time. Indeed, since the 1990s, ECEC at both provincial and national levels has experienced wild swings in direction across Canada as new policy and increases were replaced by downsizing and expansion, then, in some instances, growth again. The previous edition of this chapter stated that:

> In the years between the 1970 recommendation of the Royal Commission on the Status of Women for a national child care program and the present, there were four efforts to begin this process by three successive federal governments. Each announced that a national strategy for child care would be developed but each of the first three attempts failed to materialize. (Friendly, 2000, p. 347)

In 2003, the Multilateral Framework Agreement (MFA) on Early Learning and Care had finally broken through the "anything but child care" approach of the last decade to presage a national ECEC strategy. This multilateral agreement, in which all provinces/territories except Quebec (which had already begun to put its own program in place) participated, was depicted by then-Human Resources Minister Jane Stewart as "the first step to a national child care program." The MFA restricted use of federal funds to regulated child care and committed to public reporting in a number of specific areas. There were, however, no national goals, legislation, targets, and timetables, or implementation plans.

The "next step" came in the 2004 election campaign when the federal Liberals promised to develop a national early learning and child-care system based on four principles—Quality, Universality, Accessibility, and Developmental [programming] (QUAD)—promising to transfer $5 billion to the provinces to build the system. After the Liberals won the 2004 election with a minority, they began negotiations to secure co-operation from the provinces based on several federal conditions: (1)

Box 9.2: Mr. Harper, leave the child-care program alone
Maureen McTeer

Almost 30 years ago, as a pregnant law student, I joined the fight for a national, high-quality and publicly funded child-care program. Today, about to become a grandmother, I am forced to do so again.

Most of my generation spent our children's young lives balancing motherhood and work responsibilities—including those at home. We breathed a sigh of relief last year when the federal Liberals kept a promise made by every government during every successive election campaign over the past three decades. Finally, working (or studying) Canadian families who needed quality care for their children would have systems of care with specific safety and educational standards.

But now, less than a year later, the Conservatives want to turn back the clock for working Canadian families. In place of a child-care program, they plan to mail a $1,200 cheque to each family with a child under six to do with as they please.

In his first press conference last week as prime-minister-designate, Stephen Harper made clear that his party's political ideology would trump the needs of Canadian children. He insisted that "Canadian parents and families expect Parliament as a whole to deliver them that benefit." Who wouldn't? Such a taxable direct payment may appease his own conservative constituency, at the expense of a program for the seven out of 10 mothers in the work force who have children under six, but that ideologically driven decision is not about providing or improving child care.

Mr. Harper and his Conservatives have choices.

In this case, if they so want to keep this anti-child-care election promise, then do so. Send every Canadian with a child under six a cheque. Heaven knows, they can always use whatever is left after the taxes on that $1,200. But leave the bilateral child-care agreements with the provinces in place. Better still, work to improve them so all Canadians with children benefit from publicly funded programs and child-care options, and systems of the highest quality. Certainly, this is a vision worthy of our families and children across Canada.

If he does this, Mr. Harper wins on both counts. He pays back his political constituency and also shows he is capable of real vision and leadership for the benefit of our children and grandchildren.

Source: McTeer, Maureen. (2006). "Mr. Harper, leave the child-care program alone." *The Globe and Mail* (February 6), p. A15.

provinces were to consult on and publish Action Plans before five-year funding agreements were finalized; (2) federal funds were to be used only for regulated child care; (3) provinces would publicly report on the use of funds. Thus, by the end of 2005, each province had an agreement with the federal government to move forward on ECEC. There was enormous anticipation of improvements to come as these agreements marked the first time that a national government had followed through with an election commitment to improve child care across Canada.

However, by the beginning of 2006, a fourth attempt had come and gone as the 2006 federal election brought another powerful shift for child care. The minority Conservative government elected in January 2006 announced that it was cancelling the agreements with provinces and that the federal ECEC transfers would end March 31, 2007. The government promised instead an individual taxable cash payment of $100/month to all parents of children under age six and a tax credit for capital funds to encourage child care in workplaces.

Following the announcement that the federal ELCC transfers would be short-lived, Action Plans in some of the provinces/territories were put aside, although in some instances, provinces continued some expansion or improvements. But the idea of a national program with principles, with provinces following a public Action Plan, reporting on spending and accomplishments, and working together to develop a national curriculum framework and a national strategy for data and research was—for the time being, at least—at an end.

Conclusion

This chapter has discussed how and under what circumstances ECEC programs can be an important social determinant of health through their impact on children, their families, and communities. Although ECEC outside the family is only one of a number of factors that have an impact on children during early life, high-quality ECEC is known to provide a platform for adult employment, education, income, status, and lifestyle. These are, in turn, well linked to adult health.

Some would argue, given our knowledge today about its multiple impacts, that ECEC is so fundamental to well-being that it should be a human right. In addition to including early childhood education and child care in such United Nations' compacts as the Convention on the Rights of the Child, the Convention on the Elimination of All Forms of Discrimination against Women, and Education for All, UNICEF (the United Nations Children's Fund) calls on world government leaders to take action on ECEC in order to "make children—the youngest especially—the priority at all policy tables … and to ensure that this has the necessary political and financial support" (United Nations Children's Fund, 2001, p. 3) no matter what the ideological stripe of the government in power. For Canada, this will require the mustering of vision, commitment, and political will to ensure that the "first step" leads to the next steps and, ultimately, to the goal of high-quality early childhood education and care for all.

Notes

1. It is important to note that while there have been multiple Canadian rationales for ECEC over the years, a key point of view that has become central to the mainstream discourse about children elsewhere—that entitlement to ECEC is connected to children's citizenship rights and that children should be valued as children, not simply for what they may become later on—has not really been part of the debate in Canada.

2. It should be noted that these services are all publicly funded, although—with the exception of full school-day programs for children aged 2.5 to six, which are usually free to the user—there are parent fees in most cases. However, affordability isn't a significant issue in most countries even outside the older preschool group.

3. The $5 a day fee was increased to $7 a day for all income groups in the fall of 2003.

Critical Thinking Questions

1. Before reading this chapter, had you thought about how the availability, affordability, and quality of ECEC programs are connected to the idea of social determinants of health? Has the chapter contributed to your ideas about this?
2. Thinking about your familiarity with ECEC policy and programs, do things that you learned from reading this chapter—for example, that Canada is the lowest spender per capita on ECEC programs or that access to good-quality ECEC programs is so low—surprise you?
3. Look for newspaper or other media stories about ECEC for a period of time. How do the topics they cover relate to what you've read in this chapter?
4. Why do you think Canada's provision of ECEC programs is so poor compared to other countries?

Recommended Readings

Friendly, M., Beach, J. & Doherty, G. (2005). *Quality in early learning and child care: What we know and what we think.* Working documents from Quality by Design. Toronto: Childcare Resource and Research Unit.

Organisation for Economic Co-operation and Development. (1998–2006). The more than 50 documents generated by the OECD's Thematic Review of Early Childhood Education and Care include *Starting Strong* (2001) and *Starting Strong 2* (2006), the Review's two summary documents, the Canada Background Report, and *Canada Country Note* (2004), as well as reports on the reviews of the other 19 countries and several reports from seminars on special topics. These documents form perhaps the most extensive body of comparative policy analysis in the field. Links to all documents can be accessed through the Child Care Resource and Research Unit's online Issue File on the project at action.web.ca/home/crru/rsrcs_crru_full.shtml?x=108172 or directly through the OECD's Web site at www.oecd.org

> Key documents:

> Organisation for Economic Co-operation and Development (OECD). (2001). *Starting strong: Early childhood education and care.* Education Division. Paris: OECD.

> Organisation for Economic Co-operation and Development (OECD). (2004). *Canada country note.* Thematic Review of Early Childhood Education and Care Education Division. Paris: OECD.

> Organisation for Economic Co-operation and Development (OECD). (2006). *Starting strong 2: Early childhood education and care.* Thematic Review of Early Childhood Education and Care Education Division. Paris: OECD.

Related Web Sites

Campaign 2000—www.campaign2000.ca

Campaign 2000 is a cross-Canada public education movement to build Canadian awareness and support for the 1989 all-party House of Commons resolution to end child poverty in Canada by the year 2000. Universal early childhood education and care is a key objective for Campaign 2000.

Child Care Advocacy Association of Canada—www.child careadvocacy.ca

The Child Care Advocacy Association of Canada (CCAAC), founded in 1982, advocates for high-quality, publicly funded child care accessible to all. The Web site provides links to position papers, news releases, and other key documents. Some content is available in French.

Child Care Human Resources Sector Council—www.ccsc-cssge.ca

The Child Care Human Resources Sector Council is a pan-Canadian, non-profit organization dedicated to moving forward on the human resource issues in child care. It brings together national partners and other sector representatives to develop a confident, skilled, and respected workforce valued for its contribution to early childhood care and education. Web site includes council publications, press releases, and projects, and is also available in French.

Child Care Resource and Research Unit (CRRU)—www.childcarecanada.org

The Child Care Resource and Research Unit is Canada's premier early childhood care and education research and policy institute. The comprehensive Web site includes links to a wide range of documents on the topic, online versions of CRRU reports, and current developments in ECEC in Canada. It is updated weekly and sign-up for an email notification of additions is available on the site.

SpeciaLink—www.specialinkcanada.org

SpeciaLink's goal is to expand the quality and quantity of opportunities for inclusion in child care, recreation, education, and other community settings for young children with special needs and their families. It provides referrals to other organizations, and information and technical assistance. Also provides newsletters, fact sheets, books, videos, and a speakers bureau.

Chapter 10

EARLY CHILDHOOD EDUCATION AND HEALTH

Brenda L. Smith-Chant[1]

Introduction

In 1938, two psychologists by the name of Skeels and Dye were assessing infants and children for placement into an orphanage and inadvertently came across an interesting phenomenon (Skeels, 1966). They had initially assessed two infant girls (15 and 18 months of age) as profoundly mentally retarded. Because they were considered so low functioning, the girls were deemed ineligible for adoption, removed from the orphanage, and placed in a long-term care facility for the mentally retarded, a common practice at that time. Six months later, Skeels and Dye were shocked when they visited the facility and found two very active, well-functioning little girls. Initially, they were very concerned about the possibility that they had made a grievous error in their assessments. However, over time they became convinced that the caring attention, one-on-one interaction, and diverse experiences the girls received from both the adult residents and the nursing staff in the facility had dramatically and positively impacted their development.

Skeels and Dye (1939, cited in Skeels, 1966) were inspired to explore their ideas on the impact of attention and care on child development. They designed an intervention comparing two groups of children: (1) an experimental group, consisting of 13 children, were placed as "house guests" in the wards of the mental institution; and (2) a contrast group, consisting of 12 children, remained in the orphanage. All of the children

in the study were between the ages of seven and 30 months. The study lasted for three years, after which it was terminated due to changes in management and the Second World War.

The children in the experimental group were distributed across the wards of the institution and allowed to interact freely with the residents and staff. In this setting, the children quickly developed caring relationships with undesignated foster parents and were provided with opportunities to go on trips outside the facility with the staff. Alternatively, the children in the contrast group lived in the orphanage that, by modern standards, would be considered overcrowded and understaffed. Thirty to 35 children lived in a cottage with one matron, who was assisted by three or four untrained assistants. There was limited time for the caregivers to interact with the children due to the high adult-to-child ratio (1:7–8).

At the initial stages of the study, the children in the experimental group had a considerably lower average IQ than the children in the contrast group (see Table 10.1). This inequality was due to the reluctance of the orphanage officials to allow "higher functioning" children to be removed from the orphanage and placed in the long-term residence with mentally retarded adults. However, by the end of the study, the children in the experimental group had gained an average of 27 points in intelligence whereas the contrast group had fallen by an average of 26 points. All of the children in the experimental group improved so dramatically that they were eventually adopted. None of the children in the contrast group were ever adopted.

Skeels (1966) had the opportunity to return 30 years from the beginning of the study to see if the changes in the children's functioning had been maintained into adulthood. Also, Skeels hoped to see if these children had continued the generation-to-generation cycle of poverty that they had been born into or if any of their children showed the same development problems that their parents had. To assess quality of life, Skeels looked at a variety of measures, including educational attainment, occupation, income, marital status, residential type, various socio-economic scores, spouse occupation and education, and number of dependants (children residing with the parent).

Skeels's (1966) results could not have been more dramatic. The individuals in the control group did not do well. Almost all remained in institutional care their entire lives, and those who worked had menial, low-paying jobs. Only two of the contrast group ever married. One of these individuals had four children who were of typical IQ; the other divorced quickly and had one child who was classified as moderately mentally retarded. Alternatively, most of the experimental group finished high school and some completed college. Their general level of employment was higher, resulting in higher average incomes than those in the contrast group. All but two of the members of the experimental group married and among the group they had 38 typically developing children. By any measure, the experimental group was significantly higher functioning than the contrast group.

In his summary, Skeels (1966) attributed the dramatic changes exhibited by the children in the experimental group to the warm, responsive relationships and the enriched environment they were exposed to. Correspondingly, he attributed the poor outcome of the children in the contrast group to the extreme deprivation of their early environment. Although Skeels cautioned about the need for further research to identify the causal links

Table 10.1: Descriptive measures from Skeels (1966)

Measurement characteristics	Group Experimental	Contrast
Number	13	12
Percent males	23	67
Initial study		
Average age (months)	18.3	16.6
Average IQ score	64.3	86.7
Final study		
Average IQ score	91.8	60.5
Average IQ change from initial to final	+27	−26
30-year follow-up		
Average grade attained	13.4	4.0
Average annual income ($)	4,224	1,200
Average number of dependants*	2.7	0
Number of low-functioning children	0	1

*Dependants are defined as children of the study group members who are living under their care. Children not in residence (due to family breakdown and/or divorce) were not included as dependants.

Source: Skeels, H.M. (1966). "Adult status of children with contrasting early life experiences." *Monographs of the Society for Research in Child Development, 31*(105).

between the early environment and child development, he noted that future researchers should "recognize that the child interacts with his environment and does not merely passively absorb its impact" (1966, p. 57). He advocated the need for enriched and attentive early environments to promote optimal child development and learning.

What is remarkable about Skeels (1966) is not merely the illustration of the impact of the early environment on the children in the study. This study identified the key components of a successful early educational intervention with the potential to dramatically change the life course of a child at risk. In this chapter, we will explore the factors underlying effective early educational initiatives. We will use an interdisciplinary approach summarizing developmental theory from biology and neuropsychology to explain why early development is such a critical social determinant of health. Based on these theories, we propose that well-designed education interventions that are early, intensive, and systematic have the potential to alter lifelong health and well-being, just as Skeels observed.

Early Childhood as a Social Determinant of Health

The social factors present during early childhood are powerful direct and indirect predictors of lifelong health and well-being (see Galobardes, Lynch & Smith, 2004, for a review). For example, social factors such as poverty, illiteracy, domestic violence, family dysfunction, illness and disease, and other factors associated with socio-economic deprivation have long been identified in research as major predictors of lifelong health. To mitigate the negative impact of early social factors, governments around the world have invested considerable economic resources into early childhood education initiatives. As of 2004, the US government alone had invested $66 billion over four decades in the Head Start preschool early education program (Kafer, 2004). The focus of these early education initiatives is to provide children, often from impoverished backgrounds, with enriched social experiences and learning opportunities to compensate for the lack of these resources in their environment. The goal of this enrichment is to mitigate the negative impact of their early environment, maximize their potential to become contributing citizens, and reduce the generation-to-generation cycles of poverty.

The rationale for the early education intervention approach is based on research exploring the role of the environment and experience on neural development before age eight. According to theory, exposure to an early education program not only provides a child with foundational skills for later learning, but also has the capacity to permanently change brain development and improve cognitive (i.e., thinking) abilities (Bauer & Boyce, 2004; McCain & Mustard, 1999). Consistent with this idea, the renowned economist Heckman (Heckman & Masterov, 2005) estimated that every dollar spent on early intervention would return between $7–$10 on investment by reducing need for special education, welfare, unemployment, and prison expenditures.

In reality, the success of these early education intervention programs is a contentious issue in both academic and policy domains (Kafer, 2004; Lefebvre & Merrigan, 2002; Magnuson, Ruhm & Waldfogal, 2007; Ramey & Landesman-Ramey, 1998). For example, Ramey and Landesman-Ramey (1998; see also Nelson, Westhues & MacLeod, 2003) noted that frequently, the size of the initial short-term gains observed in children who experience early education programs are moderate to very small. When gains are made, they are frequently not maintained over the long term (Magnuson, Ruhm & Waldfogel, 2007). Often the positive impacts identified in one study have not been replicated in other studies and some negative impacts of early learning initiatives have been reported (Lefebvre & Merrigan, 2002).

The observation that researchers have not consistently found substantial, long-lasting effects of early learning and care initiatives on children's cognitive ability (and hence long-term health and well-being) is in conflict with the theory that an early education permanently and dramatically changes the neural pathways required for cognition. It might be expected that early gains would be somewhat washed out over time by the cumulative effects of an impoverished environment. However, a child who experienced improved brain development as a result of early intervention should retain at least some long-term benefit from the permanent effects of this enrichment (Rutter, 2002). This leads to two possibilities: Either many early education interventions are not as effective at permanently changing cognitive development as hoped, or they are effective but other factors mitigate or alter the efficacy of the intervention afterwards. There is considerable evidence supporting the view that early interventions are frequently not early, intensive, or systematic enough to be effective.

Why Must an Effective Intervention Be Early?

In the early stages of human development, biological processes, environmental conditions, and social factors interact so that a relatively malleable newborn child is shaped into one that is adapted to a specific environment. As a result of this malleability, a human is born ready to acclimatize to a diverse range of environments and social conditions. One unfortunate implication of this malleability is that the process of adapting to a specific environment is not always productive for the long-term success and well-being of the individual. This is particularly true if the early environment is associated with socio-economic deprivation. If the child is born into social poverty or neglect, the adaptive processes will ensure that that child fits that environment. The implications of the early environment for long-term health and well-being are significant. The early environment fundamentally alters an individual's physiology, impacting how he or she perceives, thinks, and reacts to the world (Black, 1998). Understanding these processes is critical for understanding the features of a successful intervention.

There are a number of biological processes impacting development and supporting a child's adaptation to his or her environment during the early stages of life. One of the first influences is genetic inheritance. Even before scientists identified the role of genes, humans have long observed that certain traits ran in families. The science of quantitative genetics is concerned with measuring heritability (ranging from 0 percent to 100 percent). Heritability ranges widely across different types of characteristics. For example, Rutter (2002) noted that the majority of psychological characteristics (both normal and abnormal)—including IQ, personality traits, and even parenting qualities—have heritability rates in the range of 20–40 percent. However, some behavioural characteristics—such as schizophrenia, attention deficit hyperactivity disorder, and autism—can have heritability rates of 70 percent or more, and some physical characteristics, such as height, have heritability rates over 90 percent.

It is quite important, from a developmental perspective, that children are born highly related to their parents. This relation increases the likelihood that the parents will provide their child with optimal stimulation and a supportive environment because many characteristics and predispositions are inherited (Rutter, 2002). For example, parents who are extroverted are much more likely to provide an environment conducive to their child's disposition if their child is extroverted as well. This is known as the shared environment impact on development. Unfortunately, this means that parents with characteristics that predispose them to poverty or social deprivation (e.g., mental illness, cognitive deficits) are also more likely both to have children who inherit these conditions and to create an environment that fosters the development of this characteristic (Rutter, 2002).

However, the interaction between genes and the environment in human development is not merely a case of genetic heritability and shared environments. Certainly, some of the genes that a child inherits from the parents directly determine an aspect of development, but most other genetic contributions work more as a guideline or a set of probabilities for development (Black, 1998; Rutter, 2002). For example, Gottesman (1963) identified that genetic input sets a range of reaction for development. One of the key factors determining the final form that genetic input takes is the environment. The range of reaction principle is one of the biological mechanisms that allow a child to adapt to the conditions that he or she experiences.

A common example used to describe the principle of range of reaction is height. Even though height has a heritability rate of 90 percent, there is still the potential for the environment to have significant impact on these attributes (Rutter, 2002). A male child might inherit the genetic potential to reach a range of heights between 5′9″ and 6′ from his parents. However, his eventual height within this range is determined by environmental conditions. If this boy has a nutritious, healthy, and active childhood, he could potentially reach his maximum height. If this child is malnourished, unhealthy, or inactive, he may reach only the lower limits of his possible range. Gottesman (1963) noted that genetic inheritance sets limits on the possible outcomes of development. Accordingly, the boy in the example could not naturally attain a height of 6′6″ regardless of how optimal his environment was. Nor could he become 4'9" even with the impact of illness or malnutrition because this is outside his range of reaction. Much of development operates within this simple principle of a range of reaction, including such characteristics as intelligence, personality, language, and even sex (Dennis, 2004). In this way, the expression of genetic inheritance is modified and altered by the environment.

One major practical limitation with the range of reaction principle is that the genetic potential carried by an individual is not visible or measurable (Skeels, 1966). For example, at one time in history it was assumed that a child's potential could be determined by observing the characteristics of biologically related family members. Although it is true that many characteristics are genetically inherited, potential cannot be determined from such observations. This is because the adults in a child's family have had their range of reaction limited to the lower end of their potential by experiences of poverty, deprivation, and neglect. Currently, there is no sure way to measure potential. As a result, providing individuals with an enriched environment so that social deprivation does not limit their potential to the lower end of their range of reaction is a major rationale for preschool and educational interventions for children from impoverished backgrounds.

The reason why the early environment has such a major impact on every aspect of later development, including health and well-being, is also attributable to other processes guiding brain development. Biologically, human infants are born at a relatively premature state of development and their brain is only 30 percent the size of an adult's (Thatcher, Lyon, Rumsey & Krasnegor, 1996). From birth, the brain grows rapidly both in size and density of brain cells (neurons) until age two, when it is 70 percent the size of an adult brain. Much of this development is not guided by genetic encoding, mainly because there isn't enough room in the genome to contain all of the instructions that would be necessary (Black, 1998). Black (1998) identified that much of brain development relies on the environment to trigger and stimulate growth of neurons and neural pathways, a feature termed "neural plasticity." There are two main types of neural plasticity processes: Experience-expectant and experience-dependent (Black, 1998; Rutter, 2002).

Experience-expectant neural development is a process by which the neural pathways of the brain undergo a fine-tuning or alteration process that is triggered by environmental conditions at key points in development. During infancy, the brain has more connections between neurons than it will have at any other point in development (Kolb & Whishaw, 2003, p. 616). Once a part of the brain matures, a process begins to reduce the number of potential connections. This is known as synaptic pruning (Janowsky & Finlay, 1986; Thompson & Nelson, 2001). The rationale seems to be that by eliminating unproductive or unnecessary neural connections, energy can be focused on productive ones, allowing the brain to be more efficient. As well, as one part of the brain becomes more organized and efficient, it serves as a foundation and organizational support for the development of other areas of the brain (Black, 1998; Rutter, 2002). For example, it would be logical to expect that the developmental of language would be facilitated and supported by having an efficient and organized auditory cortex for processing sound.

Synaptic pruning relies on developmentally timed experiences that are commonly experienced by children. For example, in the normal course of development, almost all children experience a wide range of visual stimuli as they interact with their environment; they experience touch as they interact with their caregivers; and they hear the sounds of the language that the people in their environment direct at them. As a result, these common experiences trigger optimal synaptic pruning in the associated areas of the brain. A failure to trigger the process would not only result in a failure of the synaptic process to appropriately fine-tune that aspect of the brain, but would also result in a domino effect as other areas of the brain relying on that aspect of the brain development as a foundational support would be undermined. This failure is usually unlikely to occur because the experience-dependent processes rely on common experiences; it is only in extremely impoverished conditions that these triggers are not present, such as in Skeels's orphanage cottages of the 1930s.

The timing of synaptic pruning varies dramatically across the parts of the brain (Kolb & Whishaw, 2003, p. 617). Notably, some areas of the brain, such as those responsible for breathing, sleeping, and circulation, go through the process of synaptic pruning before birth as these areas of the brain are critical for the survival of the newborn. Other areas of the brain undergo synaptic pruning shortly after birth and during infancy, such as the sensory systems that serve as foundations for other cognitive processes that develop later, such as hearing or vision. Some areas of the brain, notably the frontal lobe, which is responsible for higher forms of logical thought, are not completely pruned until puberty and beyond to adulthood. In fact, neural plasticity periods extend well into maturity (Rutter, 2002).

Experience-dependent neural plasticity is associated with what we recognize as learning and memory (Black, 1998; Rutter, 2002). As an individual encounters new experiences, there is an increase in the synaptic density of the brain in the corresponding areas. Synaptic density refers to the number of connections between neurons. Generally, the more connections there are between neurons, the greater the cognitive potential (Kolb & Whishaw, 2003, pp. 624–625). Experience-dependent neural plasticity is not dependent on developmental timing and occurs throughout life. Unlike the experience-expectant neural plasticity, experience-dependent processes encode idiosyncratic aspects of experiences that can differ dramatically from person to person. According to Black (1998), it is novelty that drives this process, not simply intensity or frequency of an experience. Not surprisingly, infancy and early childhood is typically the most active time for experience-dependent neural growth. Most of the experiences an infant has are new, stimulating an increase in synaptic density. As people age, they generally encounter fewer new experiences.

The neurological processes that allow children to adapt to their early environment have some implications for early educational programs. For example, there has been a recent focus on providing children with enriched preschool (i.e., ages three to five years) environments. However, this enrichment happens after large portions of the brain have already been synaptically pruned, particularly those areas involved in processing information from the outside world (i.e., touch, taste, smell, hearing, vision). The impact of this earlier setting of the neural pathways restricts the range of reaction possible for other, later developmental processes that rely on these systems for their development.

The research on Head Start supports the notion that earlier intervention is generally better for children at risk.

For example, in the US Department of Health and Human Services (2005) found that the positive effects of the Head Start program were greatest with the youngest children. Another intervention that depends on early timing is the Intensive Behavioural Intervention (IBI), developed by Lovaas (1987) to treat children born with autism.

Autism and autism spectrum disorder are a category of pervasive developmental disorders describing individuals who have extreme deficits in processing social information. The degree of deficit ranges across a spectrum. At the less-impaired ranges, children with autism may behave very similarly to other children, but have difficulty processing the social cues and the non-verbal information that facilitates social exchanges (i.e., knowing the subtle signs that your conversational partner is getting annoyed with you). In the most extreme ranges of the continuum, children with autism cannot seem to process language (both verbal and non-verbal) and often find social contact (e.g., touching, hugging) uncomfortable.

Lovaas (1987) developed the IBI program based on behaviourist principles (i.e., classical and operant conditioning using punishments and rewards) to treat children with moderately severe symptoms of autism. However, he cautioned that for this intervention to work, the child must be younger than four years of age. He indicated that older children are not as likely to benefit from this type of treatment because older children are already too discriminating and harder to integrate into mainstream classes (1987, p. 3). Other researchers exploring the efficacy of IBI have confirmed that age is an important factor to the success of the intervention (Eikeseth, 2001; Harris & Handleman, 2000).

Unfortunately, there is a tendency to overstate the importance of early brain development for the long-term outcome (Bailey, 2002; Bruer, 1999; Rutter, 2002). Specifically, experience-expectant systems are triggered by events that are common to all children as it would not be adaptive to have the development of the brain dependent on an experience that is optional for the species. Thus, it is only in conditions of extreme deprivation that early intervention is needed to ensure the brain pathways are triggered (Bailey, 2002), such as in a crowded orphanage or when there is a difficulty processing information from the environment, such as autism.

Accordingly, the observation that earlier intervention is more effective than later does not imply that interventions after some developmental window has closed are pointless (Currie, 2001). In fact, Black (1998) identified that the experience-dependent synaptic plasticity process continue throughout life, which is a good thing for those of us who are no longer children. Nor should this observation be taken to mean that once an effective early intervention is delivered, there is no need to continue support beyond the preschool and early primary grades. For example, Nelson et al. (2003) identified that educational interventions continuing throughout school were significantly more effective than interventions that were only preschool-based. Although early childhood seems to be a time where the the brain is particularly open to developing new pathways to process information as opposed to using existing ones, this does not imply that later experiences are unimportant (Bailey, 2002; Black, 1998).

Why Must an Intervention Be Intensive?

An early intervention does not necessarily result in an effective intervention. In order for an early intervention to be effective, it must also be intensive (Ramey & Landsman-Ramey, 1998). Simply put, the more frequently a child is exposed to an intervention, the more likely the intervention will alter development in a permanent way. How intensive does an intervention need to be? This depends on a number of factors, such as how malleable this aspect of development is at the time the intervention occurs, and how targeted (i.e., direct) the intervention activities are. Generally, it seems that in order for an intervention to be effective, it must be more prominent than other, potentially competing experiences that are shaping development.

There has been considerable research done to determine the intensity of various interventions necessary to permanently change or alter a developmental outcome. For example, Lovaas (1987) hypothesized that his IBI intervention could improve an autistic child's functioning if it was the dominant experience they had "during most of their waking hours for many years" (pp. 3–4). The IBI intervention experimental group involved 40 hours of one-on-one time per week, during which well-trained therapists use behaviour-modification techniques to get the children to attend to social information, interact with others, and initiate social contact. One control group consisted of children who received identical therapy, but for only 10 hours per week (minimal training group). Parents from both of these groups were also fully trained in the technique with the expectation that they would provide the children with IBI beyond the time the children spent with the trained therapists. Finally, Lovaas included a third control group consisting of children who received no IBI training at all (no training group).

Typically, children with autism require considerable assistance and a modified program to attend school. However, Lovaas (1987) reported that 47 percent of the children who experienced IBI for 40 hours a week attained average/above-average intelligence scores, were able to attend regular school, and were promoted from first to second grade. Alternatively, none of the children from the minimal training group and only one child in the no-training group met these criteria. Essentially, 10 hours of training had a similar impact as never having IBI at all. In his conclusion, Lovaas attributed the success of the intervention to: (1) the young age of the children; (2) the intensity of the intervention; and (3) the systematic structure of IBI (i.e., following his detailed manual on the technique and using highly trained staff). Lovaas's (1987) study has been highly debated and critiqued over the years and many researchers who have assessed the impact of other IBI initiatives have failed to replicate his 47 percent recovery rate (Eikeseth, 2001; Shea, 2004). However, many of these later studies note that although they cannot attain the same degree of success, the IBI program can be effective in improving the outcome of children with autism if the criteria of early and intensive are met.

Ramey and Landesman-Ramey (1998) identified the principle of program intensity as a major factor for the effectiveness of early interventions. They conclude that programs that are more intensive in terms of hours of treatment and number of sessions are, as a rule, more effective than those that are less so. For example, they summarize evidence that home-visiting interventions for high-risk families with newborns that were offered once a week or less were generally not effective as programs operating with three visits per week. Alternatively, daily interventions during the first three years of life had a strong and positive impact on children's cognitive development.

Unfortunately, very few early educational programs are intensive enough to alter the development of a high-risk child who has been encountering an impoverished environment. According to the research, in order to be maximally effective, an intervention must be experienced virtually daily while the child is at an early stage of development. This is quite difficult to achieve due to the time and cost involved. There are attempts to reduce the cost by having parents do the intervention (Lovaas, 1987; Ramey & Landesman-Ramey, 1998), but this indirect method of intervention is often not as effective as a more direct approach (Ramey & Landesman-Ramey, 1998).

Early and intensive involvement by itself is not sufficient for an effective intervention (Ramey & Landesman-Ramey, 1998). For example, many parents were very surprised to hear that the number of hours their child spent watching *educational* baby videos and television programming, apparently designed to stimulate infant language development, was actually associated with slower language attainment (Zimmerman, Christakis & Meltzoff, 2007). Similarly, child care, an activity that many children experience almost daily, is not always associated with positive impacts on their cognitive development (Currie, 2001; Gagne, 2003; and Lefebvre & Merrigan, 2002).

Many researchers and advocates, as outlined in the preceding chapter by Martha Friendly, propose that this lack of an impact is attributable to the often poor quality of available child care. They contend that effective child care that incorporates an early learning program offers the potential of positively impacting development, not only for children at risk, but also for all children. One important characteristic differentiating child care from Early Childhood Education and Care (ECEC) is that ECEC is systematic; that is, it is characterized by organized guiding principles. This is the third and most important criterion for a successful intervention.

Why Must an Intervention Be Systematic?

A systematic intervention for children accommodates and supports an individual according to her or his stage of cognitive development. Unfortunately, there are many programs that fail on this account. Many of these programs err by assuming that infants and young children learn in the same way that older children and adults do, just simplified. For example, although adults can learn from educational videos, this doesn't mean that infants can similarly acquire knowledge in this way. The environment that infants and children need in order to learn is qualitatively different than at later stages of development.

First, infants and children do not have the perceptual and cognitive skills necessary for more adult-like learning environments. Notably, one of the most important requirements that must be met before an experience can have the opportunity to impact cognition is that it must be perceived (i.e., processed by the sensory system). During infancy, some of the perceptual and cognitive processes necessary for later learning have not yet developed. For example, infants cannot focus visually on objects until they are two months old, and do not have the visual acuity and visual discrimination abilities of an adult until they are one year old (Slater, 2001). With hearing, infants must learn not only to discriminate meaningful sounds like language from other sounds, but then they need to learn words and their meanings. This process is not well developed until age four. Because of their immature perceptual systems, infants rely on their caregivers to provide them with highly specialized types of stimulation that are individually tailored to their abilities, e.g., placing their face or objects within the child's area of visual focus or talking in simplified language form known as "infant-directed speech (Kuhl, 2004).

Even beyond perception, young children need adults to support their learning with one-on-one interaction to direct their attention. This need for one-on-one input is necessary because the brain pathways involved in focused attention are not well developed until the ages between five to seven (i.e., known as the five-to-seven shift; see Siegler, 1996). Before this stage, children find it very difficult to attend to the relevant information in their environment and to filter out the irrelevant. When adults interact with young children, they help the child focus on the relevant by maintaining their interest with their voice, providing eye contact, restricting distracters, and providing contextualized feedback. This process of adjusting the support to the needs of the learning child is known as "scaffolding" (see Berk & Shanker, 2006; p. 260). For young children under the age of five, instruction needs to be individualized and responsive and is optimally provided in one-on-one settings.

Why doesn't more one-on-one interaction occur in early education interventions? It is expensive. In order to make child care and early intervention services cost effective, the ratio of adults to children is relatively high (see Table 10.2). For example, in Ontario, the adult-to-child ratio in licensed child-care settings is 3:10 for infants (i.e., up to 18 months of age); 1:5 for infants up to 30 months; and 1:8 for children 30 months to five years. This relatively high adult-child ratio at such a young age affects not only the intensity of the ECEC program, but also impacts the delivery of a systematic educational program that is ideally tailored to children at this stage of development.

For example, in much of Canada at 30 months of age, the adult-to-children ratio for children is 1:8. This means that a child who spent eight hours in a ECEC centre could expect a maximum of only one hour of one-on-one time with a caregiver (8 hours ÷ 8 children = 1 hour per child). This maximum would never be achieved in a real-world setting because ECEC workers have to arrange meals, organize activities, confer with parents and colleagues, and attend to record-keeping. Even when ECEC workers attend to one child, they must remain at least partially vigilant so as not to compromise the safety of the other seven. For most toddlers, this lack of one-on-one time isn't devastating because most parents provide intensive one-on-one experiences at home. However, with high-risk children, their parents may be unable, unaware, or unwilling to provide sufficient one-on-one time.

The observation that ECEC programs do not provide sufficient one-on-one opportunities for optimal learning is not meant to imply that a high-quality ECEC program has little to offer a developing child. There are very important lessons fostered in a quality ECEC program

Table 10.2: Examples of adult-child ratios for child cares in various jurisdictions

Jurisdiction	Regulated child care	
	Age group	Adult:child ratio
Ontario	Less than 18 months	3:10
	18–30 months	1:5
	30 months–5 years	1:8
British Columbia	Less than 36 months	1:4
	30 months–5 years	1:8
New Brunswick	Less than 2 years	1:3
	2 years	1:5
	3 years	1:7
	4 years	1:10
	5 years	1:12
United Kingdom	Less than 2 years	1:3
	2–3 years	1:4
	3–5 years	1:8
Japan	Less than 1 year	1:3
	1–3 years	1:6
	3–5 years	1:20
Sweden (differs across regions)	Less than 3 years	1:3 or 1:5
	3–5 years	1:7 or 1:9
Skeels's orphanage in 1939	2 years and up	1:7 or 1:8

that children acquire during solitary play, peer interaction, and small-group, adult-led instruction. For example, in the preceding chapter, Friendly identified key goals of effective ECEC programs, including: enhancing children's well-being, healthy development, and lifelong learning; supporting parents in education, training, and employment; fostering social cohesion; and providing equity. Although these goals are exemplary social principles to embed in an ECEC program, an intervention that hopes to change the course of a specific child's life must correspond with the child's learning capabilities and support the development of more advanced skills. In order to support early learning, children require a responsive relationship with an adult.

A responsive, tailored one-on-one environment was the key to Skeels's (1966) intervention. The children who were moved from the orphanage to the institution with adults were immersed in a highly responsive environment where people interacted with them in individualized ways. Notably, the adult-child ratio in Skeels's (1966) orphanages was about 1:7 (i.e., four or five staff to 30–35 children). However, it is likely that the adult-to-child ratio in the institution was more like 7:1. According to Skeels, even though many of these adults were intellectually disabled, most of the adults in the residence were able to be highly responsive in developmentally appropriate ways with the children. This has implications for social policy. ECEC workers, who are trained to be aware of the importance of responsivity, would likely be very effective at impacting children's cognitive development if their efforts were supported with lower adult-to-child ratios.

Conclusion: Implications for Early Education as a Social Determinant of Health

The social demographic information on Canadian children shows signs that we are failing to meet their needs. For example, data from the National Longitudinal Survey of Children and Youth (NLSCY) indicates that children are increasingly more anxious and less likely to display age-appropriate social behaviours (Government of Canada, 2006). Rises in childhood obesity, diabetes, and other eating disorders have reached alarming levels (Shields, 2005). How are we failing our children?

One trend that may be having an impact is the degree to which families and children are socially isolated. In the past, we associated deprivation with poverty, poor environments, and neglect. The neglect was caused in large part by parents struggling with the ramifications and/or causes of poverty (i.e., addiction, mental illness, stress). However, the current trend is impacting children from across socio-economic boundaries. I propose that as a society, many of our children are facing a different form of deprivation: social interaction deprivation.

Increasingly, post-modern children live in settings that are relatively isolated from social contact. For example, in an extended family environment, children have the opportunity to receive attention from members of their extended family and not just their parents. Attention from a variety of adults provides two major benefits. It not only provides important relief for parents because looking after children is a very tiring and frustrating activity, but it provides multiple opportunities for the child to interact with individuals in a warm and responsive manner. Because families are smaller today than at any other point in history (Canadian Council on Social Development, 2006) and people often live away from their extended family network, many children do not have the opportunity to interact regularly with a variety of family members.

Additionally, the proportion of families where either both parents work (or single parents who work) is steadily increasing. For example, according to Statistics Canada, the percentage of children in child care in Canada has increased from 42 percent (1994–1995) to 53 percent (2000–2001; *The Daily,* February 2007). For many preschool children, this reduces their time in one-on-one interactions because eight to 10 hours are spent in sleep and nine to 10 hours are spent in child care (parent workday and commute time). Much of the remaining time is spent eating, dressing, cleaning, and other doing organizational activities. On weekends, families often catch up with shopping, cleaning, and other chores. As well, in an average week, preschoolers watch over 17 hours of television and/or videos (Media-Awareness Network, 2007).

Parents recognize the impact of time constraints on their children. According to Roberts and Gowan (2007), over 51 percent of parents indicated that work negatively impacted on the time they had with their children, and 42 percent of these families said that work had a negative impact on their relationships with their children. However, the majority of families cope with the stress and strain of balancing work and family life quite well and most children receive enough one-on-one time to meet the environmental needs for their cognitive development. Unfortunately, for some children this lack of time in one-on-one interaction with a caregiver who is scaffolding their learning environment may cause difficulties. This would be particularly true if the child had a difficulty in learning or a social-processing deficit. These children may need more intensive interaction to ensure that they develop along a typical pathway than is provided in modern families.

The impact of increasing isolation on child development creates a social dilemma: If young children require responsive and individualized attention in order to optimally learn, how does a society support this need? There are two main streams of thought on this issue: Encourage parents and family members to alter their work patterns to spend more time with their children. This perspective is often associated with a traditionalist, conservative agenda where the responsibility of child rearing is viewed as a family responsibility, but it is also associated with initiatives that support parental involvement. For example, one social program that reflects this philosophy is the Federal Parental Leave program, which allows some parents to stay at home with their children through a combination of unpaid and paid leave for up to 89 weeks through the Employment Insurance program. As well, this philosophy is evident in flexible work arrangements that allow parents to reduce the total number of hours they work outside the home (Roberts and Gowan, 2007).

Alternatively, a second philosophy is to develop social services where others support the family by providing child care and early education while parents work. This is often associated with a more liberal social agenda and is the motivation for a national ECEC program. This agenda is also associated with initiatives to increase the quality and efficacy of licensed ECEC agencies. For example, Ontario's Ministry of Children and Youth Services established an Expert Panel on Quality and Human Resources to advise policy-makers on ECEC issues (see online resources at the end of this chapter). The ministry also established an Expert Panel to develop an Early Learning Framework outlining the goals for ECEC programs supporting the development of preschool children and infants (see online resources at the end of this chapter). These documents support the need for highly responsive, low adult-child ratio learning environments in child-care settings, staffed by highly trained and valued professionals.

The optimal development of children requires the provision of early, intensive, and, most importantly, systematic early learning programs. The decisions on how to accomplish this goal is a social/political debate. In policy, there is often a focus on higher social goals and the needs of the individual are lost. However, any program or policy hoping to change outcomes for children must consider the mechanisms that will be responsible for the change at this level. With early learning initiatives, these mechanisms are the developmental processes that drive the course of development and prepare a child for his or her social context.

Note

1.   The author would like to acknowledge the support and assistance of Richard Vachon, who supported the research and writing of the chapter.

Critical Thinking Questions

1.   Some advocates have been charged with oversimplifying the developmental processes and their impact on lifelong learning and health, mainly to justify the need for preschool interventions, while others have suggested that this overstatement was necessary to mobilize policy-makers and generate public support. Critics have suggested that

this overstatement has led to an emphasis on preschool interventions at the expense of education and interventions for older children and young adults. Is oversimplification necessary or a manipulation of social policy?

2. Skeels's (1966) study was initiated in 1938 and incorporated a very controversial methodology that would not meet modern ethical standards. What does this study reveal about the attitudes and beliefs about the causes of social deprivation prevalent at that time? Have those ideas changed? What does this study reveal about historic attitudes toward people who are intellectually disabled? Have these attitudes changed for better or worse in our current society?

3. The social cost of meeting the need for intensive and systematic interventions that will be effective for young children is quite high. Although the potential cost savings are substantial, the major benefits are not realized for years. Given the public's reluctance for increased social costs and the need for governments to have measurable results of their policy initiatives in the four- to five-year election cycle, what are some political strategies for implementing initiatives with long-term benefits?

Recommended Readings

Hewlett, S.A. (1991). *When the bough breaks: The cost of neglecting our children.* New York: Harper Perennial.

This book provides a very insightful perspective on the impact of neglect and social trends on the development and well-being of children in the latter part of the 20th century. Although the book is now somewhat historic, many of the social trends and their impact are still pertinent today.

McCain, M.N. & Mustard, J.F. (1999). *Early years study: Reversing the real brain drain.* Toronto: Ontario Children's Secretariat. Online at www.childsec.gov.on.ca

This report provides a compelling rationale for the focus on early intervention as a social strategy for the health and well-being of society. The authors reference a huge body of evidence describing biological, neurological, and social evidence supporting the efficacy of early intervention.

Skeels, H.M. (1966). "Adult status of children with contrasting early life experiences: A follow-up study." *Monographs of the Society for Research in Child Development, 31*(3), 1–56.

In this comprehensive review of his research on the children living in orphanages and long-term residences for the mentally retarded, Skeels outlines the progression of his suspicions about the role of attention and enriched social experiences during his early work with Dye, which culminated in the study contrasting two groups of children. He describes in great detail the follow-up study conducted 20 years later when the children were adults. This study illustrates the potential of early interventions for children in impoverished conditions, and also details the limits of early assessments of potential.

Werner, E.E. & Smith, R.S. (2001). *Journey from childhood to midlife: Risk, resilience, and recovery.* Ithaca: Cornell University Press.

Werner and Smith provide a comprehensive overview of the development of resilience among children born in poverty on the island of Kauai. This study is remarkable in that it followed the children for 40 years.

Related Web Sites

Centre of Excellence for Early Childhood Development—www.excellence-earlychildhood.ca

The centre provides summaries of high-quality empirical and theoretical work in early child development. The centre's focus is on mobilizing knowledge to support the development of evidence-based policy in the form of reports, linkages, and bulletins. The centre also has compiled a very useful and informative online encyclopedia on early child development and a directory of researchers in the field.

Human Early Learning Partnership (HELP)—www.earlylearning.ubc.ca

HELP is an interdisciplinary group of faculty and researchers across universities in British Columbia who work on creating new knowledge in the area of early child development and on developing tools for communities, policy-makers, and researchers to develop effective interventions. A very interesting aspect of HELP's work is the development of interactive mapping to illustrate population patterns in school readiness and other social factors to support program planning.

Report by the Expert Panel on Early Learning—www.children.gov.on.ca/NR/CS/Publications/en_elf.pdf

In this document, the expert panel on early learning outline a framework describing milestones in key domains of development from birth until age six. The early learning framework provides a detailed perspective on the goals of early learning programs that is developmentally appropriate. This document is designed to support the development of high-quality ECEC programs.

Report by the Expert Panel on Quality in Human Resources—www.children.gov.on.ca/NR/CS/Publications/QHRReport_en.pdf

This report outlines the issues concerning the development and maintenance of high-quality human resources in the area of early child education (ECE). The expert panel makes recommendations for policy-makers around the need to address low wages and other working conditions to improve recruitment and retention of ECE professionals.

—●—

Chapter 11

THE STATE AND QUALITY OF CANADIAN PUBLIC ELEMENTARY AND SECONDARY EDUCATION

Charles Ungerleider, Tracey Burns, and Fernando Cartwright

Introduction

Since its inception in the late 19th century, universal public schooling in Canada has responded to forces arising beyond its borders as it has prepared the young for the responsibilities of adult citizenship. This chapter explores the impact of demographic, social, and political forces on the state and quality of Canadian public elementary and secondary schools.

Notwithstanding their considerable successes, Canadian public schools struggle to respond to the challenges posed by changes to Canadian society. Failure to respond to the challenges puts public schools at risk. In turn, because of the centrality of public schooling in the transmission of core Canadian values, the failure of public schooling puts Canada at risk.

Canada Transformed

Social, demographic, and economic changes have transformed Canada and Canadian families with consequences for the education and educability of school-age children. People are marrying later in life, having fewer children, and delaying childbirth (Statistics Canada, 2007). High rates of separation and divorce have created new family relationships: Common-law marriages, single-parent households, step-families, and blended families have brought about changes affecting the education of the children living in those families (Statistics Canada, 2006).

Children from More Advantaged Families Perform Better in School

Those who delay parenthood tend to have more formal education and higher family incomes. The reverse is true for those who have children early. Children living in families with two parents have more favourable behavioural, psychological, and school outcomes than children living in lone-parent or step-families, even when socio-economic conditions are controlled (Kerr & Beaujot, 2001), but more than one-third of all marriages end in divorce. Children of families that have experienced disruption are more likely to leave home at an earlier age because of family conflict and less likely to return home after they have left (Ravanera, 2000). Adolescents whose parents divorced were more likely to remain unmarried, and if they did marry, were likely to marry later and have their own marriages end in divorce or separation (Corak, 1999).

Child poverty remains a significant Canadian problem. Over the past quarter century, income inequality between families with children has worsened (Ross, Roberts & Scott, 2000, pp. 51–54).

Average market income in the bottom decile fell by 18.7 percent from 1979 to 1989 and by a further 10.7 percent from 1989 to 2004. Average market income in the top decile rose by 12.7 percent in the 1980s and by 21.6 percent in the 1989–2004 period (Heisz, 2007, p. 23).

Estimates indicate that 22 percent of the approximately 1.4 million children 15 years of age or younger in Canada were living in low-income families in 1996 (Canadian Education Statistics Council, 2000, pp. 17–18).

Socio-economic status has a direct impact on higher levels of achievement and superior academic focus. Young children who live in families with lower incomes and children living in single-parent families face more challenges than older children and children in two-parent families. Children living in poor families have higher rates of emotional and behavioural disorders, are less likely to perform well in school, and may experience a lower level of social acceptance by others (Canadian Education Statistics Council, 2000; Phipps & Lethbridge,

2006). For children living in single-parent families, the situation is considerably worse—more than half live below the Statistics Canada low-income cut-off.

Children in low-income families differ from children in moderate or high-income families in ways that affect their socialization and education both directly and indirectly. They are more likely to live in poorly functioning families; live in neighbourhoods where drug use and alcohol consumption is prevalent; be in the top 10 percent in frequency of delinquent behaviours; have high delinquency scores; have a problem with one or more basic abilities such as vision, hearing, speech, or

---

Box 11.1: Participation in post-secondary university education and family income: 1993–2001

Most young people have aspirations of attending university and, according to the 2002 *Survey of Approaches to Education Planning*, over 80 percent of Canadian children had parents whose aspirations for them included going to university (Shipley et al., 2003, cited in Drolet, 2005). Yet the chances that young people will be able to realize this goal are strongly linked to family income: Young people from high-income families were two times as likely as those from low-income families to have participated in university education in the period 1993–2001. In 2001, 45.6 percent of youth from high-income families ($100,000 or more) have completed or were enrolled in university, compared to only 19.5 percent of youths from the lowest-income families (less than $25,000).

Participation in post-secondary university education and family income, 1993-2001

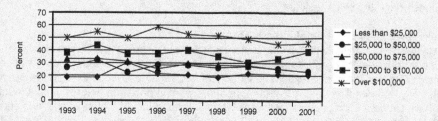

Source: Drolet, M. (2005). Statistics Canada. Data are from the *Survey of Labour and Income Dynamics* (SLID), 1993–2001. Online at www.statcan.ca/english/research/11F0019MIE/11F0019MIE200543.pdf.

As the above graph demonstrates, university participation rates generally rise with family income. However, from an equity perspective, there is one troubling detail: The participation rates for youth from families with modest incomes are little different from those with the lowest incomes. As mentioned above, in 2001 only 19.5 percent of youth from families in the lowest-income bracket participated in university compared to 23 percent of youth from families with incomes between $25,000 and $50,000, and 25 percent from families with incomes between $50,000 and $75,000. Compared to the 46.5 percent of youth from families with incomes of $100,000 or more, this is worrying.

Also worrying is the lack of change in these patterns over the eight years under consideration. In 1996 youth from high-income families had university participation rates that were 37.1 percent higher than the rates for youth from the lowest-income families; in 2001 this difference was 26.1 percent. Although reduced, the gaps are not statistically significant from one another. The pattern remains essentially unchanged.

Source: Drolet, M. (2005). Statistics Canada. Data are from the *Survey of Labour and Income Dynamics* (SLID), 1993–2001, online at www.statcan.ca/english/research/11F0019MIE/11F0019MIE200543.pdf.

mobility; and exhibit delayed vocabulary development (Ross, Roberts & Scott (2000, pp. 51–54). In addition, socio-economic status has an indirect influence on achievement. Higher socio-economic status is correlated with lower levels of parental depression, which, in turn, diminishes the incidence of family dysfunction, lowering

---

Box 11.2: Factors related to adolescents' self-perceived health, 2000–2001

While the majority of Canadian adolescents considered themselves to be in "very good" or "excellent" health in 2000–2001, nearly one in three 12- to 17-year-olds rated their health as no better than "good," according to a new study. Adolescents who considered their own health to be poor, fair or good were more likely to smoke, drink, or be obese. They were also less likely to live in a relatively high-income household. The study also found that the lower the educational level in the adolescent's household, the worse his or her self-rated health is likely to be.

Boys' self-perceived health tends to be better than that of girls. According to data from the 2000–2001 *Canadian Community Health Survey* (CCHS), girls' perceptions of health become less favourable in mid- to late adolescence. At ages 12–14, 73 percent of boys and girls reported very good or excellent health. But by ages 15–17, the proportion for boys remained about the same, while it dropped to 66 percent for girls.

Girls Are Vulnerable to Depression
Mental health is a major factor in overall health. Previous studies have shown that adolescents, particularly girls, are vulnerable to depression. According to the 2000–2001 CCHS, nearly 6 percent of 12- to 14-year-old girls had a high risk of having had a major depressive episode in the year before the survey, compared with 2 percent of boys the same age. Among 15- to 17-year-olds, the proportion of girls who had had such an episode was much higher (11 percent).
     By contrast, 15- to 17-year-old boys were no more at risk of depression than those aged 12–14.
     Depression was significantly associated with reduced odds of reporting excellent or very good health for both older and younger adolescents, even accounting for other factors such as chronic conditions, socio-economic status, obesity, and health behaviours.

Knowledge of Risks Doesn't Prevent Smoking and Drinking
Smoking and drinking were associated with the way that adolescents rate their health. Even after accounting for other contributing factors, the 15- to 17-year-olds who were daily smokers or episodic heavy drinkers had lower odds of reporting very good or excellent health, compared with those who did not drink or smoke. "Episodic heavy drinking" is defined as having five or more drinks on one occasion at least once a month.
     Other studies have suggested that adolescents may be aware of the health effects of smoking and excessive drinking. Nonetheless, 14 percent of 15- to 17-year-olds were daily smokers, with girls slightly more likely than boys to smoke daily. About the same proportion of adolescents in that age group also reported episodic heavy drinking, although in this case, the practice was more common among boys.

Obesity Also Key Factor in Self-Perceived Health
Being obese lowered the odds of an adolescent reporting very good or excellent health, even when the effects of other potential factors were taken into account. The study also found that adolescents who reported relatively low fruit and vegetable consumption or being physically inactive had lower odds of reporting very good or excellent health.

Chronic Conditions
In 2000–2001, a substantial number (29 percent) of 12- to 17-year-olds reported having at least one chronic condition, most commonly asthma, bronchitis, back pain, or migraine. For boys, the prevalence of chronic conditions did not differ by age. For girls, however, the prevalence of chronic conditions was significantly higher for the older age group (36 percent).

Source: Statistics Canada, *The Daily*, October 31, 2003.

the amount of hostile parenting. Lower levels of hostile parenting contribute to better academic focus, which, in turn, influences higher achievement (Ryan & Adams, 1999, pp. 30–43).

Changing Patterns of Socialization

Schools attempt to address problems that have their origin in unsuccessful socialization prior to the youngster entering school. More Canadian children have relatively little supervision than at any previous time. Initial socialization that was once provided directly by family members is now provided by a combination of parents, caregivers, a child's peers, and the media. Access to media has exposed them to values and experiences that children a half-century ago would not have acquired until they attended school for some time. Though still eager to learn when they come to school, today's youngsters are equally eager to be entertained.

The Aggression Trap

Aggression among young people is creating stress in schools. Although they are reputed to underreport, about 15 percent of Canadian students say their peers abuse them. This figure is consistent with reports from other countries (e.g., in 2007 10 percent of students reported being bullied in Norway, with similar numbers in the Slovak Republic and Germany (International Network on School Bullying and Violence, oecd-sbv.net/Templates/MainSubject.aspx?id=16. In 1997, the National Crime Prevention Council of Canada interviewed 6,000 Canadian students from grades one to eight. Six percent of the students admitted to bullying other children more than once or twice in the previous six weeks. Twenty percent admitted to being involved as either a bully or victim more than once or twice during the school term (Pepler & Craig, 1997).

Richard Tremblay, chair of Child Development at the University of Montreal, points out that children who do not learn alternatives to physical aggression early in life are more likely to be: hyperactive and inattentive; less likely to respond when others need help; often rejected or isolated by their classmates; more disruptive in school; more likely to leave school before graduation; more likely to have serious accidents; more likely to engage in violent

behaviour; and more likely to be charged under Canada's Young Offenders Act. Such children have lower grades, are more susceptible to substance abuse, and have sexual intercourse earlier and more frequently than children who have learned to solve conflicts peacefully (Tremblay, 2000, pp. 19–24).

According to Tremblay (2000), studies following aggressive children into their adult years have shown that there are extremely negative consequences for the aggressive individuals, for their mates, their children, and for the communities in which they live. These consequences include early parenthood, unemployment, family violence, and poverty. "From this perspective," says Tremblay, "failure to teach children to regulate violent behaviour during the early years leads to poverty much more clearly than poverty leads to violence" (2000, p. 14).

Scholars from the University of Guelph and the University of Toronto who analyzed data from the *National Longitudinal Survey of Children and Youth* found that "children who were less committed to schools were more likely to be involved in aggressive behaviour" (Sprott, Doob & Jenkins, 2001). Children who report disliking school are three times more likely to say they have been involved in aggressive acts than children who say they like school a lot. In general, "children who do not like school, think they are not doing well, think grades are not important, and do not want to go far in school are more likely to be involved in aggressive acts." The social relationships that students had in school were related to their involvement in aggressive acts. Children are more likely to be involved in aggressive behaviours when they "feel unsafe at school, that they are being bullied, that other children say mean things to them, and that they feel like an outsider."

Youth involved in delinquent acts involving property are, similarly, more likely to have low educational aspirations. In general, "children who do not like school, whose school progress is poor and think that grades are not important are more likely to be involved in delinquent acts involving property." Low educational aspirations, the belief that teachers do not like them and do not treat them fairly, and skipping classes are also associated with delinquent acts involving property.

School academic and social factors are not the only things leading to delinquent and aggressive behaviour.

Risk factors in the family and environment are also associated with such behaviours. Basically, the more risk factors children and youth face, the more likely they are to say they are engaged in aggressive and delinquent behaviours.

Demographic Changes

Changing sources of immigration, increasing linguistic diversity, growing numbers of Aboriginal children, the survival of low birth-weight babies, and a growing proportion of children with special needs make demands upon public schooling that were less evident 50 years ago. The number of children with learning disabilities is increasing. New medical technologies have saved the lives of children who, even a decade ago, would not have survived birth, resulting in a dramatic increase in the number of children with severely impaired cognitive abilities entering public schools (c.f., Behnia & Duclos, 2003). Deinstitutionalization in the health and social services sectors has resulted in retention in the community of students who, in previous generations, would have been "out of sight, out of mind." More sophisticated diagnosis of learning and behavioural problems has led to parents' higher expectations that the diagnosed conditions will be addressed.

Approximately one-tenth of students receive some form of special education because of learning disabilities, emotional or behavioural problems, problems at home, speech impairment, intellectual or physical disabilities, language problems, or other problems that limit their ability to do school work. Children living in low-income families are more likely to receive special education. Children living in single-parent families (17 percent) are twice as likely as children from two-parent families (9 percent) to receive special education assistance and to have "problems at home" (63 percent vs. 37 percent). Children receiving special education (24 percent) are more likely to have a parent who did not finish high school than children who are not receiving special education (14 percent) (Bohatyretz & Lipps, 1999, pp. 7–19). They are also more likely to be boys (60 percent) than girls (40 percent) (Organisation for Economic Co-operation and Development, 2007b).

Over the course of the past 25 years, Canadian students have also become more diverse in terms of their ethnocultural backgrounds. At any given time, Canada's population includes 15 percent born elsewhere. Diversity is also evident in the presence of languages other than French or English. Linguistic diversity poses challenges to public schools. Because immigrant integration depends upon the education of children and youth, public schools play a central part in helping those who do not speak English or French to acquire one of Canada's official languages and in ensuring that children learn about respectful treatment of people from backgrounds different from their own. Once ignored, addressing the differences among students from differing backgrounds and the challenges those differences sometimes produce is central to ensuring the success of all students and ameliorating inequalities that threaten Canada's social cohesion.

Aboriginal and First Nations Learners

People of Aboriginal ancestry make up approximately 4.4 percent of the Canadian population. The birth rate among Aboriginal Canadians exceeds that of non-Aboriginals. In 2004 the birth rate for Status (i.e., registered) Indians was 22.6 per 1,000 population, compared to 10.5 per 1,000 for the Canadian population as a whole. Status Indians have a median age of 25 compared with a median age of 35 for the Canadian population as a whole.

The First Nations population in Canada is young, growing, and moving more toward band-centred education. The proportion of children enrolled in band-operated elementary and secondary schools is increasing (from 44 percent in 1990–1991 to 61 percent in 2000–2001). The remaining 39 percent of children are enrolled in schools under the jurisdiction of provincial (37 percent) or federal (1 percent) governments (Department of Indian Affairs and Northern Development, 2002). The decline in attendance at federal and provincial schools signals a change in the role of the band in First Nations education. While this trend is positive in terms of band self-determination and identity, it also raises the possibility of greater variance in the quality of instruction and education between schools of different bands and social circumstances. Lowering the variance among band schools becomes crucially important in light of Chandler's findings that the prevalence of adolescent suicides and other correlated social variables were directly (and inversely) linked to the level of band self-determination across BC communities (Chandler & Lalonde, 1998, pp. 191–219).

Graduation rates for Aboriginal and First Nations are well below levels for the rest of Canada. In 2001, 48 percent of Aboriginal youth aged 20–24 had incomplete secondary school as their highest level of schooling (Statistics Canada, 2003b). Aboriginal students attending provincial public schools are much less successful than their non-Aboriginal classmates.

One of the factors that may account for the low performance of Aboriginal and non-Aboriginal students is the mismatch between the world views of Aboriginal students and the world view that permeates the subjects taught in elementary and secondary schools. For example, Aikenhead (2001) has described most Aboriginal students' experience with science education "as an attempt at assimilation into a foreign culture." These world view differences are illustrated by the experience of Kickapoo Indian children studying in off-reserve schools: Kickapoo students prefer co-operative learning rather than the competitive learning environment fostered in Western classrooms. They tend to think holistically about the natural world, whereas the Western science approach explains things by reducing complex systems to simpler parts. Kickapoo students view time and space as cyclical in nature while these concepts are treated more linearly in Western science. Kinship, harmony, co-operation, and spiritualism with respect to the natural world are highly valued by Kickapoo students, while the corresponding Western values are more exploitative, competitive, decontextualized, rational, and materialistic. In Western science classrooms, Kickapoo students were unengaged and showed little evidence of learning; however, the very same students faced with the very same lessons in a different context (i.e., in their own village) were active, engaged, and showed evidence of learning by enthusiastically answering questions (Canadian Council on Learning, 2007).

The cultural mismatch between Aboriginal and Western science world views forces many Aboriginals to choose between three problematic strategies for coping with science education:

1. They can learn Western science by adopting a Western science world view and abandoning or allowing the marginalization of their Aboriginal values and ways of knowing.

2. They can acquire enough superficial knowledge of the material presented in science classes to achieve a passing grade without acquiring a meaningful understanding of the concepts, thus avoiding potential threats to their Aboriginal identity.

3. They can avoid learning any science at all and accept the consequent failing grades and/or lack of participation in science education. (Canadian Council on Learning, 2007)

None of these choices is a satisfactory approach to developing an interest in, and capacity for, understanding science.

The significant gap between Aboriginal and non-Aboriginal students is evidence that public schools have a long way to go in addressing the factors that impede the progress of Aboriginal learners. Until recently (Canadian Council on Learning, 2007), public schools have done relatively little to address racism, low expectations, and the neglect that produces low academic achievement, poor grade-to-grade transitions, student mobility, and abysmal failure rates, especially for Aboriginal learners.

Canadians' Expectations for Learning Are Changing

In 2006, the Canadian Council on Learning published the results of the first of its annual surveys of Canadian opinion about various dimensions of learning. Administered to more than 5,000 Canadians on behalf of the Council by Statistics Canada, the survey asked respondents how critical the various stages of learning were to success in life. The majority of respondents agreed or strongly agreed that learning at each stage—first five years (87 percent), elementary school (95 percent), high school (93 percent), and post-secondary (83 percent)—is critical to success in life (Canadian Council on Learning, 2006a).

Between 92 percent and 96 percent of respondents agreed that teaching students the basics (reading, writing, and arithmetic), preparing students for work and for education after high school, and teaching students to be good citizens and to love learning were important goals. A strong majority of Canadians agreed that schools were doing a good job achieving the goals, but the response patterns indicated that people with recent experience with

Canadian elementary or secondary schools (i.e., those who attended or have a child who attended school within the last five years) felt there was considerable room for improvement. While 80 percent of the respondents agreed that schools did a good job with the basics and 79 percent felt similarly about preparation for citizenship, only about two-thirds of the respondents were as satisfied with the way that schools were preparing students for work and for the love of learning (Canadian Council on Learning, 2006b).

Canadian Public Elementary and Secondary Students Do Well

Canadian public elementary and secondary students do well. The educational attainment of Canadians has risen steadily over the years. According to Statistics Canada, more Canadians are graduating from high school (Statistics Canada, 2002; Canadian Council on Learning, 2005), and continuing on to post-secondary education (Statistics Canada, 1998). In 1991, 25 percent of men and 21 percent of women aged 25–34 did not have a high school diploma. By 2001, this figure had declined to 15 percent (Statistics Canada, 2003a). During the same period, the percentage of Canadians in this age group who had earned university degrees rose from 17 percent to 26 percent (Statistics Canada, 2000).

In 1995, Canada had the highest percentage of the population (48 percent) with some post-secondary education compared with an average of 23 percent for the member nations of the Organisation for Economic Co-operation and Development (OECD). However, in 2005 Canada ranked slightly below the OECD average for enrolment rates for both 15–19-year-olds and 19–29-year-olds (Organisation for Economic Co-operation and Development, 2007a). Although Canada has been a high performer internationally in the past, it has not kept pace with the advancement of other countries in this area.

In addition, Canada's ratio of graduates to population aged 18 (75 percent) is the second lowest among G-7 countries. Another troubling statistic is the number of years Canadian children expect to stay in school. Among all the countries surveyed by the OECD from 1995–2002, only Canada showed a decrease in the number of expected years in school across the time period (Canadian Education Statistics Council, 2000). Unfortunately,

more recent data were not available (Organisation for Economic Co-operation and Development, 2007a).

One of the many success stories of Canadian education is the improvement Canadian women have made in educational attainment (Statistics Canada, 2000). In fact, among the population between the ages of 25–29, women now achieve higher levels of educational attainment than men (Canadian Education Statistics Council, 2000; Statistics Canada 2003a).

Canadian students perform well in reading, mathematics, and science, according to an OECD study that assessed the performance of 15-year-olds in these subjects. Canadian students were among the best-performing students in reading, science, and mathematics among the 32 countries that participated in the OECD's Programme for International Student Assessment (PISA) (Organisation for Economic Co-operation and Development, 2000b, 2003, 2006).

There are, however, sizable differences among the provinces, with Alberta, Quebec, and British Columbia obtaining significantly higher scores than other provinces and territories. In addition, Canada was one of only three countries (along with Germany and France) where gender was significant in the performance on the math test, with boys outperforming girls in all three countries. Science was the main focus for PISA 2006. Mathematics and reading were assessed, but not to the same degree. Nonetheless, gender differences in mathematics and reading were consistent with results from previous PISA assessments. Boys outperformed girls in mathematics and girls outperformed boys in reading (Bussière et al., 2007).

Canada as a whole performs well on national and international assessments, but disparities exist among populations and regions that do not seem to be diminishing with time. In addition, gender differences persist in older children, with girls outperforming boys in reading and boys outperforming girls in math. The PISA data indicate that the male advantage in math is not a worldwide trend and thus cannot be dismissed as a result of "gendered abilities." Along with the rest of the world, Canada shows a significant difference in performance on PISA literacy tests as a function of socio-economic status and immigrant status. Lower socio-economic status and second-language students perform less well than students from more advantaged and non-immigrant backgrounds, though immigrants in Canada fare better than immigrants elsewhere (Bussière et al., 2007, p. 40). Nonetheless, performance differences among identifiable groups are worrisome.

Early School Leaving

The Canadian Council on Learning commissioned Statistics Canada to analyze Canadian school attendance data from its Labour Force Survey (LFS). The school year 1990–1991 was the first year for which dropout rates were calculated using the LFS. During that year, the dropout rate was 17 percent. By 2004–2005, only 10 percent of Canadians 20–24 years of age did not have a high school diploma and were not enrolled in school. Nonetheless, that means that in 2004–2005, 212,000 Canadians between the ages of 20 and 24 had not completed high school, nor were they currently enrolled in a high school program.

Dropping out of high school is becoming less common in all parts of Canada, but the decrease in the dropout rate is most apparent in eastern Canada. For the 1990–1991 to 1992–1993 school years, close to 20 percent of 20- to 24-year-olds in Newfoundland and Labrador and in Prince Edward Island were without a high school diploma and were not attending school, the highest dropout rates in the country at the time. During the three most recent school years, the dropout rate in both of these provinces has been in the range of 8–10 percent, putting them among the lowest in Canada. Dropout rates also declined sharply in Nova Scotia and New Brunswick.

Although dropout rates have exhibited a downward trend across Canada, not all population subgroups have declined in equal proportion. Dropout rates are higher among boys than girls, Aboriginal learners, and among learners in some small towns and rural areas.

Young males leave school before graduation at higher rates than young women. In 1990–1991, 19 percent of males between the ages of 20 and 24 had not completed high school compared to 14 percent of young women. By 2004–2005, the rate for young men was down to 12 percent and to 7 percent for young women.

Although the overrepresentation of males among young dropouts is not a new phenomenon, the share of male school leavers has increased in recent years. In 1990–1991, the majority of dropouts were young men (58 percent). By 2004–2005, that proportion had increased to 64 percent. The change in proportion for males does not indicate that more young men are dropping out; in fact, there has been a decrease in the actual number of male dropouts. The proportional increase for males reflects the fact that the dropout rate for young women has fallen more sharply than for young men. Across Canada the pattern is the same: More men than women drop out. The difference is most pronounced in Quebec where, in 2004–2005, seven in 10 young dropouts were men (Canadian Council on Learning, 2005).

Despite the reduction in the dropout rate, it is still high in some populations. The *Youth in Transition Survey* provides a relatively comprehensive profile of dropouts and graduates: Dropouts are more likely than graduates to live in "mixed" (vs. nuclear) families and single-parent families. Twice as many graduates (57 percent compared to 28 percent of dropouts) had at least one parent who completed post-secondary education, and three times as many graduates had at least one parent who completed a university degree (Bowlby & McMullen, 2002, see Table 11.1).

In terms of work, there is a bimodal distribution for dropouts. They were both less likely than graduates to have worked in their last year of high school and more likely to have worked at a job more than 30 hours a week. Dropouts are also more likely to have children (14 percent of dropouts vs. 2 percent of graduates). For women, 28 percent of all dropouts had children (compared to 5 percent of male dropouts). More than half of the female dropouts with children were single.

Overall, the data on graduation rates are positive in that they show declining rates of dropping out. However, they also reveal that students in danger of dropping out generally fit a well-established demographic profile. They exhibit readily identifiable behaviours at school and in the community, which is characterized primarily by non-involvement. These patterns of behaviour have remained constant in the last 15 years. Most troubling is the finding that over a quarter of female dropouts had children, and half of those were single parents, making the possibility of returning to school less likely. These data suggest that more resources for at-risk adolescents and teen parents would further decrease the dropout rate and increase dropouts' likelihood of returning to complete their studies (c.f., Ontario, 2007).

Table 11.1: Selected findings from the Youth in Transition Survey (developed from Bowlby & McMullen, 2002)

	Graduates	Dropouts
Family Structure		
• Two-parent family	81%	66%
• Single-parent family	16%	33%
Parental Education		
• University degree	31%	11%
• Post-secondary certificate or diploma	26%	17%
• High school	45%	34%
• Less than high school	9%	27%
Father's Occupation		
• Management	17%	9%
• Business, finance, and administration	9%	4%
• Health, natural, and applied science	12%	6%
• Social science, government, art, culture, and recreation	9%	4%
• Sales and service	13%	13%
• Trades, transport, and equipment operators	25%	41%
• Primary processing, manufacturing, and utilities	16%	23%
Academic Grades (Overall GPA final year)		
• 80–100% A	42%	13%
• 70–79% B	43%	35%
• 60–69% C	14%	35%
• 50–59% D	1%	14%
• < 50% F	—	4%
Hours worked for pay each week during the last year of high school		
• 0–No job	37%	48%
• 1–9	17%	11%
• 10–19	23%	13%
• 20–29	17%	16%
• 30 or more	5%	13%
Peer Influence and Behaviours		
• Most or all close friends planning to further education or training beyond high school	79%	52%
• Skipped class once per week	21%	58%
• Drank alcoholic beverages one a week or more during the last year of high school	29%	38%
• Used marijuana or hash once a week or more during the last year of high school	9%	28%
Educational Aspirations		
• University degree	65%	23%
• College, CEGEP, trade, vocational, or business school	26%	45%
• Some post-secondary	1%	4%
• High school completion	2%	20%
• Less than high school completion	—	4%
• Undecided	6%	6%

Gender and Educational Achievement

Recent reports indicate that there is still a trend for girls to encounter difficulties when transitioning between elementary and high school, and for boys to have more difficulty transitioning between high school and post-secondary education. There are also continuing differences in academic achievement in math and reading related to gender and age, as discussed above (McCall, 1998; Organisation for Economic Co-operation and Development, 2003).

In addition, teachers had higher expectations of future educational attainment for girls compared to boys. The role of teachers' expectations and behaviour is highlighted here as there is an urgent need for more research into how teachers' expectations translate into behaviour in the class. We need clearer data on the correlation between teacher evaluation, parent evaluation, and future academic and workplace performance.

Immigration

International data indicate that Canada is one of the few OECD countries whose first- and second-generation immigrants in the aggregate perform on the same level as native-born students. In fact, for some populations, immigrant students *outperform* their Canadian-born counterparts (Organisation for Economic Co-operation and Development, 2003, 2007a).

In addition, the 1994–1998 *National Longitudinal Survey of Children and Youth* indicate that: (1) children born in Canada of immigrant parents do at least as well as the children of Canadian-born parents; (2) children born in Canada of immigrant parents whose language is either English or French have especially high outcomes; (3) children born in Canada of immigrant parents whose language is neither English or French have problems in kindergarten, although by elementary school these problems remain only for reading. As would be expected, the longer the child stays in the school system, the less the difference between children of native- and non-native-born Canadians. By the age of 13, children born in Canada of immigrant parents perform at least as well as children of Canadian-born parents by the age of 13 (Lipps & Yiptong-Avila, 1999).

However, this analysis does not include data on children who themselves are immigrants to Canada, nor those who enter the Canadian school system after the age of 11. Using BC Ministry of Education data to examine the academic trajectories of different ethnocultural and English-proficient subsets of ESL students from the BC grade eight cohort of 1997, Garnett and Ungerleider (2008) found that Chinese-speaking ESL students fare very well in the school system even with limited English proficiency, whereas students from other linguistic groups exhibit weaker academic trajectories that are further diminished by limited English proficiency. Furthermore, given what we know about increasing difficulty of language acquisition after puberty, there is a real possibility that students who speak neither English nor French who enter Canadian schools after their elementary years will continue to have problems in scholastic performance, especially in reading and writing.

The Vulnerability of Public Schools and Students at Risk

Canadians can take pride in the accomplishments of their public schools. At the same time, they should be worried about their vulnerabilities and about the inequalities among students distinguished by socio-economic, ethnocultural, and gender differences. As Box 11.3 makes clear, education is fundamental to the well-being of society.

Most of human history is the story of political, social, and economic inequalities based upon accidents of birth or group membership. While there was gradual improvement in equality over time, largely following the Industrial Revolution, most of the significant improvements occurred after the Second World War. The Depression and the Second World War made Canadians conscious of the importance of fairness, human rights, and the need to diminish inequalities.

People who had suffered the privations of the Depression helped to forge policies that would ameliorate the most severe consequences of the accidents of birth, place of residence, or plain bad luck. People who had survived the nationalisms that permitted the extermination of people on the basis of their group membership helped to create institutions to protect human rights. People who had fled societies in which basic human rights and well-being were primarily determined by economic and social standing helped to create institutions that tempered the

Box 11.3: The Composite Learning Index

Learning, which occurs within formal settings such as public schools and in other informal and non-formal situations, has far-reaching consequences in spheres of social and economic activity that may appear disconnected from learning activities such as health.

The Composite Learning Index (CLI), developed by the Canadian Council on Learning, is the first index of its kind in the world, providing an annual measure of Canada's performance in a number of areas related to lifelong learning. The CLI 2007 is an aggregation of 27 indicators related to the pervasiveness and quality of learning in Canada. The single index score is composed of four sub-indices labelled "Learning to Know," "Learning to Do," "Learning to Live Together," and "Learning to Be" (Delors et al., 1996). Each of these sub-indices is an aggregation of indicators related to their respective domains. The indicators are aggregated in such a way that the composites have strong links to the social and economic well-being of communities in Canada. Social and economic well-being is measured by five variables:

1. the proportion reporting excellent or very good self-perceived health
2. the voter participation rate
3. the proportion of children who are vulnerable in at least one domain of the Early Development Inventory
4. the unemployment rate of adults 25–64 years old
5. the average income

The breadth of these outcomes eclipses the traditional scholastic outcomes of formal learning. Although successful learning is certainly not the primary factor influencing each of these outcomes, *it is one of the only factors affecting all of them*.

The correlations between the CLI index and sub-indices and each of these five outcomes, calculated across economic regions in Canada, are shown in Table 11.2 [economic regions (ER) are the unit of analysis because the majority of variation in the CLI and its indicators is between the 74 ERs for which data are available].

The Composite Learning Index and social and economic well-being of communities*

	Proportion reporting excellent or very good self-perceived health	Voter participation rate	Proportion of children who are vulnerable in at least one domain of the Early Development Inventory	Unemployment rate of adults 25–64 years old	Average household income
CLI	0.24	0.30	0.57	−0.70	0.73
To know	0.33	0.13	0.30	−0.35	0.65
To do	0.22	0.17	0.59	−0.64	0.62
To live together	-0.03	0.34	0.43	−0.61	0.30
To be	0.20	0.31	0.48	−0.62	0.66

*Note: All correlations in this table are significant at the $p < 0.01$ level. n = 74.

Given that the CLI is composed of indicators related to learning rather than variables explicitly related to each of these five outcomes, these correlations, which are moderately large for social research, are evidence of the pervasive impact of learning across macro-level social activity.

The Focus on Health

Although the CLI is constructed to maximize its relationship with all five outcomes simultaneously, it is possible to construct it to maximize the relationship with a single outcome, such as self-perceived health. Such a health-oriented CLI would not necessarily be the optimal measure of the impact of learning on general community well-being, but it would be a more accurate measure of the impact of learning on health specifically. The relationship of the health-oriented CLI and sub-indices with all outcomes is shown in Table 11.3.

The health-oriented Composite Learning Index and social and economic well-being of communities*

	Proportion reporting excellent or very good self-perceived health	Voter participation rate	Proportion of children who are vulnerable in at least one domain of the Early Development Inventory	Unemployment rate of adults 25–64 years old	Average household income
CLI[h]	0.43	0.16	0.21	−0.29	0.69
To know	0.35	0.10	0.19	−0.23	0.59
To do	0.31	0.28	0.41	−0.56	0.73
To live together	0.30	-0.14	-0.32	0.40	0.17
To be	0.37	0.20	0.19	−0.30	0.58

*Note: All correlations in this table are significant at the $p < 0.01$ level. n = 74.
This composite has been created to have an optimal relationship with self-perceived health.

The correlations in the table above indicate that all domains of learning have a non-trivial impact on the health of communities. The magnitude of the relationships is surprisingly similar across all four sub-indices despite the apparent dissimilarity between the indicators underlying each separate sub-index. Furthermore, although these composites are optimized for health, all remain moderately strong predictors of the other broad measures of social and economic well-being.

These results support the notion that learning—which happens in a variety of formal, informal, and non-formal situations—has far-reaching consequences in spheres of social and economic activity that may appear superficially disconnected from learning activities.

most egregious consequences of inequalities. But these changes, largely occurring after the Second World War, seem to have been relatively short-lived.

Conclusion

Today, strong forces are at work to alter the relationship between citizens and government in order to diminish the part that government plays in our lives. The still malleable citizenship that was created in the postwar period is devolving into something "old" and "worn out." Canada is becoming a country that wants to make individuals responsible for looking after themselves, rather than a country that says we create institutions to look after each other.

From Whalley to Whitehorse, from Hazelton to Halifax, and from Saanich to St. John's, the trends are the same: As most of the population ages, concerns have changed. Interest in child care, education, and the part that education plays in ameliorating inequalities has been replaced by interest in pension protection and health care. For those who have remained interested in child care and education, orientations have changed. The balance between concern for the well-being of one's own children and for children generally has shifted to an emphasis on one's own children to the exclusion of other children.

Public schools are the institutions that we rely upon to bind us together as Canadians. They do it by communicating the values—fairness, respect for people, and a sense of social justice—that Canadians share. At a time when selfishness and individualism are increasing, ethnocentrism and alienation are growing, petty regionalisms divide us, and politicians describe concerned citizens as "special interests" and are capable of uniting only in opposition to their central government, we need an institution that can remind us of the values that we share and can help us to preserve our communities and our country. Canadian public schools are not perfect. There are many ways in which they can be and should be improved. But, like Canadian singer-songwriter Joni Mitchell wrote, "You don't know what you've got till it's gone."

If we allow public schools to fail those most in need of their services, it won't be long before our communities disintegrate and Canada comes undone. Make no mistake about it: If our public schools fail, Canada fails.

Critical Thinking Questions

1. What does Richard Tremblay mean when he says, "failure to teach children to regulate violent behaviour during the early years leads to poverty much more clearly than poverty leads to violence"?

2. How should children be taught to regulate their violent behaviour during the early years? Does the evidence support your contentions?

3. Why might a community's level of self-determination be linked to the suicide of adolescents living in that community?

4. What factors might limit the ability of public schools to retain students until graduation? How might these factors be overcome?

5. Do significant educational inequalities pose a threat to Canadian society?

Recommended Readings

Bowlby, J.W. & McMullen, K. (2002). *At a crossroads: First results for the 18- to 20-year-old cohort of the Youth in Transition Survey*. Online at www.hrdc-drhc.gc.ca/sp-ps/arb-dgra/publications/books/yits-encov.pdf.

The *Youth in Transition Survey* (YITS), designed to collect a broad range of information on the education and labour market experiences of youth, is a longitudinal survey developed by Human Resources Development Canada and Statistics Canada. *At a Crossroads* presents findings from the first cycle of the YITS 18–20-year-old cohort, a survey of more than 22,000 Canadian youth conducted between January and March 2000.

Canadian Council on Learning. (2008). *Lessons in Learning*. Online at www.ccl-cca.ca/CCL/Reports/LessonsInLearning?Language=EN.

Published to provide Canadians with independent information about what works in learning, each *Lesson in Learning* is approximately 2,000 words, and focuses on a specific topical issue.

Statistics Canada, Census Operations Division. (2003). *Education in Canada: Raising the standard.* Online at www12.statcan.ca/english/census01/products/analytic/companion/educ/pdf/96F0030XIE2001012.pdf.

Education in Canada: Raising the standard provides information on the changes in the education profile of the Canadian population over the past 10 years.

Ungerleider, C. (2003). *Failing our kids: How we are ruining our public schools.* Toronto: McClelland & Stewart.

Drawing on the latest research and using examples from across the country, Ungerleider describes what's right and what's wrong about our public schools system and provides solutions for making them better.

Wiegers, Wanda. (2002). *The framing of poverty as "child poverty" and its implications for women.* Online at www.swc-cfc.gc.ca/pubs/0662322177/index_e.html.

Examines the sources and implications for women of a focus on child poverty in discussion of Canadian state policy.

Related Web Sites

Canadian Centre for Policy Alternatives (CCPA)—www.policyalternatives.ca

The CCPA describes its mission as offering "an alternative to the message that we have no choice about the policies that affect our lives." The CCPA produces research reports, books, opinion pieces, fact sheets, and other publications about issues of social and economic justice.

Canadian Council on Learning—www.ccl-cca.ca

This is an independent, not-for-profit, pan-Canadian organization whose work is focused on three key areas: (1) research and knowledge mobilization; (2) monitoring and reporting on progress in learning; and (3) exchange of knowledge about effective learning practices among learning stakeholders.

Institute for Research on Public Policy (IRPP)—www.irpp.org/indexe.htm

The mission of the IRPP is to be an independent, national, non-profit organization "to improve public policy in Canada by generating research, providing insight and sparking debate that will contribute to the public policy decision-making process and strengthen the quality of the public policy decisions made by Canadian governments, citizens, institutions and organizations."

Organisation of Economic Co-operation and Development (OECD)—www.oecd.org/edu

The OECD is one of the world's largest and most reliable sources of comparable statistics, and economic and social data. The OECD monitors trends, analyzes and forecasts economic developments, and researches social changes or evolving patterns in numerous areas, including education.

Statistics Canada—www.statcan.ca

Canada's central statistical agency publishes a variety of documents and reports about nearly every facet of Canadian society, including demographics, health, education, resources, economy, and culture.

Vanier Institute for the Family—www.vifamily.ca

Its mission is "to create awareness of, and to provide leadership on, the importance and strengths of families in Canada and the challenges they face in their structural, demographic, economic, cultural and social diversity." The institute provides information and analysis-based research, consultation, and policy development "to elected officials, policy makers, educators and researchers, the business community, the media, social service professionals, the public and Canadian families themselves."

—⬤—

Chapter 12

Literacy and Health Literacy:
New Understandings about Their Impact on Health

Barbara Ronson and Irving Rootman

Introduction

Large-scale national and international literacy testing in recent decades has spurred academic interest in the meaning of "literacy" and its relation to other variables such as income, educational attainment, social engagement, and health. A number of social trends have resulted in special interest in the relationship between literacy and health and in the mediating construct "health literacy." Social trends prompting this interest include rising health care costs, an aging population, an increase in chronic diseases, and a growing need for consumers to manage their own care. Without the ability to understand health care information in print and electronically, many patients face possible danger in the short term and decreased quality of life from indirect effects of low reading, writing, understanding, and communication skills in the long term. This chapter presents empirical evidence regarding the importance of literacy and "health literacy" as social determinants of health and considers the role of policy in determining the level of literacy within jurisdictions.

Evolving Definitions of Literacy and Health Literacy

Today, literacy is more often considered as a continuum of skills rather than a set of skills that one either has or doesn't have. Tests have moved beyond the old method of assessing people's ability to read a passage from a book (as immigration authorities have been known to do) as well as beyond looking at people's ability to sign a marriage or baptismal certificate with more than an X (as historians have done to estimate literacy levels in times past). International literacy tests today assess skills on five levels with scores ranging from 0–500 points. Experts consider level 3 necessary to function in today's society with everyday reading and writing tasks. The definition of literacy used for the 1994 *International Adult Literacy Survey* (IALS) was "the ability to understand and employ printed information in daily activities—at home, at work and in the community—to achieve one's goals and develop one's knowledge and potential." The IALS test consisted of three components: (1) prose literacy (reading and comprehending text in sentence and paragraph form); (2) document literacy (the ability to use forms, graphs, charts, etc., effectively); and (3) quantitative literacy (the ability to use numerical information effectively). The more recent (2003) *International Adult Literacy and Skills Survey* (IALSS) enhanced the quantitative component, renaming it "numeracy." A problem-solving component was also added to the survey, although it was not considered as a literacy measure.

Some scholars, especially those in the education sector, are now speaking of "literacies" rather than "literacy" and use multiple terms such as "media literacy," "computer literacy," "information literacy," and "health literacy." New understandings from Aboriginal Canadians and immigrants about how literacy is culturally defined and how literacy, health, and culture are inextricably

Box 12.1: Relative importance of education/literacy as a determinant of health

A number of statistical analyses that have controlled separately for the effects of education and income indicate that, while both are associated with ill health, lack of education is the predominant factor. For example, an analysis of the *Health Promotion Survey* found that when controlled for education, the initial relationship between income and self-reported health drops out. In other words, apparent effects of income on self-reported health in this survey are actually a result of education/literacy. Similarly, a reanalysis of Statistics Canada's 1976 *Survey of Fitness, Physical Recreation, and Sport* found that education accounted for a much larger share than did income or other factors of the differences in physical activity rates. In other countries, Slater and Carlton (1985) have indicated that "the education differentials probably provide more reliable indicators of socio-economic differentials in mortality in the United States than do income differentials." Grossman (1987), following a review of a variety of studies, concluded that "schooling is a causal determinant of the two other components of socioeconomic status: income and occupation" and cites 10 separate studies in the United States that all indicate that "schooling is a more important correlate of health than occupation or income."

Source: Perrin, B. (1989). *Literacy and health: Making the connection: The research report of the literacy and health project phase one: Making the world healthier and safer for people who can't read.* Ontario Public Health Association and Frontier College. Online at www.opha.on.ca/resources/literacy1research.pdf. More recent studies that reinforce this finding include a Montreal study on "Effect of neighbourhood income and maternal education on birth outcomes" by Z. Luo, R. Wilkins, M. Wilkins, and M. Kramer, *Canadian Medical Association Journal, 174*(10) (2006), 1415–1421, and A. Carp et al., "Relation of education and occupation-based socioeconomic status to incidence of Alzheimer's disease," *American Journal of Epidemiology, 159*(2) (2004), 175–183.

connected lend insight into the need for open, evolving definitions with input from the populations to be served by our education and health care systems.

The term "health literacy," like literacy, is defined most precisely by the tests that try to measure it. Still, the creators of such tests normally start with a guiding definition. The US Institute of Medicine Expert Committee on Health Literacy adopted a definition of health literacy as "the degree to which individuals have the capacity to obtain, process, and understand basic health information and services needed to make appropriate health decisions" (Ratzan & Parker, 2000). In 2006, the Canadian Public Health Association (CPHA) formed an Expert Panel on Health Literacy, which agreed to use the following definition of health literacy: "the ability to access, understand, evaluate and communicate information as a way to promote, maintain, and improve health in a variety of settings across the life course" (Rootman & Gordon-El-Bihbety, 2008). The Rapid Estimate of Adult Literacy in Medicine (REALM) and the Test of Functional Health Literacy in Adults (TOFHLA) have been the main tests for health literacy. Recently, however, Statistics Canada, the Educational Testing Service, the US National Center for Educational Statistics, and the School of Public Health at Harvard

University developed a measure of health literacy using a subset of the questions on the Adult Literacy and Skills Survey (IALSS). The results showed that 55 percent of Canadians of working age fall below level 3 for health literacy (thought to be the threshold of skills needed to manage one's health without compensatory help) whereas only 42 percent do so on the IALSS prose scale (Canadian Council on Learning, 2007b). This makes sense conceptually since for most of the health-related items, respondents needed proficiency in the other domains of literacy (prose, document, and numeracy) and not just one domain as in the prose scale. As might be expected, the score for health literacy in this measure is predominantly accounted for by the underlying literacy score, with prose literacy the most important predictor. Still missing in all the above tests of literacy and health literacy are oral and aural skill assessment, which are needed if one is true to the functional definitions on which these tests are based. Also lacking in the health literacy test is a measure of the underlying attitudes, values, and beliefs needed to use one's skills for health improvement (Canadian Council on Learning, 2008). Nevertheless, this measure of health literacy is more rigorous than any of the other measures in common use and it is the only one available at the national level. Figure 12.1 shows the evolution of the study of Canadian literacy and health in Canada.

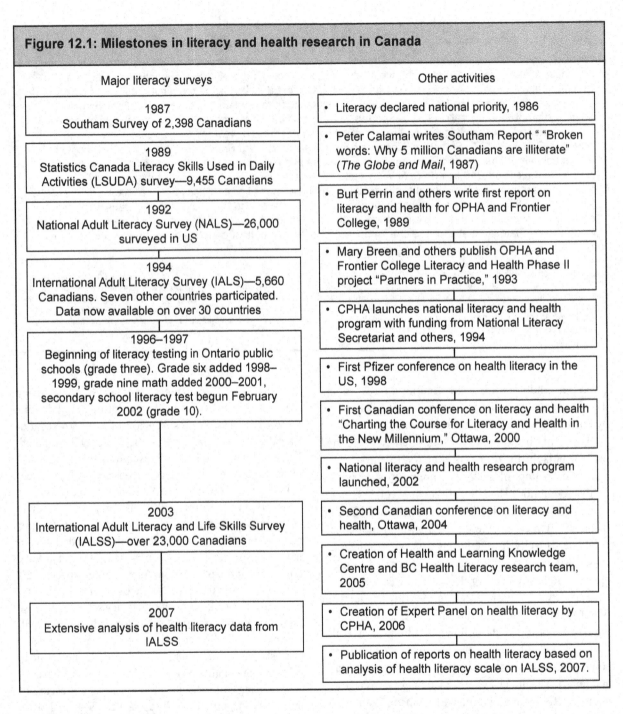

Figure 12.1: Milestones in literacy and health research in Canada

Major literacy surveys

1987
Southam Survey of 2,398 Canadians

1989
Statistics Canada Literacy Skills Used in Daily
Activities (LSUDA) survey—9,455 Canadians

1992
National Adult Literacy Survey (NALS)—26,000
surveyed in US

1994
International Adult Literacy Survey (IALS)—5,660
Canadians. Seven other countries participated.
Data now available on over 30 countries

1996–1997
Beginning of literacy testing in Ontario public
schools (grade three). Grade six added 1998–
1999, grade nine math added 2000–2001,
secondary school literacy test begun February
2002 (grade 10).

2003
International Adult Literacy and Life Skills Survey
(IALSS)—over 23,000 Canadians

2007
Extensive analysis of health literacy data from
IALSS

Other activities

- Literacy declared national priority, 1986
- Peter Calamai writes Southam Report " "Broken
  words: Why 5 million Canadians are illiterate"
  (*The Globe and Mail*, 1987)
- Burt Perrin and others write first report on
  literacy and health for OPHA and Frontier
  College, 1989
- Mary Breen and others publish OPHA and
  Frontier College Literacy and Health Phase II
  project "Partners in Practice," 1993
- CPHA launches national literacy and health
  program with funding from National Literacy
  Secretariat and others, 1994
- First Pfizer conference on health literacy in the
  US, 1998
- First Canadian conference on literacy and health
  "Charting the Course for Literacy and Health in
  the New Millennium," Ottawa, 2000
- National literacy and health research program
  launched, 2002
- Second Canadian conference on literacy and
  health, Ottawa, 2004
- Creation of Health and Learning Knowledge
  Centre and BC Health Literacy research team,
  2005
- Creation of Expert Panel on health literacy by
  CPHA, 2006
- Publication of reports on health literacy based on
  analysis of health literacy scale on IALSS, 2007.

Mechanisms and Pathways by Which Literacy Influences Health

Direct Effects of Literacy on Health

There is evidence in the research literature that literacy is directly related to both overall health status and possibly to mental health status as well (though more study is needed to confirm the latter) (Baker et al., 1997, 2002; Roberts & Fawcett, 1998). Literacy is also directly related to the co-morbidity burden (Guerra & Shea, 2003) and life expectancy (OECD & Statistics Canada, 2000). In addition, there is evidence that low-literate consumers and their families are at risk of harm due to their difficulty in reading medication prescriptions, baby formula instructions, and other written material (Kalichman et al., 1999). The direct effects of literacy on health are a matter of concern for all health care providers. If their communications and instructions are not helpful and are potentially harmful for large numbers of their clients, addressing the problem should be a priority. Concerns relate not only to health service providers' professional effectiveness but also to the costs to the system of drug-benefit plans and medical insurance when prescription drugs are misused and patients are unable to follow directions properly (Friedland, 1998). Particularly unsettling is the fact that seniors are among the least literate groups in society and also the most heavily dependent on medications and health services (Roberts & Fawcett, 1998; Statistics Canada & OECD, 2005).

Literacy should also be of concern to employers, manufacturers, and retailers who handle potentially dangerous products and processes. Direct effects of literacy on health also occur in workplaces and other settings where safety may be dependent on one's ability to read rules, signs, and manuals. A Manitoba study, for example, indicated that "difficulty comprehending precautions on farm and recreational machinery such as all-terrain vehicles, watersleds, snowmobiles and farm equipment of all sorts, makes rural life more dangerous" (Sarginson, 1997). Edwards (1995) found that the Workplace Hazardous Materials Information System (WHIS) consists of text often written at the college level. In addition, there is evidence that occupational injuries, the degree of awareness of the dangers in the workplace, and installation of home safety features are associated with limited literacy (Health Canada, 2003).

Indirect Effects of Literacy on Health

Research also suggests that literacy is related to lifestyle practices. For example, an Australian study of students in primary schools found that low literacy predicted tobacco use among both boys and girls and alcohol use among boys (Hawthorne, 1997). Similarly, a study in the United States found that low literacy was associated with choice of contraceptive methods as well as knowledge about birth control (Gazmararian et al., 1999). In addition, there is much evidence that education has a powerful influence on a range of personal lifestyle choices. The higher the level of education, the less likely Canadians are to smoke or be overweight (Federal, Provincial, and Territorial Advisory Committee on Population Health, 1999). The higher the literacy levels, the more likely people are to participate in voluntary community activities or belong to community groups and the higher the representation of females in government (OECD & Statistics Canada, 2000; Canadian Council on Learning, 2007b).

People with limited literacy also have less knowledge about medical conditions and treatment (Parker et al., 2003) and they have trouble understanding health issues generally (Rudd et al., 1999). They also have more difficulty with practitioners' verbal communications (Schillinger et al., 2002) and they tend to have higher stress levels and feelings of vulnerability (Health Canada, 2003). People with lower literacy levels also tend to be less aware of and make less use of preventive services (Scott et al., 2002). They are also less likely to seek care (Scott et al., 2002), but have higher rates of hospitalization (Baker et al., 2002) and experience more difficulties using the health care system (Davis et al., 1996).

Undoubtedly, health has a strong impact on literacy just as literacy impacts on health. Children who are hungry, tired, and stressed by poor or abusive home lives do not learn well (Anderson, 2003). They are absent more often and leave school earlier. Canadians with lowest health literacy scores are 2.5 times more likely to be in fair or poor health as those with skills at the top levels, even after removing the impact of age, gender, education, mother tongue, immigrant, and Aboriginal status (Canadian Council on Learning, 2008).

The link between literacy and the following other determinants of health will be discussed below: culture, income and socio-economic status, living and working conditions, educational attainment, gender, and early life.

Culture

Literacy is closely linked to culture. Literacy tests, like intelligence tests, are not value neutral. They are usually composed by representatives of the dominant language and culture in society—the same group that writes and enforces the laws, controls the commerce, and has the most power to hire, fire, resolve conflicts, and make decisions. The Centre for Literacy, Quebec, recognizes culture centrally in its definition of literacy as "a complex set of abilities to understand and use the dominant symbol systems of a culture for personal and community development" (Shohet, 2002). In her article on "Micmac Literacy and Cognitive Assimilation," First Nations author Marie Battiste writes that "Literacy is a social concept more reflective of culture and context than of formal instruction and can be used for cultural transmission within a society or for cultural imperialsm when imposed from the outside" (Battiste, 1984). Aboriginal peoples and immigrants tend to have lower literacy scores in Canada (Statistics Canada, 1996; Statistics Canada & OECD, 2005). For the francophone community, results are also lower (though they write their own tests in their own language), but differences tend to disappear among the younger generations (Statistics Canada, 1996; Statistics Canada & OECD, 2005). In the US, racial and ethnic minority populations, including Aboriginals and Spanish-speakers, are more likely than others to have lower literacy scores (Kirsch et al., 1993).

Literacy studies have drawn attention to the importance of first-language acquisition before or along with studies in one of Canada's official languages. Aboriginal literacy practitioners have found Native language studies to be an important precursor or complement to literacy studies in English or French. The reasons for this are likely related to the influence of culture, social connectedness, and support networks on health and well-being, and the impact of health on learning. The lack of social connectedness and belonging is known to be a primary barrier to well-being and learning (Department for International Development, 2005; Galabuzi, 2004; DeWit et al., 2002). Conceivably, then, when one feels more grounded, included, and connected in one's own culture, language, and traditions, literacy will improve. Literacy in English or French, moreover, is a means of learning about Aboriginal culture due to the growing number of books by First Nations authors that have captured Native history and culture in these languages. Aboriginal researcher Eileen Antone defines "health literacy" for Aboriginal people as "a way of life with a holistic world view balancing mind, body, heart and spirit as in the four components of the medicine wheel.... Aboriginal people still experience cultural poverty and want access to their own gentler systems of health and literacy" (Antone, 2004). As Kofi Annan, seventh secretary-general of the

United Nations, said, literacy can be a vehicle for the promotion of cultural and national identity as well as a platform for democratization, a bulwark against poverty, and a building block of development—"an essential complement to investments in roads, dams, clinics and factories ... the road to human progress and the means through which every man, woman and child can realize his or her full potential" (Annan, 1997).

Income and Social Status

Literacy is clearly linked to income. People with limited income are more likely to have limited literacy skills (Weiss et al., 1994). The larger the proportion of adults at the highest literacy levels, the larger the GDP per capita; and the higher the proportion of adults with the lowest literacy levels, the lower the GDP per capita (OECD & Statistics Canada, 2000). Furthermore, literacy skills were highly correlated with wages in 22 of 23 countries that participated in the *International Adult Literacy Survey* (IALS), as well as in the majority of countries who participated in the IALSS study. The data suggested that the role literacy plays in the determination of wages is greater in economies that are more flexible and open (e.g., the US and Canada), i.e., the economic returns of literacy (when controlling for education) are largest in open economies. As well, in all participating countries in the Programme for International Student Assessment (PISA) study, students from higher socio-economic backgrounds performed better than those from lower socio-economic backgrounds. People with limited literacy or health literacy are more likely to be unemployed, receiving income support, and working for minimum wage in unskilled jobs (Statistics Canada, 1996; Canadian Council on Learning, 2007b; Canadian Council on Learning, 2008). They are also more likely to be working in older industries (Statistics Canada, 1996). Literacy is also related to type of employment. Highest literacy levels in the *Survey of Literacy Skills Used in Daily Activities* (LSUDA) study were found in the teaching, science, engineering, social science, and managerial professions. The greatest proportion of respondents testing at the lowest levels were in the product fabricating, service, and farming sectors (Statistics Canada, 1996).

There is evidence that countries with a wide gap between income levels of the rich and the poor also have the widest gaps between highest and lowest literacy levels of the top and bottom quarter of the population. In Denmark the range of scores between the 5th and the 95th percentile is 120 points. In the US it is almost twice as large (231 points). In Canada the range of scores between the 5th and the 95th percentile is also large on all three IALS scales (prose, document, and quantitative). On the prose scale it is 219 points (the 3rd largest discrepancy of all IALS countries). A similar range is found in the UK, Poland, Portugal, and Slovenia as well as the US.

In the most recent international test, Canadians whose parents had completed 12 years of schooling scored 24 points higher than young people whose parents completed only eight years. In contrast, the difference was only 13 points in Norway, showing that it was more successful at reducing the disadvantages of skills typically associated with low levels of parental education (Statistics Canada, 2005). The fact that literacy outcomes vary in some countries by socio-economic status more than in others suggests that the problem can be addressed through policy and quality of the education system. For example, Sweden, which has a strong income-security system, also has the highest scores on all three IALS scales, ranging from 301–306 points for each out of 500. Chile has the lowest (from 209–221 points). Canada ranks 5th on prose (279) behind Sweden, Finland, Norway, and the Netherlands; the US ranks 10th; and the UK 13th. On the document scale, Canada ranks 8th (279), and on the quantitative scale Canada is 9th with 281 points. In Sweden even those who did not complete secondary

education do better than their counterparts in other countries with 59 percent scoring above level 2 compared to 27 percent without secondary education above level 2 in Canada, and 51 percent in Germany (OECD & Statistics Canada, 2000).

Further evidence that policy may affect literacy levels comes from the PISA study. Students in Canada from the 25 percent of families with the lowest SES scored above the average for all students in OECD member countries with an average of 503 compared to the overall average of 500. This contrasts to the US where the poorest quartile averaged 466. The wealthiest quarter of students in both countries scored more comparably: 568 on reading, math, and science for Canadians and 554 for US students (Totten & Quigley, 2003).

Though it appears that performance on literacy tests reflects the quality of the education system and/or social safety net, this needs further study. Other factors may be the number and background of immigrants and whether or not the First Peoples of a country are the dominant culture.

Living and Working Conditions

Between 22 percent and 50 percent of adults with lower levels of literacy live in low-income households, compared with only 8 percent of those with high-level literacy skills (Roberts & Fawcett, 1998). Those at health literacy level 1 are 2.5 times more likely to be receiving income support (EI or social assistance) than those at level 4 or 5, even after removing the impact of

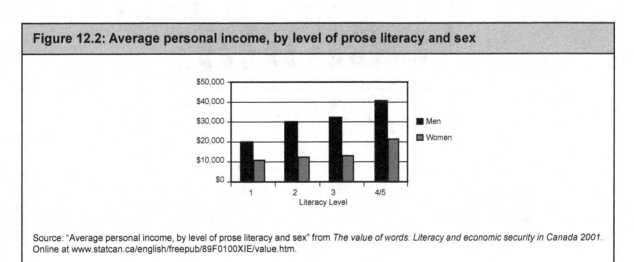

Figure 12.2: Average personal income, by level of prose literacy and sex

Source: "Average personal income, by level of prose literacy and sex" from *The value of words: Literacy and economic security in Canada 2001*. Online at www.statcan.ca/english/freepub/89F0100XIE/value.htm.

Figure 12.3: Comparative distribution of literacy levels

Figure 12.3a: Percentage of adult population aged 16–65 at each *prose* literacy level, 1994–1995

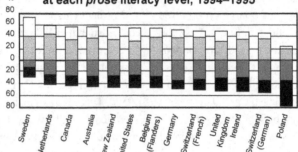

Figure 12.3b: Percentage of adult population aged 16–65 at each *document* literacy level, 1994–1995

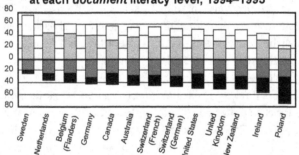

Figure 12.3c: Percentage of adult population aged 16–65 at each *quantitative* literacy level, 1994–1995

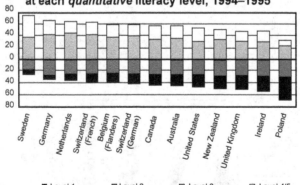

■ Level 1   ▨ Level 2   ▨ Level 3   ☐ Level 4/5

Countries are ranked by the proportion in levels 3 and 4/5.

Source: International adult literacy survey, 1994–1995.

Figure 12.3 shows the proportion of adults at each level of literacy for each country. Level 1 is the lowest; level 5 is the highest.

age, gender, education, mother tongue, immigrant, and Aboriginal status (Canadian Council on Learning, 2008). Violence and abuse are key threats to learning capacity. Women in literacy programs have identified men's violence (or its threat) as the greatest barrier to their learning (Davies, 1995). Violence and abuse undoubtedly affect children's capacity for learning as well, and are key reasons why young people do not complete high school and/or run away from home. According to the *National Longitudinal Survey of Children and Youth* (NLSCY), students who reported bullying behaviours "sometimes" or "often" scored significantly lower in math and reading scores than those who reported no bullying behaviour (Totten & Quigley, 2003).

Non-abusive workplaces can provide opportunities for literacy. Since the mid-1980s when literacy was declared a national priority, a growing number of workplace literacy programs have been provided. The Conference Board of Canada found that at least one-third of employers had problems in their workforces attributable to low literacy and basic skills (Darville, 1992). There is increasing attention being paid to healthy school environments as the "workplace" for approximately one-fifth of the population. Improving school environments has proven to be important for improving student health and achievement (WHO, 2003). With growing knowledge of the inextricable relationship between health and learning, the World Health Organization has made much progress with its Global School Health Initiative and its support for health-promoting schools and/or coordinated school health initiatives around the world (WHO, 2003).

Educational Attainment

There is a strong positive relationship between educational attainment and skills on all domains measured in IALSS, but there are substantial variations of performance within each level of education. For example, surprisingly, 25 percent of adults who completed post-secondary education score less than 25 percent of those who did not complete high school (Statistics Canada & OECD, 2005). One-fifth of university graduates scored below level 3, the desired threshold for coping with the increasing demands of a knowledge society (HRSDC & Statistics Canada, 2005). Moreover, the average prose literacy proficiency of university graduates has decreased between the IALS (1994) and the IALSS (2003) studies (HRSDC &

Statistics Canada, 2005). On an early literacy survey of Canadians sponsored by Southam Inc. in 1989, one in five high school graduates tested as functionally illiterate (Calamai, 1999). Such figures show the potential for serious error bias in literacy estimates based on years of schooling that do not control for a wider set of socio-demographic factors and the quality of years of schooling (Charette & Meng, 1998). Though educational attainment is the strongest predictor of prose and document literacy, the most significant factor related to health literacy in the IALSS was reading practices in daily life (Canadian Council on Learning, 2008). This includes reading books, newspapers, magazines, and letters, notes, or emails. Educational attainment was only the second strongest factor explaining health literacy proficiency. An above-average level of educational attainment by one's parents had a moderate effect on one's health literacy proficiency (Canadian Council on Learning, 2008). Though education level appears to have a strong, persistent effect on skills over time, it is well documented that literacy scores decrease after age 16 more than educational level can account for. In other words, most adults either "use it or lose it" in terms of reading and writing skills.

Gender

In less-developed countries, women tend to have lower levels of literacy than men (Weiss, 2001). One of the strongest predictors of life-expectancy among developing countries is adult literacy, particularly the disparity between male and female adult literacy, which explains much of the variation in health achievement among these countries after accounting for per capita GDP. For example, among the 125 developing countries with per capita GDP less than $10,000, the difference between male and female literacy accounts for 40 percent of the variation in life expectancy after factoring out the effect of per capita GDP (Daniels et al., 2000).

Most recent Canadian surveys of adult literacy show comparable literacy rates for men and women (Statistics Canada, 1996; Calamai, 1987), however, men tend to display an advantage in numeracy and document literacy skills, while women tend to display an advantage in prose literacy (Statistics Canada & OECD, 2005). This finding is consistent with that of tests of school-age children such as the IEA Reading Literacy Study and the Programme for International Student Assessment (PISA)

(Statistics Canada & OECD, 2005). Mandated literacy tests in Ontario schools show that girls in grades three, six, and 10 consistently score higher than boys in reading with an average score of 548 compared to 418 for boys (Education Quality and Accountability Office, 2003). Forty percent of Canadian girls report reading at least 30 minutes a day for enjoyment compared to about 25 percent of boys. Still, both genders scored at level 3 on a scale of one to five, "capable of solving reading tasks of moderate complexity such as locating multiple pieces of information, making links between different parts of a text, and relating it to familiar everyday knowledge" on the PISA (Totten & Quigley, 2003, p. 27).

Among immigrants to Canada there are higher numbers of women with low literacy (Boyd, 1991). Nearly one-third (32 percent) of foreign-born women have extreme difficulty dealing with printed material or can use printed words only for limited purposes compared to over one-fifth (24 percent) of foreign-born men and approximately one-tenth of Canadian-born women and men (Boyd, 1991).

Early Life

Children of parents with reading problems are more likely to have reading problems themselves (Puchner, 1993). In the 2000 PISA, parental attitudes toward academic study were a key variable: Students with a home environment that stimulated learning did better than all students across all countries. Students with parents who took them to a variety of cultural events and who discussed current affairs outperformed other students in all countries. As well, students who enjoyed reading, borrowed books from a library, and had high career aspirations did better than other students (Totten & Quigley, 2003). However, the impact of parents' education on literacy level is not as profound in Denmark, Finland, Norway, and Sweden as it is in Canada, Australia, Ireland, New Zealand, the UK, and the US (OECD & Statistics Canada, 2000). This suggests that the quality of education and life outside the family for children of the lowest SES play a strong role.

Recent research in brain development has drawn attention to findings that indicate the highest capacity for learning is in the early years. Studies show a "hard wiring" of the brain over time that affects capacity for future learning, lifelong attitudes, and problem-solving approaches (Mustard & McCain, 1999; Halfon, Shulman & Hochstein, 2001; Koller & Hertzman, 2006). Early child-development programs, moreover, have proven capacity for breaking intergenerational cycles of disadvantage and dramatically improving chances of high school graduation and workplace participation (Schweinhart et al., 1993). The critical period for learning a first language is thought to be between zero and three years. Learning a second language becomes more difficult after 10 years of age (Begley, 1996).

Such findings have led to a relatively new trend in literacy programs—the recent proliferation of family literacy classes. These classes readily span the literacy and health arenas since health concerns and interventions during the early years are particularly frequent. Programs such as Rhymes That Bind, Books for Babies, and Health for Two have been developed in Canada, in part to apply new knowledge on healthy development of children from the attachment literature within the medical/psychiatric field. Preliminary research indicates that retention is higher in family literacy than in traditional literacy programs; that the goal of supporting their children's learning is a powerful motivator for adults; and that embedding literacy in activities connected to daily life leads to greater sustainability (Shohet, 1997). There is also much to be learned from the highly successful intergenerational nature of many Aboriginal programs. Unfortunately, according to Dr. Eileen Antone, there is very little understanding of or funding support for Aboriginal adult education programs that include intergenerational literacy participation and practices (Antone, 2003).

Other Factors

A National Literacy and Health Research Program was launched in Canada in 2002. As a preliminary step, a conceptual diagram of the pathways linking literacy and health was developed and field-tested in focus groups across the country. In addition to the factors discussed above, factors of aging and personal capacity were deemed important determinants of literacy, which, in turn, is a determinant of health. The conceptual diagram also suggested five kinds of actions that can improve literacy: health communications, capacity development, community development, organizational development, and policy development. In this chapter, policy development approaches to improve health through improving literacy will be discussed, and policy development will be looked to as a means of encouraging the other kinds of actions that can improve literacy.

The Role of Policy in Determining the Level of Literacy within Jurisdictions

Policy plays a crucial role in affecting levels of literacy across countries around the world.

Rootman (1991) summarizes the policy recommendations arising from the LSUDA study. Among other things, the study authors recommend that governments improve the educational system for young people; develop an adult education and training system; create policy and funding commitments to ensure that adults have access to a variety of literacy and learning opportunities in their home communities; support public participation in the health care system; strengthen community health services; develop and coordinate public health policies in a variety of sectors; ensure that information and materials provided by the government are written in plain language; provide incentives to organizations that attempt to make information more accessible to people with low literacy skills; encourage and fund projects aimed at increasing accessibility of information; and ensure that attention is given to literacy when health-promotion strategies are developed (Rootman, 1991).

Box 12.2: School libraries are threatened, despite powerful evidence they're key to student achievement

VANCOUVER—Roch Carrier, Canada's National Librarian and author of the beloved children's classic *The Hockey Sweater*, has declared October 27 to be National School Library Day in an effort to raise awareness about the erosion of school libraries across the country. Today teachers throughout British Columbia are echoing his call for a major reinvestment in libraries.

"As governments cut education budgets, school libraries are declining and librarians are struggling to maintain collections and meet students' needs," said Neil Worboys, president of the BC Teachers' Federation. "We've got to turn this trend around, because it has serious consequences for children's opportunities to learn."

Research shows that students who attend schools with well-funded, properly stocked libraries managed by qualified teacher-librarians have higher achievement, improved literacy, and greater success at the post-secondary level. For detailed information, see Dr. Ken Haycock's report *The Crisis in Canada's School Libraries: The Case for Reform and Reinvestment,* online at www.peopleforeducation.com/librarycoalition/ Report03.pdf.

Worboys noted that most Canadian students attain high levels of literacy, consistently performing near the top on international testing. "However, we must not allow the continued deterioration of our school libraries, especially as governments in the US, Europe and Asia are aggressively investing in school libraries and literacy programs," he said.

"Given all we know about the links between quality school libraries and high student achievement, it's disturbing to see the decline in BC school libraries," Worboys said. "In the past two years, 91 school libraries have closed altogether and many more are open only part-time. So many teacher-librarians have been cut due to funding shortfalls, we're afraid that they are practically becoming an endangered species in BC schools!"

"I encourage parents to inform themselves about the health of the library at your children's schools," Worboys said. "Is your library staffed by a qualified teacher-librarian? Does he or she have to work at more than one school? What about the condition of your library's collection: Are the classics there? Are the science books up-to-date? What about electronic resources? Is your library open throughout the day, every school day? If not, why not?"

Worboys urged parents, students and other concerned citizens to speak out for a strong school library. "The library is the heart of every school," he said. "It's the place where reluctant readers become avid ones, where children's imaginations can take them anywhere in the universe."

Source: Canada NewsWire, General News, October 27, 2003.

Similar policy recommendations continue to be advocated by Canada's expert panel on health literacy, particularly in their discussion of "barriers and enablers" (Rootman & Gordon-El-Bihbety, in press). Previously in this chapter, we have seen how literacy appears to be influenced by quality of education and the social safety net as there are wide variations in literacy levels among countries that cannot be accounted for by years of education alone.

In this section the following kinds of policy recommendations for the improvement of literacy will be discussed: (1) policies to encourage more research; (2) re-examining policies that define accountabilities and goals in our education system; and (3) policies that encourage interministerial collaboration.

Encouraging More Research

More research needs to be done on the effectiveness of various kinds of actions to improve health through improving literacy. In particular, various studies have identified the following research needs as priorities: the costs of health care delivery related to direct and indirect impacts of literacy (Health Canada, 2003; Rudd et al., 1999; American Medical Association Ad Hoc Committee on Health Literacy, 1999); longitudinal studies of potential changes in health status following changes in literacy skills (Breen, 1998); effective communication approaches (including the use of multimedia) for health providers (Health Canada, 2003; American Medical Association Ad Hoc Committee on Health Literacy, 1999); evaluation of promising approaches and practices (e.g., community development and participatory education) addressing literacy, lifelong learning, and health issues (Health Canada, 2003; Canadian Public Health Association, 2003); the role of literacy and other factors in enabling people to feel more confident and empowered to take action regarding their own health (Health Canada, 2003); understanding the causal pathway of how literacy influences health (American Medical Association Ad Hoc Committee on Health Literacy, 1999); and studying literacy and health within the unique circumstances of the Aboriginal and francophone communities, and culturally diverse and challenged groups (Canadian Public Health Association, 2003).

In addition, more research needs to be done on the effectiveness of capacity-development approaches such as education and training. Much research supports the need to design programs based on learners' interests and motivations. Mary Norton, Pat Campbell, Tammy Horne, Priscilla George, Eileen Antone, and Mary Breen are some of the Canadian literacy specialists who have written about literacy, health, and participatory education based on practical experience. Participatory approaches involve learners in issue selection and content development. Numerous examples of participatory development of health information were found in a recent assessment of Canadian research needs in literacy and health (Rootman et al., 2003). One example is a video and discussion guide called *A Better You: The Benefits of a Healthy Lifestyle*, produced by the Dartmouth Literacy Network in Nova Scotia. Another example is Heart Health Nova Scotia's work on *Literacy and Health Promotion: Four Case Studies*. A third example is Canadian Public Health Association's *What the Health! A Literacy and Health Resource for Youth*. A more recent example is the development of videos on navigating the health system developed in British Columbia for the Farsi-speaking community (Poureslami, Murphy, Balka, Nicol & Rootman, 2007). The quality of these products suggests that it is well worthwhile to do more such participatory development and evaluation within literacy classes.

As noted above, Health Canada suggested that there is a need for evaluating a wider range of promising approaches and practices such as community development (Health Canada, 2003). A number of resources have recently been developed that can enhance literacy practitioners' skills and knowledge of effective community development approaches. Grass Roots Press's adult literacy resources include the following: R. Arnold, B. Burke, C. James, D. Martin, and B. Thomas, *Educating for a Change*; New England Literacy Resource Center's *Civic Participation and Community Action Sourcebook: A Resource for Adult Educators*; Carmen Rodriguez, *Educating for Change: Community-Based/Student-Centred Literacy Programming with First Nations Adults*; Pat Campbell and Barbara Burnaby, *Participatory Practices in Adult Education*; and NWT and Nunavut Literacy Council's *Tools for Community Building: A Planning Workbook for Northern Canadian Community-Based Literacy*.

At minimum, it would be worthwhile to evaluate the usefulness of these resources.

A better understanding of the unique situation of new Canadians interested in literacy programs is needed as well. We also need to better understand what are the effective messages and methods of delivery in terms of different ethnic groups (Canadian Public Health Association, 2003). Foreign-born women and men with low literacy are less likely to be burdened by stigma about low skills in English or French, but more likely to work long hours and be unable to participate in programs outside the workplace. A large percentage of foreign-born Canadians with low literacy skills participate in the workforce. Of all women in the workforce testing at the lowest levels of literacy, 52 percent are foreign-born, although they represent only 17 percent of the female workforce. Foreign-born males represent 18 percent of the workforce and 34 percent of the men in the workforce who have low literacy levels 1 and 2 (Boyd, 1991).

Encouraging a Re-examination of Goals and Accountabilities of Education

One reason it is important to have continuous dialogue about the definition of literacy and numeracy is that our public education systems are commonly held accountable for these measures above any other goals. Large-scale testing of literacy and numeracy in schools, moreover, has caused much concern that such tests have narrowed the work of schoolteachers in a way that is less helpful (if not harmful) to many students, especially those who, despite success in many other aspects of schooling, are unlikely to pass the secondary school literacy test regardless of how many times they try or how hard they study, with reasons ranging from cultural factors to the quality of early education and care to dyslexia (Clarkson, 2004; Kohn, 2004). Students with a natural ability in reading and writing may also be less well served by a school that spends an inordinate amount of time preparing students for literacy and numeracy tests at the expense of activities not deemed to be the "core business of schools," such as arts, sports, and theatre. A better understanding of literacy testing itself on the health and literacy levels of children and youth is important given that hundreds of thousands of Canadian students are being tested for literacy level every year. From Ontario's Education Quality and Accountability Office, which administers the tests, we know that scores have been rising significantly over the past five years. The fact that more students are achieving grade-level expectations in reading, writing, and numeracy sounds promising. We need to know more about whether such results can be achieved without sacrificing other important outcomes of public education.

Research in health literacy can help encourage schools to think beyond narrow definitions of literacy and numeracy. It can influence schools to work more effectively toward improving the well-being of each child and graduate. The development of measures of health literacy may help broaden our thinking about the goals of education and put Canadian schools more in line with international models of health-promoting schools through comprehensive school health programs that include more physical activity and less seatwork, and more attention to curriculum, school environment, and support systems based on what makes people healthy.

While it is important to provide every child with the opportunity to become as highly skilled as possible in reading and writing in English and/or French in Canada, it may not be necessary for every child to reach a certain level in these skills, so much as it is necessary to give them all a sense of belonging and connectedness with abilities to compensate for any skills they may lack. Some students may be able to express themselves with video and computer skills, for example, though they may always need assistance from proofreaders, spell-checkers, writers, and editors. In Ontario a literacy course can now be substituted for passing the secondary school literacy test, which is an important step. If tests of health literacy and/or other kinds of literacy were administered on a similar scale (smaller) as tests of traditional reading and writing literacy, there may be a "healthy" shift away from narrow definitions of what public schools are accountable for.

In addition, there is a need to think more systemically about a lifelong learning strategy for schools. As Burt Perrin, author of the original OPHA and Frontier College report on literacy and health explained, a lifelong learning strategy "would establish a drop-in drop-out philosophy allowing people to acquire the skills they need when they need them" (Perrin, 1989, p. 34). Peter Calamai, who put literacy on the Canadian map with his *Globe and Mail* reports (Calamai, 1987) based on the early Southam survey of literacy levels, concurs. More recently, he wrote a publication on literacy called *The Three L's: Literacy and Life-long Learning* (Calamai, 2000). The recent National Workshop on Literacy and Health Research supported this direction in concluding that "studying the impact of literacy and life-long learning on health" was one of the top four priorities (Canadian Public Health Association, 2003). CPHA's Expert Panel on Health Literacy recommends a pan-Canadian strategy on health literacy in collaboration with other current initiatives such as the Movement for Canadian Literacy's National Literacy Action Plan, which is grounded in lifelong learning. The Ontario Ministry of Education defines literacy education as:

> ... part of a process or cycle of lifelong learning, based on life experience, shared knowledge, and decision-making by learners supported by their instructors. Literacy education contributes to the development of self knowledge and critical thinking skills. In turn, this development empowers individuals and communities. (Parkland Regional College, 1998, p. 9)

An agenda for lifelong learning may better address new understandings about multiple literacies and encourage learners previously held back by stigma. An agenda for lifelong learning could begin to treat adults and teenagers on more similar terms and make high schools or community education centres welcoming and appealing to the young and old who are ready to learn. It would allow for healthy mixed-age groupings in classes, perhaps breaking the current stronghold of peer pressure that too often leads to disrespect of elders and immature behaviour. It would also go some way toward reducing the stigma of dropping out, and reducing the number of students who are not engaged in their school work, if alternatives such as extended co-op placements can be found for them.

Encouraging New Mechanisms for Interministerial Collaboration

This chapter, like the others in this book, highlights the degree to which health status is affected by areas of jurisdiction of government ministries other than health. Sectors such as education, social services, culture and immigration, justice, and social security are thought to have primary influence on health. Yet when it comes to the health of individuals, too often, front-line people from every sector decide that the problem is within the jurisdiction of another sector. Fragmentation in our communities exacerbates problems with the health of our children. For example, many schools are empty after school and on weekends while children and youth in the neighbourhood have no safe places to play and no constructive activities to do. Many recreation centres now charge user fees, which discourage participation of at-risk children and youth who are most in need of constructive outlets. Children and youth who need special services are bounced from one provider to another with little communication between them. Over 40,000 children and youth remain on waiting lists for mental health services in Ontario, and many schools do not have specialist teachers or access to professional support staff.

Clearly, a higher level of support for community collaboration among multiple sectors is needed. Nowhere is this more evident than within our school communities. But progress is certainly being made, especially by public health units working together with schools on a "healthy school" framework. Healthy schools were recognized as a direction to pursue at the "Realizing the Promise of Public Education" forum held by the Ontario Teachers' Federation in the spring of 2003. Healthy schools have been subsequently endorsed by the Council of Ministers of Education and by ministers of health from across the country. Healthy schools continually strive for healthy physical and social environments, a strong health and physical education curriculum, and increased community support services (as advocated by most international frameworks).

They may also be more likely to have built-in lifelong learning opportunities with mixed-age as well as peer groupings with authentic learning formats that enhance a broad definition of literacy and multiliteracies. The field of health promotion has a history of advocating for and studying interministerial and intersectoral co-operation, and holds promise for continuing to shed light on how diverse groups and sectors can collaborate better to improve the well-being of the population. The healthy school movement is truly a success story in this regard.

Canada's literacy and health research program appears to be reaping considerable success as well, particularly as it has spurred collaboration between the adult literacy and public health sectors.

Conclusion

Much progress has been made in defining and measuring literacy and "health literacy" and understanding the relationship between them and health. New policies and efforts involving interministerial and intersectoral co-operation such as "healthy schools," participatory development of health information in adult literacy classes, and literacy awareness and plain language workshops for health care providers are most promising. More needs to be done, however, to improve our understanding of the relationship between literacy and health so that we can better understand how our health care providers and educators can adapt to changing needs in modern society. What we learn in this regard promises to help our citizens better manage their own health and lead healthier lives in their communities and schools.

Note

1. For more information on the history, definition, and measurement of literacy as a concept, see the paper written by Rootman and Ronson (2003).

Critical Thinking Questions

1. Compare and contrast education and literacy as social determinants of health.
2. Before reading this chapter, how aware were you of the number of Canadians whose daily activities were compromised by limited reading and writing skills? How would it impact your life if you did not have these skills?
3. What kinds of actions are suggested as a result of our improved understanding of the impact of literacy on health?
4. Make a case for investing significant health care dollars in issues related to literacy and health.
5. How would you recommend that the literacy community respond to our increased understanding of the impact of literacy on health?
6. Speculate as to how literacy testing in schools impacts health and quality of life outcomes for students.

Recommended Readings

Canadian Council on Learning. (2008). *A healthy understanding: Health literacy in Canada.* Ottawa: Canadian Council on Learning.

   This report builds on the report *Health Literacy in Canada* (Canadian Council on Learning, 2007a), which provides a summary of the initial results related to health literacy from the International Adult Literacy and Skills Survey (IALSS). *A Healthy Understanding* offers a detailed analysis of what health literacy is and how it is different from literacy; why health literacy matters; the levels of health literacy across the country and across subgroups; and the factors that can influence health literacy levels. We learn, for example, that the incidence of diabetes is related to health literacy levels in different regions of the country. We also learn that daily reading habits have the single strongest effect on health literacy proficiency: Adults who read various material most frequently score up to 38 percent higher than average, and seniors score up to 52 percent higher than average.

OPHA & Frontier College. (1989). *Literacy and health project phase one: Making the world healthier and safer for people who can't read.* Ontario Public Health Association and Frontier College. Online at www.opha.on.ca/resources/ literacy1summary.pdf.

This report describes the methods, findings, and recommendations of the first phase of the Ontario Literacy and Health project, sponsored by the Ontario Public Health Association and Frontier College.

Rootman, I. & Ronson, B. (2005). "Literacy and health research in Canada: Where have we been? Where should we go?" *Canadian Journal of Public Health*, Supplement 2, S62-77.

This article reviews the literature and research on literacy and health and identifies priorities for research on this topic. The information was analyzed using a conceptual framework. Determinants of literacy discussed are education, early childhood development, aging, living and working conditions, personal capacity/genetics, gender, and culture. Actions advocated for improving literacy and health include health communication, education and training, community development, organizational development, and policy development. The kinds of research particularly recommended are more evaluations of existing initiatives, more cost-benefit analyses, more culturally specific studies, and greater attention to current social trends and needs.

Rootman, I. & Gordon-El-Bihbety, D. (2008). *A vision for a health literate Canada.* Canadian Public Health Association.

This report is intended to inform policy-makers and practitioners about the concept of health literacy, the levels of health literacy in the Canadian population, and barriers and approaches to improving health literacy. It reviews recent research on literacy and health literacy, including adverse costs to society of low health literacy. It makes a strong case for more awareness and investment in improving health literacy and improving health care providers' communications with consumers. It proposes a pan-Canadian strategy for health literacy, including a framework for action.

Shohet, L. (2002). *Health and literacy: Perspectives in 2002.* Online at www.staff.vu.edu.au/alnarc/ onlineforum/ AL_pap_shohet.htm.

This paper discusses the links between literacy and health as they are currently represented in the discourse communities of the medical profession and of adult literacy. After comparing the positions taken by the medical field and the adult literacy field, and examining some selected government policies, the author outlines some directions for the future.

Related Web Sites

Canadian Council on Learning Health and Learning site—www.ccl-cca/CCL/AboutCCL/KnowledgeCentres/ HealthandLearning/

The health and learning knowledge centre of the Canadian Council on Learning serves as a national network linking expertise about the vital connections between learning and the health of Canadians. It features requests for proposals for applied research in this area and summaries and reports from funded projects. It is frequently updated with new developments in the field.

Communities and Schools Promoting Health—www.safehealthyschools.org

This Web site is designed as a gateway to many resources in school health promotion. It is also a home for the Canadian School Health Centre and the Canadian School Health NGO Network. There is also a reference to the School Health Research Network as another part of the school health-promotion community in Canada. These organizations, as well as many other initiatives, are linked in an effort to create the Canadian School Health Knowledge Network.

This site contains links to information on school-based health promotion with connections worldwide.

Communities and Schools Promoting Health—www.safehealthyschools.org

Extensive background information is provided, as well as tools such as lesson plans, webquests, sample policies, evaluation tools, and practical advice.

CPHA Literacy and Health Program—www.nlhp.cpha.ca

This Web site describes the National Literacy and Health Program and its associated services and projects, including the National Literacy and Health Research Program.

Harvard School of Public Health, Health Literacy Studies—www.hsph.harvard.edu/healthliteracy

This site contains introductions to health literacy, PowerPoint presentations, videos, literature reviews, annotated bibliographies, research reports, health education materials, guidelines on creating and evaluating written materials, curricula, highlights of talks and presentations, news items, insights, and links to related Web sites.

National Adult Literacy Database—www.nald.ca

This Web site describes the National Adult Literacy Database, lists literacy organizations in Canada, presents information about what's new and events in the field, as well as awards and contacts. It also provides access to literacy discussion groups and to expert advice, newsletters, a literacy collection, full-text documents, a resource catalogue, and links to internal resources and data.

Part Four

FOUNDATIONS OF LIFELONG HEALTH:
FOOD AND SHELTER

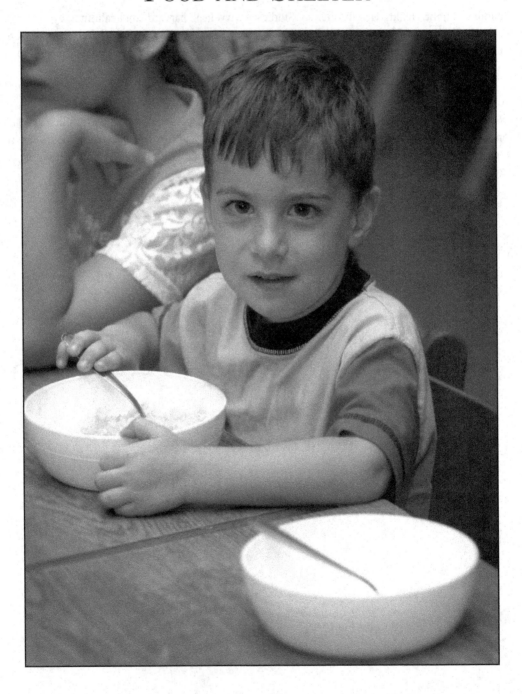

Canada is the signatory to a number of international agreements that guarantee the provision of basic needs such as food and shelter. Yet, one of the most shocking developments in Canada over the past 20 years has been the increasing incidence of food and housing insecurity. Canadian policy decisions related to the provision of adequate income and shelter have greatly weakened the state of these social determinants of health. In its most extreme but not particularly rare manifestation, these policy decisions have led to frightening levels of hunger and homelessness among Canadians. The explosive growth in the number of Canadians forced to rely upon food banks for food and temporary shelters for housing are the most obvious indicators of this situation. In its less extreme but more pervasive forms, the effects of food and housing insecurity are associated with increasing numbers of Canadians being unable to acquire quality diets and spending disproportionate amounts on shelter. What is particularly disturbing about this image of Canadians being unable to meet the basic needs of food and shelter is that this is occurring during a time when economic resources in Canada have never been at higher levels. This section details the extent of food and housing insecurity in Canada and the factors that have led to this situation. The health effects of the situation are reviewed and policy options to alleviate these crises are presented.

Lynn McIntyre and Krista Rondeau provide a history of food insecurity in Canada. They then provide the latest available information on the incidence of food insecurity, including hunger, in Canada. They identify who is most at risk for food insecurity and relate these factors to a lack of available income resources. Factors leading to food insecurity are primarily due to lack of money; issues of financial management and lack of nutritional knowledge of the food insecure are of minor importance. Nutritional implications are presented, as are a number of policy options to address food insecurity in Canada, which highlight the contribution and interrelationship of other social determinants of health such as income, housing, and employment to food insecurity.

Valerie Tarasuk shows how food insecurity threatens healthy nutritional status, interferes with chronic disease management, and can lead to body-weight problems. Food insecurity is related to the health of children, youth, adults, and the elderly. It increases the likelihood of emotional and health problems among the elderly, leads to poor academic and psychosocial development of younger children, and to depressive disorders among adolescents. Since health issues of food-insecure Canadians are similar to those associated with low income and other indicators of material deprivation, policy solutions require providing people, especially those out of work, with enough income to cover the costs of meeting basic needs.

Michael Shapcott outlines the scope of the housing crisis in Canada today and how it is a result of a number of policy decisions by the federal and provincial governments. Data are provided on the increasing number of housing-insecure and homeless Canadians. The Aboriginal situation and the barriers faced by Canadian women to acquire adequate housing are especially problematic. Canada has gone from a leader in providing adequate housing to its citizens to one whose housing crisis has drawn critical and negative international attention. The latest developments in housing policy are outlined and policy solutions presented. The contrast between government statements and actions on housing issues is particularly interesting.

Toba Bryant details the health effects of homelessness and housing insecurity. Traditional epidemiological approaches to studying housing and health are limited and new ways of conceptualizing the relationship are required. Federal and provincial housing policies threaten health by increasing homelessness and housing insecurity. The stresses associated with increasing housing insecurity also threaten health. Housing insecurity affects other social determinants of health by leaving fewer resources available for food, education, and recreation. Bryant provides a model of the policy change process that can be applied to provoke action on housing and other social determinants of health. Areas of further inquiry are outlined.

Chapter 13

Food Insecurity

Lynn McIntyre and Krista Rondeau

Introduction

Food used to be called a basic human need along with water, peace, shelter, education, and primary health care. It has also been called a prerequisite for health. Food security is a determinant of a lot of things: life, health, dignity, civil society, progress, justice, and sustainable development. In this chapter, food security is considered as a determinant of health.

This chapter is organized to first present a conceptual framework of hunger and food insecurity in higher-income countries. It then outlines a brief social history of food insecurity in Canada, describes its current status, and offers several policy recommendations. While presenting a high-level analysis of food insecurity, the specific situation of women and their children is explored in some detail.

Understanding Hunger and Food Insecurity

The World Health Organization Commission on Social Determinants of Health explains the difference between inequities that are unfortunate and those that are unjust. Outcomes that are unjust are avoidable because of an inequitable distribution of social conditions (Commission on Social Determinants of Health, 2007, p. 9). Another way of presenting the same idea is to say that there are things that are bad and things that are wrong. We would contend that food insecurity is wrong, yet it is treated as though it were merely bad.

Food insecurity, as experienced in higher-income countries, results from social conditions and policies that limit the resources available to a household to purchase adequate, nutritious food. The generally accepted definition of food insecurity is "the inability to acquire or consume an adequate diet quality or sufficient quantity of food in socially acceptable ways, or the uncertainty that one will be able to do so." The word "hunger" has recently been redefined by a United States Department of Agriculture (2006) panel to refer to "a potential consequence of food insecurity that, because of prolonged, involuntary lack of food, results in discomfort, illness, weakness, or pain that goes beyond the usual uneasy sensation." For a comparative discussion of hunger and food insecurity in lower- and middle-income countries and higher-income, industrialized countries, see Box 13.1.

The experience of food insecurity is dynamic. It occurs at both the level of households and individuals. Household members may have different experiences of food insecurity and hunger due to intra-household food provisioning that favours the needs of one or more family members over those of others. Mothers, in particular, may experience more severe food insecurity than their children. The sequence of stages that defines the experience for individuals reflects graded levels of severity, ranging from food anxiety to qualitative

---

Box 13.1: Comparing hunger in lower- and middle-income and higher-income countries

Food and Agriculture Organization of the United Nations report, *The State of Food Insecurity in the World* (2006), chronicled the 854 million people who were undernourished in 2001–2003, of whom 9 million or 1.1 percent lived in higher-income/industrialized countries; the remaining 845 million resided in lower-income countries (820 million) and transition or middle-income countries (25 million). Clearly there is difference in scale and severity of hunger in higher-income versus lower-income countries. Malnutrition is synonymous with hunger in lower-income countries.

Malnutrition is defined as the failure to achieve nutrient requirements, which can impair physical and/ or mental health. "Hidden hunger" is the popular term used for developing country-acquired micronutrient deficiencies. Iron, iodine, and vitamin A deficiencies are subtle and go unnoticed, although they are terribly health-damaging. Lower-income countries measure hunger through indicators of chronic energy deficiency; mild, moderate, and severe malnutrition; growth retardation; and serious key nutrient deficiencies at the population level. Sometimes absolute poverty and low per capita energy consumption are cited as indirect measures of hunger in the poorer countries of the world. In both higher-income and lower- and middle-income countries, hunger and food insecurity occur through a combination of individual through to international factors.

In both contexts, nutritional adequacy is an essential and arguably the single most important determinant of health. Those with too little food, regardless of place, have too little because they are very poor or destitute; with adequate resources, they could acquire food. Hunger in lower-income and higher-income countries is starkly different in three ways. Firstly, hunger is lethal in lower-income countries. It is not obviously so in higher-income countries. In lower-income countries, food needs are a priority for both short-term and long-term survival. Secondly, in higher-income countries, the food budget is the most elastic, i.e., the most discretionary of all essential expenditures. Shelter needs come first. Thirdly, in lower-income countries we are seeing rapid increases in obesity and chronic diseases associated with dietary preference change from even modest economic development, while at the same time gross malnutrition persists. In North America, obesity and chronic diseases are the overriding nutrition problems of the poor.

---

compromises in food selection and consumption, to quantitative compromises in intake, to the physical sensation of hunger. At its most severe stage, food insecurity is absolute food deprivation (i.e., individuals not eating at all). Only insufficient intake in this model is equated with classical hunger.

Validated instruments such as the *United States Household Food Security Survey Module* (which was adapted for use in the 2004 *Canadian Community Health Survey*), the Cornell-Radimer questionnaire, and the Community Childhood Hunger Identification Project questionnaire directly measure the occurrence and severity of food insecurity. Food insecurity is also measured through smaller sets of indicator questions administered as part of both Canadian and American national surveys. These survey instruments usually classify respondents as food-secure, moderately food-insecure, and severely food-insecure. Sometimes adult hunger and child hunger are reported as components of severe food insecurity. Indirect measures of hunger and food insecurity include food-bank use, adequacy of income, and homelessness.

The persistence of food insecurity in Canada raises the issue of whether it is perceived to be a consequence of absolute or relative poverty. Relative poverty relates to both material and social deprivation—a deprivation of resources required for a dignified participation in society. Severe food insecurity, including hunger, would likely be regarded as wrong if it were an outcome of absolute poverty, i.e., people being genuinely destitute and not having enough food to eat, but the situation could be perhaps regarded as only bad or unfortunate if people did not have enough money to buy nutritious food. At issue is the meaning of "hunger" in Canada.

Hunger, the "H" word, conceptually has three elements: it is about suffering; it is about absolute poverty and the consequences of relative deprivation; and it is about political dismissal of a fundamental abrogation of human rights. Hungry individuals are illegal. Canada recognized the right to food as a fundamental human right in 1948 when it signed and adopted the Universal Declaration of Human Rights (Rideout, Riches, Ostry, Buckingham & MacRae, 2007). Since then, Canada has recognized the right to food through a number of international and domestic agreements (Rideout et al., 2007). Many international covenants have deemed that adults and children have "an inalienable right to adequate nutritious food" (United Nations, 1996); and "the fundamental right of everyone to be free from hunger" (World Food Summit, 1995). Graham Riches speaks most eloquently in Canada about the "right to food" as a way to conceptualize our approaches to food insecurity. He asserts that the media's social construction of hunger as a matter of charity (hence the perception of food drives and food banks as a panacea for the unfortunate) is detrimental to the argument for a "right to food" that would need to be realized through social justice action (Riches, 2002; Rideout et al., 2007). Indeed, there is a lively literature critiquing food banks and other charitable food-distribution systems as not meeting food needs of the disadvantaged while serving the benevolence and corporate needs of the volunteers and donors respectively (Raine, McIntyre & Dayle, 2003; Tarasuk & Eakin, 2003, 2005).

Household and individual food insecurity differs from community food security in that they are about income-related food access and not the broader food system (Tarasuk, 2005). Similarly, individual and household food insecurity is linked with societal issues of food security and sustainable food production and distribution, topics that are beyond the scope of this chapter. However, it is important to recognize that globalized food systems, the international trade of food commodities, the agri-food industry, agricultural policies that support or disadvantage local domestic producers, marketing boards' supply management of food staples, grocery-distribution systems, processed-food marketing and distribution, school food policies, and labour protections for agricultural workers are just some of the factors that make up a complex web of supra-individual and -household factors that create or diminish conditions of individual and household food insecurity.

So why is it important that we understand that hunger and food insecurity not only exist but persist in Canada? Because to deny that among those with food insecurity in Canada are people who are truly hungry is to deny that we have gone too far.

A Brief Social History of Food Insecurity in Canada

A very brief social history of food insecurity in Canada would read simply: Poverty increased, then it deepened. Food insecurity emerged, then it increased in severity. While poverty is a long-standing area of social study in Canada, food insecurity is relatively new. Canada has had its food problems before: decades of malnutrition before the First World War; drought and the Depression; charitable food-delivery systems operating between the world wars; and a famine among the Inuit as late as 1950. Ostry's recent book on the history of nutrition policy in Canada recounts the Depression-era findings of compromised intake among women in Canada: "As well, these dietary surveys showed that men in poor families were the most well fed followed by children, and that mothers may have been cutting back on their own consumption to ensure that these other family members were more adequately fed" (Ostry, 2006, p. 87). But food insecurity, a child of the 1980s, was rediscovered when food banks emerged, and children's feeding programs in schools could be counted. Child poverty was on the map with the passage of the famous 1989 House of Commons resolution committing the government to the elimination of child poverty by the year 2000.

Globally Canada is a rich country, ranking first in the United Nations' Human Development Index between 1994 and 2000 (United Nations Human Development Report Office, 2008). Nonetheless, the 1990s were marked by a fundamental restructuring of Canadian social programs. Global recession shifted federal spending priorities away from social union programs. Provincial deficit reduction or cost-control strategies concurrently reduced social expenditures in health, education, and community services. Although Canada has experienced federal budget surpluses since 1997, this has been due in part to reductions in provincial transfer payments and subsequent reductions in social spending at the provincial level (Rideout et al., 2007). Combined federal spending on post-secondary education and welfare/social services decreased by 3.3 percent between 1989–1990 and 2004–2005 (Rideout et al., 2007). The result has been increased levels of food insecurity as one manifestation of growing poverty and inequity. Food security is named as a central issue in the call for domestic action in Canada's Action Plan for Food Security. Despite this call to action, in its 2006 review of Canada's progress in implementing the provisions of the International Covenant on Economic, Social, and Cultural Rights, the United Nations Committee of the same name expressed concern that food security was an ongoing problem in Canada: "Recommendations from [previous reviews] had also been neglected, and some situations had actually got worse, in particular the extent of poverty and the concomitant lack of food security" (United Nations Office at Geneva, 2006, p. 13).

Over the past two decades, communities across the country have initiated a host of food programs in an effort to alleviate food insecurity locally, signalling that citizens across the country recognize that people are experiencing hunger in Canada. A recent national representative survey revealed that 71.0 percent of Canadians believe that hunger is a serious problem in Canada (Heimann, 2004). Responses to food insecurity in Canada have been community-based, ad hoc, and largely focused on the provision of free or subsidized food (e.g., food banks, targeted meal programs). Health promotion and community-development initiatives have typically been small in scale and focused on either enhancing food shopping and preparation skills (e.g., community kitchens, targeted education programs) or on alternative methods of food acquisition (e.g., community gardens, farmers' markets, field-to-table programs, "good food" boxes). Children's feeding programs have been implemented throughout the country, representing a social movement predicated on Canadians' beliefs that virtually all poor children would go to school hungry without them.

Food supplement and coupon programs for poor pregnant women and their children are run through federally funded national networks. In 1997, there were 905 emergency food programs in Canada; in 2002, 620 food banks distributed food through 2,912 affiliated agencies (Wilson & Tsoa, 2002); and in 2007, 673 food banks were operating through 2,867 agencies in every province and territory in Canada (Canadian Association of Food Banks, 2007). Today, food banks have become entrenched in Canada's food-security landscape. For a discussion of how food banks have discomforted the comfort food, Kraft Dinner, see Box 13.2.

It is generally conceded that food banks are stop-gap measures, offering important immediate assistance, but not yielding sustainable solutions. Similarly, the implications (positive, negative, or neutral) of other community-based strategies for those who are severely food-insecure are not well studied, but such programs have not been shown to significantly reduce food insecurity or improve nutritional status among vulnerable populations (Broughton, Janssen, Hertzman, Innis & Frankish, 2006; Fano, Tyminski & Flynn, 2004; Raine, McIntyre & Dayle, 2003; McLaughlin, Tarasuk & Kreiger, 2003). The lack of demonstrated effectiveness of such programs is likely because they maintain a focus on *food* as the problem rather than *income* (Tarasuk, 2005). There is evidence that some community-based programs can shift food needs among those with milder degrees of food insecurity. For example, a recent study of collective-kitchen programs in Saskatoon, Toronto, and Montreal found that insofar as the participant did not experience severe food insecurity, collective kitchens were perceived as a tool to help stretch the food budget and avoid using a food bank or other charitable food-distribution systems (Engler-Stringer & Berenbaum, 2007).

Since 1989, the year used for most comparisons, we have sadly counted the poor, poor children, hungry children, emergency food-bank users, the homeless, and in 2004, we counted the numbers and proportions of food-insecure individuals and households in all of Canada. The results of local, regional, and national food-insecurity studies have been released with similar shameful results. We have launched and relaunched child-poverty initiatives. This brief social history of food insecurity in Canada concludes that since 1989, we have failed to eliminate or even significantly reduce hunger and food insecurity despite a high level of public activity, awareness, and sympathy for those who do not have enough to eat. How can that be? Perhaps it lies in the numbers, which are alternately considered too low or too high.

Prevalence of Hunger and Food Insecurity in Canada

In 2007, Health Canada released national and provincial estimates of the income-related food-security status of Canadian households in 2004 based on the data collected in the *Canadian Community Health Survey*, Cycle 2.2, Nutrition. The *Household Food Security Survey*

Box 13.2: Kraft Dinner: The iconic food bank donation

Kraft Dinner has a long history as a comfort food. Its consumption is also associated, however, with low income and poverty. This dichotomy is exemplified in the common practice of donating Kraft Dinner (and its imitators) to food banks. While food-secure Canadians tend to associate Kraft Dinner with *comfort* and voluntary consumption, food-insecure Canadians tend to associate Kraft Dinner with *discomfort* and obligatory consumption.

Food-secure Canadians perceive Kraft Dinner as an ideal food donation because it is seen as a complete and palatable meal that is easy to prepare, easy to store, and ultimately easy to donate. Kraft Dinner is cheap (often less than $1 per box), making it possible to donate in large quantities, while recognizing that the eventual recipients may also purchase it themselves. As a result, Kraft Dinner provides comfort to food-secure Canadians through both physical and vicarious consumption.

For food-insecure Canadians, consuming Kraft Dinner is discomforting because it is often a food of last resort, obtained as a result of serious financial constraint; it is monotonous and it is an additional source of milk stress. Contrary to the perception of food-secure Canadians that Kraft Dinner is a complete meal, the reality is that fuel, water, butter or margarine, and milk are all required to make Kraft Dinner according to package directions. Ironically, these fresh ingredients are not frequently found in food bank hampers. Furthermore, fresh milk is one of the most precious commodities in a food-insecure household and is carefully distributed among family members. It is likely that the Kraft Dinner consumed in food-insecure households across Canada toward the end of the month, when financial crises most often occur, is watered down and prepared with little or no milk.

The disconnect between these two perspectives shows that food-secure Canadians are generally quite ignorant of what it is like to be food-insecure in Canada. This likely accounts, at least in part, to the perpetuation of food banks and food charity as Canada's dominant response to food insecurity. Understanding the discomfort that results from the obligatory consumption of Kraft Dinner, whether it has been obtained from a food bank or purchased under financial duress, requires an effort to see the world through food-insecure eyes and understand what it is like to be poor amidst plenty.

Source: Rock, M., McIntyre, L., Rondeau, K. (In press). Discomforting comfort foods: Stirring the pot on Kraft Dinner in Canada. *Agriculture and Human Values*.

Module was administered to determine the food-security status among adults and children in the household; a household's food-security status was then determined from that of adults and children (if present). The food-security module will be used in subsequent cycles of the *Canadian Community Health Survey*, allowing for comparison of food-security dimensions over time (Health Canada, 2007). Households were categorized as food-secure, moderately food-insecure, and severely food-insecure, based on the number of affirmative responses to food-insecure conditions outlined in the food-security module (Health Canada, 2007).

From the results of the survey (see Table 13.1), it is estimated that more than 1.1 million households (9.2 percent of Canadian households) were food-insecure at some point during 2004 as a result of financial difficulties accessing food. This represents 2.7 million Canadians (8.8 percent of the population in 2004) living in food-insecure households. Among households with children, 5.2 percent reported child-level food insecurity (Health Canada, 2007). The province with the highest prevalence of food insecurity was Nova Scotia, where 14.6 percent of households experienced food insecurity, significantly higher than the national prevalence (Health Canada, 2007). Aboriginal households experienced greater and more severe food insecurity than non-Aboriginal households (only off-reserve people were studied): More than 33 percent of Aboriginal households were food-insecure, including 14.4 percent who were severely food-insecure (Health Canada, 2007).

Other food insecurity counts add to a comprehensive picture of the extent of food insecurity in Canada. The annual *HungerCount Survey*, a national survey of food-bank use in Canada, conducted by the Canadian Association of Food Banks (CAFB), is the most consistent, albeit indirect, measure of hunger and food

Table 13.1: Numbers and proportions of Canadian households experiencing income-related food security and food insecurity, CCHS 2.2, 2004

Household type	Food secure n (%)	Food insecure n (%)		
		All	Moderate	Severe
All households	11,089,200	1,123,600	769,900	353,700
	(90.8)	(9.2)	(6.3)	(2.9)
Households with children	3,542,000	412,300	317,100	95,200
	(89.6)	(10.4)	(8.0)	(2.4)
Households without children	7,547,200	711,200	452,800	258,800
	(91.4)	(8.6)	(5.5)	(3.1)
All Aboriginal households	132,200	66,300	37,700	28,600
	(66.7)	(33.4)	(19.0)	(14.4)

Source: Adapted from Health Canada. (2007). Canadian Community Health Survey, cycle 2.2, Nutrition (2004)—Income-related household food security in Canada. Ottawa: Office of Nutrition Policy and Promotion, Health Products and Food Branch.

insecurity in Canada. It was initiated in 1989 by the Canadian Association of Food Banks and has been conducted annually since 1997. In March 2006, the CAFB reported that its annual count of emergency food-program users for the month was 753,458 or 2.4 percent of the total Canadian population, a 99.3 percent increase in food-bank use since 1989 (Canadian Association of Food Banks, 2006). Forty-one percent of food-bank users or 268,774 were children under the age of 18 years. Although food-bank use underestimates the true prevalence of food insecurity, it is highly sensitive to the hunger state (i.e., few people who use a food bank are not truly hungry).

Further insight into the scope of food insecurity in Canada has emerged from analyses of limited sets of indicator questions included in some recent population surveys (see Table 13.2).

Child hunger is an extreme manifestation of household food insecurity and it was the first food-insecurity indicator measured in Canada. Our earliest data on child hunger come from the 1994 and 1996 cycles of the *National Longitudinal Survey of Children and Youth* (NLSCY), in which 22,000 and 16,000 households were asked respectively, "Has your child ever experienced hunger because there was no food in the house or money to buy food? If yes, how often?" In the study reporting on the 1994 survey, hunger occurred in 1.2 percent or 57,000 Canadian families with children under 11 years of age, 35.0 percent of whom reported that their child experienced hunger at least every few months (McIntyre, Connor & Warren, 2000). The adjusted rate for 1994 and 1996 comparisons was 1.3 percent. In 1996, 1.6 percent of the sample reported child hunger, representing 75,615 Canadian families of children under 13 years of age. In 1996, 37.5 percent of these families reported frequent hunger, which was defined as hunger experienced at least every few months. Among these, hunger most often occurred regularly at the end of the month (McIntyre, Walsh & Connor, 2001).

The first adult- and child-level population data on food insecurity in Canada came from the 1998–1999 *National Population Health Survey*, which included three screening questions for food insecurity. Survey results revealed food insecurity among 10.2 percent of Canadian households representing 3 million people (Che & Chen, 2001). Additionally, the most severely food-insecure, termed the food poor, represented 4.1 percent of households, and 4.9 percent or 338,000 children (Rainville & Brink, 2001).

The 2000–2001 *Canadian Community Health Survey* had three screening questions for food insecurity. If respondents reported having been in at least one of the

Table 13.2: Estimates of food insecurity in Canada

Survey	Question to assess food insecurity	Prevalence of food insecurity %
CCHS 2.2, 2004	Household Food Security Survey Module (HFSSM), 18 questions	9.2[1]
CCHS, 2000/2001	"In the past 12 months, how often did you or anyone else in your household: • Not eat the quality or variety of foods that you wanted to eat because of a lack of money?" • Worry that there would not be enough to eat because of a lack of money?" • Not have enough food to eat because of a lack of money?"	14.7[2]
NPHS, 1998/1999	"In the past 12 months, did you or anyone in your household: • Worry that there would not be enough to eat because of a lack of money?" • Not eat the quality or variety of foods that you wanted because of a lack of money?" • Not have enough food to eat because of a lack of money?"	10.4[3]

NPHS, 1996/1997	1. "Thinking about the past 12 months, did your household ever run out of money to buy food?" Yes/No (If yes, respondent was asked the next two questions.)
	2. "In the past 12 months, has anyone in your household received food from a food bank, soup kitchen or other charitable agency?" Yes/No
	3. "Which of the following best describes the food situation in your household?
	  a. Always enough food to eat."
	  b. Sometimes not enough food to eat."
	  c. Often not enough food to eat."
		4.0[4]

NLSCY, 1996	"Has your child ever experienced hunger because there was no food in the house or money to buy food?"	1.2[5]
NLSCY, 1994	"Has your child ever experienced hunger because there was no food in the house or money to buy food?"	1.6[6]

Source: Adapted from Tarasuk, V. (2005). "Household food insecurity in Canada." *Topics in Clinical Nutrition*, 20, 299–312.

1. Health Canada (2007)
2. Ledrou & Gervais, (2005)
3. Che & Chen, (2001)
4. Vozoris & Tarasuk, (2003)
5. McIntyre, Walsh & Connor, (2001)
6. McIntyre, Connor & Warren (2000)

three situations because of a lack of money, they were considered to be living in a food-insecure household (Ledrou & Gervais, 2005). Based on these criteria, an estimated 3.7 million (14.7 percent) Canadians aged 12 years and older had experienced food insecurity (Ledrou & Gervais, 2005).

Local and regional studies also provide insights into the extent of food insecurity among vulnerable populations. A recent study examined the food insecurity and hunger of 141 low-income lone mothers with children in Atlantic Canada over the past year and during the course of one month. Virtually every household experienced food insecurity over the past year (96.5 percent). This was reduced only modestly to 78 percent over the past four-week period. Maternal hunger was reported by 42 percent of mothers over the previous year and 23 percent over the month of the study. Child hunger was very similar to maternal hunger over the study period (McIntyre, Glanville, Officer, Anderson, Raine & Dayle, 2002). Using the *Food Security Core Module* to assess food insecurity in women attending Metropolitan Toronto food banks, Tarasuk and Beaton (1999) found that 94 percent reported some degree of food insecurity, with 70 percent reporting quantitative compromises in food intake ("hunger") over the past year and 57 percent reporting such problems in the past 30 days. Both studies documented the problem of food insecurity among low-income women with children, and both identified variation in the severity of food insecurity. As with other studies, it is difficult to compare the prevalence of hunger and food insecurity without using comparable measures.

It is impossible to know whether these survey rates represent an improvement or a worsening of food insecurity in Canada. Prior to the *Canadian Community Health Survey 2.2*, every study of hunger and food insecurity in Canada used slightly different measures and terms according to the food-insecurity spectrum. Surveys measured food anxiety, food insufficiency, food poverty, compromised diet quality, and child hunger. A comparison of Canadian and American food-insecurity rates could not be assessed before the use of the *Household Food-Security Survey Module* in both countries. While the classification system used in Canada differs somewhat from the United States, Nord and colleagues have produced the first synthetic chart comparing food insecurity in the two countries (see Figure 13.1). Using this comparison, adult food insecurity is substantially less prevalent in Canada than in the US (9.0 percent versus 14.1 percent), but, as is also seen in Figure 13.1, rate disparities vary by household type (Nord, Hooper & Hopwood, 2007).

This discussion of the "true" rate of food insecurity in Canada brings us back to the concern that the numbers do not seem to trigger social action. While we do not make a distinction in heart attack counts by percent cardiac muscle damage or in stroke counts by density of paralysis, it seems that with food-insecurity reporting, what exactly is being measured and how that translates into a palatable (pardon the pun) number seems to matter a lot. National child-hunger rates seem too low, and national population food-insecurity rates seem too high to mobilize Canadians or their policy-makers into action.

Risk Factors for Hunger and Food Insecurity in Canada

While it may be impossible to determine whether there has been an improvement or a worsening of food insecurity in Canada, surveys such as the *Canadian Community Health Survey*, the *National Population Health Survey*, and the *National Longitudinal Survey of Children and Youth* (NLSCY) can be used to identify those who may be vulnerable to hunger and food insecurity in Canada (Health Canada, 2007). The socio-demographic characteristics of hungry families are similar from study to study. Risk factors for hunger and food insecurity are also similar from one study to another—there are few surprises left among the descriptive and analytic studies of food insecurity and hunger in Canada. These misery surveys need not be reproduced again and again. Instead, intervention studies targeted at reducing the determinants of food insecurity are required.

In 1994, NLSCY families headed by lone mothers were eight times more likely to report that their children were hungry compared to other families. Children from families receiving welfare or social-assistance income were 13 times more likely to experience hunger than non-welfare or social-assistance income earners (McIntyre et al., 2000). In 1996, NLSCY families with hungry children were six times more likely to be lone parent-led than other families with over half of such families reporting hunger (McIntyre et al., 2001). While 54 percent of

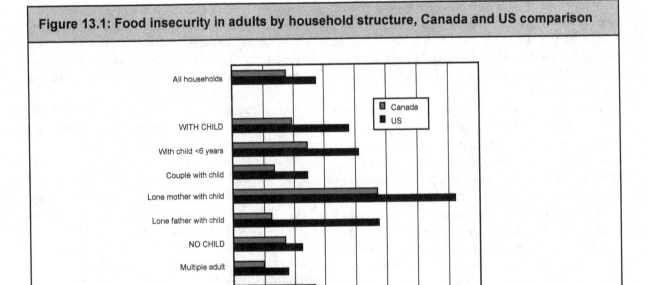

Figure 13.1: Food insecurity in adults by household structure, Canada and US comparison

Percent of households

Data sources: Canadian Community Health Survey cycle 2.2; Current Population Survey Food Security Supplements, 2003–2005.

Source: Adapted from Nord, M., Hooper, M. & Hopwood, H. (2007). *Food insecurity in Canada and the United States: An international comparison.* Presented at the 19th IUHPE World Conference on Health Promotion & Health Education, Vancouver, BC, June 10–15.

all hungry families received their main income from employment in the 1996 survey, families whose incomes included social assistance had greater than an eightfold risk for child hunger and half of such families reported hunger. The only ethnic group that had significantly higher hunger rates was people of Aboriginal descent, who were four times more likely to report hunger than other respondents (this survey includes only off-reserve Aboriginal people).

In 1996, NLSCY logistical regression models identified the following predictors of hunger in addition to low household income: There was a fourfold risk of hunger when the mother reported that her health was fair or poor. When the family was led by a lone parent, the risk increased threefold, and Aboriginal status increased the risk by 60 percent. We also found that a higher total number of siblings in the household independently increased the risk of hunger by 40 percent (McIntyre et al., 2001).

According to both the 1998–1999 *National Population Health Survey* and the 2000–2001 *Canadian Community Health Survey*, the odds of reporting food insecurity increased with declining income adequacy and reliance on social assistance; prevalence was also greatest among lone mothers with children and off-reserve Aboriginal peoples (Che & Chen, 2001; Ledrou & Gervais, 2005).

The data from the *Canadian Community Health Survey 2.2* has been consistent with previous national surveys. There is strong evidence of the relationship between household income adequacy (lowest income is equivalent to lowest income adequacy) and household food insecurity. Figure 13.2 provides a compelling visual depiction of this trend: As a household's income adequacy declines, the prevalence of household food insecurity increases. Indeed, 48.3 percent of households in the lowest-income adequacy category experienced food insecurity; 29.1 percent of households in the lower middle-income adequacy category experienced food insecurity; and 13.6 percent, 5.2 percent, and 1.3 percent of households in the middle-, upper middle-, and highest-income adequacy categories experienced food insecurity. Again, food insecurity was much more prevalent in households whose main source of income was social assistance (59.7 percent) or workers' compensation/employment insurance (29.0 percent) than in those whose main source of income was salary/wages (7.3 percent). In particular, 84.0 percent of Alberta households for whom social assistance was their main source of income experienced food insecurity, the highest rate in the country (Health Canada, 2007).

The *Canadian Community Health Survey 2.2* also revealed that the prevalence of food insecurity was greater in households with children (10.4 percent) than in households without children (8.6 percent). As we have seen in previous national surveys, households led by lone mothers were especially vulnerable (24.9 percent). In all circumstances, Aboriginal households experienced significantly more food insecurity than non-Aboriginal households. Recall from Figure 13.1 that US policy also contributes to the finding that lone mother-led households

are the most disadvantaged of all household types with respect to food insecurity.

Most research on food insecurity has focused upon the experiences of domiciled families; however, homeless individuals are a particularly vulnerable segment of the population for food insecurity. Homeless individuals are excluded from national surveys and, until recently, little has been known about their food-insecurity experience. An ethnographic study of homeless youth in Toronto (Dachner & Tarasuk, 2002) found that their food access was insecure as youth relied primarily on limited and often unsafe charitable food donations and food purchases that were made in the context of poverty. As seen with domiciled families, the amount of money available to homeless individuals for food after shelter and other expenses are considered is severely constrained; added to that is the instability of their daily life and their need for survival, which further jeopardizes their access to food (Dachner & Tarasuk, 2002). The same research team also documented a "disturbingly high prevalence" of nutrient inadequacy and some indications of chronically compromised energy intakes among homeless youth (Tarasuk, Dachner & Li, 2005).

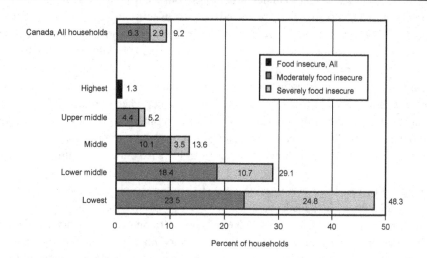

Figure 13.2: Income-related household food security status in Canada by income adequacy category, 2004

Data source: *Statistics Canada, Canadian Community Health Survey, Cycle 2.2, 2004 - Share File*, Household Weights
E: Data with a coefficient of variation (CV) from 16.6 percent to 33.3 percent; interpret with caution.

Source: Health Canada. (2007). Canadian Community Health Survey, Cycle 2.2, *Nutrition (2004)—Income-related household food security in Canada*. Ottawa: Office of Nutrition Policy and Promotion, Health Products and Food Branch.

In summary, the major risk factor for hunger and food insecurity in Canada is lack of sufficient income. Income-related food insecurity in Canada affects those most vulnerable to policies that perpetuate poverty: lone mothers, particularly those on social assistance or welfare; Aboriginal peoples living off-reserve; and workers who are low-waged or on employment or workers' compensation benefits.

Coping and Management Strategies

For very low-income and food-insecure families, the food budget is often the most elastic, meaning that it is the most flexible component; shelter costs and child care often take budgetary priority (Dietitians of Canada, 2005). Williams, Johnson, Kratzmann, Johnson, Anderson, and Chenhall (2006) attempted to determine whether households earning minimum wage would be able to afford a nutritious diet using food-costing data in Nova Scotia. Basic monthly costs included shelter, power/heat/water, telephone, transportation, child care, clothing and footwear, and food. The amount allotted for food was assessed from the National Nutritious Food Basket. In 2006, a family of four with one adult working full-time and the other part-time would experience a projected financial shortfall of $295.89 to meet its basic monthly costs, including food. However, a lone female-parent family with two children would experience a projected financial shortfall of $7.77 *before purchasing food*. Once the cost of the food basket was factored in, this shortfall increased to $385.07. Reports outlining the ability of low-income households to purchase a nutritious diet in Alberta (Alberta Provincial Community Nutritionist's Group, 2005), British Columbia (Antonishak, Bennewith, Lutz, Macdonald, Raja & Sheppard, 2004), and Newfoundland and Labrador (Ewtushik, 2004) have shown similar results.

Management strategies that have been reported by those who experience food insecurity include: purchasing food on credit, sending a child to a friend or relative's home for a meal, selling or pawning possessions, giving up services such as telephone or cable television, delaying bill payments, working odd jobs to increase income, using coupons, comparison shopping, returning bottles, borrowing money and/or food, stealing food, eating less-expensive food, skipping meals or eating less, seeking food from charitable sources (e.g., food bank, soup kitchen), joining community kitchens or food-buying clubs, and planting gardens (Dietitians of Canada, 2005; Hamelin, Beaudry & Habicht, 2002; McIntyre, Glanville, Officer, Anderson, Raine & Dayle; 2002; Tarasuk, 2001). It appears that even within a single month, there is a direct impact of resource depletion on reducing the energy and nutrient intakes of women who live in food-insecure households (Tarasuk, McIntyre & Li, 2007).

The national surveys have also asked food-insecure families how they coped when they had insufficient food. The *National Population Health Survey* analysis of all age groups found that among those reporting food insecurity, 22 percent sought food from charitable sources, almost half reduced the quality of their foods, and about a quarter skipped meals or ate less. Similar to the 1994 survey, among 1996 NLSCY respondents, 21.2 percent reported that they reduced the variety of foods usually eaten when the family had run out of food or money to buy food; 33.2 percent of hungry families reported that the parent skipped meals or ate less; and 4.9 percent reported that the child skipped meals or ate less.

The *Canadian Community Health Survey 2.2* revealed that adults are more likely to experience food insecurity than children in a food-insecure household, especially as the severity increases (Health Canada, 2007). This is consistent with the Atlantic Canadian study of 141 women and children, which examined not only the food-security status, but also the dietary intake of the mother and her children weekly for a month (McIntyre, Glanville et al., 2003). Figure 13.3 depicts caloric intake of mothers and children over the month. At the first of the month when the family has the most money to buy food, mothers' and children's intakes are quite close, but mothers' consumption declines over time. Children have an increase during the third week of the month—what was called the T3 or second cheque of the month effect. This second cheque is often the Child Tax Credit or Goods and Services Tax refund. The same pattern was found for minerals and vitamins (Figure 13.3). Children's dietary intake was consistently better than their mothers, and generally exceeded adequacy levels in comparison with their mothers, whose prevalence of inadequacy was high.

A subsequent analysis of the data from this study (Glanville & McIntyre, 2006) was conducted to

Figure 13.3: Selected dietary intakes of Atlantic Canada lone mothers and their children over one month

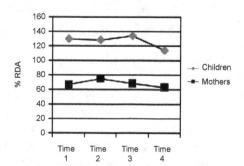

Figure 13.3a: Vit A consumed by mothers and children over time as % RDA of median intake

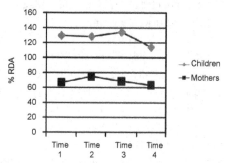

Figure 13.3b: Calcium consumed by mothers and children over time as % adequate intake (AI)

Source: Adapted from McIntyre, L., Glanville, N.T., Raine, K.D., Dayle, J.B., Anderson, B., and Battaglia, N. (2003). "Low-income lone mothers compromise their nutrition to feed their children," *Canadian Medical Association Journal* 168, 686–691.

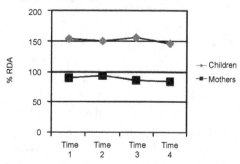

Figure 13.3c: Zinc consumed by mothers and children over time as % RDA of median intake

Source: Adapted from McIntyre, L., Glanville, N.T., Raine, K.D., Dayle, J.B., Anderson, B., and Battaglia, N. (2003). "Low-income lone mothers compromise their nutrition to feed their children," *Canadian Medical Association Journal* 168, 686–691.

determine the diet quality among household members using the *Healthy Eating Index*, which was adapted for the Canadian context. The *Healthy Eating Index* is a tool developed by the United States Department of Agriculture (2007). It is used to measure the quality of diets based on federal nutrition recommendations and dietary guidelines. Both mothers and older children (four to eight years) had significantly poorer diets than younger children (one to three years) (Glanville & McIntyre, 2006). The diet quality of mothers was poor (35.5 percent) or in need of

improvement (64.5 percent), and in fact, no mother in the study had a good diet. It seems that the youngest children are protected from poor-quality diets in food-insecure households (Glanville & McIntyre, 2006).

Assuming these results are generalizable to other vulnerable mothers, the implications are clear. In the Atlantic Canada study, mothers' dietary intakes were consistently poorer than their children's intakes. The difference in adequacy of intake between mothers and children widened from the beginning to the end of the month concurrent with the depletion of income resources. Dietary improvement occurred in children when a small amount of cash was infused into the home and, in fact, except for a few nutrients, children attained dietary adequacy.

Recently, a dietary modelling study (McIntyre, Tarasuk & Li, 2007) was conducted to see if nutrient inadequacies observed in 226 food-insecure women from the Atlantic Canada study (McIntyre, Glanville, et al., 2003) and the Toronto food bank study (Tarasuk, 2001) could be lessened by adding typically chosen healthy foods (fruit, vegetables, and milk) to their reported dietary intake. After adding women's personal food preferences, and adjusting for the effects of food insecurity with hunger, the prevalence of nutrient inadequacy was reduced by more than 50 percent for calcium, iron, magnesium, niacin, riboflavin, thiamin, vitamin B12, vitamin A, vitamin C, vitamin B6, and zinc (McIntyre, Tarasuk & Li, 2007). By providing access to their preferred healthy foods, i.e., the financial resources to do so, food-insecure women could see significant improvements in their nutritional status, insomuch as these resources would be directed toward the purchase of fruit, vegetables, and milk for their own consumption.

These studies demonstrate how both gender and age act as moderators of food insecurity as mothers compromise their own nutritional intake in order to preserve the adequacy of their children's diets, particularly their youngest children's diets.

The 1996 *National Population Health Survey* revealed that 35 percent of respondents sought help from food banks; seeking help from relatives and friends was reported by 31 percent and 29 percent respectively. Clearly, food-bank use grossly underestimates the number of food-insecure families, although food-bank visitors are distinct from other food-insecure families. From the 1996 NLSCY analysis, the independent predictors of food-bank use were lone parenthood, a higher number of siblings in the household, and income from social assistance (McIntyre et al., 2001). Tarasuk (2001) also found that food-bank use was related to a higher number of children in the family. These families are the poorest, the most isolated, and among the most severely food-insecure. The Atlantic Canada study of lone mothers and their children asked the mothers about sources of free food. Less than 10 percent of mothers *did*

not receive free food and a startling 54 percent visited the food bank. Another four in 10 received food from relatives. Reflective of a rural population, some women had their own hunting licences to acquire food, and they gardened (McIntyre et al., 2002). Again, for such a complex social phenomenon, socio-demographic and behavioural results from one food-insecurity study to another are remarkably similar.

Nutritional Implications

It is well documented that low-income Canadians have poorer health than others. Low income has also been associated with increased likelihood of suboptimal nutrient intake and decreased likelihood of food-consumption patterns consistent with "healthy eating" (Power, 2005); however, it is unclear what role long-term food insecurity plays in observed health inequities. Tarasuk's accompanying chapter in this volume further discusses the relationship among food insecurity, its nutritional implications, and health.

Hunger and Food-Insecurity Dynamics

Another food-insecurity descriptor is the dynamics of hungry households. While persistent hunger is a problem, hunger transitions are also worthy of study. There were 358 families in the NLSCY cohort for both 1994 and 1996 who ever reported hunger. Only 22.6 percent of them reported persistent hunger, i.e., hunger in both time periods. Families with persistent hunger were remarkable for their lack of any meaningful change in circumstance. But that does not mean that these families were in some type of equilibrium. They reported the highest levels of family dysfunction (McIntyre et al., 2001).

There were many factors that could tip a family into the hunger state (Table 13.3). They are categorized as another mouth to feed (one or more siblings added to the household; a change in the number of parents in the household); job loss (the father lost full-time work; the mother's unemployment status changed); and health problems (the mother's health status worsened; the child's health status changed for either better or worse). Getting out of hunger depended upon one change only: The mother gets a full-time job, and the family's income rises accordingly (McIntyre et al., 2001). Annual income changes were calculated for families by hunger state. The total family income needed to increase by $3,827 in 2001 dollars in order for a family to leave the hunger state, but a loss of only $2,690 could tip a family into hunger, indicating that these families are fragile already. These results related to change in hunger status underscore not only the fluidity of hungry families but their predictability.

Conclusion

The data presented support the fact that hunger and food insecurity are real issues in Canada created by social policies that increase rather than reduce disparities. Policy recommendations required to address food insecurity and hunger are easy to name, but they do require the political will to address them.

1. Real incomes must rise, whether from minimum wage or social assistance. Food insecurity results from anything that limits household resources or the proportion of those resources available for food acquisition. Limited employment opportunities; low minimum-wage scale and social assistance benefits; and increases in non-discretionary, non-food expenditures such as the cost of housing, utilities, and child care all contribute to insufficient income to purchase food.

2. Healthy foods must be affordable, particularly the food staples such as milk. Food must meet not only caloric needs but provide essential nutrients for optimal health. Community-based food-assistance programs such as food banks do not support the achievement of healthy diets among recipients. These initiatives represent a poor policy alternative to the family purchase of healthy foods.

Many lower- and middle-income countries monitor and support the price of food staples, e.g., tortilla flour in Mexico. Canada's marketing board policies protect the supply of staples and the incomes of producers, but not the affordability of food staples for consumers. Fluid milk is one example. Despite its superior nutritional value, inadequate consumption of milk products is consistently observed in low-income populations; particularly for low-income, mother-led families, lack of milk security can be a preoccupation (McIntyre, Williams & Glanville, 2007). It may be time for Canada to adopt a food-staples policy that supports opportunities for healthy eating among its most vulnerable citizens.

Table 13.3: Risk factors among NLSCY families who report hunger in 1996 and no hunger in 1994

Risk factor	Odds ratio (95% confidence interval)
Another mouth to feed	
>1 new sibling in home	5.75 (2.18–16.03)
Change in number of parents in household	2.06 (1.02–4.21)
Job loss	
Father lost full-time work	5.64 (1.15–26.57)
Mother unemployment status change	2.57 (1.58–4.21)
Health problems	
Mother health status worse	3.45 (1.27–8.52)
Child health status change	2.25 (2.09–5.70)

Source: Adapted from McIntyre, L., Walsh, G. & Connor, S.K. (2001). *A follow-up study of child hunger in Canada*. Working paper W-01-1-2E. Applied Research Branch. Strategic Policy. Ottawa: Human Resources Development Canada.

3. Because food needs give way to shelter needs in the poorest households, affordable housing is urgently required.

4. In families with children, lack of affordable, quality daycare is often a significant barrier to employment.

5. Some self-sufficiency demonstration projects have shown the promise of work-related supports, health and recreation provision, and other transition assistance. These types of employment-support programs should be widely disseminated.

This grouping of recommendations speaks to the determinants of food insecurity and together, they are the subjects of wide policy debate. There is strong evidence supporting their contributions individually and collectively to poverty reduction and improved life quality.

6. There should be a consistent monitoring system for hunger and food insecurity—not to survey misery but to determine progress, deterioration, or shifts among those affected. In turn, a food-security policy lens must be applied to social policies to ensure that they reduce genuine hunger rather than exacerbate it.

The data presented for this paper have been assembled by individual effort and through the retrieval of disparate sources. Canada's Nutrition Plan of Action and other documents and lobbying efforts by non-governmental bodies call for a systematic monitoring of food insecurity with an eye to rapid policy translation. Now that we have established the household food-security module as the standard measure for population-level food insecurity in Canada, it is disappointing that the 3.1 cycle of the *Canadian Community Health Survey* cannot be compared to the 2.2 cycle because several provinces opted out of collecting the information.

Food security is perhaps the most precious of all determinants of health. If Canada is prepared to make the necessary investments, it can reap a food-security dividend that enriches all of society with payoffs in health, social capital, sustainability of our physical and social environments, justice, and both cost savings and wealth creation.

Critical Thinking Questions

1. From your understanding of food insecurity in Canada, is it bad or is it wrong (unfortunate or unjust)?

2. Why is the charitable response (e.g., food banks) rather than a social justice response (e.g., poverty-reduction policies) the dominant response to food insecurity in Canada?

3. Should food insecurity be considered in the list of social determinants of health or is there a better way of conceptualizing how it relates to health?

4. Why are the rates of food insecurity reported in national surveys insufficient to lead to policy change to alleviate the problem?

5. Will increased income truly reduce food insecurity in poor households or will the money be diverted to other essential household needs?

Recommended Readings

Engler-Stringer, R. & Berenbaum, S. (2007). "Exploring food security with collective kitchens participants in three Canadian cities." *Qualitative Health Research, 17*, 75–84.

This is a recent study that examines the experience of participants in collective-kitchen programs in Saskatoon, Toronto, and Montreal. In groups that cooked large quantities of food (upwards of five meals per month), the study found that insofar as the participant did not experience severe food insecurity, collective kitchens were perceived as a tool to help stretch the food budget and avoid using a food bank or other charitable food-distribution systems. Nonetheless, the authors conclude that long-term strategies to improve food security are needed.

McIntyre, L., Glanville, N.T., Raine, J.D., Dayle, J.B., Anderson, B. & Battaglia, N. (2003). "Do low-income lone mothers compromise their nutrition to feed their children?" *Canadian Medical Association Journal, 168*, 686–691.

The objective of this study was to document whether or not low-income lone mothers compromise their own dietary intake so that their children have an adequate food intake. The study did find that mothers' intakes failed to meet their requirements for total kilocalories and a number of essential nutrients, and that children's intakes were consistently more adequate than their mothers'. A weekly follow-up for one month of the nutrient consumption showed that the infusion of extra resources in the third week led to improved consumption among children, but not their mothers.

Rideout, K., Riches, G., Ostry, A., Buckingham, D. & MacRae, R. (2007). "Bringing home the right to food in Canada: Challenges and possibilities for achieving food security." *Public Health Nutrition, 10*, 566–573.

This article covers the international legal agreements proclaiming the right to food. It then focuses upon Canada's policy infrastructure for food security, tracing the history of the social safety net in Canada from the 1996 Canada Assistance Plan to the federal surpluses that have been recorded annually since 1997. The paper also comments on the institutionalization of food banks and argues that charitable food-distribution systems have led to a shift in the policy debate on solutions from one based on rights to one based on benevolence. As a result, Canada lacks a comprehensive food and nutrition policy directed at the optimal nourishment of the population.

Tarasuk, V. (2001). "A critical examination of community-based responses to household food insecurity in Canada." *Health Education and Behaviour, 28*, 487–499.

Over the past two decades, household food insecurity has emerged as a significant social problem and serious public health concern in the First World. This article reviews the recent emergence of hunger as a Canadian concern and the development of responses to this problem. The author provides a critical examination of the community development strategies that attempt to respond to food insecurity.

Tarasuk, V., McIntyre, L. & Li, J. (2007). "Low-income women's dietary intakes are sensitive to the depletion of household resources in one month." *Journal of Nutrition, 137*, 1980–1987.

In food-insecure households, food supplies are more limited and individuals have less varied diets; less consumption of fruits, vegetables, and milk products; and lower energy and nutrient intakes in the context of food insufficiency and food insecurity. This study examined the impact of resource depletion on the dietary intakes of women who experienced various levels of food insecurity. As household resources were depleted, women with moderate or severe food insecurity exhibited declines in energy, carbohydrate, vitamin B6, and fruit and vegetable intakes. No similar patterns were apparent in those classed as food-secure or marginally food-insecure. The study concluded that the daily food intakes of women in deprived circumstances are sensitive to the state of their household resources, declining as resources become depleted.

Related Web Sites

Canadian Association of Food Banks (CAFB)—www.cafb-acba.ca/english/EducationandResearch-ResearchStudies.html

The Canadian Association of Food Banks represents food banks in every province. While providing member food banks with groceries for people in daily need, they ultimately work toward a hunger-free Canada. This site provides information on CAFB, public education and research, finding a member food bank, and supporters. This site provides access to the annual HungerCount publication, which documents food-bank use in Canada.

Centre for Studies in Food Security (CSFS) at Ryerson University—www.ryerson.ca/foodsecurity

The purpose of the Centre for Studies in Food Security is to facilitate research, community action, and professional practice to increase food security by focusing on the issues of health, income, and the evolution of food systems. The Web site provides links to the work of the centre, publications, conferences, and affiliated organizations.

Food Secure Canada (FSC)—www.foodsecurecanada.org

Food Secure Canada is a new Canadian organization that unites people and organizations working for food security nationally and globally. The organization sponsors conferences and events, has initiated a plan for action, and includes a site for publications.

Health Canada Office of Food and Nutrition—www.hc-sc.gc.ca/fn-an/index_e.html

This site hosts the latest in Health Canada news and reports. Perhaps its most important holding is *Income-Related Household Food Security in Canada*, the second report in a series related to the *Canadian Community Health Survey*, Cycle 2.2, Nutrition (2004). The full report can be viewed at the Health Canada Web site at: www.hc-sc.gc.ca/fn-an/surveill/nutrition/commun/cchs_focus-volet_escc_e.html.

United Nations Food and Agriculture Organization—www.fao.org/docrep/009/a0750e/a0750e00.htm

The State of Food Insecurity in the World 2006 presents the latest estimates of the number of chronically hungry people in the world and reports on global and national efforts to reduce that number by the year 2015. Detailed information is provided on the prevalence of undernourishment in developing countries and countries in transition and on food availability, dietary diversification, poverty, health, and child nutritional status.

——————●——————

Chapter 14

HEALTH IMPLICATIONS
OF FOOD INSECURITY

Valerie Tarasuk

Introduction

Food security is commonly defined as the state that "exists when all people, at all times, have physical and economic access to sufficient, safe and nutritious food to meet their dietary needs and food preferences for an active and healthy life" (Agriculture and Agri-Food Canada, 1998), but household food security typically focuses on households' financial ability to access adequate food. Rooted in the breakdown of Canada's social safety net, household food insecurity is a serious social problem (Riches, 1997a, 2002) and a violation of the basic human right to food (Rideout, Riches, Ostry, Buckingham & MacRae, 2007). It is also a public health problem in Canada (Power, 2005; Joint Steering Committee, 1996).

This chapter examines the health and nutrition implications of household food insecurity for Canadians. The chapter begins with an overview of the measurement of household food insecurity. The relationship between food insecurity and nutrition is then examined, and the associations between food insecurity and various indicators of poor health are reviewed. A discussion of the policy implications of food insecurity in Canada is presented by Lynn McIntyre and Krista Rondeau elsewhere in this volume.

Measuring Food Insecurity in Canada

Since the inclusion of three questions about child hunger on the 1994 *National Longitudinal Survey of Children*

and Youth (McIntyre, Connor & Warren, 1998), indicator questions on household food insecurity have been included on several national surveys. In most instances, however, the measurement properties of the questions used have not been assessed, so it has been unclear what exactly they were measuring and how well they captured it. In addition, the questions used to assess food insecurity on Canadian population health surveys have been altered from one survey to the next, precluding the examination of trends in household food insecurity over time (Tarasuk, 2005). However, with the inclusion of the *Household Food Security Survey Module* (HFSSM) on Cycle 2.2 of the *Canadian Community Health Survey* in 2004 (CCHS 2.2), we now have food-security prevalence estimates that are based on a well-researched, standardized, multiple-indicator measure of food security (Health Canada, 2007b).

CCHS 2.2 sampled individuals of all ages living in private dwellings in the 10 provinces, excluding full-time members of the Canadian forces and individuals living in the territories, on First Nations reserves, and in some remote areas (Health Canada, 2007b). From this survey, an estimated 1.1 million households (9.2 percent) were found to be food-insecure at some point in the previous year because of income-related barriers to food access. Expressed another way, 2.7 million Canadians lived in food-insecure households in 2004.

Understanding what it means for 1.1 million Canadian households to be classed as food-insecure requires a review of the survey questions and responses that

Table 14.1: Reponses to items in the Household Food Security Survey Module, Canada, 2004[1,2]

	Households affirming item[3,4]					
	All households		Households with children		Households without children	
	n	%	n	%	n	%
Adult Food Security Scale						
You and other household members worried food would run out before you got money to buy more	1,224,700	10.0	468,100	11.8	756,600	9.2
Food you and other household members bought didn't last and there wasn't any money to get more	936,200	7.7	331,800	8.4	604,400	7.3
You and other adults in your household couldn't afford to eat balanced meals	1,030,900	8.4	325,100	8.2	705,900	8.6
You or other adults in your household ever cut size of meals or skipped meals	530,000	4.3	162,200	4.1	367,700	4.5
You or other adults in your household ever cut size of meals or skipped meals in 3 or more months	406,100	3.3	116,900	3.0	289,200	3.5
You (personally) ever ate less than you felt you should	561,500	4.6	179,300	4.5	382,200	4.6
You (personally) were ever hungry but did not eat	317,800	2.6	79,900	2.0	237,900	2.9
You (personally) lost weight	198,000	1.6	44,000	1.1	154,000	1.9
You or other adults in your household ever did not eat for whole day	113,100	0.9	26,000	0.7	87,100	1.0
You or other adults in your household ever did not eat for whole day in 3 or more months	93,900	0.8	19,400	0.5	74,400	0.9
Child Food Security Scale[5]						
You or other adults in your household relied on only a few kinds of low-cost food to feed children	337,400	2.8	337,400	2.8	...	...

	n		n			
You or other adults in your household couldn't feed children a balanced meal	230,500	1.9	230,500	1.9	...	...
Children were not eating enough	98,800	0.8	98,800	0.8	...	...
You or other adults in your household ever cut size of any of the children's meals	25,300	0.2	25,300	0.2	...	...
Any of the children were ever hungry	21,100	0.2	21,100	0.2	...	...
Any of the children ever skipped meals	14,900	0.1E	14,900	0.1E	...	...
Any of the children ever skipped meals in 3 or more months	10,500	0.1E	10,500	0.1E	...	...
Any of the children ever did not eat for the whole day	F	F	F	F	...	...

Legend
n Weighted sample size, rounded to nearest 100
E Data with a coefficient of variation (CV) from 16.6 percent to 33.3 percent; interpret with caution
F Data with a coefficient of variation (CV) greater than 33.3 percent or a cell size <30; data suppressed
... Not applicable

Footnotes
1. Territories and First Nations reserves are not included.
2. The wording of each question as read to the respondent includes explicit reference to resource limitation (e.g., "because there wasn't enough money for food").
3. Bootstrapping techniques were used to produce the coefficient of variation (CV) and 95 percent confidence intervals (CI).
4. Households for which the item was "not applicable" were excluded from the denominator.
5. Results from the Child Food Security Scale were obtained only from households with children. Children are defined as individuals younger than 18 years of age.

Source: Health Canada. (2007). Canadian Community Health Survey, Cycle 2.2, Nutrition (2004)—Income-Related Household Food Security in Canada. Reproduced with the permission of the Minister of Public Works and Government Services Canada, 2007.

underpin this statistic (Health Canada, 2007b, Table 14.1). The questions focus on concrete experiences of diminished diet quality and reductions in food intake, differentiating the experiences of adults from those of children in the household. Ten questions comprise the Adult Food Security Scale, and eight comprise the Child Food Security Scale. When asked on the survey module, each question specifies a lack of money or ability to afford food as the reason for the condition or behaviour. All of the questions are referenced to the previous 12 months, so food insecurity over the previous year is captured.

In examining the proportion of households that reported experiences of food insecurity on CCHS 2.2, two patterns are apparent in Table 14.1:

1. The items and the proportion of households responding affirmatively to them follow a pattern that reflects the graded severity of these experiences. People in 1.2 million households worried that they would run out of food before they got money to buy more, for example, but a somewhat smaller number (1,030,900) said they could not afford to eat balanced meals. A much smaller number (113,100) reported that one or more adults did not eat for a whole day because there wasn't enough money for food. This is consistent with our understanding of the sequence of events that characterize food insecurity among domiciled individuals and

families; food-related anxiety typically precedes compromises in food intake, and compromises in the quality and variety of foods eaten occur long before the situation becomes so dire as to result in absolute food deprivation.

2. Among households with children, the experiences of food insecurity captured on this questionnaire are more common among adults than children. For example, adults in 79,900 households reported the experience of being hungry but not eating because they couldn't afford enough food, but this condition was reported for children in only 21,100 households. This is consistent with a vast array of research (discussed in more detail later in this chapter) suggesting that parents typically do whatever they can, including compromising their own food intakes, to minimize constraints on their children's food intakes.

For a household to be classed as food-insecure, two or more items on either the adult or child scale needed to be affirmed. As indicated in Table 14.1, the experiences that most commonly characterized food-insecure households in Canada were worrying about running out of food; running out of food and not having the money to get more; and not being able to afford balanced meals. However, more extreme levels of dietary compromise and food deprivation were reported by hundreds of thousands of households. Households were considered to have experienced severe food insecurity if they reported disrupted eating patterns and reduced food intake among adults and/or children, as well as multiple problems with food access. This was determined by the affirmation of six or more items on the adult scale and/or five or more items on the child scale. Approximately 353,700 households (2.9 percent) fell into the category of severe food insecurity.

Food Insecurity among Some Extremely Vulnerable Groups

Although most of our understanding of household food insecurity in Canada comes from the results of large population surveys such as CCHS 2.2, it is worth noting that some extremely vulnerable population subgroups were not included in CCHS 2.2: on-reserve Aboriginal

peoples, people living in the territories and some remote regions, and homeless people. Although these groups comprise relatively small proportions of the total population, they are at a particularly high risk of food insecurity and nutritional vulnerability.

The results of CCHS 1.1, conducted in 2000–2001, shed some light on the vulnerability of people living in Yukon, Northwest Territories, and Nunavut. On that survey, food security was assessed in terms of three indicator questions, so the results are not directly comparable to the prevalence estimates from CCHS 2.2. Nonetheless, the results are concerning; food-insecurity prevalence estimates of 21 percent, 28 percent, and 56 percent were reported for Yukon, Northwest Territories, and Nunavut respectively (Ledrou & Gervais, 2005). All of these estimates were well above those observed in the 10 provinces and above the national prevalence of 14.7 percent (Ledrou & Gervais, 2005), highlighting the pervasiveness of household food insecurity in Canada's North. Further evidence of this comes from recent studies in three northern Aboriginal communities documenting prevalences of food insecurity in excess of 60 percent (Lawn & Harvey, 2003, 2004a, 2004b). These estimates are based on the same food-security questionnaire used in CCHS 2.2. The findings reflect the extraordinarily high rates of poverty and high food costs in these communities (Willows, 2005).

Reports of food scarcity and food deprivation among homeless groups also abound (Hagan & McCarthy, 1997; Tarasuk, Dachner & Li, 2005; Khandor & Mason, 2007). While it is impossible to know the magnitude of problems of homelessness in Canada, the abject poverty that characterizes homelessness means food insecurity and extreme levels of nutritional vulnerability are integral to this existence (Tarasuk et al., 2005).

The exclusion of particularly vulnerable groups like homeless individuals, Canadians living in remote northern communities, and First Nations peoples living on reserves from national population surveys mean that the food-security prevalence estimates generated from these surveys underestimate the true extent of this problem in Canada.

Household Food Insecurity: The Dietary Manifestation of Acute Financial Insecurity

The inclusion of indicators of food insecurity on population surveys in Canada has facilitated a clear delineation of the socio-demographic factors associated with a vulnerability to household food insecurity in this country. The risk of food insecurity escalates as the adequacy of household income declines (Health Canada, 2007b). Furthermore, income adequacy is by far the strongest predictor of household food insecurity in Canada (Che & Chen, 2001; Vozoris & Tarasuk, 2003). Other markers of vulnerability to food insecurity include Aboriginal status; lone parenthood; reliance on social assistance, workers' compensation, or employment insurance; and renting rather than owning one's dwelling (Health Canada, 2007b)—all factors that are closely linked to household income. Problems of household food insecurity are primarily problems of financial insecurity, not problems arising because of a lack of food-preparation skills, poor budgeting skills, or the lack of motivation to prepare foods from scratch (McLaughlin, Tarasuk & Krieger, 2003; Travers, 1995).

Inadequate income poses a major barrier to healthy eating. An analysis of household food-expenditure data in Canada indicates that households' purchases of milk products and fruits and vegetables fall precipitously as income declines (Ricciuto, Tarasuk & Yatchew, 2006). Not surprisingly, the nutritional quality of foods purchased also declines (Ricciuto & Tarasuk, 2007). Household food insecurity occurs in the context of low incomes, but it denotes particularly extreme constraints on food purchasing. Families who receive income on a regular basis, but typically cannot make ends meet, often describe their food restrictions as cyclic, with food shortages most acute at the end of the month, when household resources are exhausted (Hamelin, Beaudry & Habicht, 2002; Hamelin, Habicht & Beaudry, 1999; Tarasuk, 2001).

Within low-income households, the kinds of restrictions on individuals' food intakes that are assessed on survey instruments are tightly intertwined with the deterioration of household resources. This is illustrated in a recent examination of changes in dietary intake over the month in a sample of low-income, predominantly food-insecure women with children, drawn from two earlier Canadian studies (McIntyre, Tarasuk & Li, 2007; Tarasuk, McIntyre & Li, 2007). Almost all (97 percent) of the 182 women included in the analysis relied on welfare for most of their income, and all had incomes well below the Statistics Canada Low-Income Cut-offs

(the poverty line). Sixty-five percent had experienced moderate or severe adult food insecurity over the month (Tarasuk, McIntyre & Li, 2007). As the days since their receipt of a cheque increased, women's food intakes systematically declined (as indicated by a fall in their energy intakes). In particular, they consumed fewer servings of milk products and vegetables. When the women's food-security status was taken into account, the food intakes of those with moderate or severe food insecurity appeared most sensitive to the depletion of household resources over time.

Our study was limited insofar as we were able to examine changes in women's intakes only over time. More research is needed to understand how others in households like these are affected. Given the research suggesting that women in severely resource-constrained circumstances will deprive themselves of food to spare their children from deprivation (Campbell & Desjardins, 1989; McIntyre et al., 2003; Dowler & Calvert, 1995; Power, 2006), women's food intakes may be more sensitive to dwindling household resources than are the intakes of other family members. However, it would be naive to assume that the food intakes of children in these households were completely unaffected. A recent study of Hispanic children in California showed significant declines in their energy intakes and meat intakes in food-insecure households as payday approached (Matheson, Varady, Varady & Killen, 2002).

It is noteworthy that we documented significant declines in food intake in relation to time since the receipt of income among a sample of women with children, 97 percent of whom depended on social assistance for their income. Among low-income Canadians, those on welfare are particularly vulnerable to food insecurity (Health Canada, 2007a, 2007b; Che & Chen, 2001; Vozoris & Tarasuk, 2003; McIntyre, Connor & Warren, 2000). In the 2004 CCHS, 60 percent of households that relied on welfare were food-insecure, and half of these households were classed as severely food-insecure (Health Canada, 2007b). This reflects the impoverishment that has come to define welfare programs in Canada. Although welfare income levels are set by the provincial and territorial governments and these rates vary by household type, incomes rarely exceed two-thirds of the Statistics Canada Low-Income Cut-offs, and they are often much, much lower (National Council of Welfare, 2006). Furthermore,

Box 14.1: The best medicine money can buy
Carol Goar

Medical schools didn't spend much time on malnutrition when David McKeown trained to be a doctor. Hunger wasn't considered a health problem.

Today, it is one of McKeown's major preoccupations. As Toronto's medical officer of health, he sees the consequences of malnutrition daily—in underweight babies; children with developmental problems; adults with diabetes, anemia, high blood pressure, osteoporosis, and obesity.

"When people don't have enough money to buy healthy food, they get sick. It's that simple," McKeown says. "Eliminating poverty is the best medicine money can buy."

More than 300,000 Torontonians need that medicine.

It strikes McKeown as odd that the Ontario government has developed a sophisticated tool to diagnose hunger, yet refuses to treat it.

Each of the province's 36 public health units uses a rigorous formula handed down by the Ministry of Health and Long-Term Care to calculate how much it costs to provide a healthy basic diet. In Toronto, a family of four needs $576.06 a month to fulfill its nutritional requirements.

But the maximum welfare payment available to such a family is $1,291 a month. An average two-bedroom apartment in Toronto rents for $1,073 a month. That leaves $218 for food, clothing, heat, hydro, transportation and everything else. Eating properly is just not possible.

"Once you decide, as a matter of public policy, that the state should be providing support to people in need, your purpose should be to provide a modest, dignified, healthy life," McKeown says. "That's all I'm asking."

Although the numbers are not quite as stark, Ontario's minimum wage also forces many families to skimp on food. The maximum a parent with a minimum-wage job could earn is $1,408 a month. It would require a feat of financial wizardry to pay the rent, provide a well-balanced diet and buy other essentials. Usually, it is the food that gets cut.

"We must bring their incomes up to a level where they have enough to eat," McKeown says.

He has called on the province several times to raise social assistance rates and increase the minimum wage. He renewed his appeal during last month's election campaign.

It appears to have had no impact on the government's plans. The Liberals, who breezed back into power, said they'd proceed, as outlined in last spring's budget, to boost welfare rates by 2 per cent in November and raise the minimum wage to $8.75 in March. But they offered nothing else.

If McKeown is discouraged, it doesn't show. He is encouraging other medical officers of health across the province to speak up and work with community groups in Toronto to fight poverty neighbourhood by neighbourhood.

"We are getting better at articulating these issues in a way that grabs people," says Nick Saul, executive director of The Stop Community Food Centre in the city's west end. "We're trying to create some kind of tipping point."

Right now, there's not a lot of visible momentum, McKeown admits. "But tipping points are hard to see before you get to them."

It would be helpful if more of McKeown's medical colleagues stood with him. But he sees little prospect of that happening. "I don't think this is high on the agenda of the health-care system."

It would also be helpful if medical schools paid more attention to root causes of chronic illness. But McKeown is not counting on that either. "It's on the curriculum, but it has to compete with all the technical knowledge and clinical skills students want."

So he is turning to the public to help him make food a basic human right. That's what Toronto's medical officer of health has always done.

The public health office celebrates its 125th anniversary next year. In preparation for the event, McKeown has been poring over the records kept by Toronto's first medical officer of health, Dr. Charles Hastings.

"His biggest challenges were housing, poverty and access to food," McKeown says.

He lets the comment hang in air, eloquent and damning.

Source: *The Toronto Star*, October 17, 2007, www.thestar.com/article/267732

welfare incomes have declined over the past decade in most provinces and territories (National Council of Welfare, 2006). Income-expense comparisons indicate that, for many recipients, welfare incomes are insufficient to cover the costs of basic needs.[1] These findings highlight the policy origins of problems of household food insecurity in Canada.

Nutritional Implications of Food Insecurity

The prevalence of household food insecurity in Canada is an important indicator of population health because this condition reflects the nutritional health and well-being of household members. What follows is an overview of research examining the food and nutrient intakes of adults and children in the context of household food insecurity, and a discussion of the implications of such dietary intake patterns for longer-term health.

Dietary Compromises and Heightened Nutritional Vulnerability

The dietary compromises associated with household food insecurity in the US have been extensively documented (Bhattacharya, Currie & Haider, 2004; Dixon, Winkleby & Radimer, 2001; Rose, 1999), but given the limited nature of nutrition monitoring in Canada, we have much less research on the nutritional implications of household food insecurity for Canadians. Prior to CCHS 2.2, Canadian research into the nutritional consequences of food insecurity comprised dietary assessments of small samples of individuals in particularly vulnerable circumstances. These included studies of low-income, lone-parent women and children (Badun, Evers & Hooper, 1995; McIntyre, Raine, Glanville & Dayle, 2001; McIntyre et al., 2002; McIntyre et al., 2003), food-bank users (Jacobs Starkey, Gray-Donald & Kuhnlein, 1999; Jacobs Starkey, Kuhnlein & Gray-Donald, 1998; Jacobs Starkey & Kuhnlein, 2000; Tarasuk & Beaton, 1999a, 1999b; Tarasuk, 2001), and homeless youth (Tarasuk et al., 2005). While the studies yielded some disturbing evidence of nutritional vulnerability, the generalizability of the research was severely limited by the small, community-based nature of the samples. Furthermore, because the studies lacked food-secure comparison groups, there was no way to estimate the toll of household food insecurity on the nutritional health

and well-being of Canadians. The collection of data on both dietary intake and household food security from a nationally representative sample of 35,000 Canadians in CCHS 2.2 has finally enabled an examination of the nutritional implications of household food insecurity in this country.

To examine the effect of household food insecurity on individuals' dietary intakes, we conducted a series of comparison using the data from CCHS 2.2 (Kirkpatrick & Tarasuk, 2008). Considering individuals' intakes in relation to the four food groups of Canada's Food Guide (Health Canada, 2007c), we found that, on average, adults and children of all ages in food-insecure households consumed fewer servings of fruits and vegetables and milk products when compared to those in food-secure households (figures 14.1 and 14.2). There were fewer differences in the consumption of meat and alternatives and grain products by household food-security status (figures 14.3 and 14.4). While many of the observed differences for adults' and adolescents' intakes were statistically significant (as denoted by the asterisks in these figures), few significant differences in the mean intakes of children in relation to household food-security status were detected.

Consistent with the observed differences in food-intake patterns, the nutritional quality of individuals' intakes also differed systematically by food-security status (Kirkpatrick & Tarasuk, 2008). Adults in food-insecure households had lower intakes of most vitamins and minerals, although the statistical significance of observed differences varied somewhat by age and sex. Differences were also noted in the nutrient intakes of adolescents, and adolescents and adults in food-insecure households also generally exhibited lower dietary-fibre intakes. Very few significant differences in children's nutrient intakes were observed in relation to household food-security status.

To assess whether the observed differences in nutrient intakes were of sufficient magnitude to increase the vulnerability of individuals in food-insecure households to problems of nutrient inadequacy, we compared individuals' intakes to current estimates of nutrient requirements (Kirkpatrick & Tarasuk, 2008). Higher prevalences of inadequacy were observed among adults and adolescents in food-insecure households for several nutrients, including protein, vitamin A, vitamin C,

Figure 14.1: Consumption of fruits and vegetables (servings/day) by Household Food-Security Status

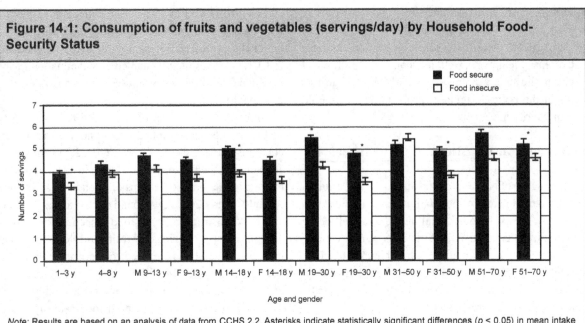

Note: Results are based on an analysis of data from CCHS 2.2. Asterisks indicate statistically significant differences ($p < 0.05$) in mean intake by food-security status.

Source: Kirkpatrick, S. & Tarasuk, V. (2008). Food insecurity is associated with nutrient inadequacies among Canadian adults and adolescents. *Journal of Nutrition, 138*, 604–612.

Figure 14.2: Consumption of milk products (servings/day) by Household Food-Security Status

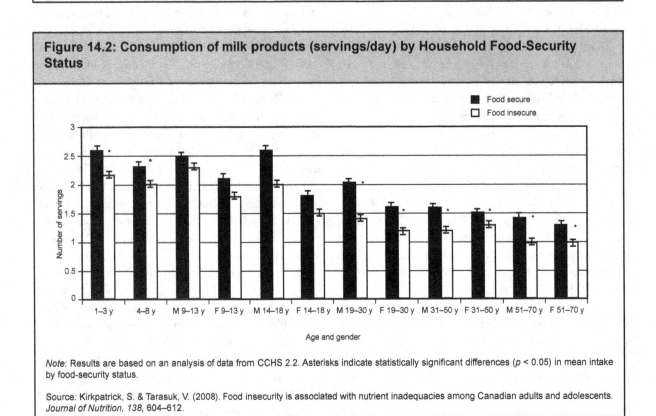

Note: Results are based on an analysis of data from CCHS 2.2. Asterisks indicate statistically significant differences ($p < 0.05$) in mean intake by food-security status.

Source: Kirkpatrick, S. & Tarasuk, V. (2008). Food insecurity is associated with nutrient inadequacies among Canadian adults and adolescents. *Journal of Nutrition, 138*, 604–612.

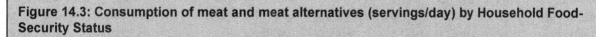

Figure 14.3: Consumption of meat and meat alternatives (servings/day) by Household Food-Security Status

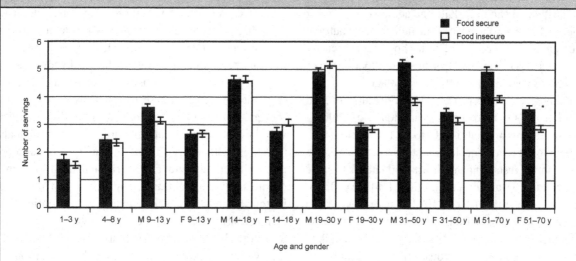

Note: Results are based on an analysis of data from CCHS 2.2. Asterisks indicate statistically significant differences ($p < 0.05$) in mean intake by food-security status.

Source: Kirkpatrick, S. & Tarasuk, V. (2008). Food insecurity is associated with nutrient inadequacies among Canadian adults and adolescents. *Journal of Nutrition, 138,* 604–612.

Figure 14.4: Consumption of grain products (servings/day) by Household Food-Security Status

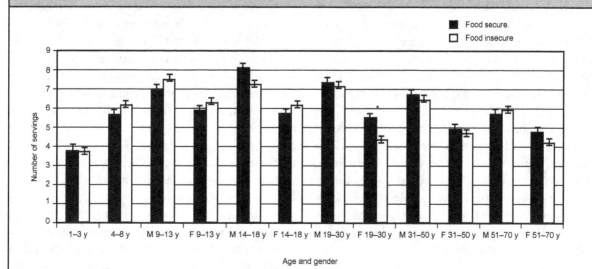

Note: Results are based on an analysis of data from CCHS 2.2. Asterisks indicate statistically significant differences ($p < 0.05$) in mean intake by food-security status.

Source: Kirkpatrick, S. & Tarasuk, V. (2008). Food insecurity is associated with nutrient inadequacies among Canadian adults and adolescents. *Journal of Nutrition, 138,* 604–612.

thiamin, riboflavin, vitamin B6, folate, vitamin B12, magnesium, phosphorus, and zinc. These results suggest that household food insecurity poses a very real threat to the nutritional health of adults and adolescents. Among children, however, there was little indication of nutrient inadequacy, irrespective of household food-security status, and thus no evidence that children in food-insecure households were nutritionally disadvantaged.

The observation that household food insecurity exerted less effect on the food and nutrient intakes of children than adolescents or adults in CCHS 2.2 is consistent with the findings of several qualitative studies in which adults have reported restricting their own food intakes to spare their children (Hamelin et al., 2002; Radimer, Olson, Greene, Campbell & Habicht, 1992). Our results are also consistent with those of other Canadian and American researchers who have compared the intakes of children and adults in food-insecure households. For example, in their study of 141 lone-parent, low-income women in the Atlantic provinces, McIntyre et al. (2003) found that most women had inadequate intakes of folate and vitamin C, and over one-third had inadequate intakes of iron and vitamins A and B6, but the nutrient intakes of most of the children in these households appeared adequate. The findings suggest that women compromised their own nutritional intake in order to preserve the adequacy of their children's diets (McIntyre et al., 2003). The inference is supported by the results of several US studies in which children's dietary intakes generally appeared to be less affected by household food insecurity than adults' (Bhattacharya et al., 2004; Cristofar & Basiotis, 1992; Knol, Haughton & Fitzhugh, 2004; Rose, 1999; Rose & Oliveira, 1997a, 1997b). It should be noted, though, that most of these studies have focused on young children. As children grow older, there are some indications that their experiences of household food insecurity more closely resemble those of adults. This is certainly suggested by our finding from CCHS 2.2 that adolescents in food-insecure households exhibited greater levels of dietary compromise than young and school-aged children in that study (Kirkpatrick & Tarasuk, 2008).

Implications for Nutritional Status
The evidence of higher prevalences of nutrient inadequacies among adolescents and adults in food-insecure households in Canada (Kirkpatrick & Tarasuk,

2008) implies that these individuals are at increased risk of nutrition-related health problems. The nature of the health consequences, however, depends on the duration and severity of the dietary compromises. This is because episodic, short-lived compromises in dietary intake can be inconsequential. However, there is increasing evidence that for many nutrients, chronically low intakes may heighten individuals' risk of major chronic diseases (e.g., cardiovascular disease, osteoporosis, some types of cancer). In addition, the chronic consumption of a diet very low in essential nutrients predisposes individuals to nutrient deficiencies. Thus, the consequences of food insecurity for individuals' nutritional health depend on the frequency, duration, and severity of the food insecurity and the specific dietary manifestations of this insecurity. Such detail cannot be derived from the measure of household food insecurity included in CCHS 2.2. Moreover, we have no data on the proportion of Canadian households who experience severe, income-related compromises in diet quality month after month, year after year.

Given the limitations of cross-sectional dietary assessments, clinical and biochemical measures of nutritional status provide important insight into the impact of food insecurity on individuals' nutritional status and long-term health. Unfortunately, only one Canadian study has examined food-security status in relation to biochemical indices of nutritional status: a study of a convenience sample of 142 children, two to five years of age, in Vancouver (Broughton, Janssen, Hertzman, Innis & Frankish, 2006). The authors found that serum zinc levels were lower among children in food-insecure households, but they found no differences in iron depletion (as measured by serum ferritin) in relation to household food-security status. The results of this small study are provocative, but not generalizable.

Insofar as we can generalize from US research, food insecurity would appear to compromise nutritional status among at least some age/sex groups. Results from one large US population survey indicated that adults in food-insufficient[2] households had lower concentrations of several serum nutrients (Dixon et al., 2001). A US population-based survey of elderly, disabled women found that those women who reported food insufficiency were three times more likely than food-sufficient women to have iron-deficiency anemia (Klesges, Pahor, Shorr

& Wan, 2001). They also tended to have lower serum albumin and lower total cholesterol (measures that, in other studies, have been linked to increased risk of coronary heart disease and non-cardiovascular diseases respectively among older people), although these differences were not statistically significant. In contrast to these findings, an analysis of children's data from the US *National Health and Nutrition Examination Survey III* revealed no association between iron deficiency and household food insufficiency among preschool and school-aged children once other risk factors (i.e., socio-demographic and family characteristics, past health risk, health care risk, and environmental risk) were taken into account (Alaimo, Olson, Frongillo & Briefel, 2001). This study did report a significantly increased risk of iron deficiency among children in low-income families, but no independent effect of food insufficiency could be detected.

Implications for Long-Term Health and Disease Management

Irrespective of whether the food insecurity experienced by Canadian households is severe enough to impact the nutritional status of individuals, chronic food insecurity must pose a serious barrier to healthy eating. In affluent countries such as ours where problems of nutrient deficiency are generally rare, attention is increasingly focused on the identification and promotion of dietary practices that will reduce risk of heart disease and other diet-related conditions of public health significance. Healthy eating includes an emphasis on fruits and vegetables (particularly dark green and orange vegetables), whole-grain breads and cereals, low-fat milk products, fish, and foods low in sodium (Health Canada, 2007c). Yet the low fruit and vegetable intakes, limited consumption of milk products, and relatively low fibre content of the dietary intakes observed among adults, adolescents, and, in some cases, children in food-insecure households in CCHS 2.2 (Kirkpatrick & Tarasuk, 2008) indicate that individuals in food-insecure settings are much less likely than other Canadians to follow healthy-eating practices.

Insofar as household food insecurity poses a barrier to healthy eating, it presents a particular hazard for individuals with heightened dietary needs. These include pregnant and lactating women, as well as children and adults suffering from diet-related chronic diseases. An analysis of Canadian data from the 1996–1997 *National Population Health Survey* revealed significantly higher odds that individuals in food-insufficient households would report heart disease, diabetes, high blood pressure, and food allergies compared to those in food-sufficient households (Vozoris & Tarasuk, 2003). These associations persisted even after adjusting for age, sex, income adequacy, and education. More recently, a cross-sectional analysis of US population data from 1999–2002 revealed that participants with severe food insecurity were two times more likely to have diabetes than those without food insecurity, even after adjusting for socio-demographic factors, physical activity level, and body-mass index (Seligman, Bindman, Vittinghoff, Kanaya & Kushel, 2007). Because the observed associations are cross-sectional in nature, it is impossible to infer causality. Regardless of why the associations exist, however, the fact that individuals in food-insecure households are more likely to report chronic health conditions such as diabetes is worrisome because they clearly face a serious obstacle to the effective management of their conditions through dietary modifications. While Canadian research in this area is sparse, there is some American research indicating poorer disease management among adults with diabetes who are food-insecure (Nelson, Brown & Lurie, 1998; Nelson, Cunningham, Andersen, Harrison & Gelberg, 2001).

Food Insecurity and Body Weight

Over the past decade, research into the relationship between food insecurity and body weight has burgeoned. However, the question of whether food insecurity predisposes adults or children to weight gain remains. Several cross-sectional studies have reported increased prevalence of overweight and obesity among women in food-insecure households (Adams, Grummer-Strawn & Chavez, 2003; Harrison et al., 2005; Kaiser, Townsend, Melgar-Quinonez, Fujii & Crawford, 2004; Lyons, Park & Nelson, 2008; Olson, 1999; Seligman et al., 2007; Townsend, Peerson, Love, Achterberg & Murphy, 2001; Wilde & Peterman, 2006). Others have reported significant associations for adults not differentiated by sex (Che & Chen, 2001; Sarlio-Lahteenkorva & Lahelma, 2001). Some study findings suggest that men in food-insecure households are not at increased risk of overweight or obesity (Lyons et al., 2008; Seligman et al., 2007; Townsend et al., 2001), and still others report no association for either men or women (Laraia, Siega-Riz & Evenson, 2004; Vozoris & Tarasuk, 2003).

Examinations of the association between household food-security status and overweight and obesity among children have also yielded inconsistent results. Two Canadian studies of preschool children, one in Vancouver and the second in Quebec, have found higher odds of overweight among children in food-insecure households (Broughton et al., 2006; Dubois, Farmer, Girard & Porcherie, 2006), but there has been little other Canadian research in this area and research from the US has yielded inconsistent results. A recent analysis of data from a large, well-designed, population-based cohort of young children in the US (including measured heights and weights and food security measured using the HFSSM) found that children in food-insecure households were 20 percent less likely to be overweight than their food-secure counterparts (Rose & Bodor, 2006).

Methodologic problems may be partly to blame for the inconsistent results arising from investigations of the association between food insecurity and body weight. Data limitations have caused most authors to treat food insecurity as a dichotomous, household-level variable, but there is some evidence to suggest that among adults, severe food insecurity may increase the risk of thinness, while less severe food insecurity increases the risk of obesity (Olson, 1999; Sarlio-Lahteenkorva & Lahelma, 2001; Seligman et al., 2007). A recent examination of Canadian data from CCHS 1.1 and CCHS 2.2 extends this analysis even further by drawing attention to the bias associated with analyses using self-reported rather than measured height and weight data (Lyons et al., 2008). Lyons et al. (2008) found that when self-reported height and weight data were used in calculating obesity-prevalence rates, rates were significantly higher among both food-insecure men and women than among food-secure men and women in CCHS 1.1. When measured data from CCHS 2.2 were used, the only significant difference observed in the Canadian data were greater odds of obesity among women in households classed as food-insecure with mild hunger (i.e., moderate food insecurity).

The observed associations, albeit inconsistent, have spawned considerable speculation about possible mechanisms by which dietary choices or patterns of food intake characteristic of chronic food insecurity might predispose people to weight gain. One hypothesis is that food insecurity predisposes people to a "feast and famine" pattern of eating, whereby they overeat when resources are replete and then endure periods of relative food deprivation as they await their next influx of income or food stamps (Dietz, 1995; Kaiser et al., 2004; Olson, 1999; Townsend et al., 2001). Yet apart from anecdotal reports (Dietz, 1995; Kempson, Keenan, Sadani, Ridlen & Rosato, 2002) and some evidence of disordered eating patterns among women in food-insecure settings (Kendall, Olson & Frongillo, 1996; Olson, Bove & Miller, 2007; Olson, 1999), there is little empirical evidence of this phenomenon (Tarasuk et al., 2007). A second hypothesis is that food insecurity leads to the consumption of inexpensive foods that are high in energy density, which in turn leads to weight gain (Drewnowski & Specter, 2004). Consistent with this hypothesis, we found food insecurity to be associated with higher energy density among women and girls in CCHS 2.2 (Kirkpatrick & Tarasuk, 2008), but whether this dietary pattern results in weight gain remains to be determined.

Cross-sectional associations and compelling hypotheses are insufficient to conclude that food insecurity contributes to problems of overweight or obesity. Longitudinal studies are required to determine whether there is a causal association between food insecurity and weight gain. One recent study of 1,700 US women with preschool children found no significant association between baseline food-security status or change in food-security status and weight gain (based on measured heights and weights) over a two-year period of follow-up (Whitaker & Sarin, 2007). These results are consistent with those from a second US study in which a nationally representative sample of 5,303 women aged 18–74 were followed over a two-year period (Jones & Frongillo, 2007). Working with self-reported weight data, these authors found no differences in weight gain between those women who remained food-secure and those who were food-secure at baseline but not at follow-up. They also found that food-security status at baseline was unrelated to increased risk of gaining weight over the next two years. While these studies are not without limitations and more longitudinal research is needed to definitively rule out a causal association between food insecurity and weight gain, the results seriously challenge the notion that food insecurity leads to overweight or obesity.

Implications for Health

Several studies in Canada have documented significant relationships between indicators of household food insecurity and the likelihood of individuals reporting poor or fair self-rated health and multiple chronic health conditions (Che & Chen, 2001; McIntyre et al., 2000; Vozoris & Tarasuk, 2003). In an analysis of data from the 1996–1997 NPHS, Vozoris and Tarasuk (2003) found that individuals in households characterized by food insufficiency had significantly higher odds of reporting poor/fair health, of having poor functional health, restricted activity, and multiple chronic conditions, of suffering from major depression and distress, and of having poor social support (Figure 14.5). Given the broad spectrum of health indicators for which associations were observed, it seems unlikely that the effect of food insecurity on health is condition-specific.

The robustness of the association between indicators of household food insecurity and poor health is reminiscent of another particularly robust relationship—the relationship between income and health. In the general population, health tracks income across a wide variety of indicators. The observed associations between food insecurity and health may be an extension of the income-health gradient. Measures of household food insecurity are essentially measures of the dietary manifestations of acute financial insecurity. In this sense, food insecurity denotes a more extreme level of material deprivation than that identified by conventional measures of low income (Rose, 1999; Tarasuk, 2001). As such, indicators of household food insecurity may be functioning as markers of the population subgroup at the extreme end of the poverty-wealth spectrum. The extraordinary disadvantage associated with this social position is exemplified in the increased likelihood of poorer physical, mental, and social health among this group when compared even to others with low incomes.

Increasingly, researchers are endeavouring to identify the pathways through which household food insecurity may impact individuals' health. Obviously one route is through the nutritional compromises associated with chronic food insecurity. Chronically poor nutrition can predispose individuals to problems like hypertension, hypercholerolemia, diabetes, and some types of cancer, for example. However, the extraordinary stress that individuals endure as they struggle to cope with food insecurity may also impact their health. Several studies have linked food insecurity to increased likelihood of depression among adults (young and old) (Kim &

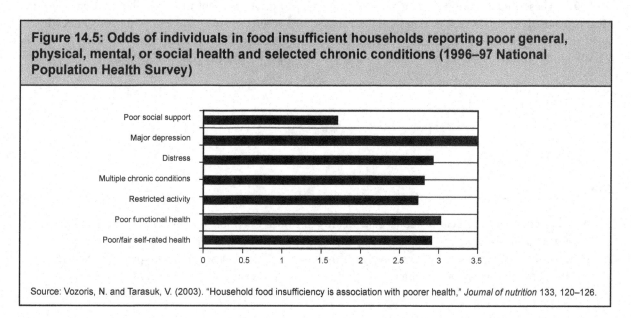

Figure 14.5: Odds of individuals in food insufficient households reporting poor general, physical, mental, or social health and selected chronic conditions (1996–97 National Population Health Survey)

Source: Vozoris, N. and Tarasuk, V. (2003). "Household food insufficiency is association with poorer health," *Journal of nutrition* 133, 120–126.

Frongillo, 2007; Klesges et al., 2001; Siefert, Heflin, Corcoran & Williams, 2001; Vozoris & Tarasuk, 2003; Whitaker, Phillips & Orzol, 2006). Food insecurity has also been found to be associated with depressive disorder and suicidal symptoms among adolescents in the US (Alaimo, Olson & Frongillo, 2002). The results of a recent US prospective survey of women who were welfare recipients extend this research even further, providing evidence that food insecurity may be a causal or contributing factor to women's depression (Heflin, Siefert & Williams, 2005).

Insofar as food insecurity leads to depression among adults, it can have both profound implications for their children's health. Parental depression linked to food insecurity has been associated with poor infant health (Bronte-Tinkew, Zaslow, Capps, Horowitz & McNamara, 2007). The results of a recent US population-based case-control study indicate that food insecurity is associated with increased likelihood of birth defects (Carmichael, Yang, Herring, Abrams & Shaw, 2007). While the findings may relate to compromised maternal nutrition, they may also reflect the potential negative effects of stress on maternal and child health.

Several studies have documented an increased prevalence of behavioural, emotional, and academic problems among children in food-insecure versus food-secure households (Kleinman et al., 1998; Murphy et al., 1998; Wehler, Scott & Anderson, 1992; Alaimo et al., 2001). These findings are particularly interesting when juxtaposed against the results from CCHS 2.2 and other surveys suggesting that children in food-insecure households do not have markedly poorer dietary intakes than other children. Although parents may buffer children from the nutritional impacts of food insecurity, it would appear that they are less successful in protecting their children from the negative psychological impacts of household food insecurity.

Conclusion

Household food insecurity in Canada is a serious public health problem. It is clearly associated with increased nutritional vulnerability among both adults and adolescents, and there is growing evidence that food insecurity jeopardizes individuals' mental health. While the dietary consequences of household food insecurity for Canadian children are less apparent, there are indications that this problem exacts a toll on children's psychological health and well-being. Moreover, the long-term health impacts of household food insecurity for the adults, adolescents, and children affected can only be negative.

Given the implications of household food insecurity for nutritional health and well-being, this problem needs to be addressed. As discussed by Lynn McIntyre and Krista Rondeau elsewhere in this volume, problems of food insecurity are rooted in the failure of our social programs to protect low-income families from abject poverty. There is an urgent need for concerted policy action by both the national and provincial/territorial levels of government to ensure that all Canadians are food-secure. There is also a need for food insecurity to be systematically monitored across the country, so that progress toward this goal can be tracked.

Notes

1. A recent report on food security and income security in British Columbia provides an excellent illustration of this sort of analysis of the adequacy of welfare benefits (Kerstetter & Goldberg, 2007).
2. Food insufficiency is a measure of relatively severe food insecurity. Households are typically considered food insufficient if they reported "sometimes" or "often" not having had enough to eat over the past year.

Critical Thinking Questions

1. Most individuals and families on welfare in Canada are food-insecure, but few provincial and territorial governments are taking any action to improve welfare benefit levels. Why not? Should Canadians on welfare be food-secure or is food security a privilege to be enjoyed only by Canadians who can afford it?
2. Given the associations between household food insecurity and problems of physical and mental health, should we add food insecurity to the list of modifiable risk factors for conditions like diabetes and depression? What could health care providers do to treat this risk factor?
3. Food banks have long been the primary public response to problems of household food insecurity in Canada, but Riches has argued that their positioning of food insecurity "as a matter of charitable concern rather than of social justice" has effectively depoliticized this issue, facilitating the erosion of income-support programs for those at the bottom and leading to increased need for charitable food assistance (Riches, 1997b). What do you think of this argument? Are food banks part of the problem or part of the solution?
4. There are reports of an increasing number of university students turning to food banks for help to meet their food needs. What would it take to make universities hunger-proof?
5. Some people have proposed instituting publicly funded meal programs in schools as a way to improve the food security of low-income families, but others have argued that such programs are missing the mark. What do you think? Would giving children free or low-cost meals in school help to offset the negative health effects of household food insecurity for them?

Recommended Readings

Hamelin, A.M., Beaudry, M. & Habicht, J.-P. (2002). "Characterization of household food insecurity in Quebec: Food and feelings." *Social Science & Medicine, 54*, 119–132.

Drawing on data from in-depth interviews with a sample of 98 low-income households, Anne-Marie Hamelin and colleagues present a graphic portrait of the lived experience of food insecurity among Quebec families.

Health Canada. (2007). *Canadian Community Health Survey Cycle 2.2, Nutrition (2004)—Income-Related Household Food Security in Canada.* Ottawa: Office of Nutrition Policy and Promotion, Health Products and Food Branch, Health Canada. Online at www.hc-sc.gc.ca/fn-an/surveill/nutrition/commun/income_food_sec-sec_alim_e.html.

This report provides a comprehensive description of the assessment of income-related food insecurity in Canada on CCHS 2.2. The socio-demographic characteristics of food-insecure households are presented. The supplementary tables (also available on this Web site) provide a detailed breakdown of the results by province and by several socio-demographic characteristics.

Heflin, C.M., Siefert, K. & Williams, D.R. (2005). "Food insufficiency and women's mental health: Findings from a 3-year panel of welfare recipients." *Social Science & Medicine, 61,* 1971–1982.

In the US as well as Canada, welfare recipients are particularly vulnerable to food insecurity, but there is also extensive research linking food insecurity to poor mental health. Heflin and colleagues examine whether a change in household food insufficiency is associated with a change in women's self-reported mental health in a sample of current and recent welfare recipients over a three-year period. Their research provides a disturbing account of one way in which problems of food insecurity appear to erode poor women's lives.

Riches, G. (2002). "Food banks and food security: Welfare reform, human rights, and social policy: Lessons from Canada?" *Social Policy and Administration, 36*, 648–663.

Food banks remain the primary response to food insecurity in Canada. In this paper, Graham Riches critically examines the growth of food banking in Canada from three perspectives: (1) the role of food banking in terms of advancing the human right to food; (2) its effectiveness in achieving food security; and (3) the extent to which food banking contributes to and/or counters governments' increasing emphasis on welfare reform policies informed by a neo-conservative ideology.

Whitaker, R.C. & Sarin, A. (2007). "Change in food security status and change in weight are not associated in urban women with preschool children." *Journal of Nutrition, 137,* 2134–2139.

Although there is a plethora of studies examining the association between food insecurity and body weight, this research by Whitaker and Sarin is exemplary. In overcoming many of the very serious limitations of previous research, they provide the most compelling analysis of food insecurity and body weight yet. Their results raise serious questions about the widely held belief that obesity is a problem of food insecurity.

Related Web Sites

Canadian Association for Food Studies (CAFS)—www.foodstudies.ca

The Canadian Association for Food Studies (CAFS) includes academics, students, professionals, and others interested in food studies research. Formed in 2005, the goal of this association is to promote critical, interdisciplinary scholarship in the broad area of food systems: food policy, production, distribution, and consumption. CAFS encourages research that promotes local, regional, national, and global food security, but the organization does not advocate or endorse specific policies or political platforms. The Web site provides up-to-date information on publications, conferences, and other resources related to food studies in Canada.

Canadian Association of Food Banks (CAFB)—www.cafb_acba.ca/public_e.cfm

The Canadian Association of Food Banks (CAFB) conducts an annual survey of food-bank use in Canada, as well as periodic surveys of public opinion on the problem of hunger in this country. As well, the CAFB occasionally releases position papers on policy issues of particular relevance to problems of food insecurity and hunger in Canada. These reports can be viewed and downloaded on their Web site.

Food Secure Canada—www.foodsecurecanada.org

Food Secure Canada was established to unite people and organizations working for food security nationally and globally. It works toward three interconnected goals: (1) zero hunger; (2) a sustainable food system; and (3) healthy and safe food. Food Secure Canada develops working papers related to these three goals, and they can be downloaded from this Web site. The Web site also contains news and information on upcoming events related to food-security issues in Canada.

Health Canada, Food and Nutrition—www.hc-sc.gc.ca/fn-an/

This Web site includes links to a number of government reports on food and nutrition issues affecting Canadians. As well as the recent report on income-related food insecurity in Canada (discussed above), the Web site includes a map depicting the geographic distribution of food insecurity in this country.

National Council of Welfare (NCW)—www.ncwcnbes.net

The National Council of Welfare (NCW) is a citizens' advisory body to the minister of Human Resources Development Canada on matters of concern to low-income Canadians. The NCW monitors the individual welfare programs in the provinces and territories, producing regular reports on welfare incomes in relation to poverty lines and average incomes as well as policy analyses and public statements on policy developments of particular relevance to poverty and welfare in Canada. Their reports and statements can be viewed or downloaded from this Web site.

Chapter 15

———◆———

HOUSING

Michael Shapcott

Introduction

Canada is, in global terms, a very rich country. There is plenty of money and other resources to ensure safe, good-quality, affordable housing for all. However, more than one in five Canadian households are unable to find affordable and healthy homes, and more than 300,000 people will experience homelessness every year.

The roots of this crisis lie in the federal, provincial, and territorial governments' decisions to cut funding and programs for new social housing and cancel programs over the past two decades, which set the stage for the nationwide housing crisis and homelessness disaster.

Elected officials in most parts of the country opted to rely on private markets in ownership and rental housing to provide new homes for Canadians. The markets responded, especially from 2000–2004, with a near-record number of new homes. But almost all of those homes were pitched to middle- and upper-income households, dividing the country along increasingly deep divisions: The housing "haves" and the "have-nots" (Hulchanski, 2001). In the decade starting in 1980, an annual average of 11 out of every 100 new homes in Canada were affordable (social). In the decade ending in 2007, the annual average slipped to less than one in 100 (Shapcott, 2007).

Renter households have, on average, less than half the annual income of owner households. As upper-income renter households took advantage of low mortgage rates

and new supply to move into home ownership in the late 1990s and early part of the 21st century, the income gap between owners and tenants has grown wider. In addition, renters have a mere fraction of the household wealth of owners, which makes it much harder for renter households to make a down payment on an ownership home. While there are some poor households that own their own homes, most low- and moderate-income households are in the rental market and, with the cancellation of national affordable housing programs in the early 1990s, most of them are forced to rent from private landlords.

Canada's national government has been preaching housing globally, but back home has been setting in place policies that ensured growing homelessness. At the same time that the federal housing minister was at Habitat II, the United Nations-sponsored global housing summit in Istanbul in 1996, to join with countries around the world in proclaiming the goal of "housing for all," the federal government announced plans to transfer responsibility for its housing programs to provincial and territorial governments. It had locked in place a plan for annual cuts to housing spending that will see national funding shrink to zero over the next three decades.

By the late 1990s, the federal government had signed housing-transfer deals with the provinces and territories, abandoning a national role in affordable housing. Canada became one of the few countries in the world without a national housing strategy.

In 1998, the federal government "commercialized" the Canada Mortgage and Housing Corporation (CMHC), shifting the mandate of the national housing agency away from its historic role of encouraging the development of a range of housing. CMHC now generates profits of hundreds of millions of dollars on its mortgage-insurance program, but housing developers report that the high cost of the premiums is blocking development of new affordable units.

In 2001, in response to effective political advocacy and growing housing need across Canada, the federal, provincial, and territorial governments signed the Affordable Housing Framework Agreement, which was supposed to deliver $2 billion in new homes over five years. However, by 2007, federal housing spending was up only by $234 million, or about one-quarter of the amount promised in 2001; combined provincial/territorial housing spending was actually down by $210 million in 2007 compared to 2001 despite a commitment to increase spending by $1 billion (Shapcott, 2008). The "bad boy of Confederation" was Canada's biggest and richest province, Ontario, which had promised to increase housing spending by $358 million and had actually cut spending by $732 million.

As governments abandoned their housing policies and programs, they believed or hoped that private markets would pick up the slack. After all, the majority of Canadians live in homes that were built by the private sector, so why not turn over the entire housing sector to corporate development interests?

However, the private sector had already started to abandon affordable rental housing in the early 1970s, and that trend picked up in the 1990s. There is, quite simply, no big profit to be made in building housing for low-, moderate-, and middle-income households. With the potential for return on investments relatively low for new development in rental housing (versus, for instance, commercial properties or ownership developments), private money flowed out of the sector.

By the late 1990s, some smart operators had created a profitable niche in the rental market. Real estate investment trusts bought existing buildings with moderate rents. Taking advantage of lax rent-regulation laws in most parts of the country, they drove up the rents and banked significant returns on investment. This was good for wealthy investors, but bad for tenants as rents rose and moderate-priced units were lost.

With no new government funding and a declining private role, Canada's rental housing sector has slipped from one crisis to another in terms of both supply and affordability (Canada Mortgage and Housing Corporation, 2007):

- Vacancy rates for affordable units are extremely low and in some parts of Canada, the tiny amount of new rental housing has been outpaced by demolition and conversion of existing stock, leading to a net loss of affordable homes at a

---

Box 15.1: UN reports on housing in Canada

Everywhere that I visited in Canada, I met people who are homeless and living in inadequate and insecure housing conditions. On this mission I heard of hundreds of people who have died, as a direct result of Canada's nation-wide housing crisis. In its most recent periodic review of Canada's compliance with the International Covenant on Economic, Social and Cultural Rights, the United Nations used strong language to label housing and homelessness and inadequate housing as a "national emergency." Everything that I witnessed on this mission confirms the deep and devastating impact of this national crisis on the lives of women, youth, children and men. Canada has ratified numerous international human rights instruments that not only recognize the right to housing, but also create an obligation on the Government to take steps for the progressive realization of these human rights with the maximum of its available resources. In recent reviews by United Nations' authorities, including—most recently—the May 2006 period review of Canada's compliance with the International Covenant on Economic, Social and Cultural Rights, Canada's continuing failure to incorporate these international legal standards into Canadian domestic law has been noted with growing concern.

Source: Miloon Kothari, United Nations' special rapporteur on the right to adequate housing, Preliminary Observations of Mission to Canada, October 22, 2007.

time when the population, and the need for new affordable housing, is growing.

- Rents are increasing much faster than stagnant renter household incomes, creating an affordability squeeze that has generated a growing number of evictions.
- The existing housing stock is aging and much of it has been poorly maintained, and there are significant concerns about declining quality of the units, including appalling conditions in almost half the housing in Aboriginal communities.
- Supports and services for people who need special assistance to access and maintain housing due to physical or mental health concerns are fragmented or non-existent, forcing many vulnerable people into overcrowded homeless shelters or onto the streets.
- Two, three, or sometimes more families are crowded into homes designed for only one family, swelling the ranks of the "hidden homeless."

The rental housing crisis has triggered a big increase in homelessness, not just in big urban areas, but in small towns, and in remote, rural, and northern communities. The mayors of the country's biggest cities gathered in Winnipeg in 1998, declared that homelessness was a "national disaster," and called on senior levels of government to restore funding for housing programs. In 2008, a new report from the Federation of Canadian Municipalities (FCM) confirmed the deep and persistent housing and homelessness crisis across the country (Federation of Canadian Municipalities, 2008a), prompting the FCM to renew its call for a comprehensive national housing strategy (Federation of Canadian Municipalities, 2008b).

In response to growing political pressure, the federal government, and all the provinces and territories, signed the Affordable Housing Framework Agreement at a national summit in Quebec City in November 2001. Under that deal, the federal government agreed to spend $680 million in new dollars for new affordable housing and the provinces and territories agreed to match the federal dollars with new money of their own. The federal government added $320 million in 2003 to bring the total promised to $2 billion (including provincial and territorial matching shares).

However, as of 2006, the national government had increased housing spending by only $234 million, or about a quarter of what they committed. The provincial and territorial governments promised to match the federal dollars with $1 billion of their own money, but by 2007, combined provincial and territorial housing spending was actually down by $210 million. The main culprit was Ontario, which cut housing spending by $732 million.

Box 15.2: Housing in Canadian cities

It's an all too-familiar scene in Canada's big cities: the weather turns steadily colder until temperatures dip well below freezing and the city's shelters quickly fill to capacity. Social service agencies work frantically with municipal officials to find extra spaces for dozens of people who normally sleep on the streets. Sometimes it can mean collecting homeless people in city buses and adapting empty buildings as emergency shelters. Winter in Canada is not the time for anyone to be without shelter. It's when homelessness becomes an emergency and adequate shelter a matter of life and death. It's also when many of us understand most clearly why having adequate shelter is a necessity, not a luxury. But stark homelessness is not our only housing problem. As this report shows, many people in Canada's large cities struggle to find decent, affordable housing as they move from living on the street, living in emergency shelters, and living in short-term transitional housing.... Municipalities deal with the immediate human consequences of inadequate housing and homelessness. Increasingly, they must use their strained resources to help individuals and families that cannot find adequate shelter. Municipal governments have programs and strategies to assist people that need housing, but they do not have the resources to solve the housing problem. That requires the co-operation and support of other orders of government.

Source: Gord Steeves, president, Federation of Canadian Municipalities, 2008.

Remove Ontario, and the increase in housing spending by provinces and territories is $522 million, just over half the amount committed (Shapcott, 2008).

A Nationwide Housing Crisis

Canada's national affordable housing crisis is hidden behind a picture of relative comfort.

Owner households in most parts of Canada have incomes that are, on average, about double the household income of renters (Hulchanski, 2001). Mortgage rates are relatively low, the supply of new and existing housing is generally good, and there are a number of government funding programs to assist homeowners, including direct subsidies and tax incentives. The tax-based programs to help homeowners are many times more costly than the affordable housing programs for lower-income Canadians.

Even as the sub-prime mortgage crisis in the United States threatened to drag that economy into a recession in early 2008, conditions remained relatively stable for homeowners, although affordability was eroding in late 2007 as house prices continued their speculative increases. This relative prosperity obscures the housing crisis facing millions of low- and moderate-income tenant households.

Canada's renter households have incomes, on average, half of the income of owners. While owner incomes have increased since the recession of the early 1990s, tenant household incomes have been stagnant. Some of the poorest households, including families living on social assistance (welfare), have seen their income drop in real terms.

Low income makes it increasingly difficult for tenant households to move into ownership, especially in the biggest cities. But about one-third of Canadians are renters (a total of 4.8 million households, or about 13 million women, men, and children) and for them, the affordable housing crisis and homelessness disaster is a devastating reality. Median incomes for renter households are less than half those of owner households, and they have been falling since 1984. In a research bulletin for the University of Toronto's Centre for Urban and Community Studies, Dr. David Hulchanski analyzed this "tale of two Canadas" and concluded that:

The household income and wealth of renters is dramatically below that of owners, and the gap is growing. Renter households may find it increasingly difficult to move into home ownership. Government policies that focus on incentives for home ownership (such as tax-exempt savings plans or the Ontario government's waiver of land transfer taxes) do not address the housing needs of the vast majority of renter households. The federal government has not provided new social housing for low- and moderate-income renters since 1993.

A comprehensive national housing policy, with complementary regional policies, must address the very low income and wealth of renters. Canada, more than most Western nations, relies on the private sector to provide housing. Renters must find adequate housing in housing markets in which prices are driven by the income and wealth levels of homeowners.

Social policies and traditional income assistance programs (social assistance, unemployment, disability pensions, and so forth) must better address the growing income inequality between owners and renters.

Federal and provincial/territorial housing policies must recognize that very few renters have incomes high enough to pay the rent levels required by unsubsidized new construction.

Increased supply—the construction of new rental housing—is the only answer to low vacancy rates. Given the income and wealth profile of Canada's renters, only significant public-sector intervention will increase the supply of affordable rental housing.

In summary, there is a growing *social need* for affordable housing among renters. As the data from the Statistics Canada survey of financial security demonstrates, there is very limited *market demand*. The income and wealth levels of most renter households are much too low— and continuing to fall relative to homeowners. (Hulchanski, 2001, p. 4)

Many tenant households cannot afford conventional rental units, or can't find them in the tight urban markets, and turn to the "non-conventional" or secondary rental market. These are condominiums (ownership housing bought by investors and rented to tenant households), illegal and substandard housing (basement apartments and other units that don't meet building and safety codes), and other rented units. But the secondary market is providing no relief for tenant households. Much of the housing is illegal and unregulated, and there are serious concerns about security of tenure for low-income tenants.

The housing crisis has grown so severe that even the big banks have started to notice. TD Economics, the research division of the TD Bank Financial Group, released a major study on housing in June 2003. TD noted in their introduction that:

> Housing is a necessity of life. Yet, after ten years of economic expansion, one in five households in Canada is still unable to afford acceptable shelter—a strikingly high number, especially in view of the country's ranking well atop the United Nations human-development survey. What's more, the lack of affordable housing is a problem confronting communities right across the nation—from large urban centres to smaller, less-populated areas. As such, it is steadily gaining recognition as one of Canada's most pressing public-policy issues....
>
> We are used to thinking of affordable housing as both a social and a health issue. This is not altogether surprising, given the fact that many social housing tenants receive their main source of income from government transfer payments. As well, in study after study, researchers have shown that a strong correlation exists between neighbourhoods with poor quality housing and lower health outcomes.
>
> However, working to find solutions to the problem of affordable housing is also smart economic policy. An inadequate supply of housing can be a major impediment to business investment and growth, and can influence immigrants' choices of where to locate. Hence, implementing solutions to resolve this issue ties in well with the TD goal of raising Canada's living standards and overall quality of life. (TD Economics, 2003, p. i)

Growing Homelessness Disaster

Nowhere is the housing crisis more visible than in the huge and growing number of homeless people living—and dying—on the streets of Canada. There are no reliable numbers on the number of homeless people in the country. Even figures for the number of people taking shelter in temporary hostels and other facilities for the homeless are not collected on a consistent basis. The National Housing and Homelessness Network released a comprehensive overview of homelessness in Canada in 2001 (National Housing and Homelessness Network, 2001). The following material is taken from the report *State of the Crisis, 2001* (National Housing and Homelessness Network, 2001).

During the International Year of Shelter for the Homeless in 1987, the Canadian Council on Social Development estimated that 100,000 people would experience homelessness during that year.

By 1999, the Finance Committee of the Canadian House of Commons had accepted an estimate that there were 250,000 people who would experience homelessness during that year.

A survey of eight Ontario communities in 1998 found that there were 1.5 million overnight stays in homeless shelters. Other studies suggest that the number of homeless people "sleeping rough"—that is, outside of shelters—is often as high or higher than the number sleeping inside.

Toronto, the largest city in Canada, has the biggest number of homeless people and that number is staggering. Almost 32,000 people stayed in homeless shelters in that city in 2002, an increase of 21 percent from 1990.

In recent years, Toronto has reported that the biggest increase among the homeless is among children. About 6,200 children took shelter in Toronto in 1999, up 130 percent from the 2,700 in 1988. One-third of those children were under the age of four. The city's housing crisis is forcing people to stay longer in the emergency-shelter system. More households are moving in and out of homelessness. The city is also reporting a growing number of seniors in city homeless shelters.

One measure of the serious state of the homelessness disaster in Toronto is the crowded shelters. Average occupancy in Toronto's homeless shelters has been over 90 percent for years. That means that every available bed is filled, and even the mattresses on the floor are mostly occupied. In the winters, hundreds of mats are placed in church basements to accommodate homeless people who cannot find room in the regular shelters.

Almost everywhere in the country, the numbers are up.

Muskoka, a rural area in central Ontario known as "cottage country" since it provides vacation homes for many people in southern Ontario, reported that in 1998 there were 219 admissions at Interval House, 38 emergency-housing vouchers, and 43 motel rooms used by homeless people.

The main homeless shelter in London, Ontario, saw a 22 percent increase in homeless admissions from 4,319 people in 1995 to 5,269 in 1999.

The Peterborough (Ontario) Social Planning Council surveyed 206 homeless or near-homeless households (a total of 502 family members) in March 2000. They found that:

- As many people were staying temporarily with friends or on the streets as in shelters.
- Nine families (18 children) were homeless.
- One in four homeless were employed.
- Two-thirds of homeless are not on waiting lists for social housing.
- Among the near-homeless, 70 percent could not afford basic necessities such as food, clothing, personal hygiene products, telephone transportation, or recreation.
- The lack of affordable rents is the biggest barrier to finding housing.

Among those surveyed, the top solutions were more supply of affordable housing (77 percent) and better income (59 percent) through improved wages and social-assistance programs.

Sudbury, a mid-sized city in northern Ontario, has the highest rental vacancy rate in the country. In theory, its rental market should provide plenty of vacant, lower-cost rental units as the market adjusts to meet demand. In fact, Sudbury is trapped in the same homelessness cycle as other communities. An October 2000 study by the regional municipality found that during a seven-day period, 407 people were identified as homeless in the region. More than a quarter (28 percent) were children

or adolescents. During that time, there were only 68 available beds in homeless shelters.

The study reported that the most frequent cause of homelessness in Sudbury was related to employment, followed by problems with social assistance (in particular, the inadequacy of social-support payments), a lack of affordable housing, and domestic violence.

"Homelessness is one of the most pressing social issues affecting communities across the country today, and unfortunately, the Sudbury Region is no exception," said regional councillor Doug Craig.

In London, Ontario, a prosperous community in the province's southwestern region, there are about 400 households per month using shelters, up by 13 percent from 1995. In nearby Windsor, the only hostel for the homeless had a licensed capacity for 90 beds in 1998, but it commonly sheltered 150–165. Hamilton, Ontario, has over 230 beds for homeless people and families escaping domestic violence. Shelter usage in Hamilton jumped by 35 percent between November 1998 and March 2000.

In Saint John, New Brunswick, a comprehensive review in early 2001 found that "the high rate of poverty in the city (27 percent) and the numbers of people who can't afford adequate housing (56 percent of unattached individuals and 18 percent of all families living in Saint John), along with the lack of affordable, adequate housing (low vacancy rates, long waiting lists, and the ghettoizing of subsidized housing)" were among the key factors in generating housing and homeless problems. "Those in highest needs are lone-parent families and non-elderly singles," according to the study.

A tour of the rest of the country shows the following:

- There was a 97 percent occupancy rate at shelters for the homeless in Edmonton, Alberta. Shelters for abused women were so full that they had to turn away 3,000 families in 1997. About 1,980 families used shelters in the city during 1998.
- Shelters in Montreal, Quebec, offered space to about 12,660 people in 1996. Most of the centres report that they have reached a saturation point and often turn people away.
- Regina, Saskatchewan, in Canada's prairies, has a relatively small number of homeless people (there were only 60 beds in the city in

1998), but staff report a large increase in the number of "repeat" clients who use the shelters as "permanent" housing rather than temporary relief.

- The other major city in Saskatchewan, Saskatoon, reports that 68 percent of the people using its homeless shelters are First Nations peoples, even though they represent only 8 percent of the city's population. A total of 6,700 people stayed in shelters in 1998, with 28 percent of them children.
- St. John's, Newfoundland, on Canada's eastern coast, reports a major problem with "hidden" homeless; that is, people living in illegal and substandard housing.
- On Canada's West Coast, there are about 300–400 people who sleep in homeless shelters every night, and another 300–600 people who "sleep rough" in Vancouver. City shelters are almost always full. From 1995–1998, the number of people sleeping on the floor in one shelter tripled from 3,887 to 10,758.

A study of hostels by the Toronto Disaster Relief Committee (TDRC) in the winter of 2000 provided a grim list of the conditions in the shelters. It documents overcrowding, poor food quality, lack of hygiene facilities, theft and violence, disease, and death both in the shelters and on the streets.

The study concludes that shelters in the rich city of Toronto fail to meet the emergency shelter standards set by the United Nations High Commissioner for Refugees (Toronto Disaster Relief Committee, 2000).

First Nations People

First Nations people, the original inhabitants of Canada, make up a disproportionately large share of the number of those experiencing homelessness or living in substandard housing. Conditions on Native reserves (often in rural, remote, or northern locations) are desperate. Some First Nations peoples leave the appalling conditions on reserves for urban areas, only to have a large number of them join the ranks of homeless people.

"The single most critical issue currently facing the Assembly of First Nations, Department of Indian and Northern Affairs, and First Nation leadership is on-reserve housing," according to the Assembly of First Nations (AFN), one of the national groups representing First Nations peoples. The AFN estimates that almost one-third of the existing on-reserve housing stock requires major repair or replacement.

In cities and towns, First Nations peoples face poverty and discrimination. Aboriginal households are three times more likely to be living in poverty than non-Aboriginal households. Combined with the lack of rental vacancies and rising rents throughout Canada, it adds up to a major crisis.

In the 1970s and 1980s, the federal government set targets for urban Aboriginal housing projects. About 10,000 units were developed before the federal programs were cancelled in 1993, according to the National Aboriginal Housing Association.

A 1998 study using Statistics Canada data found that Aboriginal women experience higher levels of unemployment than other women, have lower average earnings, tend to have less formal education, and have a shorter life expectancy than other women (National Housing and Homelessness Network, 2001).

Women and Children

About 3 million women live in poverty in Canada. Single-women-led families are among the poorest in the country. "A significant proportion of Canadian women live on low incomes, on their own or with others. [Women] have serious housing difficulties and are suffering because of them," according to Reitsma-Street et al. (2001). "Most discouraging is the realization that the scope and depth of the housing concerns of women living on low incomes have not changed much, despite years of housing policies, laws, and programs by all levels of government, and despite successful strategies to assist people with moderate income to find and keep suitable accommodation" (Reitsma-Street et al., 2001, p. 2).

Canada's housing crisis and homelessness disaster also puts children at risk: "Lack of reasonably priced housing in and of itself poses risks to positive outcomes for children, primarily via the enabling condition of adequate income. Parents stressed by overcrowding, for example, may not parent as well as they might if conditions were more favourable. Similarly, neighbourhoods in which poor housing is the norm are also likely (not necessarily) neighbourhoods with few services, higher than average levels of violence and so on" (Cooper, 2001, p. 7).

The Private Sector

As federal and provincial governments in Canada have cut funding for non-market housing in the past decade, they have expected the private sector to take the lead in developing new affordable housing.

This represents a big change from the first 40 years after the Second World War, when Canada relied on a strong and successful social housing program to deliver more than 600,000 social housing units for low-income households.

The Ontario government established a Housing Supply Working Group in the late 1990s to advise on this strategy. They tried to put a positive spin on the lack of new affordable development. The government's own advisers noted that the only possibility for new private housing is at the upper end of the rental scale, then said, "even rental development at the high end increases affordability, because it adds to the overall stock, putting downward pressure on rents and freeing up more affordable units as higher income tenants move into the new supply" (Ontario Housing Supply Working Group, 2001). In other words, they claimed that wealthy tenants would abandon existing units to move into the newly built, even more expensive private housing, and

then the vacancies would eventually trickle down to the lowest-income households.

The Ontario government called this "filtering" and it was the cornerstone of provincial housing policy from 1995–2003, but there are three main barriers to "filtering" as a means of delivering new affordable housing:

- Even with massive public subsidies, low-income households still don't have enough money to pay the rents required by private developers to make a "reasonable" return on investment after covering the high costs of developing and managing housing.
- In most parts of the country, even if new high-end rental housing is created, the vacancies created down the rental spectrum by filtering will result in massive rent increases across the board due to lax or non-existent rent-regulation laws.
- Recent trends in the rental market show increasing vacancies at the high end. The rental market is flooded with expensive rental units that are sitting empty. No investor would want to build even more units that would remain vacant.

The cost of building a new housing project, or acquiring and renovating an existing building, is

---

Box 15.3: Public solutions to the crisis

Obviously the most convenient and economical way of providing the community with an adequate supply of decent accommodation is through the economic market for new housing. If those who can afford to own or to rent new housing could maintain such a volume of production that every family could be well-housed and obsolete housing could be successfully removed, then in the process of time there would be no housing problem.... Unhappily, any study of the economic factors involved seems to lead inevitably to the conclusion that a balance of incomes and housing costs is most unlikely to be established at a level which would produce an adequate supply of housing. This has certainly been the experience of all other industrialized nations and there are no factors peculiar to our economy which indicate that Canada is likely to be an exception to this experience. In fact, the requirements of shelter in our stern climate are likely to make the economics of housing in Canada especially intractable. If this conclusion is well founded it will be necessary to devise a means whereby a larger proportion of the national income may be directed into the production of housing. It will be necessary to supplement the supply of housing created by the private market.

Source: Carver, Humphrey. (1948). *Houses for Canadians: A study of housing problems in the Toronto area* (p. 3). Toronto: University of Toronto Press.

high, especially in the big cities of Canada. A review of construction costs prepared by the Federation of Canadian Municipalities (FCM) in 2001 range from a low of $47,000 to acquire an existing building in Halifax (on Canada's East Coast) to a high of $132,000 to construct a new building in Vancouver (on Canada's West Coast).

While conventional lenders (such as banks or credit unions) will lend a portion of the costs, the amount of capital grant required ranges from $26,000 for the Halifax unit to a high of $93,000 per unit for a new housing project in downtown Toronto.

Without a large capital subsidy (including free or low-cost land, waiving of taxes and fees and outright grants), the rent for the new or renovated housing would be $1,300 or more per month, well beyond the affordable range. Even with a subsidy, rents would still be in the $600 or $700 range in most major urban areas, which is not affordable for the lowest-income households (Federation of Canadian Municipalities, 2002).

The Swinging Pendulum

Canada has a record of success in delivering a national social housing program that funds affordable social housing units. From the late 1940s to 1993, the federal government (with some cost-sharing from the provinces) funded about 650,000 social housing units. The Ontario government, in Canada's most populous province, funded a social housing program from the mid-1980s to 1995.

In recent years, the federal government has posted annual surpluses of more than $10 billion. The two reasons for the large surplus are:

- spending cuts over the past decade, including cuts to housing programs
- increased revenues in recent years from an upturn in the economy

Canada's federal government began to cut housing spending with the election of the Conservative government of Brian Mulroney in 1984. By 1993, the federal government had cut almost $2 billion from housing programs and had cancelled development of new social housing.

In opposition during this time, the Liberal Party created a housing task force headed by two members of Parliament, Paul Martin and Joe Fontana. In May 1990, they issued a scathing indictment of the federal withdrawal from housing. The Liberals promised to restore funding for social housing, including new housing co-ops (Martin & Fontana, 1990).

In the fall of 1993, the Liberals were elected to the government of Canada and remained the governing party until 2006. MP Martin was promoted to finance minister, the second most powerful position in the government next to the prime minister.

Although Finance Minister Martin controlled the books, he refused to implement the recommendations of his own task force of three years earlier. Not only did he fail to keep his promise to bring in a new national housing strategy, but in his 1996 budget, he announced plans for the federal government to abandon entirely its responsibility for social housing.

The federal government has signed housing-transfer agreements with most of the provinces and territories. While the federal government will continue to fund existing housing projects after administration has been shifted to the provinces and territories, it has locked itself into a steady and growing decline in housing spending.

The federal government currently spends about $1.7 billion subsidizing the hundreds of thousands of social-housing units built until the program was cancelled in 1993. Funding will start to decline by 2010, falling to about $800 million by 2024 and then to zero by 2036. The annual drop is fairly small, but the cumulative amount represents the complete withdrawal of all federal funding for housing over three decades (Canadian Housing and Renewal Association, 2003).

In addition to an overall budgetary surplus, the federal government is also running a large surplus with its national housing agency, the Canada Mortgage and Housing Corporation (CMHC). The agency sells commercial insurance services and it is a lucrative business, especially the return on investments of the assets. CMHC's annual surplus is expected to grow to $1.3 billion by 2011 and its retained earnings will grow to $5.3 billion, but not one penny of that surplus in the housing agency budget will go to desperately needed new housing (Shapcott, 2007).

In 1996, the federal housing minister was in Istanbul to commit her government to support the principles of the Habitat Agenda, with its goal of "housing for all." At home, the same minister was presiding over a rapidly deteriorating housing policy.

During the 1990s, the federal government has:

- cancelled all spending on desperately needed new social housing
- cut spending from existing housing programs
- transferred its responsibility for administration of housing programs to the provinces and territories
- locked itself into a downward spiral of decreasing spending

All this in a decade that ended with the first of a growing number of budgetary surpluses.

Tenant households across the country face a patchwork of laws offering a diminishing amount of legal protection. Ontario started the decade with the strongest tenant-protection laws in the country. The province had laws to protect rental housing from conversion to non-rental uses (to protect affordable housing), rent-regulation laws to protect tenants from sharp practices by landlords, security of tenure, and a package of anti-discrimination laws. Most of those laws have been gutted or cut entirely.

Canada's vanishing housing policies have attracted critical comments from two separate United Nations' committees in recent years. Both the UN Human Rights Committee and the UN Committee on Economic, Social, and Cultural Rights have called on governments in Canada to take positive steps to correct violations of international commitments.

A fact-finding mission to Canada in October 2007 by Miloon Kothari, the United Nations special rapporteur on the right to adequate housing, produced a devastating assessment of Canada's failures to meet its international housing obligations. He set out a series of practical action to bring Canada back in compliance with international housing rights laws (Kothari, 2007).

The federal government has taken several positive steps in recent years in response to growing political pressure from national and local advocacy groups, along with opinion polls that show housing is a key issue for a majority of Canadians.

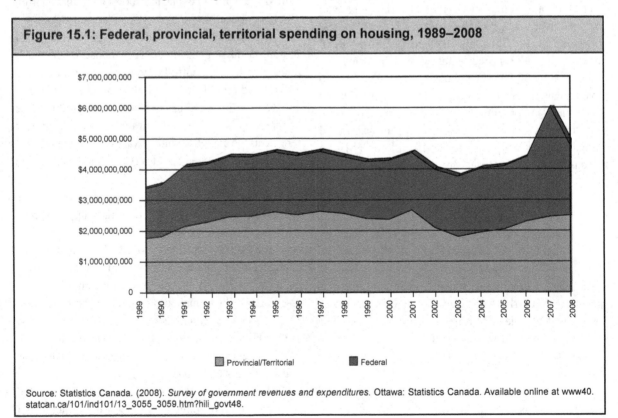

Figure 15.1: Federal, provincial, territorial spending on housing, 1989–2008

Source: Statistics Canada. (2008). *Survey of government revenues and expenditures*. Ottawa: Statistics Canada. Available online at www40.statcan.ca/101/ind101/13_3055_3059.htm?hili_govt48.

In December 1999, it announced a national homelessness strategy, including the Supporting Community Partnerships Initiative (SCPI)—$753 million over three years. Using SCPI and other funding, innovative projects have created transitional housing and services in several cities.

In November 2001, the federal government signed the Affordable Housing Framework Agreement with every province and territory. The federal government agreed to provide $1 billion over five years. Provinces and territories agreed to match the federal dollars. However:

- Most provinces are not paying their matching share. The definition of "affordable" has been changed to "average market rents," so the new housing will be rented at existing market. However, as many as two-thirds of renters cannot afford average rents, which puts the housing out of the reach of those who need it the most.
- Even if the framework agreement was fully funded, the total number of units would be well short of the amount required to meet the massive and growing need for affordable rental housing.

The combined impact from the withdrawal of the private sector in the 1970s, and the government in the 1990s, led to a serious and growing shortfall in the supply of affordable housing by the end of the 20th century. At the same time, the gap between rich and poor Canadians was growing more extreme, exacerbating the affordability crisis.

As the national and most provincial economies were booming in the years following the recession of 1991, an increasingly slender portion of that economy was directed to meeting the housing needs of low-, moderate-, and middle-income Canadians. This created the troubling phenomenon of growing poverty, growing income inequality, and growing housing insecurity in the midst of growing prosperity.

Economists and policy experts make the case that housing investment makes good economic sense—it generates jobs and tax revenues for the government, stimulates the economy, and helps to create inclusive and sustainable communities (Maclennan, 2008).

One Percent Solution

In 1998, the Toronto Disaster Relief Committee (TDRC) launched a national campaign called the One Percent Solution. The campaign grew out of an observation by Dr. David Hulchanski, a leading Canadian housing scholar, who noted that in the early 1990s, the federal, provincial, territorial, and municipal governments spent about 1 percent of their overall budgets on housing. The TDRC figured that doubling that amount—or adding an additional 1 percent—would create an envelope to fund a comprehensive, national housing strategy (Toronto Disaster Relief Committee, 1998).

In its 2000 pre-budget submission to the House of Commons Standing Committee on Finance, the Toronto Disaster Relief Committee joined with the National Housing and Homelessness Network (NHHN) to renew the call for implementation of the One Percent Solution. The enhanced funding envelope, combined with existing housing spending, would allow the federal government to adopt a comprehensive national housing strategy with these key elements:

- supply (increase the number of rental units)
- affordability (ensure the new units are affordable to the households that need the new housing the most)
- supports (programs for those who require special services)
- rehabilitation (funding to maintain housing to a proper standard)
- emergency relief (special support for people who are already homeless)

The first four are prevention strategies, aimed at ensuring that everyone has access to good-quality, affordable housing. The fifth is relief, aimed at providing a basic level of comfort for those who are on the streets and also assistance to help them secure permanent homes (National Housing and Homelessness Network, 2002).

The NHHN and its housing partners on the national stage—the Federation of Canadian Municipalities, Co-operative Housing Federation of Canada, and the Canadian Housing and Renewal Association—have been successful in convincing the federal government to commit a limited amount of new funding for affordable housing. But the latest national housing report card from the Wellesley Institute, released in February 2008, noted that the federal government and most provinces and territories have failed to meet the commitments that they made in 2001 (Shapcott, 2008).

In September 2005, the federal, provincial, and territorial housing ministers met in White Point, Nova Scotia, and released a set of "principles for a new Canadian Housing Framework" (Shapcott, 2007). The housing ministers promised in 2005 that they would "accelerate work" on the new housing framework, but then didn't even schedule another meeting until February 2008, more than two and a half years later. The federal housing minister boycotted the meeting, but, facing significant political pressure, announced on the day that the provincial and territorial ministers were meeting that he would meet with his counterparts within 60 days.

The emerging patchwork of housing and homelessness funding and programs that federal, provincial, and territorial politicians announced in the first few years of the 21st century failed to replace the massive cuts of the 1990s and fell far short of the growing housing needs of Canadians. Funding was short-term and program rules were inconsistent, leaving community-based housing and service providers to spend significant time and resources to cobble together housing solutions in the absence of a comprehensive national housing strategy.

The One Percent Solution calls for an additional $2 billion in annual federal spending on top of the $2 billion currently being spent. Other recent national housing proposals, including the January 2008 plan from the Federation of Canadian Municipalities, call for a similar scale of response (the FCM target is $3.35 billion).

Conclusion

The devastating reality of the nationwide housing crisis concerns Canadians, even though two-thirds are comfortably housed by global standards. Numerous opinion polls starting in the late 1990s show growing public concern for housing and homelessness issues, and support for increased government funding for solutions. This polling, combined with effective political advocacy, is creating a powerful political dynamic.

The housing history of Canada over the past 100 years shows a cycle of rising concerns, which are eventually met by limited government responses.

The outbreak of disease in Toronto's slums in the early 1900s led to the development of the country's first affordable housing projects, Spruce Court and Bain Co-op, two townhouse developments built in 1913 that continue to provide good-quality homes even today.

The appalling conditions in many communities in 1930s led to large-scale development of government-managed public housing starting in the late 1940s.

Concerns about conditions in the public housing projects, along with a more general housing crisis in the late 1960s, led to the national co-op and non-profit housing program of 1973, which generated hundreds of thousands units until the program was cancelled in 1993.

The affordable housing crisis and homelessness disaster of the late 1990s have led to an emerging patchwork of responses from senior levels of government starting in 2001. Housing advocates are trying to break this pattern with the One Percent Solution, a permanent, fully funded comprehensive national housing strategy.

A manufactured response, they argue, is the only solution to a manufactured housing crisis and homelessness disaster.

Critical Thinking Questions

1. Some economists say that "a rising tide lifts all boats." Why has the relatively robust Canadian economy in the period since 1991 not delivered good-quality and affordable homes for all Canadians?

2. Humphrey Carver wrote in 1948 that the private market is not able to deliver affordable housing for low- and moderate-income households. Explain why private developers have delivered near-record numbers of new homes since the year 2000, but only a tiny fraction have been truly affordable.

3. Miloon Kothari, the United Nations' special rapporteur on the right to adequate housing, has concluded that Canada has fallen short of its international obligations when it comes to housing and homelessness. Why is the right to housing considered one of the most important and fundamental human rights?

4. Even as Canada's economy has boomed in recent years, the percentage of the gross domestic product (one measure of economic activity) devoted to affordable housing has fallen. Should Canadians expect that a rising economy will mean growing spending for affordable housing?

5. The One Percent Solution calls for the federal government to double its housing spending to approximately $4 billion. Should housing spending be considered an important investment for governments?

Recommended Readings

Carver, H. (1948). *Houses for Canadians: A study of housing problems in the Toronto area.* Toronto: University of Toronto Press. Online at www.urbancentre.utoronto.ca/pdfs/policyarchives/1948HumphreyCarver. pdf.
    This is a classic in Canadian housing literature, especially Chapter 6, the "ultimate housing problem."

Crowe, Cathy et al. (2007). *Dying for a home: Homeless activists speak out.* Toronto: Between the Lines.
    Cathy Crowe, a Toronto "street nurse" has been a leading advocate for affordable housing.

Hulchanski, J.D. & Shapcott, M. (2004). *Finding room: Policy options for a Canadian rental housing strategy.* Toronto: Centre for Urban and Community Studies, University of Toronto Press.
    This is a collection of current research and advocacy on key elements of the affordable housing crisis.

Layton, J. & Shapcott, M. (2008). *Homelessness: How to end the national crisis.* Toronto: Penguin.
    Jack Layton and Michael Shapcott have been leaders in Toronto and nationally in the struggle for more affordable housing. This book provides a lively overview of the crisis and solutions.

Okpala, Don et al. (2006). *State of the world's cities: 2006/07; The millennium development goals and urban sustainability: Thirty years of shaping the Habitat Agenda.* Nairobi: United Nations Human Settlements Program (UN Habitat).
    This is a global review of housing and human settlements.

Related Web Sites

Canada Mortgage and Housing Corporation—www.cmhc-schl.gc.ca
    The federal government's national housing agency publishes market data and research, including the annual *Canadian Housing Observer.*

Centre for Urban and Community Studies—www.urbancentre.utoronto.ca
    The University of Toronto research centre publishes policy-relevant research on local, national, and international housing and urban issues.

Homeless Partnering Strategy—www.homelessness.gc.ca
    The major federal homelessness program supports transitional housing and support services in more than 60 communities across Canada.

Toronto Disaster Relief Committee—www.tdrc.net

The is a local housing and homelessness advocacy group with online resources from the TDRC, Housing and Homelessness Network in Ontario, and the National Housing and Homelessness Network.

Wellesley Institute—www.wellesleyinstitute.com

The Wellesley Institute is a community-centric policy and research institute dedicated to advancing the social determinants of health, including housing and homelessness.

Chapter 16

Housing and Health: More Than Bricks and Mortar

Toba Bryant

Introduction

The *Ottawa Charter for Health Promotion* recognizes shelter as a basic prerequisite for health (World Health Organization, 1986). Yet, Canadian political leaders and the housing policies they offer fail to meet the housing needs of many Canadians. In the first edition of this book, I noted that federal NDP leader Jack Layton's book on homelessness had documented how the number of Canadians who sleep in the streets, use temporary shelters, or spend more than 30 percent or 50 percent of their income on housing had been increasing at alarming levels (Layton, 2000). In 2008, this situation has continued to deteriorate (see Shapcott's chapter in this volume, as well as Layton & Shapcott, 2008). These developments have clear implications for the health of Canadians.

The first objective of this chapter is to provide the available evidence on how housing issues affect health. The first and most obvious question to be considered is: What is the effect of homelessness on health? The second question is: What is the effect of poor housing conditions on health? The third question is: How does spending an excessive amount of income on housing influence the quality of other social determinants of health? Tying all of these issues together is the concept of housing insecurity and its effects on health.

The second objective of this chapter is to consider why health researchers and policy-makers have neglected housing as a health issue. Given the existence of a housing crisis, it would be expected that housing and health would be well-developed areas of Canadian research and policy concern. This does not appear to be the case. There is housing and health research in Canada, but much of it is carried out within rather limited models that examine how physical aspects of dwellings affect health. The role that housing plays in relation to other social determinants of health is rarely considered, nor do these models consider how public policies contribute to the housing crisis in Canada. New ways of thinking about and researching how housing and health are related are presented.

The third objective of this chapter is to consider how policy-makers can be influenced to address housing and health issues. There are policy options than can improve housing, thereby improving health. To see successful implementation of these options requires understanding how policy-makers use different forms of evidence to develop housing policies to support health.

The Housing Crisis in Canada

A key issue in Canada, particularly in urban areas, is the lack of affordable private rental accommodation and the private rental market's inability to produce affordable units. Rental housing affordability emerged as a major issue in the 1980s. It has remained largely unaddressed through the 1990s, and so far, also the 2000s. Many analysts attribute the growing number of homeless and housing-insecure in Canada to reduced state provision of social housing.

Indeed, Canada has the most private sector-dominated, market-based system of any Western nation (Freeman, Holman & Whitehead, 1996). It also has the smallest social housing sector of any Western nation with the exception of the US (see Hulchanski, 2002, for a history of Canadian housing policy from the 1940s to the present).

Other contributing factors to the crisis are lack of affordable rental accommodation and growth of low-paying jobs or precarious employment that are both insecure and low paying (Jackson, 2005). Canada has one of the highest levels of low-paying jobs at 23 percent and among the highest family poverty rates among Western nations (Innocenti Research Centre, 2001). The result is increasing numbers of families and individuals with insecure housing. Growing numbers of Canadians are underhoused, living in motels, dependent on the shelter system, or living on the street (Layton, 2000; Layton & Shapcott, 2008). Three aspects of the housing crisis have implications for health: homelessness, the experience of poor living conditions, and the effects of housing insecurity on other social determinants of health.

Homelessness

Shelter use continues to increase across Canada. Of all the provinces, Ontario had the highest shelter occupancy with 6,100 in 2001 (Statistics Canada, 2002). Of 32,700 people in emergency shelters in Toronto in 2005, 4,600 were children (Homelessness Action Group, 2007). According to some reports, over 30,000 women, men, and children crowd into emergency shelters annually in Toronto (City of Toronto Planning Policy & Research, 2006). Although there has been a slight decrease in shelter occupancy since 2002, some attribute the decline to fewer sheltered families as a result of tightened federal immigration rules. When more recent data is available, sharp increases are apparent (City of Calgary, 2002). Official counts do not capture all the people who are homeless because they have other options than shelters or are unable to find space in emergency shelters.

Increased Incidence of Poor Living Conditions

CMHC devised the term "core need" to track the number of households experiencing housing difficulties. Core-housing need exists when one or more of the following issues are present (Layton, 2000):

Box 16.1: Women and housing in Canada: Barriers to equality

Women and children are the fastest growing group using shelters. The increasing number of women in shelters is only a small fraction of women across Canada experiencing housing crises and homelessness in diverse ways—living with the threat of violence because there are no other housing options; sacrificing other necessities such as food, clothing, and medical needs to pay rent or to make mortgage payments or moving into overcrowded accommodation with family or friends.

The homelessness crisis facing women is also a poverty crisis and cannot be understood merely in relation to scarcity of appropriate housing. It is important to consider the interconnections between housing programs, subsidy eligibility and allocation, income security, access to credit, security of tenure, transportation, and service needs.

The withdrawal of federal funding for new social housing, culminating in the 1993 freeze in federal contributions to social housing and the cancellation of funding for any new social housing (except for on-reserve Aboriginal housing), had a particularly adverse effect on women, who are most likely to be in need of housing subsidies.

In most provinces and territories, the National Child Benefit Supplement is clawed back from social assistance recipients by agreement with the federal government. Despite the fact that women on social assistance may be most in need of this benefit and most unable to pay for housing and related expenses, they are excluded from the federal government's only initiative to address child (family) poverty.

Changes that have been put in place to Employment Insurance eligibility have placed many women at increased risk of eviction when dealing with loss of a job, pregnancy or disability. This is an area of direct federal responsibility for protecting the needs of women for income and housing security.

Source: *Women and housing in Canada: Barriers to equality.* (2002). Ottawa: Women's Program, Centre for Equality Rights in Accommodation. Online at www.equalityrights.org/docs/barriers_exec_summary.doc

- *Affordability:* Tenants pay more than 30 percent of their gross income on their housing.
- *Suitability:* Tenants live in overcrowded conditions, whereby household size exceeds recommended actual space.
- *Adequacy:* Tenants' homes lack full bathroom facilities, or require significant repairs.

In a recent report on housing conditions in Canada, CMHC reported that suitability and adequacy are less likely to be reported as issues than affordability (Engeland, Lewis, Ehrlich & Che, 2005). Most cases of core-housing need pertain to affordability. This finding is not surprising. Figure 16.1 shows that low-end incomes have failed to keep pace with low-end market rents in virtually every Canadian municipality.

Indeed, recent CMHC data shows that over 1.7 million Canadian tenant households are in core-need situations (Engeland, Lewis, Ehrlich & Che, 2005). Renters are at greater risk of being in core-housing need. The figures in 2001 are 30.1 percent of renters and 8.6 percent of homeowners (Dunning, 2007; Engeland, Lewis, Ehrlich & Che, 2005). Core-housing need is more widespread in the three territories. Among the provinces, British

Columbia, Nova Scotia, and Ontario have the highest incidence of core-housing need. British Columbia and Ontario are major reception areas for new immigrants.

Other populations are also at risk of having core-housing need. For example, lone-parent families, most of whom are female-led, have a 30 percent incidence of core-housing need, which is twice that of other Canadian households. For households that have recently immigrated to Canada, the incidence of core-housing need is three times that of non-immigrant households. Moreover, for households whose primary source of income comes from government transfers, the incidence is almost 40 percent. Aboriginal households are much more likely to have core-housing need (24 percent) than non-Aboriginal households (13.5 percent). These are all striking findings that show the depth of need for affordable housing in Canada.

Weakening of Other Social Determinants of Health as a Result of Housing Insecurity

In 2000, almost 40 percent (39.6 percent) of Canadian tenant households spent 30 percent or more of their

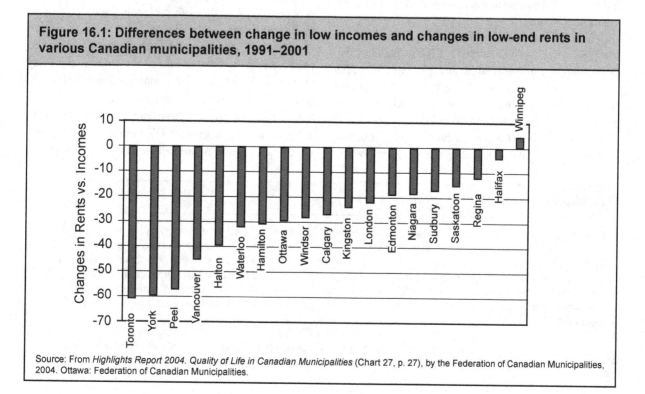

Figure 16.1: Differences between change in low incomes and changes in low-end rents in various Canadian municipalities, 1991–2001

Source: From *Highlights Report 2004. Quality of Life in Canadian Municipalities* (Chart 27, p. 27), by the Federation of Canadian Municipalities, 2004. Ottawa: Federation of Canadian Municipalities.

incomes on housing (Engeland et al, 2005), down from 39.2 percent of renter households in 1995 (Statistics Canada, 1995). And 18.6 percent of Canadian households spent more than 50 percent of their income on rent. This percentage is down from 21.6 percent of renter households in 1995. Tenants paying more than 50 percent of incomes on rent are in a revenue/expense structure that makes losing their housing a real possibility (Layton, 2000). Such conditions have both direct material effects on health and increase stress and insecurity, another established determinant of health (Brunner & Marmot, 1999).

Housing and Health

A recent review of the housing and health literature concluded that research has focused on and identified findings in four key areas (Dunn, 2000): (1) homeless people experience poor health status and have limited access to health care; (2) problematic dimensions of dwellings are associated with adverse physical and mental health outcomes; (3) stresses linked with unaffordable and/or inadequate housing can affect health status; and (4) unhealthy individuals are often disadvantaged in the housing market and are directed into substandard housing conditions.

The focus here is on three variants of these issues: (1) the health effects of homelessness; (2) how poor housing conditions influence health; and (3) how spending excessive amounts of available income on housing influences health. The experiences of homelessness and poor housing conditions are placed in a broader context of how individuals in Canada systematically differ in their access to economic and social resources. Poor housing

is one indicator of potential disadvantage in Canadian society.

The link between one's housing situation and health seems obvious (see Box 16.2). Homelessness and inadequate and insecure housing have effects on health and well-being. While most of those who are homeless appear to be men, most of those living in poor housing conditions or insecure situations are women with children.

Homelessness and Health

It would hardly seem necessary to argue the case that housing—and homelessness in particular—are health issues, yet surprisingly few Canadian studies have considered it as such. In the UK, where the housing and health research tradition is more established, numerous studies have shown strikingly high incidences of physical and mental health problems among homeless people as compared to the general population. Homelessness is understood as directly attributable to structural inequalities and housing policies (Shaw, 2004). Several studies have shown that homeless people have poorer health outcomes compared to the larger population. They experience respiratory disease; alcohol and drug dependence; mental health problems; and are prone to suicide, accidents, and violence.

Among 1,280 homeless people in the UK who used hostels, bed-and-breakfast accommodation, day centres, and soup runs, numerous problems were more common than among the general population (Bines, 1994). Table 16.1 shows these data as comparisons with a representative sample of UK residents whose rates are calculated as standardized—taking into account age

---

Box 16.2: *Three evils of inadequate housing*

A pamphlet published in 1944 quotes the Chief Medical Officer at the then new Ministry of Health in United Kingdom at the time on the three "evils" of inadequate housing: "There is *diminished personal cleanliness and physique* leading to debility, fatigue, unfitness, and reduced powers of resistance. A second result of bad housing is that the *sickness rates* are relatively high, particularly for infectious, contagious, and respiratory diseases. Thirdly, the general *death-rates* are higher and the expectation of life is lower. The evidence is overwhelming, and it comes from all parts of the world—the worse people are housed the higher will be the death rate."

—J.N. Morris, *Health, No. 6: Handbooks for discussion Groups.* London: Association for Education in Citizenship. Reprinted in M. Shaw, "Health and housing: A lasting relationship," *Journal of epidemiology and community health* 55(2001), p. 291.

and gender—morbidity ratios with a value of 100. All rates were higher than the general population with those sleeping on the street having the highest likelihood of experiencing these afflictions.

Many other studies find much greater incidence of a variety of conditions and ailments among the homeless population (see Hwang, 2001). These include greater incidence of mental illness, HIV infection, and physical violence (Dunn, 2000). A Toronto survey of homeless people found much higher risk than the general population for chronic respiratory diseases, arthritis or rheumatism, hypertension, asthma, epilepsy, and diabetes (Ambrosio et al., 1992). Tuberculosis is more common among the homeless in the UK (Ramsden et al., 1988) and Canada (Hwang, 2001).

Few studies examine the life expectancy of homeless people. A UK study found that homeless people are at greater risk of premature death (Shaw et al., 1999). It showed that male street sleepers in London had an average age at death of 42 years and residents of hostels for the homeless have a life expectancy of 63 years. The primary causes of death for this group were drug overdoses, AIDS, and suicide. A Danish study also showed an increased probability of early death for homeless hostel residents (Nordentoft & Wandall-Holm, 2003).

In the US, being without housing shortens life expectancy by 20 years (Hwang et al., 1997). The average age of death of homeless people in Boston is 47 years

and in Georgia, 46 years. In the UK, it is 42 years. In Toronto, homeless people die at a younger age than the general population. Between 1979 and 1990, 71 percent of homeless people who died were less than 70 years old as compared to 38 percent in the general population (Kushner, 1998). A study of 9,000 men who used shelters in 1995 showed that young homeless men in Toronto were eight times more likely to die than men of the same age in the general population (Hwang, 2001). Another Canada study found that mortality rates were a very high 515 per 100,000 person-years for homeless women aged 18–44 years and 438 per 100,000 person-years for homeless women aged 45–64 years in Toronto (Cheung & Hwang, 2004). These risks of premature death were ten times greater for younger homeless women than women in the general population. They were 20 percent higher for older women. The mortality rate of younger homeless women was similar to that of younger homeless men.

It is sometimes argued that these health outcomes cannot be clearly attributed to being homeless as their presence may precede the experience of homelessness. It is clear that "while some health conditions may precede homelessness, it certainly is the case that the daily conditions of homelessness, both material and psychosocial, compound existing health problems, cause additional problems (such as problems with feet and respiratory illness) … " (Shaw, Dorling & Davey Smith, 1999, p. 232). Not surprisingly, homeless people also experience barriers to accessing health care services.

Table 16.1: Standardized morbidity ratios[1] for reported health problems for hostel users and rough sleepers (Bines, 1994)

Health problem	Hostels and B and Bs	Sleeping rough day centres	Soup runs
Musculoskeletal problems	153	185	221
Wounds, skin ulcers or other skin complaints	105	189	298
Chronic chest or other breathing problems	183	259	365
Fits or loss of consciousness	651	2109	1892
Frequent headaches	264	338	365

[1] SMRs for the general population are 100.

Source: Bines, W. (1994). *The health of single homeless people*. York: Centre for Housing Policy, University of York.

Poor Housing Conditions and Health

An extensive review of the health effects of housing conditions categorized findings as either definitive, strong, possible, or weak (Hwang et al., 1999). *Definitive* findings were seen for health effects associated with the presence of lead, asbestos, poor heating systems, and lack of smoke detectors. *Strong/definitive* findings were seen for presence of radon, house dust mites, cockroaches, and cold and heat. *Strong* findings were seen for environmental tobacco smoke. *Possible* findings were seen for dampness and mould, high-rise structures, overcrowding and high density, poor ventilation, and poor housing satisfaction. This review used a narrow set of criteria for isolating the effects of these factors independent of the presence of other factors, an issue discussed in the following sections.

Many studies have investigated the effect of poor housing conditions such as inadequate heating and dampness on health. A UK survey of older people reported that 25 percent were not using as much heat as they would have liked because of cost (Savage, 1988). Studies have confirmed that dampness in homes contributes to, and exacerbates, respiratory illness. Strachan (1988) found children living in homes with damp and mould in Edinburgh had increased risk of developing wheezing and chesty coughs. Another study found higher levels of several symptoms for both child and adults in damp and mouldy houses as compared to those living in dry dwellings (Platt et al., 1989).

It is difficult to separate the effects of any single variable or sets of variables upon health as indicators of disadvantage—poverty, poor housing, pre-existing illness—frequently cluster together. One study was able to do this. In *Home Sweet Home: The Impact of Poor Housing on Health*, Marsh and colleagues (1999) used a lifespan approach to examine the link between housing and health and, using longitudinal data, showed the link between housing and health among more than 13,000 citizens. Housing conditions played a significant and independent role in health outcomes.

Greater housing deprivation shows a dose-response relationship—the worse the conditions, the greater the health effects—to severe/moderate ill health at age 33. Those who experienced overcrowded housing conditions in childhood to age 11 had a higher likelihood of infectious disease as adults. In adulthood, overcrowding was also linked to increased likelihood of respiratory disease. Living in poor housing in the past and in the present make independent contributions to the likelihood of poor health.

Another study of childhood housing conditions and later mortality showed poorer housing conditions to be generally associated with increased adult mortality in selected areas in the UK (Dedman et al., 2001). Statistically significant associations were found between lack of private indoor tapped water supply and increased mortality from coronary heart disease, and between poor ventilation and overall mortality.

The Effects of Excessive Spending on Shelter on Other Social Determinants of Health

When spending on housing becomes excessive, there is less money available for other needs. In a recent study on housing conditions in Census metropolitan areas between 1991 and 2001, the Canada Mortgage and Housing Corporation reported that the main issue for most households is finding affordable housing, particularly for households that rent (Engeland et al., 2005). Indeed, a comparison of incomes compared to rents shows that many people spend more than 30 percent of their incomes on housing.

The average monthly gross welfare income in Ontario in 2005 for a single adult with one child aged one to 12 years was $1,204 (National Council of Welfare, 2006), and the average rent was $889 for a one-bedroom apartment. This left about $315 to cover food and other expenses (City of Toronto Planning Policy & Research, 2006). For two adults with two children, gross welfare income was $1,608, and rent for a two-bedroom apartment was $1,060. This left about $550 to cover food and other living expenses. Clearly, having little after-rent income makes it difficult to cover other important expenses such as food, thereby contributing directly to food insecurity as well as housing insecurity, malnutrition, and consequent poor health. Excessive spending on housing reduces amounts to be spent on other social determinants of health.

This situation was clearly described in a recent report on the impacts of housing insecurity on children's health (Watt, 2003). Thirty percent of Canadian families who rent have affordability (less money than needed for other expenses) problems. Fifty-eight percent of lone-parent—usually female-led—families who rent have affordability issues and if the parent of these lone-parent families is under 30 years of age, the figure rises to 76 percent. The striking rise in food-bank use in Canada has also been attributed to continuing housing inadequacy and its impacts upon available monetary resources among the working and non-working poor (Daily Bread Food Bank, 2002). Figure 16.2 shows how housing insecurity and housing inadequacy impacts upon other social determinants of health.

Little housing research places the experience of homelessness or insecure housing into this broader context (Bryant, 2003). There is little research that considers how insecure housing and related health effects are integral to issues related to inequalities in material resources that exist among the population. Another way of putting this is to ask the question: How does the experience of poor housing reflect the general experience of being materially deprived within a society? This places the issue of the clustering of disadvantage among individuals into focus and how poor housing is part of a common pathway to poor health together with other indicators of economic and social disadvantage (Dunn & Hayes, 1999; Hwang et

al., 1999; Shaw, Dorling, Gordon & Davey Smith, 1999). As Shaw argues, "Housing, health, and poverty are still empirically related and conceptually interconnected" (Shaw, 2004, p. 413).

There are significant health inequalities across the entire socio-economic spectrum in Canada. These inequalities are related to differences in access to material resources necessary for health, including housing. Housing research has tended to focus narrowly on the concrete aspects of housing, such as homelessness and material aspects of housing poverty (Dunn, 2000). There is a need for research that recognizes that housing is both part of and a contributor to the social gradient in health by which Canadians of different income levels differ in health status. The goal is to understand the sources of disadvantage that manifests itself across the socio-economic spectrum.

Reasons for the Neglect and Narrow Focus of Housing and Health Research

A recent analysis of research needs, gaps, and opportunities in the housing and health area (NGOA) identified opportunities for "high-impact, longitudinal and quasi-

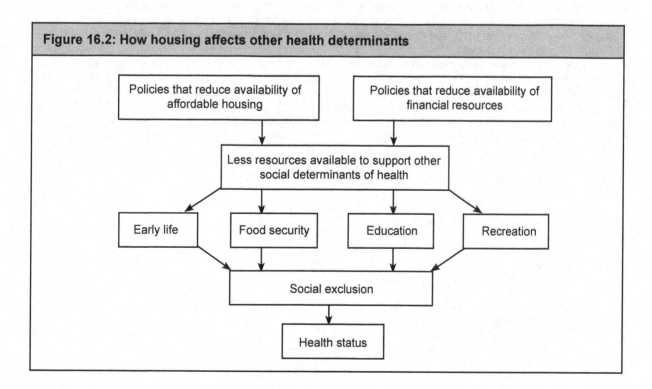

Figure 16.2: How housing affects other health determinants

Policies that reduce availability of affordable housing

Policies that reduce availability of financial resources

Less resources available to support other social determinants of health

Early life   Food security   Education   Recreation

Social exclusion

Health status

experimental research" (Dunn et al., 2006). This review points to opportunities for enhancing the understanding of the effects of social environments on health and reducing inequalities in health. This review fails to acknowledge, however, the influence of public policies on housing conditions and in increasing inequalities in health. The review is primarily an epidemiological approach to understanding the impact of housing on health.

Despite such calls for an expanded analysis of housing and health issues, such research is uncommon in Canada. One reason may be the difficulties that such research presents for those trained in traditional epidemiological methods. Epidemiological models attempt to understand the relationships between housing and health, but existing models may be insufficient to capture the complexity of

these relationships. Epidemiologists argue it is necessary to isolate specific causes of an outcome such as poor health status. In the case of housing and health, this can be difficult, if not impossible, as housing disadvantage is associated with numerous other indicators of disadvantage (see Box 16.3).

The model presented in Figure 16.3 identifies the material conditions of housing such as mould and draft as the area of interest. Studies attempt to control for the effects of personal characteristics of research participants. It then separates the unique effects of housing conditions from other potential variables that may influence health. To confirm such associations and identify causal relationships between variables, experiments or controlled trials would generally be carried out. Such

---

Box 16.3: Traditional epidemiological model of housing effects on health

Epidemiology is the study of the distribution and determinants of diseases and injuries in human populations. Epidemiologists frequently aim to identify the unique causal effects of single variables upon health outcomes through various analytical procedures. Identifying unique health effects of housing does not easily lend itself to such a model. Living in disadvantaged housing circumstances is associated with other indicators of disadvantage. Indeed, Shaw et al. argue that: "health inequalities are produced by the clustering of disadvantage—in opportunity, material circumstances, and behaviours related to health across people's lives" (1999, p. 65).

Epidemiologists therefore have tended to focus on aspects of housing and health that can be isolated for measurement such as the presence of mould and the development of respiratory infections in children, or overcrowding and its impact on mental health. But its models attempt to identify the effects of these factors independent of the contextual variables associated with disadvantage in general. Many problems are associated with this methodology.

Many studies have investigated the relationship between housing and health and have pointed to the confounding factors that make such research difficult. People in poor housing suffer many deprivations rendering it difficult to assess any one risk factor. In addition, the direction of cause and effect is often unclear. People with pre-existing ill health tend to live in substandard housing because of their low income. All of these factors contribute to methodological difficulties in designing and conducting appropriate research. Figure 16.3 is an example of a traditional epidemiological model that could be deployed to examine the relationship between housing and health.

Figure 16.3: Traditional epidemiological model

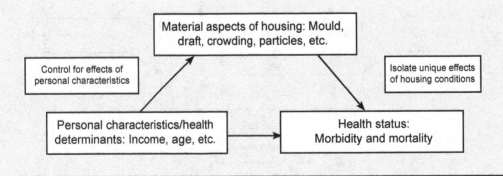

activities are usually not possible for investigating housing and health.

Moreover, the relationships investigated in such models do not explain how people end up in poor housing and the effects of housing on the other determinants of health. Attempts to identify the unique effect of poor housing are unable to measure or capture the complexity and interaction among the social determinants of health. "Some of these problems occur as a result of the rigid criteria of biomedical research, particularly in establishing causal mechanisms, which contradicts the more ethnographic nature of research on the social causes of illness" (Wilkinson, 1999, p. 3). These models also focus on individuals instead of considering the effects of various policies and programs on groups in society. They rarely consider the effects of income on both housing quality and health, and may tend to blame individuals for their poor housing conditions instead of addressing larger structural issues, such as housing policy, which may contribute to their housing circumstances.

Income affects the type of housing people have. If people have low income, they are likely to live in poor housing. High income increases choices for housing and influences general living conditions. Income and housing insecurity also create stress.

An Expanded Model of the Housing and Health Relationship

There is overwhelming evidence that social and environmental conditions determine the presence of health-damaging stress (Brunner & Marmot, 1999). Especially important conditions are the availability of adequate housing and income. Lack of monetary resources is frequently related to public policy decisions that reduce the availability of both affordable housing and monetary resources. Figure 16.4 shows how these factors come together to influence health.

Researchers in Britain are leaders in investigating how material deprivation creates health-damaging stress (Davey Smith, 2003). Brunner and Marmot (1999) report that social and psychological circumstances can "seriously damage" health in the long term. Chronic anxiety, insecurity, low self-esteem, social isolation, and lack of control over home and work weaken mental and physical health. The human body has evolved to react to emergencies. This reaction triggers a whole range of stress hormones that affect the cardiovascular and immune systems.

The ability to respond to a crisis is highly adaptive and can save life in the short term. However, if the biological stress-reaction system is triggered too often and for too long, as it is for people living in poor or insecure housing and on low income, it results in considerable health damage. This includes depression, vulnerability to infection, diabetes, high blood pressure, and the related risks of heart attack and stroke. Individuals who are materially disadvantaged and experience income, housing, and food insecurity experience greater stress with associated increased risk of morbidity and premature death.

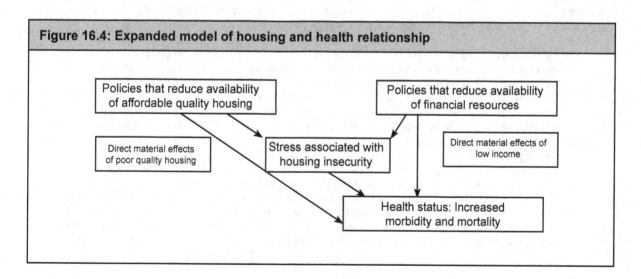

Figure 16.4: Expanded model of housing and health relationship

Toward the Future: Understanding the Complexities of the Housing and Health Relationship

There are many innovative models for examining the relationship between housing and health. Box 16.4 provides one example. Interrelationships among housing and other determinants of health must be considered as should policy decisions that affect the presence of material resources such as income and affordable housing. Ethnographic studies of people's housing experiences could document the meaning that housing provides to people and how these affect health. Finally, geographic studies are necessary to consider the spatial dimensions of housing and how these interact with other health determinants to influence health.

Introducing the Policy Dimension into Housing and Health Studies

As shown earlier in figures 16.2 and 16.4, the availability and cost of housing have direct material effects on health. But the availability of both affordable housing and other economic resources are directly influenced by governments' policy decisions. Both types of policy decisions contribute to housing insecurity, increased stress, morbidity and mortality, and increased incidence of social exclusion, illness, and disease.

Housing advocacy groups have brought forward solutions to the housing crisis, in particular to increase the availability of affordable housing and eradicate homelessness. The Toronto Disaster Relief Committee (TDRC) developed the One Percent Solution to end the housing crisis (Toronto Disaster Relief Committee, 1998). The TDRC argues that if all governments increased their spending on housing by 1 percent of overall spending, the homelessness crisis could be eliminated in five years. The One Percent Solution calls for three actions by government:

1. Annual funding for housing of $2 billion federally, and another $2 billion among provinces and territories
2. Restoring and renewing national, provincial, and territorial programs to resolve the housing crisis and homelessness disaster
3. Extending the federal homelessness strategy with immediate funding for new and expanded shelter and services across the country

---

Box 16.4: Housing as a socio-economic determinant of population health: A research framework

Canadian geographer James Dunn and others identified knowledge gaps in the understanding of the housing and health relationship (Dunn et al., 2002). Dunn argues that, "Housing, as a central locus of everyday life patterns, is likely to be a crucial component in the ways in which socio-economic factors shape health" (p. iii). The framework identifies three dimensions of housing relevant to health.

1) "Material dimensions" refer to the physical integrity of the home such as the state of repair; physical, biological, and chemical exposures in the home, and housing costs. Housing costs are critical because they are one of the largest monthly expenditures most people face. When housing costs eat up most of people's income, it affects other aspects of their lives.
2) "Meaningful dimensions" refer to sense of belonging and control in the home. Home is also an expression of social status—prestige, status, pride, and identity—all of which are enhanced by home ownership. These dimensions also provide for the expression of self-identity, and signify permanence, stability, and continuity in everyday life.
3) "Spatial dimensions" refer to a home and its immediate environment. For example, the proximity of a home to services, schools, public recreation, health services, and employment. This also includes systematic exposure to health hazards—toxins in the environment, asbestos insulation, etc. This dimension introduces the need for understanding geographic aspects of neighbourhoods and the kind of housing that is found within them. These concepts should stimulate new ways of Canadian thinking about and studying the role that housing plays in health.

Diverse policy strategies must be explored to address the housing crisis. Layton (2000) outlines several strategies developed as part of a Federation of Canadian Municipalities task force. A healthy housing sector should have four components: (1) rental housing; (2) ownership housing; (3) social housing with mixed incomes; and (4) support for people with special needs to enable them to live independently. The National Affordable Housing Strategy should consist of the following:

1. *Flexible capital grant program for housing*, a locally designed and administered program of initiatives financed by a federal or joint federal/provincial/territorial capital fund

2. *A private rental program* to stimulate private rental production

3. *An investment pool of money* to create affordable housing by attracting new funding for the development, acquisition, or rehabilitation of affordable housing

4. *Provincially administered income-supplement programs* to assist tenants who cannot afford private market rents; the program would complement capital grants to reach those most in need

Recent Policy Developments

In 2001, the federal and provincial governments signed housing agreements that commit them to building more social housing units. On the first anniversary of the signing of that agreement in November 2002, the National Housing and Homelessness Network (NHHN) reported that, outside of Quebec, less than 200 new housing units have been built since the housing agreement was signed in November 2001 (National Housing and Homelessness Network, 2002). Over half of the provincial governments have yet to fulfill their commitments to build more social housing units. Quebec and the three territories have taken action to match the federal commitment of $680 million over five years. The network expressed concern that the definition of "affordable housing" has been undermined in the bilateral housing agreements. This weakening of the term will make the rents of many new units unaffordable.

Indeed, Canadians see little governmental activity to address these social determinants of health besides policy proclamations on housing and the other social determinants. Governments are not seriously addressing social and health inequalities and the role that housing policy plays in widening these inequalities.

Understanding the Policy Change Process

An understanding of how these developments came about would help to identify some means of influencing new policy approaches toward housing. The policy framework presented in the next section can be used to consider how policy-makers use evidence to inform their housing decisions regarding housing and other related public policy.

This framework was devised to guide case studies on housing policy and health policy changes in Ontario since 1995 (see Figure 16.5). It incorporates elements of different forms of knowledge, the means by which this knowledge can be applied, and those who are likely to apply such knowledge. This framework can serve as a template for analyzing the policy change process on a case-by-case basis. It also provides insights into a government's general approach to policy change over time. Fuller presentations of the model and its applications are available (Bryant, 2002, 2003, 2004).

Government policy is affected by civil society actors such as professional policy analysts (PPA) and citizen activists (CA). PPAs are university-based academics and policy analysts associated with think tanks such as the Caledon Institute or the Canadian Policy Research Networks. CAs are usually volunteers. Different ways of knowing about a social issue refers to the different types of knowledge. Traditional or instrumental knowledge is derived from scientific or social science studies. Interactive knowledge is knowledge developed through dialogue. It can be local knowledge that residents have about their community such as its history and customs. Critical knowledge raises questions about social justice and begins to address how social structures influence the distribution of power and resources, questioning the organization of society, and challenging the distribution of wealth and political power.

Different ways of using knowledge about a social issue are reflected in the different strategies devised to present knowledge. Four strategies can be used to influence government policy and each of these strategies may be necessary to influence policy change in the housing area:

- Legal approach refers to the use of legal knowledge, argumentation, and judicial rulings to convey knowledge about a social issue.
- Public relations is marketing knowledge in order to target a message to a specific audience.
- Personal stories are the use of anecdotal evidence or the stories of individuals to illustrate the effects of specific policies and programs or of a public issue.
- Political-strategic is knowledge of how to use the political system to achieve particular policy change goals and objectives.

Finally, the last segment of the model identifies three different patterns of policy change. Routine or normal policy change is a change in policy instruments or policy settings such as a change in rental increases allowed (Howlett & Ramesh, 1995). In normal policy change, the overall policy goals and objectives remain the same. In contrast, paradigmatic policy change is a radical shift in the overall goals and objectives of a policy area, such as a shift from rent regulation such as rent control to vacancy decontrol or other methods of rent deregulation. Gradual policy change can be a series of routine policy changes over time that, taken together, signify paradigmatic policy change (Coleman et al., 1997). The framework attempts to address the following questions relevant to the consideration of housing policy and health in Canada:

- Who is trying to influence policy change?
- What type of knowledge can be used to communicate concerns and issues?
- How can this knowledge be used to influence policy change?

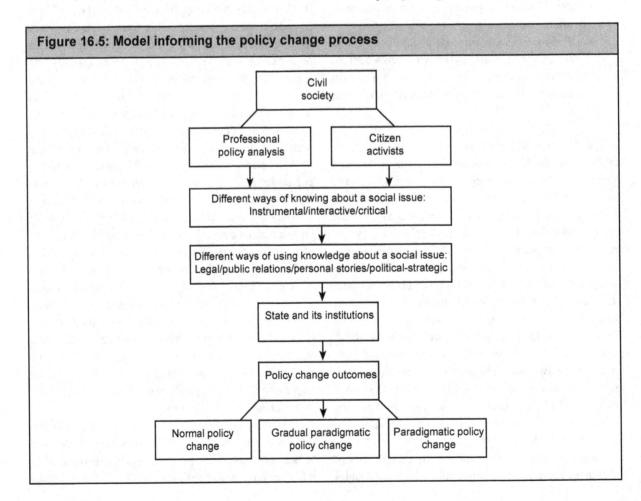

Figure 16.5: Model informing the policy change process

- How receptive is the government to these messages and to the messengers?
- What dynamics affect the government's receptivity to the messengers and the perspectives they present?
- What is the likelihood of achieving policy change?

In the case of Canadian housing policy, governments' political ideologies are significant barriers to progressive housing policy change. Housing policy appears to be especially sensitive to political ideology. Since federal and many provincial governments now have a strong pro-privatization and marketization agenda, housing is vulnerable to this agenda since it can be privatized and the public perceives it as a market issue (Bryant, 2004).

Also important is the extent to which governments subscribe to neo-liberal approaches that see the market economy as the best allocator of resources and wealth (Coburn, 2000). This view is consistent with the Harper government's policies and those of most of the provincial governments. The ideology of individualism espoused by Canadian governments and most Western nations is strongly associated with notions of "deservingness." Jenkins (1982) argues that individualism can be defined as "a way of looking at the world which explains and interprets events and circumstances mainly in terms of the decisions, actions and attitudes of the individuals involved" (p. 88). In other words, this ideology pathologizes individuals with social problems. This is relevant in the case of people living under conditions of poor or no housing.

The notion of collective social responsibility for vulnerable populations is no longer part of the political discourse. Although some consider neo-liberalism to be extreme and therefore temporary, the development of social policy that addresses the housing crisis and other social policy issues has yet to be seen. To date, only municipal governments have taken a strong stand to address housing and homelessness in Canada (see Sandeman et al., 2002; City of Calgary, 2002).

Also influencing housing policy are public perceptions of housing. Housing is an expense that most people are expected to cover themselves. Many low-income Canadians will be lifelong tenants. These populations are particularly vulnerable to policy changes in housing and policies that affect other social determinants of health. They also tend to have poorer health than the general population and homeowners in particular. The current political environment is not receptive to their concerns and impedes action on the social determinants of health such as housing from which these groups would benefit.

Conclusion

In spite of the ample evidence on the relationship between housing and health, government actions at times are at odds with a social determinants approach to health. Canadian governments are not seriously addressing the role that housing policies play in creating health inequalities. Educational and community mobilization strategies are needed to communicate to Canadians how housing policies threaten, either directly or indirectly, the health of all Canadians.

Governments should renew their commitment to housing provision. A range of policy responses have been articulated by housing activists and others to address the housing crisis in Canada. All levels of government must respond to the crisis by implementing policies that will ensure an affordable housing sector and relieve the pressures on individual households. A significant percentage of the most economically insecure Canadians—those who live in rental accommodations—are spending between 30 percent and 50 percent of their incomes on housing. Many of these tenants are at risk of losing their homes because they are unable to pay the rent.

Both the federal and provincial governments must re-enter the housing sector. Reliance on the private sector to fill the role left by government clearly does not meet housing needs. In light of this, provinces without rent controls need to restore these to ensure an affordable rental housing sector and begin to build social housing to ensure shelter for these vulnerable Canadians.

The need for government action is particularly acute in larger urban centres such as Vancouver, Montreal, and Toronto. These cities are major reception areas for recent immigrants and refugees with significant housing needs. The federal government should work in tandem with the provinces and territories by establishing a national housing strategy.

Similarly, despite the ample evidence concerning the importance of researching housing as a determinant of health in a broader perspective, most research remains narrowly focused on the physical aspects of housing. Changes wrought by neo-liberal policies have reduced investment in cities and have contributed to the housing crisis. Reduced federal and provincial housing expenditures have burdened cities with diminished revenues to address the problems of housing, which interacts with increasing depth of poverty to threaten health. This is a fundamental need for social investment to address the social determinants of health and improve population health.

Future research should consider these macro-level issues through an analysis of what might be termed a new political economy of housing. What is the relationship between general government social provision, housing policies, and population health? Do nations whose political economies reflect commitments to governmental intervention in the marketplace provide greater housing security for citizens than those nations where the market dominates policy discussions (Esping-Andersen, 1990)? Does the percentage of national resources devoted to housing support correlate with incidence of homeless and insecure housing? Do these differences in national commitments translate into differing population health profiles? And if this the case, what political strategies can be applied to promote such governmental activity?

Critical Thinking Questions

1. How can citizens be mobilized to influence public policies on housing?
2. What are some of the factors influencing the housing crisis in Canada and how are they related to health?
3. Consider the information on housing provided by the media, your courses, family, and friends. How much of this discusses decisions that governments make to address housing need in Canada?
4. What would be the difference in housing availability if housing issues were treated as health issues?
5. What are some of the effects of having so many working Canadians, particularly those with precarious employment, having core-housing need? What should be done to address core-housing need?

Recommended Readings

Hulchanski, J.D. (2002). *Housing policy for tomorrow's cities*. Ottawa: Canadian Policy Research Networks. Online at: www.cprn.com/doc.cfm?doc=161&l=en.

This report examines the role of the federal government in housing provision. It focuses on major urban centres in Canada where the housing crisis is most acute. The report explores how increasing non-market social housing units would address the urgent need for affordable rental housing.

Hulchanski, J.D. & Shapcott, M. (2004). *Finding room: Policy options for a Canadian rental housing strategy*. Toronto: Centre for Urban and Community Studies, University of Toronto.

This volume brings together several housing issues—including housing and health, the right to housing, housing affordability, and public policy solutions—to address the housing crisis in Canada. The contributors are all active researchers and/or activists in the housing field.

Marsh, A., Gordon, D., Pantazis, C. & Heslop, P. (1999). *Home sweet home? The impact of poor housing on health*. Bristol: Policy Press.

This study looks in detail at the impact poor housing has on health using data from the National Child Development Study. It provides important information on how housing influences health.

Shaw, M. (2004). "Housing and public health." *Annual Review of Public Health, 25*, 397–418.

This article reviews the housing and public health research literature and considers a broad range of factors and pathways whereby housing influences health. The author specifically considers the need to recognize the influence of public policy in addressing structural inequalities in housing and health.

Watt, J. (2003). *Adequate and affordable housing: A child health issue.* Ottawa: Child and Youth Health Network for Eastern Ontario. Online at www.child-youth-health.net/Housing_Child_Health_Eng.pdf.

This report reviews the literature on housing and health with particular emphasis on the effects of housing insecurity on children. The bibliography done for the Federal National Homelessness Initiative contains numerous articles related to health.

Related Web Sites

Canadian Housing Library—publish.uwo.ca/~cforchuk/chl/index.html

The Canadian Housing Library is an online library comprising academic publications/peer-review literature on housing and homelessness. The Web site was established as part of a project to identify and classify all Canadian housing literature from 1995 to the present.

Centre for Urban and Community Studies—www.urbancentre.utoronto.ca

The centre promotes and disseminates multidisciplinary research and policy analysis on urban issues in Canada and around the world.

Toronto Disaster Relief Committee—www.tdrc.net

The Toronto Disaster Relief Committee is a diverse group of individuals who have declared homelessness a national disaster and that Canada must end homelessness by implementing a fully funded National Housing Program through the One Percent Solution.

Wellesley Institute Housing and Homelessness—wellesleyinstitute.com/issues/housing-and-homelessness/overview

The Wellesley Institute is the former Wellesley Hospital in Toronto. It is now a public policy institute concerned about a broad range of issues that affect urban health. It approaches these issues from a social determinants of health perspective to influence public debate on these issues.

World Health Organization/ Regional Office for Europe—www.euro.who.int

This Web site provides information on a wide range of topics related to housing and health. It assesses recent evidence on housing conditions and health outcomes. Although it provides little with respect to public policies to address housing issues, particularly access to affordable housing, it promotes the development of local action plans to improve existing housing.

Part Five

Social Exclusion

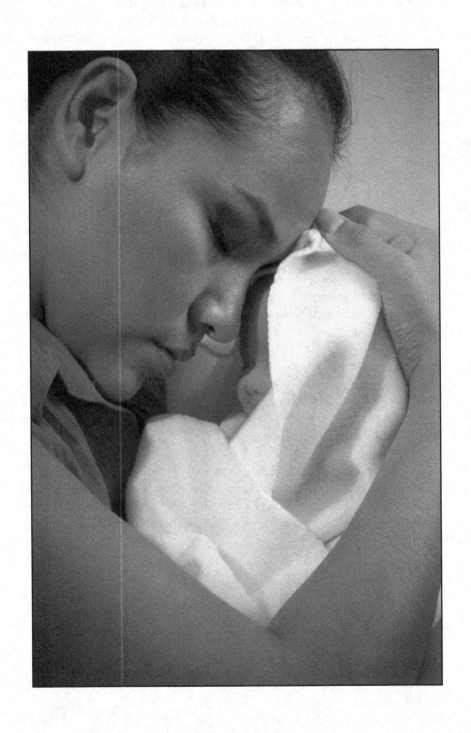

The issues raised in this volume—low income; unstable and poor-quality employment; low levels of education and literacy; and food and housing insecurity—are clearly linked to each other. They are linked in that members of a society experiencing one form of deprivation usually experience other forms of deprivation. The issues are also linked in that broad governmental policy directions tend to either produce higher-quality social determinants of health or situations in which their quality declines. In this section, the concept of social exclusion is explored as a means of understanding how this clustering comes about and why economic and social conditions in Canada appear to be under threat. Social exclusion is about the societal processes that systematically lead to groups being denied the opportunity to participate in commonly accepted activities of societal membership. It is an integrative concept that provides insights into how and why these groups experience material deprivation and how political, economic, and social conditions contribute to these conditions. In Canada, social exclusion is especially likely among Aboriginals, new Canadians, racialized groups, and women. The incidence of social exclusion has implications not only for the health of populations but also for the smooth functioning of societies. Increases in social exclusion threaten Canadian society and its institutions.

Grace-Edward Galabuzi provides an overview of social exclusion as both process and outcome. Social exclusion has four aspects: exclusion from (1) legal processes; (2) acquiring social goods; (3) social production; and (4) economic activities. He carefully outlines the components of social exclusion and the political, economic, and social forces that are driving this process in Canada. Social exclusion is a threat to individual, community, and population health, as well as to social cohesion and economic prosperity. The origins of social exclusion are primarily structural and complicated by racism and discrimination within Canadian society.

Galabuzi provides evidence of how social exclusion is especially prevalent among new Canadians and racialized groups, making them subject to all the types of material deprivation described in this volume.

Ronald Labonte reflects on how the concept of social exclusion, which is primarily focused on how society excludes people, has surfaced in Canada as an emphasis upon social inclusion. While few would dispute the need to include marginalized people from participation in Canadian life, a focus upon inclusion runs the risk of denying the sources of exclusion and placing blame for exclusion upon individuals. Labonte asks whether a society that has systematically excluded people can be expected to include those it has excluded. Social exclusion has material and economic underpinnings, and some benefit from exclusion: When racialized workers receive lower wages, employers reap rewards. Researchers, community workers, and policy-makers can use the concept of social inclusion to advantage, but should maintain a critical eye on the political, economic, and social forces that continue to promote exclusion in Canadian society.

Janet Smylie places Aboriginal health issues in the context of an Indigenous-specific and decolonizing perspective. She provides a demographic overview of Aboriginal peoples in Canada and provides a detailed history of how Aboriginal peoples' history and living circumstances have been shaped—usually not for the better—by various events and public policies. The health of Aboriginal peoples is described and these findings are placed within a social determinants of health framework. Existing health inequities between Aboriginal peoples and other Canadians can be explained by differences in living circumstances. The means by which the living situations of Aboriginal peoples can be improved, thereby reducing inequities in health, are detailed. Canada is seen as well placed to address these issues, but whether it chooses to do so remains uncertain.

Chapter 17

———●———

SOCIAL EXCLUSION

Grace-Edward Galabuzi

Perhaps health is not so much a personal matter but the aftertaste of a society's other activities, the residue of all its policies. (Fernando, 1991, p. 2)

Introduction

Poor social and economic conditions and inequalities in access to resources and services affect an individual or group's health and well-being. Groups experiencing some form of social exclusion tend to sustain higher health risks and lower health status. According to Health Canada, in Canada such groups include: Aboriginal peoples, immigrants and refugees, racialized groups, people with disabilities, single parents, children and youth in disadvantaged circumstances, women, the elderly and unpaid caregivers, gays, lesbians, bisexuals, and transgendered people (CIHR, 2002). Poverty is a key cause and product of social exclusion. Its impacts on health status are now well established (Wilkinson, 1996; Wilkinson & Marmot, 1998; Kawachi, Wilkinson & Kennedy, 1999; Raphael, 1999, 2001). Racial and gender differences in health status tend to reflect differences in social and economic conditions (Wilkinson, 1996). The "racialization of poverty" compounds inequalities in material conditions in socially excluded communities.[1] Such documented characteristics of racialized poverty as labour market segregation and low occupational status, high and frequent unemployment status,

substandard housing combined with violent or distressed neighbourhoods, homelessness, poor working conditions, extended hours of work or multiple jobs, and experience with everyday forms of racism and sexism lead to unequal health service utilization and differential health status. Recent research shows that the actual experience of inequality, the impact of relative deprivation, and the stress associated with dealing with social exclusion tend to have pronounced psychological effects and to impact health status negatively (Wilkinson, 1996; Kawachi & Kennedy, 2002).

Canadian and international research have begun to confirm the links between the minority status of ethnic, immigrant, and racialized groups and low health status (Adams, 1995; Anderson, 2000; Bolaria & Bolaria, 1994; Wilkinson, 1996; Hyman, 2001; Shaw et al., 1999; Wilkinson & Marmot, 1998). It is now generally agreed that adverse socio-economic conditions in early life lead to increased health risks in adulthood. According to Health Canada, children whose health status is most at risk tend to live in low-income families, single families, or among racialized group populations, including immigrant and refugee families and Aboriginal families (CIHR, 2002). Racialized community members, recent immigrants and refugees, women, men, and their children, experience the psychosocial stress of discrimination and racism, which contribute to such health problems as hypertension, mental health, and behavioural problems such as substance abuse. The particular vulnerability to compromised health is now documented even among recent immigrants, who have historically enjoyed higher health status because of the stringent health selection process, but research shows a loss of ground over time under conditions of social exclusion (Hyman, 2001; Noh et al., 1999; Fowler, 1998). Recent research also shows that the experience of racism and discrimination puts racialized group members and immigrants at higher risk for mental health problems (Beiser, 1988; Ontario Advisory Committee on Women's Issues, 1990; Dossa, 1999; Noh et al., 1999). Research in women's health suggests similar impacts from gender discrimination (Agnew, 2002; Adams, 1995). Canadian health research and the health system as a whole have not always appreciated the multiple influences on the health status of the affected groups imposed by these various dimensions of social exclusion. At a time when Canada's population growth and stability are increasingly dependent on immigration, with racialized group members now 13.5 percent of the population and growing (Statistics Canada, 2003), and immigrants now 18.4 percent and projected to account for 25 percent of the population by 2015, these issues are an important area of health policy and research.[2]

Social Exclusion

Social exclusion is used to broadly describe the structures and the dynamic processes of inequality among groups in society, which, over time, structure access to critical resources that determine the quality of membership in society and ultimately produce and reproduce unequal outcomes (Room, 1995; Byrne, 1999; Guildford, 2000; Shaw et al., 1999; Littlewood, 1999; Madanipour et al., 1998). Social exclusion is both process and outcome. While it has its roots in European social democratic discourse, it has been increasingly embraced by scholars in the liberal and neo-Marxist traditions, as well as by mainstream policy-makers concerned about the emergence of marginal subgroups who may pose a threat to social cohesion in industrial societies. In industrialized societies, social exclusion is a by-product of a form of unbridled accumulation whose processes commodify social relations and validate and intensify inequality along racial and gender lines (Byrne, 1999; Madanipour, 1998).

White (1998) has referred to four aspects of social exclusion. Social exclusion from civil society through

legal sanction or other institutional mechanisms is often experienced by status and non-status migrants. This conception may include substantive disconnection from civil society and political participation because of material and social isolation created through systemic forms of discrimination based on race, ethnicity, gender, disability, sexual orientation, and religion. In the post-September 11 era, racial profiling and new notions of national security seem to have exacerbated the experience of this form of social exclusion. Secondly, social exclusion refers to the failure to provide for the needs of particular groups—society's denial of (or exclusion from) social goods to particular groups such as accommodation for people with disabilities, income security, housing for the homeless, language services, and sanctions to deter discrimination. Thirdly, there is exclusion from social production, a denial of opportunity to contribute to or participate actively in society's social and cultural activities. And fourthly, there is economic exclusion from social consumption—unequal access to normal forms of livelihood and economy.

Social exclusion can be experienced by individuals and communities, communities of common bond, and geographical communities. The characteristics of social exclusion tend to occur in multiple dimensions and are often mutually reinforcing. Groups living in low-income areas are likely to also experience inequality in access to employment, substandard housing, insecurity, stigmatization, institutional breakdown, social service deficits, spatial isolation, disconnection from civil society, discrimination, and higher health risks. The resulting phenomenon is what some have referred to as one of an underclass culture (Wilson, 1987).

Social Exclusion in the Late 20th and Early 21st Century

Processes of social exclusion intensified in the late 20th century. The intensification of social exclusion can be traced to the restructuring of the global and national economies, which emphasized deregulation of markets; the decline of the welfare state; the commodification of public goods; demographic changes due to increased global migrations; changes in work arrangements toward flexible deployment and intensification of labour through longer hours; work fragmentation; multiple jobs; and increasing non-standard forms of work. These developments have intensified exploitation in workplaces, but also urban spatial segregation processes, including the gendered and racialized spatial concentrations of poverty, among others. The emergence of a neo-liberal globalized political economic order has redefined the nature of the state and redrawn the boundaries of citizenship as part of a process that institutionalizes market regulation of social relations in societies around the world (Jenson & Papillon, 2001; Gill, 1995). Under this neo-liberal order, the social exclusion framework represents a double critique of the commodification of public goods such as health care services, social services, education, and the like, brought about by the dismantling of the welfare state and the market-conditioned response to the resulting marginalization, which is euphemistically characterized simply as the individual's failure to utilize his or her opportunities in the marketplace (Yépez del Castillo, 1994). However, this atomization of social exclusion is contested. For instance, Yépez del Castillo has noted that:

> The many varieties of exclusion, the fears of social explosions to which it gives rise, the dangers of social disruption; the complexity of the mechanisms that cause it, the extreme difficulty of finding solutions, have made it the major social issue of our time. (Yepez del Castillo, 1994, p. 614)

In this policy environment, the social exclusion framework shifts the focus back to the structural inequalities that determine the intensity and extent of marginalization in society. It represents a shift of the burden of social inequality from the individual back to society, defining it as a social relation, and allows for the reassertion of welfare state-type social rights based on the concept of social protection as the responsibility of society and not the individual. It is in that respect that the policy discourse of social inclusion in response to marginalization has begun to emerge. Yet, a caution is warranted because there is not necessarily a linear relationship between social exclusion, which unravels the structures and processes of marginalization, and the more liberal conception of social inclusion, as presently constituted in policy discourse, which promises equal

opportunity for all without a commitment to dismantling the historical structures of exclusion (Saloojee, 2002).

Social Exclusion in the Canadian Context

In the Canadian context, social exclusion defines the inability of certain subgroups to participate fully in Canadian life due to structural inequalities in access to social, economic, political, and cultural resources arising out of the often intersecting experiences of oppression relating to race, class, gender, disability, sexual orientation, immigrant status, and the like. Along with the socio-economic and political inequalities, social exclusion is also characterized by processes of group or individual isolation within and from key Canadian societal institutions such as the school system, criminal justice system, health care system, as well as spatial isolation or neighbourhood segregation. These engender experiences of social and economic vulnerability, powerlessness, voicelessness, a lack of recognition and sense of belonging, limited options, diminished life chances, despair, opting out, suicidal tendencies, and, increasingly, community or neighbourhood violence. Aside from numerous health implications, the emergence of the institutional breakdown and normlessness characterized by resorting to the informal economy and community violence represents a threat to social cohesion and economic prosperity.

In Canada, the discourse on social exclusion has tended to focus on Canadians living on low incomes. Guildford's (2000) work on social exclusion and health in Canada is groundbreaking but limited because of the focus on the generic low-income experiences of social exclusion. Here, we suggest the need to interrogate the multiple dimensions of the phenomena as well as identify the subgroup dimension of the victims of social exclusion, precisely because of the extent to which their experiences are differentiated by the nature of the oppressions they suffer. This does not deter from identifying the points of convergence that can be the basis for solidarity and common struggles against marginalization. Social exclusion is an expression of unequal relations of power among groups in society, which then determine unequal access to economic, social, political, and cultural resources. The assertion of certain forms of economic, political, social, and cultural privilege, or the normalization of certain ethnocultural norms by some groups, occurs at the expense of and, ultimately, marginalization of others. This is especially true in a market-regulated society where the impetus for state intervention to reduce the reproduction of inequality is minimal as is increasingly the case under the neo-liberal regime. Social exclusion takes on a time and spatial dimension. In different societies, there are particular groups that are at higher risk of experiencing social exclusion depending on the historical social relations in the societies. In Canada, four groups have been identified as being in that category of special risk: (1) women; (2) new immigrants; (3) racialized group members; and (4) Aboriginal peoples (CIHR, 2002). The focus in this chapter is on the experiences of racialized group members and immigrants.

Social Exclusion, Racialized Groups, and Recent Immigrants

The name Chinatown continues to express the deeply embedded white desire for us to one day return from whence we came. (Pon, 2000, p. 230)

Canada welcomed an annual average of close to 200,000 new immigrants and refugees over the 1990s. Immigration accounted for more than 50 percent of the net population growth and 70 percent of the growth in

the labour force over the first half of the 1990s (1991–1996), and it is expected to account for virtually all of the net growth in the Canadian labour force by the year 2011 (Human Resources Development Canada, 2002). According to the 2001 Census, immigrants made up 18.4 percent of Canada's population, projected to rise to 25 percent by 2015. Since the shift from a European-centred immigration policy in the 1960s, there has been a significant change in the source countries, with over 75 percent of new immigrants in the 1980s and 1990s coming from the so-called Third World or global South, the majority of them falling in the category of racialized immigrants.[3]

Racialized groups and recent immigrants encounter processes of marginalization in many spheres of life. The racialization of poverty, in particular, represents two increasingly prevalent intersecting experiences of marginalization faced by Aboriginal peoples, and non-Aboriginal women and men from racialized (hereafter referred to as racialized peoples) and immigrant groups. Not only are these groups the subject of these processes of marginalization, they have received very limited treatment in the research on the social determinants of health. The preponderance of the experiences the chapter explores are those of the non-Aboriginal racialized populations whose experiences with racial and gender inequality, disproportionate low-income status, unemployment and underemployment, low occupation status, low-

Table 17.1: Selected ethnic groups in Canada, other than English, French, and Canadian, 2001

	Total population (in thousands)	As a proportion of the total Canadian population (%)
Chinese	1,094.7	3.7
South Asian	963.2	3.2
Caribbean	503.8	1.7
Arab	348.0	1.2
African	294.7	1.0
Filipino	327.6	1.1
Latin American	244.4	0.8
West Asian	205.0	0.7

Source: Statistics Canada. (2003). *2001 Census of Canada*. 2001 Census Analysis Series. The Changing Profile of Canada's Labour Force. Catalogue no. 96F0030XIE2001009, February 2003. Ottawa: Statistics Canada.

standard housing, intensified workplace exploitation, disproportionate residence in neighbourhoods with social deficits, etc., render them disproportionately vulnerable to low health status. The persistence of the racial and gender discriminatory structures, income and employment inequality, economic and social segregation, and political and cultural marginalization means that increasingly, a disproportionate number of racialized group members exist within a reality of social exclusion from the mainstream Canadian (Galabuzi, 2006).

Dimensions of Social Exclusion: The Racialization of Poverty

The racialized community is divided into Canadian-born members (roughly 33 percent) and immigrants (about 67 percent). During the last Census period (1996–2001), the growth rate of racialized groups far outpaced that of other Canadians. While the Canadian population grew by 3.9 percent between 1996 and 2001, the corresponding rate for racialized groups was 24.6 percent. Over the same period, the racialized component of the labour force grew for males (28.7 percent) and females (32.3 percent) compared to 5.5 percent and 9 percent respectively for the Canadian population. Over much of the 1990s, over 75 percent of Canada's newcomers were members of the racialized group communities, but with that shift has come a noticeable lag in social economic performance among members of the groups. These patterns seem to be holding both during and after the recession years of the late 1980s and early 1990s.

These developments have had numerous adverse social impacts, leading to differential life chances for racialized group members such as:

- a double-digit racialized income gap as high as 30 percent in 1998
- higher than average unemployment, with unemployment rates two to three times higher
- deepening levels of poverty
- differential access to housing leading to neighbourhood racial segregation
- disproportionate contact with the criminal justice system (criminalization of youth)
- higher health risks

A most significant development is the racialization of poverty, which is the emergence of structural features that predetermine the disproportionate incidence of poverty among racialized group members. What explains these trends are structural changes in the Canadian economy that conspire with historical forms of racial discrimination in the Canadian labour market to create a process of social and economic marginalization, which results in disproportionate vulnerability to poverty among racialized group communities. Racialized groups are also disproportionately immigrant communities and suffer from the impact of the immigration effect. However, current trends indicate that the economic inequality between immigrants and native-born Canadians is becoming greater and more permanent. That was not always the case. In fact, immigrants tended to outperform native-born Canadians because of their high educational levels and age advantage.

The racialization of poverty is directly linked to the deepening oppression and social exclusion of racialized and immigrant communities on the one hand and the entrenchment of privileged access to economic opportunity for a minority but powerful section of the majority population on the other. The concentration of economic, social, and political power that has emerged as the market has become more prominent in social regulation in Canada explains the growing gap between rich and poor as well as the racialization of that gap (Yalnizyan, 1998, 2007; Kunz et al., 2001; Galabuzi, 2001, 2006; Dibbs & Leesti, 1995; Jackson, 2001). Racialized community members and Aboriginal peoples are twice as likely to be poor than other Canadians because of the intensified social and economic exploitation of the racialized and Aboriginal communities whose members have to endure historical racial and gender inequalities accentuated by the restructuring of the Canadian economy and, more recently, racial profiling. In the midst of the resulting socio-economic crisis, the different levels of government have responded by retreating from anti-racism programs and policies that would have removed the barriers to economic equity. The resulting powerlessness and loss of voice have compounded the groups' inability to put issues of social inequality, particularly the racialization of poverty, on the political agenda.

Racialized Group Members Are Twice as Likely as Other Canadians to Live in Poverty

National and Census metropolitan area data now show that racialized people are two or three times more likely to be poor than other Canadians.[4] The rates are even higher among recent immigrants and some select groups such as youth, women, and seniors of Arabs, Latin Americans, Somalis, Haitians, Iranians, Tamils, East Indians, and Vietnamese origin. The levels of poverty are especially high among some racialized groups of women, youth, and seniors. While the Canadian low-income rate was 14.7 percent in 2001, low-income rates for racialized groups ranged from 16 percent to as high as 43 percent.[5]

It is, however, instructive to survey a select group of racialized communities to better establish the claim that poverty is being racialized.[6]

Some of the highest increases in low-income rates in Canada have occurred among recent immigrants. During the past two decades, as the sources of immigration shifted toward countries in the global South and a preponderance of racialized immigrants (around 75 percent), low-income rates among successive groups of immigrants almost doubled between 1980 and 1995, peaking at 47 percent before easing up in the late 1990s. In 1980, 24.6 percent of immigrants who had arrived during the previous five-year period were below the poverty line. By 1990, the low-income rate among recent immigrants had increased to 31.3 percent. After peaking at 47.0 percent in 1995, the rate fell back to 35.8 percent in 2000.[7]

This was happening at a time when average poverty rates have been generally falling in the Canadian population. Studies show that former waves of immigrants were subject to a short-term "immigration factor," which, over time (not longer than 10 years for the unskilled and as low as two years for the skilled), they were able to overcome and either catch up to their Canadian-born counterparts or even surpass them in their performance in the economy. Their employment participation rates were as high or higher than the Canadian-born, and their wages and salaries rose gradually to the level of the Canadian-born.

Recent research indicates persistent and growing difficulties in the labour market integration of immigrants,

Table 17.2: Low income by select racialized community, 2000

	Adult	Adult unattached	Children under 15
Total Canadian population	15%	38%	18%
African community	39%	56%	47%
Arab community	36%	52%	40%
Caribbean community	26%	44%	33%
Chinese community	26%	55%	27%
Filipino community	16%	48%	18%
Jamaican community	26%	41%	34%
Haitian community	39%	61%	47%
Japanese community	18%	48%	16%
Korean community	43%	72%	48%
Latin American community	28%	53%	32%
South Asian community	23%	49%	28%
Vietnamese community	27%	49%	35%
West Asian community	37%	56%	43%

Source: Statistics Canada. (2003). *2001 Census of Canada*. 2001 Census Analysis Series. The Changing Profile of Canada's Labour Force. Catalogue no. 96F0030XIE2001009, February 2003. Ottawa: Statistics Canada.

especially recent immigrants. Rates of unemployment and underemployment are increasing for individual immigrants, as are rates of poverty for immigrant families (Galabuzi, 2006; Ornstein, 2000; Pendakur, 2000; Reitz, 1988, 2001; Shields, 2002). So the traditional trajectory that saw immigrants catch up with other Canadians over time seems to have been reversed in the case of racialized immigrants. Of course the irony is that over that period of time, the level of education, usually an indicator of economic success, has been growing. A survey of the annual incomes of a select number of the groups shows these effects[8].

As Table 17.3 shows, most racialized group members experience significant income inequality in all categories, in some cases up to over $10,000. There is also a significant gender inequality both within the groups and in comparison with the average Canadian levels. These inequalities also occur when you consider the incomes of unattached earners and earners over 65 years of age.[9] A related phenomenon is the inequality in access to and retention of employment both full-time and part-time, shown below in Table 17.4 and Table 17.5.

Recent Statistics Canada analysis also show that male recent immigrants' full-time employment earnings fell 7 percent between 1980 and 2000 (Picot & Hou, 2003). This compares with a rise of 7 percent for the Canadian-born cohort. Among the university-educated, the drop was deeper (13 percent). For female recent immigrants, full-time employment earnings rose, but by less than other female full-time workers. More alarming are the low-income implications of these trends. While low-income rates among recent immigrants with less than high school graduation increased by 24 percent from 1980–2000, low-income rates increased by 50 percent among high school graduates and a whopping 66 percent among university-educated immigrants!

Recent immigrants' rates of employment declined markedly between 1986 and 1996. The result is that Canada's immigrants exhibit a higher incidence of poverty and greater dependence on social assistance than their predecessors even though the percentage of university graduates among them is higher in all categories of immigrants, including family class and refugees, as well as economic immigrants, than it is for

Table 17.3: Average income (all sources) by select racialized community, 2001

	Men	Women	Total dollars
All Canadian earners	36,800	22,885	29,769
African community	27,864	19,639	23,787
Arab community	32,336	19,264	26,519
Caribbean community	29,840	22,842	25,959
Chinese community	29,322	20,974	25,018
Filipino community	27,612	22,532	24,563
Jamaican community	30,087	23,575	26,412
Haitian community	21,595	18,338	19,782
Japanese community	43,644	24,556	33,178
Korean community	23,370	16,919	20,065
Latin American community	27,257	17,930	22,463
South Asian community	31,396	19,511	25,629
Vietnamese community	27,849	18,560	23,190
West Asian community	28,719	18,014	23,841

Source: Statistics Canada. (2003). *2001 Census of Canada*. 2001 Census Analysis Series. The Changing Profile of Canada's Labour Force. Catalogue no. 96F0030XIE2001009, February 2003. Ottawa: Statistics Canada.

Table 17.4: Unequal access to full employment: Unemployment rates (%)

	1981	1991	2001
Total labour force	5.9	9.6	6.7
Canadian-born	6.3	9.4	6.4
All immigrants	4.5	10.4	7.9
Recent immigrants	6.0	15.6	12.1

Source: Statistics Canada. (2003). *2001 Census Analysis Series*. The Changing Profile of Canada's Labour Force. Catalogue no. 96F0030XIE2001009, February 2003. Ottawa: Statistics Canada.

Table 17.5: Labour force participation (%)

	1981	1991	2001
Total labour force	75.5	78.2	80.3
Canadian-born	74.6	78.7	81.8
All immigrants	79.3	77.2	75.6
Recent immigrants	75.7	68.6	65.8

Source: Statistics Canada. (2003). *2001 Census Analysis Series*. The Changing Profile of Canada's Labour Force. Catalogue no. 96F0030XIE2001009, February 2003. Ottawa: Statistics Canada.

the Canadian-born (Citizenship and Immigration Canada, 2002).

The Ornstein Report (2000) revealed that high poverty rates are concentrated among certain groups—such as Latin American, Africans Blacks and Caribbeans, and Arabs and West Asians—with rates at 40 percent and higher in 1996, or roughly three times the Toronto rate. This research is confirmed by accounts in the popular press, which reveal a dramatic increase in the use of food banks by highly educated newcomers (Quinn, 2002).

A significant factor in these trends is the underutilization of immigrant skills within the Canadian labour market. Reitz (2001) has looked at the quantitative significance of this issue using a human-capital earnings analysis that identified immigrant earnings deficits as arising from three possible sources: (1) lower immigrant skill quality; (2) underutilization of immigrant skills; or (3) pay inequities for immigrants doing the same work as native-born Canadians. He concluded that in 1996 dollars, the total annual immigrant earnings deficit from all three sources in Canada was $15.0 billion, of which

$2.4 billion was related to skill underutilization, and $12.6 billion was related to pay inequity. He observed as well that employers give little credit to foreign education and none to foreign work experience; that discrimination specific to country of origin or visible minority status is mainly related to pay equity rather than skills utilization; and that the economic impact of visible minority status and immigrant status is very similar for both men and women. In addition, Reitz noted that race appears to be a more reliable predictor of how foreign education will be evaluated in Canada than the specific location of the origin of the immigrant from outside Europe.

Economic Exclusion in the Labour Market

The third category of the relative surplus population, the stagnant, forms a part of the active labour army, but with extremely irregular employment, hence it furnishes to capital an inexhaustible reservoir of disposable labour-power. Its conditions of life sink below that of the average normal level of the working class. This makes it at once the broad basis of the special branches of capitalist exploitation. It is characterized by a maximum of working hours, and a minimum of wages.... But it forms at the same time a self-reproducing and self-perpetuating element of the working class, taking a proportionally greater part in the general increase of that class than the other elements (Marx, 1977).

The neo-liberal restructuring of Canada's economy and labour market toward flexible labour markets has increasingly stratified labour markets along racial lines, with the disproportionate representation of racialized group members in low-income sectors and low-end occupations, and underrepresentation in high-income sectors and occupations. These patterns emerge out of a context of racial inequality in access to work and in employment income, and from the growing predominance of precarious forms of work in many of the sectors that racialized group members are disproportionately represented in and point to racially unequal incidence of low income and racially defined neighbourhood segregation. These broader processes explain the emergence of the racialization of poverty whose dimensions can primarily be identified by disproportionate levels of low income and racialized spatial concentration of poverty in key neighbourhoods.

Economic social exclusion takes the form of labour market segregation, unequal access to employment, employment discrimination, disproportionate vulnerability to unemployment, and underemployment. These are both characteristics and causes of social exclusion. Attachment to the labour market is essential for both livelihood and the production of identity in society. It determines the ability to meet material needs and also provides a sense of belonging, dignity, and self-esteem, all of which have implications for health status. Labour market-related social exclusion has direct implications for health status not just because of the impact on income inequality, but also because of the extent to which working conditions, mobility in workplaces, fairness in the distribution of opportunities, and utilization of acquired skills all have a direct bearing on the levels of stress that are generated in workplaces.

The Canadian economy and labour market are increasingly stratified along racial lines, as evidenced by the disproportionate representation of racialized group members in low-income sectors and low-end occupations, and underrepresentation in high-income sectors and occupations. These patterns emerge out of a context of neo-liberal restructuring of the economy conditioned by global competition and demands for flexible deployment of labour, persistent racial inequality in access to employment, and the growing predominance of precarious forms of work in which many of the sectors racialized group members are disproportionately represented. Labour market research shows this racial stratification is observable in the disproportionate participation of racialized groups in industries increasingly dominated by non-standard forms of work such as textiles, clothing, hospitality, retailing, and an overrepresentation of racialized group members in low-income jobs and low-end occupations. On the other hand, they are underrepresented in such high-income sectors as the public service, automobile making, and metal working, which also happen to be highly unionized.

Not only has economic restructuring polarized the labour market, it has created new forms of work and employment structures that have altered the traditional workplace relationships and exacerbated the vulnerability of racialized communities. The demands for labour market flexibility in the urban globalized economy have disproportionately exposed racialized groups to types of employment that leave them poorer than other Canadians. As a historically vulnerable group in the labour market, these changes exacerbate the impact of racial discrimination in employment.

The fastest-growing form of work in Canada is precarious work, also referred to as contingent work or non-standard work: contract, temporary, part-time, and shift work with no job security, poor and often unsafe working conditions, intensive labour, excessive hours, low wages, and no benefits. In the early 1990s, it grew by 58 percent, compared to 18 percent for full-time employment (Vosko, 2000; de Wolff, 2000). Racialized workers are disproportionately represented in this form of work as a consequence of their vulnerability to the restructuring in the economy (Galabuzi, 2001).

Most of this work is low-skilled and low-paying, and the working conditions are often unsafe. Such non-regulated service occupations as newspaper carriers, pizza deliverers, janitors and cleaners, dishwashers, and parking lot attendants are dominated by racialized group members and recent immigrants who work in conditions with little or no protection in conditions similar to low-end work in the hospitality and health care sectors, light-manufacturing assembly plants, textile and home-based garment work. Many employees are self-employed or subcontracted on exploitative contracts by temporary employment agencies, with some assigning work based on racist stereotypes.

Racialized women are particularly overrepresented in another form of self-employment—unregulated piecemeal homework. Gendered racism and neo-liberal restructuring have conditioned the emergence of what some have called Canada's sweatshops, especially in the garment and clothing industry (Yanz et al., 1999; Vosko, 2000). The intensity of the experience of exploitation imposes pressure, especially on racialized and immigrant women, who continue to carry a disproportionate bulk of housework, to go with the subcontract wage work. Many of them are single parents.

Because of the intensified exploitation characterized by demands for longer working hours and low pay and/ or multiple part-time jobs, the intensity of work under a deregulated labour market becomes a major source of stress and related health conditions. In the case of immigrants and racialized group members, the failure to convert their educational attainment and experience, whether internationally or domestically acquired, due to the structures of racial, gender inequality, or barriers in employment relating to immigrant status has been identified increasingly as a major stress generator.

Social Exclusion and Racialized Neighbourhood Selection

Space is a key function of social exclusion.
   The fact that people live in certain places can either sustain or intensify social exclusion. (Hutchinson, 2000, p. 167)

The racialization of poverty has also had a major impact on neighbourhood selection and access to adequate housing for new immigrants and racialized groups. In Canada's urban centres, the spatial concentration of poverty or residential segregation is intensifying along racial lines. Immigrants in Toronto and Montreal are more likely than non-immigrants to live in neighbourhoods with high rates of poverty, as Table 17.6 shows. Social exclusion is increasingly manifest in urban centres where racialized groups are concentrated in racial enclaves and racially segregated neighbourhoods. In what is becoming a segregated housing market, racialized groups are relegated to substandard, marginal, and often overpriced housing. These growing neighbourhood inequalities act as social determinants of health and well-being, with limited access to social services, increased contact with the criminal justice system, social disintegration, and violence engendering higher health risks.

Globalization-generated pressures have led to the state's retreat from its social obligations, leading to social deficits that impact racialized communities disproportionately. The state's diminishing commitment toward income redistribution and income supports, social services, and adequate funding for health care and education is juxtaposed to racial inequality in access to work and in employment income; the racially unequal incidence of low income; the shift toward flexible labour deployment and precarious forms of work in the urban economies, and the marked increase in South–North immigration to create isolated, racially defined, low-income neighbourhoods vulnerable to disintegration of social institutions and anti-social outcomes such as violence.

Recent studies by Hou and Balakrishnan (1996), Kazemipur and Halli (2000), Fong (2000), and Ley and Smith (1997) suggest that these areas show characteristics of ghettoization or spatial concentration of poverty, signs of concentration in urban cores, and limited exposure to majority communities. Increasingly these geographical areas represent racialized enclaves subject to the distresses of low-income communities.

A racialized spatial concentration of poverty means that racialized group members live in neighbourhoods that are heavily concentrated and "hypersegregated" from the rest of society and often with disintegrating institutions. Increasingly they deal with social deficits such as inadequate access to counselling services, life-skills training, child care, recreation, and health care

Table 17.6: Toronto area racialized enclaves and experience of high poverty rates

	Poverty rates			
	University degree	Unemployment	Low income	Single parent
Chinese	21.2%	11.2%	28.4%	11.7%
South Asian	11.8%	13.1%	28.3%	17.6%
Black	8.7%	18.3%	48.5%	33.7%

Source: Statistics Canada. (2003). *2001 Census Analysis Series.* The Changing Profile of Canada's Labour Force. Catalogue No. 96F0030XIE2001009, February 2003. Ottawa: Statistics Canada.

services (Kazemipur & Halli, 1997, 2000; Lo & Wang, 2000).

Young immigrants living in low-income areas often struggle with alienation from their parents and community of origin, and from the broader society. The social services that they need to cope with dislocation are lacking; the housing is often substandard or, if it is public housing, it is largely poorly maintained because of cutbacks; and they face unemployment, despair, and violence. They are disproportionate targets of contact with the criminal justice system.

Finally, a word about homelessness and recent immigrant and racialized groups. Homelessness is said to be proliferating among racialized group members because of the incidence of low income and the housing crises in many urban areas (Lee, 2000; Peel Region, 2000). Homelessness is an extreme form of social exclusion that suggests a complexity of causes and factors. Increasingly, recent immigrants and racialized people are more likely to be homeless in Canada's urban centres than they were 10 years ago. It compounds other sources of stresses in their lives. Homelessness has been associated with early mortality, health factors such as substance abuse, mental illness, infectious diseases, and difficulty in accessing health services. The complex interactions among these factors, homelessness, and access to health services have not received enough study and represent a key gap in the anti-racism and social determinants of health discourses.

Racialization, Social Exclusion, and Health

The importance of power relations, social identity, social status, and control over life circumstances for health status follows from the evidence upon which the population health perspective is based. This evidence can be usefully grouped into three broad categories: social inequalities in health within and between societies; social support and health; and workplace characteristics and health. (Dunn & Dyck, 1998, p. 2)

If today's immigrants have higher rates of illness than the native-born, the increased risk probably results from an interaction between personal vulnerability and resettlement stress, as well as lack of services, rather than from diseases they bring with them to Canada. (Health Canada, 1998)

There is no doubt that universal access to health care is now a core Canadian value, espoused broadly by all segments of the political elite as defining Canadian society. But beyond the policy articulation of universality of coverage, other determinants such as income, gender, race, immigrant status, and geography increasingly define the translation of the concept of universality as unequally differentiated. A review of the limited available literature indicates that the processes of social exclusion we have discussed above affect the health status of racialized and recent immigrant communities. The extent of exclusion is expressed through the gap between that promise and the reality of unequal access to health service utilization, or inequalities in health status arising out of the inequalities in the social determinants of health. It is the gap between the promise of citizenship and the reality of exclusion that represents the extent of social exclusion and the unequal impact on the well-being of members of racialized groups and immigrants in Canada. While there is limited empirical research to draw on, there is significant anecdotal evidence to make the case.

It follows, though, that given the landscape of exclusion we have painted above, a perspective based on a synthesis of a diverse public health and social scientific literature, the most important antecedents of human health status are not medical care inputs and health behaviours (smoking, diet, exercise, etc.), but rather social and economic characteristics of individuals and populations. This would suggest significant convergence between social exclusion and health status (Evans et al., 1994; Frank, 1995; Hayes & Dunn, 1998). For racialized groups and recent immigrants, power relations, identity and status issues, and life chances are influential on the processes of immigration and integration (Dunn & Dyck, 1998).

However, one of the more significant studies of immigrants and health by Dunn and Dyck (1998), using the social determinants of health approach and based on a review of National Population Health Survey data perspective, found no obvious, consistent pattern of association between socio-economic characteristics and immigration characteristics on the one hand, and health status on the other (Dunn & Dyck, 1998). Hyman (2001) has observed that neither did it find evidence to the contrary.

Racialization and Health Status

It is now generally agreed that racism is a primary source of stress and hypertension in racialized group communities. Everyday forms of racism, often compounded by sexism and xenophobia, and the related conditions of underemployment; non-recognition of prior accreditation; low-standard housing; residence in low-income neighbourhoods with significant social deficits; violence against women and other forms of domestic and neighbourhood violence; targeted policing and disproportionate criminalization and incarceration all define an existence of those on the margins of society, an existence of social exclusion from the full participation in the social, economic, cultural, and political affairs of Canadian society. They are also important socio-economic and psychosocial determinants of health. While empirical research is underdeveloped, there is significant

qualitative evidence—collected from group members, service providers, and some qualitative community-based research—to suggest that these act as determinants of the health status for socially marginalized groups such as racialized women, youth, and men; immigrants; and Aboriginal peoples (Agnew, 2002; Tharoa & Massaquoi, 2001). These conditions contribute to and mediate the experience of inequality into powerlessness, hopelessness, and despair, contributing to the emotional and physical health of the members of the groups. These conditions, in turn, negatively impact attempts by affected individuals, groups, and communities to achieve full citizenship because of their inability to claim social and political rights enjoyed by other Canadians, including the right to physical and mental well-being of residents (Government of Canada, 1984).

While there is limited literature in the Canadian context, research done internationally shows the connection between race and health more clearly. Research in the United States shows the connection between racism and health status (Randall, 1993). Wilkinson has investigated the processes of racialization, which result in the social and economic marginalization of certain social groups and has shown that "racial" differences in health status can largely be accounted for by differences in individuals' social and economic circumstances (Wilkinson, 1996; Anderson, 1987, 1991).

Institutionalized racism in the health care system—characterized by language barriers, lack of cultural sensitivity, absence of cultural competencies, barriers to access to health service utilization, and inadequate funding for community health services—has been identified as impacting the health status of racialized group members. Mainstream health care institutions are Eurocentric, imposing European and White cultural norms as standard and universal and, by extension, their cultural hegemony imposes a burden on racialized and immigrant communities. Insights from the critical race discourses help us understand that the cumulative burden of the subtle, ordinary but persistent everyday forms of racism, compounded by experiences of marginalization, also determine health status. The psychological pressures of daily resisting these and other forms of oppression add up to a complex of factors that undermine the health status of racialized and immigrant group members. They are compounded by low occupation status, low housing and neighbourhood status, high unemployment, and high levels of poverty. Health practitioners' racist stereotypes also tend to impact health status.

Social Exclusion and HIV/AIDS

> I have to worry about feeding, clothing, and housing my children. I don't have time to think about AIDS. (African-Canadian woman in Toronto study)

> A study of African-Canadian women and HIV/ AIDS, done by Women's Health in Women's Hands, respondents said that racist experiences with the health care system was one of the reasons African-Canadian women reported a reluctance to access the health care system for services like HIV/AIDS treatment, education, and care. (Tharoa & Massaquoi, 2001)

Reports on HIV/AIDS and racialized groups suggest that discrimination against people with HIV/AIDS is compounded by their racial status. A study by the Alliance for South Asian AIDS Prevention (Alliance for South Asian AIDS Prevention, 1999) found that the cultural, religious, language, and racial barriers the communities face in accessing health care services led to differential impacts in treatment between the South Asian communities and people from the majority community living with HIV/AIDS. While they had to deal with the cultural stigma imposed on those living with HIV/AIDS in the community, they were also vulnerable to racism and marginalization, which led to withdrawal and silencing and higher health risks.

Many racialized group members and immigrants with mental health issues and mental illnesses identify racism as a critical issue in their lives. The low-income, racialized group community members surveyed said that the magnitude of the association between racism and poverty and mental health status was similar to other commonly studied stressful life events such as the death of a loved one, divorce, or job loss (Across Boundaries, 1999).

Racism is a stress generator as is family separation through immigration, the intensification of work,

devaluation of one's value and worth through decredentialism, and the experience of inequality and injustice. Stress, in turn, is a major cause of a variety of health problems. It has been observed that one of the reasons the health status of immigrants declines is because of the experiences of discrimination and racism (Hyman, 2001). State-imposed barriers to family reunification through immigration policies that discourage reunification in favour of independent-class immigration lead to extended periods of family separation. Family separation and failure to effect reunification rob family members of their support network, and also engenders separation anxiety, thoughts of suicide, lack of sufficient support mechanisms, and even death.

Racism and discrimination based on immigrant status intensify marginalization and social exclusion, compounding poverty and its impacts on mental health status. The everyday hurts that arise from put-downs and diminishing self-esteem tend to undermine the mental health of racialized group members.

The stigma of mental illness often bars members from seeking treatment as some are afraid that that status would compound their marginalization. The Canadian Task Force on Mental Health Issues Affecting Immigrants identified a mental health gap between immigrants and the Canadian-born population based on the socio-economic status of immigrants. Concluding that the socio-economic status of immigrants was a determinant of mental health, it called for increased access to mental health services for immigrants, and more appropriate culturally sensitive and language-specific services to help close the gap (Beiser, 1988).

The serious gap in the research on the mental health of immigrants can benefit greatly from using a framework that recognizes the impact of racism and immigrant status on the process of social exclusion and social determination of health. Beiser et al. (1993) identify the persistence of the gap in health care utilization between immigrants and native-born Canadians, its impact on the mental health status of immigrants, and the need for research to better understand the phenomenon.

The Discrimination-Depression Relationship

Noh et al.'s study on the perceived racial discrimination, depression, and coping of Southeast Asian refugees in Canada found that the refugees who reported experiencing discrimination experienced higher depression levels than their counterparts who reported none.

The findings confirm the impact of discrimination on health status, but also suggest that forms of societal identification help reverse the process and impact of social exclusion.

Perceived racial discrimination is defined as a minority group's subjective perception of unfair treatment based on racial prejudice. The focus on the perceived nature of discrimination is to accommodate the reality of the subtle and elusive nature of certain forms of racism in the Canadian context (Noh et al., 1999).

Skill Deployment: Internationally Trained

Many skilled immigrants are experiencing mounting barriers to making full use of their skills and talents in both the economic sphere and in public life. Increasingly they are dealing with frustration at the barriers they face. Such a strong sense of inequality and injustice has implications for their mental health (Beiser, 1988). Moreover, as Anderson et al.'s (1993) study on chronic illness shows, for immigrant women living on meagre incomes and sustaining a marginal status in the labour market, the daily struggles of their meagre existence and their desire to hold onto their low-paying jobs tend to take precedence over disclosing chronic illness to ensure its active management with the support of health professionals. Along with such livelihood considerations, they often face the daunting prospect of navigating the mainstream health care system, with its barriers to access, lack of culturally appropriate services, and health care professionals' inability to understand the choices that those living in poverty and at the margins have to make to survive.

Research shows that immigrant youth sometimes find the stresses of integration on top of the challenges of adolescence overwhelming. Their feelings of isolation and alienation are linked to perceptions of cultural differences and experiences of discrimination and racism. While these are often complicated by intergenerational issues, support from friends, family, and institutions is key to overcoming the challenges. In essence, it presents them with a recreated community in response to the exclusion they face in mainstream institutions like the school system (Kilbride et al., 2000).

Conclusion: The Dearth of Research on Health and Race

I have suggested that social exclusion describes both the structures and the dynamic processes of inequality among groups in society, which, over time, structure access to critical resources that determine the quality of membership in society and ultimately produce and reproduce a complex of unequal outcomes. Social exclusion speaks both to the process of becoming and to the outcome of being socially excluded. It has received the attention of policy-makers concerned about the impact of marginal subgroups on social cohesion, and has provided them with the social inclusion framework for responding to this phenomenon. However, its use in health policy and health research is limited, although the social determinant of health approach seems to share its philosophical orientation. Its potential is especially suggestive when dealing with the complexity of issues faced by racialized and immigrant communities and their impact on health status, an area where there is limited research.

Racialized and immigrant groups are disproportionately impacted by labour market segregation, unemployment and income inequality, poverty, and poor neighbourhood selection. These differential experiences translate into health disparities and disproportionate exposure to such conditions as hypertension and diabetes for these groups. The daily experiences of discrimination based on race, gender, and immigrant status have their impact in terms of psychological pressures, which lead to a complex of factors that undermine the health status of racialized and immigrant group members. In many cases, these groups, exposed to precarious employment, are forced to take work in hazardous working conditions. It is therefore imperative that we consider racism as a social determinant of health and research the extent of its impact. This requires a shift in focus from generic notions of poverty as both generic and quantitatively based low income to understanding the differentiated, qualitative complexity of poverty and its varied impacts on the health of diverse populations within Canada. These complexities and adverse impacts of marginalization on population health can be captured through the social exclusion approach. This chapter suggests that a multidimensional approach using social exclusion as a framework to understanding the multiplicity of non-behavioural influences on health status provides a more adequate basis for assessing the health status of not just racialized and immigrant communities but other socially excluded groups such as women, people with disabilities, gays and lesbians, bisexual and transgendered, and even the "generic" poor.

Notes

1. The racialization of poverty here refers to the disproportionate and persistent incidence of low income among racialized groups in Canada.

2. There has been a significant change in the source countries, with over 75 percent of new immigrants in the 1980s and 1990s coming from the global South. Most immigrants end up in urban centres—75 percent in Toronto, Vancouver, and Montreal.

3. The term "racialized group" acknowledges the social construction of racial categories imposed on certain groups on the basis of superficial attributes like skin colour and the subsequent differential treatment endured by the identified groups. These categories carry official recognition and for the purpose of data collection at the federal level, the term "visible minority" approximates the category here termed "racialized group" and continues to be used both by Statistics Canada and in the federal employment-equity program.

4. F. Hou and G. Picot, *Visible minority neighbourhood enclaves and labour market outcomes of immigrants* (Ottawa: Statistics Canada, 2003), Research Paper Series, Catalogue no. 11F0019M1E—no. 204); K. Lee, *Urban poverty in Canada: A statistical profile* (Ottawa: Canadian Council on Social Development, 2000); M. Ornstein, *Ethno-racial inequality in the City of Toronto: An analysis of the 1996 Census* (Toronto: City of Toronto, 2000); A. Kazemipur and S. Halli, *The new poverty in Canada: Ethnic groups and ghetto neighbourhoods* (Toronto: Thompson Educational Publishing, 2000); D. Fleury, *A study of poverty and working poverty among recent immigrants to Canada* (Ottawa: Statistics Canada, 2007); G. Picot and F. Hou, *The rise in low-income rates among immigrants in Canada* (Ottawa: Statistics Canada, 2003), Analytical Studies Branch Research Paper Series, Catalogue no. 11F0019MIE#198; G. Picot, F. Hou, and S. Coulombe, *Chronic low income and low income dynamics among recent immigrants* (Ottawa: Statistics Canada, 2007), Analytical Studies Branch Research Paper Series, Catalogue no. 11F0019MIE#294.

5. C. Lindsay, *Profiles of ethnic communities in Canada* (Ottawa: Statistics Canada, 2007), Catalogue no. 89-621-XIE. Data is drawn from the 2001 Census and the 2002 *Ethnic Diversity Survey*.

6. Ibid.

7. G. Picot and F. Hou, *The rise in low income rates among immigrants in Canada* (Ottawa: Statistics Canada, 2003), Analytical Studies Branch Research Paper Series, Catalogue no. 11F0019MIE#198; G. Picot, F. Hou, and S. Coulombe, *Chronic low income and low income dynamics among recent immigrants* (Ottawa: Statistics Canada, 2007), Analytical Studies Branch Research Paper Series, Catalogue no. 11F0019MIE#294; M. Frenette and R. Morissette, *Will they ever converge? Earnings of immigrants and Canadian-born workers over the last two decades* (Ottawa: Statistics Canada, 2003), Analytical Studies Paper no. 215.

8. See C. Lindsay, *Profiles of ethnic communities in Canada* (Ottawa: Statistics Canada, 2007, Catalogue no. 89-621-XIE. Data is drawn from the 2001 Census and the 2002 *Ethnic Diversity Survey*.

9. Canadians of Japanese origin are the one racialized group with generally higher incomes than the rest of the population. In 2000, the average income from all sources for Canadians of Japanese origin aged 15 and over was just over $33,000, over $3,000 per person more than the national figure.

Critical Thinking Questions

1. What are the various components of social exclusion and how do people experience them?
2. Do you think social exclusion is increasing in Canada? On what basis do you believe this?
3. Why are people of colour especially susceptible to experiencing social exclusion?
4. How does social exclusion lead to poor health?
5. How can social exclusion be reduced?
6. What are the consequences for Canada of not addressing social exclusion?

Recommended Readings

Galabuzi, G. (2006). *Canada's economic apartheid: The social exclusion of racialized groups in the new century.* Toronto: Canadian Scholars' Press Inc.

This book calls attention to the growing racialization of the gap between the rich and poor, which is proceeding with minimal public and policy attention despite the dire implications for Canadian society. It challenges some common myths about the economic performance of Canada's racialized communities, and shows how historical patterns of differential treatment and occupational segregation in the labour market, and discriminatory governmental and institutional policies and practices, have led to the reproduction of racial inequality in other areas of Canadian life.

Guildford, J. (2000). *Making the case for economic and social inclusion.* Ottawa: Health Canada.

Groundbreaking work in Canada that brought the concept of social exclusion to Canada.

Omidvar, R. & Richmond, T. (2003). *Immigrant settlement and social inclusion in Canada.* Toronto: Laidlaw Foundation. Online at www.laidlawfdn.org/programmes/children/richmond.pdf.

This report is part of the Laidlaw Foundation Initiative on Social Inclusion.

Ornstein, M. (2002). *Ethno-racial inequality in Toronto: Analysis of the 1996 census.* Toronto: Institute for Social Research. Online at ceris.metropolis.net/Virtual%20Library/Demographics/ornstein1.pdf

A careful analysis of the growing gap in income among people of different races in Toronto, Canada's largest city.

Percy-Smith, J. (Ed.). (2000). *Policy responses to social exclusion: Towards inclusion?* Buckingham, UK: Open University Press.

A definitive UK analysis of social exclusion, its processes, and causes. It contains numerous chapters concerned with presenting possible policy solutions to this emerging problem.

Related Web Sites

Centre for Analysis of Social Exclusion (CASE)—sticerd.lse.ac.uk/case/

CASE is an ESRC Research Centre, core-funded by the Economic and Social Research Council since October 1997. CASE is a multidisciplinary research centre located within the Suntory and Toyota International Centres for Economic and Related Disciplines at the London School of Economics and Political Science.

Laidlaw Foundation—www.laidlawfdn.org

Building inclusive cities and communities is the new focus of the Children's Agenda Program of the Laidlaw Foundation. The foundation has commissioned 12 working papers that have contributed to understanding social inclusion and pointed to the importance of cities and communities as places where inclusion and exclusion are first experienced by children and families.

Social and Economic Inclusion in Atlantic Canada—www.acewh.dal.ca/inclusion-preface.htm

The Inclusion Project is a partnership project facilitated by the Maritime Centre of Excellence for Women's Health (MCEWH) and funded by the Population and Public Health Branch of Health Canada, Atlantic Region Office. The project considers the problem of poverty and the shift in thinking away from a concentration of child poverty and toward an analysis of social and economic exclusion of women and their children.

Social Exclusion Unit—www.socialexclusionunit.gov.uk

Social exclusion is a shorthand term for what can happen when people or areas suffer from a combination of linked problems such as unemployment, poor skills, low incomes, poor housing, high crime environments, bad health, and family breakdown. The Social Exclusion Unit was set up by the UK prime minister to help improve government action to reduce social exclusion by producing "joined-up solutions to joined-up problems." It provides an example of how a government is defining the problem and attempting to resolve it.

Townsend Centre for International Poverty Research—www.bris.ac.uk/poverty/

The centre was launched on July 1, 1999 at the University of Bristol. It is dedicated to multidisciplinary research on poverty in both the industrialized and developing world.

Chapter 18

———————●———————

SOCIAL INCLUSION/EXCLUSION AND HEALTH: DANCING THE DIALECTIC

Ronald Labonte

Introduction

The last decade has seen many of the "community" concepts in health (community empowerment, community capacity) replaced by "social" concepts (social capital, social cohesion). The continuous relabelling of roughly similar phenomena may be a necessary stratagem to attract attention to the economic and power inequalities that arise from undisciplined markets. "Social" concepts also have an advantage over "community" ones by directing that attention to higher orders of political systems. The latest construct being wielded by health practitioners, researchers, and policy-makers is the twinned concept of social inclusion and social exclusion. These represent sophistication over social capital and social cohesion. Like their predecessors, however, there are risks in their adoption without a critical examination of the premises that underpin them. For example, how can one include people and groups into structured systems that systematically exclude them unless the structures of exclusion are themselves altered? The cautions expressed in this article do not dissuade use of the concepts. Their utility, however, particularly at a time when not only inequalities but also their rate of growth is increasing, requires careful questioning. This chapter, then, poses two basic questions:

1. How does the social inclusion/exclusion concept advance our understanding of the social determinants of health in the broadest, deepest sense?

2. How can its uncritical use lead us to a focus on socially excluded groups rather than socially excluding structures and practices?

The chapter answers these questions indirectly by, first, exploring briefly the "community" and "social" concepts that preceded social inclusion/exclusion and then examining the embedded contradiction in the social inclusion/exclusion concept. It then discusses who is purported to be socially excluded and why, and frames this in the context of two competing social justice norms: equality of opportunity and equality of outcome. The chapter concludes with a reflection on the global aspects of social inclusion/exclusion, and the implications this new concept has for practitioners, researchers, and policy-makers.

From Society to Community to Society Once More

Thirty years ago, bristling with newly employed activists from the social movements of the 1960s and the 1970s (the New Left movement, the environmental movement, the women's movement, the civil rights movement), many rich world governments rediscovered community. From processes (community participation, community development) to attributes (community competence, community capacity) to services (community health, community education), it seemed that all we had to was drop the adjective of *gemeinschaft* ("community") in front of the noun of our particular preoccupation and the impersonal structures of *gesellschaft* ("society") disappeared. Of course, we quickly learned it was more complex than this. We confronted the vagaries of power in our workplaces, which supported communities when they weren't threatening to established rules and authority; in our assumptions, which often imposed a romantic localism on poorer people who simply wanted some of the same networked privileges we enjoyed; in communities themselves, which were far from the loving, homogeneous, always wise and self-knowing entities we contrasted against our own organizational hierarchies.[1] More fundamentally, we bumped against the lesson best expressed in the 1989 *Worldwatch Institute Report*: Small may be beautiful, but it may also be insignificant (Durning, 1989). Decisions conditioning and constraining the possibilities of local empowerment were drifting further and higher away from the purview of, and accountability to, the places where, as health promoters like to express, "people live, work, and play."

In the 1990s, our glance widened to broader social phenomena with a new, appropriately social lexicon. Community competence and capacity gave way to social capital. Community participation and development yielded to social inclusion. Social cohesion became the unstated aim of diminishing state programs and services to patch back together communities unravelling with digitized, marketized, and globalized inequalities. Even as a "new" population health research—concerned not with reproductive health in the narrow sense, but with the social production of health in the broadest sense— broached a new government slogan:

> WARNING: Inequalities may be bad for your health. Avoid excessive greed, intolerance, and poor parents.[2]

Neo-liberal economic assumptions continued their global domination, cementing their gospel of liberalization, privatization, deregulation, and welfare minimalism in the policies of the international financial institutions (the World Bank and the International Monetary Fund) and the rules of the World Trade Organization. It is in this brave, new, "history-ending world" (as conservative analysts quickly dubbed life after the fall of the Berlin Wall and the demise of the communist "other") that we need to consider whether the twinned concepts of social inclusion/social exclusion help or hinder our development of actions that will shrink the preventable differences in health, well-being, and quality of life that still demarcate and segregate our communities and nations.

An Advance on Social Cohesion and Social Capital

The twinned concept of social inclusion/exclusion is more helpful than its other social cousins, cohesion and capital. Social cohesion resides more in the realm of moral philosophy than in the grit of human relations. It is a counterfactual ideal, and perhaps even a dangerous one if we ever forget its essential idealism and let it become the driver for how we approach social change. Here it is useful to consider the school of thought known as conflict sociology, which holds, on the basis of a few thousand years of cumulative empirical evidence, that societies have always been a tenuous arrangement of fluid groupings in some degree of conflict with one another— for resources, for authority, for legitimacy; in a word, for power. Where there is no conflict, Ralf Dahrendorf once offered, there is suppression (Dahrendorf, 1959). This does not mean that we should espouse or tolerate civil or any other form of war. But it does challenge us to accept some degree of social conflict as healthy, albeit in discomforting ways. We need to retain a healthy skepticism of concepts that direct us toward a wishful desire for social harmony, however important that desire is as an ideal. Such concepts can blunt the sharp edges of mobilized criticism that has always been one of the necessary fuels for social reform.

Social capital fares little better. For one, no one can settle on a definition of what it is or what it does, apart from a mélange of psychosocial variables of differing interest to different researchers: trust, reciprocity, participation, social network density. More fundamentally, individuals and organizations with quite different visions of how societies should govern themselves can become social capital bedfellows, though perhaps with a quite different understanding of what are "means" and what are "ends." To the World Bank, social capital is the means to the end of economic growth, the necessary social glue that allows unfettered markets to work the magic of their invisible hands (Labonte, 1999). Its absence, it is conjectured, explains why liberalized market reforms (with a few Asian exceptions) have had a dismal record of delivering on their promises in Africa, Latin America, and the so-called transition economies. To others, economic growth is the sometimes necessary means to the end of building social capital. ("Sometimes necessary" because many of today's rich countries would benefit more by *developing* their economies to be more equitable and sustainable rather than simply growing them to become larger.) Economic growth provides a sufficiency of wealth required by states for universal programs and resource redistribution that, in turn, are essential to what Nobel economist Amartya Sen describes as the foundations for the capabilities that allow people "to live a life they have reason to value" (Sen, 2000). To its credit, social capital builds a linguistic bridge between those in the market and those in civil society. To its detriment, and I borrow here from how a disgruntled environmentalist once lamented the concept of sustainable development: *They* got the noun, which defines, while we got the *adjective*, which merely modifies.[3]

Social Inclusion/Exclusion: The Embedded Contradiction

Social inclusion/exclusion is more interesting and dynamic than either social cohesion or social capital, for it is poised on the very contradiction evinced by all of these terms: How does one go about including individuals and groups into a set of structured social relationships that were responsible for excluding them in the first place? Or, put another way, and in deference to Michel Foucault's brilliant essays on the positive practices of power, the seductive ways in which people internalize their own powerlessness and become their own prison guards, to what extent do efforts at social inclusion *accommodate* people to relative powerlessness rather than challenge the hierarchies that create it (Foucault, 1979, 1980)? To what degree might we consider wilful social exclusion by groups an important moment of conflict, an empowered act of resistance to socio-economic systems that, by their logic and rules, continue to replicate and heighten the material hierarchies of inequality?

I pose these questions because many who embrace the concept of social inclusion emphasize how it goes beyond simply matters of income or material inequalities

---

Box 18.1: Resistance is not futile

Many years ago I was involved in community organizing activities with single mothers receiving social assistance. Many of these women had low self-esteem. A principal reason for this was that the dominant discourse of welfare recipients was as non-autonomous, wholly dependent, and publicly accountable individuals who were, effectively, public property, objects of the state. These women had internalized their lesser eligibility; they had become lesser people. The women complained bitterly, for example, of the "spouse in the house" regulation, and of welfare workers who would call them up at all hours or drop by for surprise visits to make sure they weren't "cheating." The "spouse in the house" regulation required single mothers on family benefits allowance to remain single, which, in some instances, was interpreted to mean not having lovers stay in their apartment or house.

Some recipients claimed that they were careful to lower the toilet seat prior to welfare workers' visits in order to avoid suspicion that they may be seeing a male lover, or to trade in their double for a single bed. This is an evocative example of what Foucault described as the *modus operandi* of the "positive practice" of power: the gaze of authority that judges what it sees and, in so judging, controls the choices of those who are gazed upon. The only form of struggle against this form of power, to Foucault, was resistance to the gaze, a concealment of one's life from those with authority over the gaze and the world of judgments it creates, a deliberate act of *social exclusion*, at least from those forms of social regulation that nominally claim to promote social inclusion. Two British researchers, studying the response of poor single parents to home visitors (a hybrid public health nurse and social worker), similarly found that many of these women deliberately hid certain messy rooms, or cupboards, or ill children from the gaze of the home visitors (Bloor & McIntosh, 1990). The authors interpreted these "laconics" or acts of concealment as a rudimentary form of empowering resistance to the hegemonic power-over induced by welfare state policies and the roles they created for both welfare recipients and home visitors.

and their state-enforced redistribution (Barata, 2000), or even of securing basic human rights (Bach, 2002). Rights and redistribution, it is argued, are necessary but not sufficient conditions for people "to be accepted and to participate fully within our families, our communities, and our society," as one definition of social inclusion defines the territory (Guildford, 2000, p. 1). There is little to disagree with in these sentiments. But are there not also risks in pursuing policies and programs that assume *a priori* that income redistribution and human rights are solidly in place when most of the evidence for much of the world is that they are not?

Who Are the Excluded, and Why?

Consider, first, the list of the excluded in need of greater inclusion: women, racial minorities, the poor and the sick, those with disabilities, children and youth, especially if they face developmental challenges or disadvantaged circumstances. Like members of our previously designated "high-risk groups" for health problems, our attention turns to anyone who is not a White, middle-aged, and middle-incomed male. Conceptually, social exclusion is an improvement over its predecessor; it defines disadvantage as an outcome of social processes rather than as a group trait. But in attempting to take us away from a narrow focus on material or income inequality, the concept can falter on an even subtler victim-blaming. People are no longer at fault for their disadvantage. But their disadvantage is seen to lie in their *exclusion* rather than in *excluding structures* predicated on inequality. Let me explain.

Striding alongside social inclusion's references to acceptance by and participation in family, community, and society is social exclusion's complaint that people "do not have the opportunity for full participation in the economic and social benefits of society" (Guildford, 2000, p. 1). People are excluded from these benefits, we are told, because they are poor. But people are poor because they lack these benefits. They lack these benefits because capital and state structures allow wealth to accumulate unequally, and powerful others benefit directly and immediately from this. People are excluded from these benefits, we are also told, because they are women. But women for the past two centuries have been cast economically as a source of cheap and surplus wage labour, and of free reproductive labour. Powerful others benefit directly and immediately from women's relative exclusion from economic and social benefits. This has changed tremendously in the world's wealthier nations over the past half century. But the identical script, directed by the same cast of scriptwriters, is now being enacted globally.

People are excluded from these benefits, we are finally told, because they are Black, or Yellow, or Red, or at least "not White." But contemporary racism, though its roots may be obscured in historic competition over resources, is firmly planted in contemporary capitalism. As Brazilian writer Eduardo Galeano 35 years ago showed in his brilliant essay, *Open Veins of Latin America* (1973), only the wealth of the exploited colonies—their resources, their peoples, their enslavement—allowed Western capitalism to depose feudalism. As British novelist Barry Unsworth recounts vividly in his Booker Prize-winning novel, *A Sacred Hunger* (1993), African slavery was the fuel of both England's early capitalist and American colonial wealth. Slavery collapsed when it was no longer economically efficient, not without a bloody civil war but not because of it. Its undertow remains. Internationally, ethnic conflicts from the tribalism of Africa to the cleansings in the Balkans have powerful roots in the economic structures and political systems that allow wealth to accumulate unequally and powerful others to benefit directly and immediately from this.

This is not to say that the complexities of gender and race exclusion can be reduced to a simple stock of class and materialism. Patriarchal practices and racial exclusions predate feudal societies, much less capitalism. But every example of contemporary social exclusion based on gendered or racialized difference will also have a material and class-based component, with some people deriving benefit from it. When a recent Canadian study tells us that, all other things being equal, workers of colour earn 16 percent less than White workers, this is not only racism. This is also economic advantage for employers (*The Globe and Mail*, November 29, 2002, p. B2). Social exclusion, simply put, is not about categories of people but about the relations of power that categorize people. And uncritical use of social inclusion/exclusion can blind us to the use, abuse, and distribution of power. Power has non-zero-sum elements—the win/win empowerment of trusting, respectful relationships. So, too, does social inclusion. But power has distinctly non-zero-sum aspects—the win/lose of dominance, exploitation, and hegemony. This is manifest in social inclusion's obverse of exclusion. We should not let the warmth of our inclusive ideal smother our anger over exclusivity's unfairness. Anger is often the magnet of mobilization; mobilization is often the tool for social transformation that shifts power relations in ways that allow societies to become more inclusive.

In one sense, we can be generous about concepts, especially new and contested ones such as social inclusion/exclusion. Provided people define carefully what they mean when they use these terms, there is no problem. But people rarely do. More importantly, there is a lesson in the metaphor of a frog in a pot of water. If you throw a frog into a pot of boiling water, it immediately jumps out. It is not that stupid. If you throw it into a pot of cold water and then turn on the heat, it swims about contently as the water slowly rises to a boil and then, suddenly, it dies. It is not that smart. So it can be with certain concepts. Like cold water, we immerse ourselves in them, only to find after a time, and quite suddenly, we arrive at a place we did not originally want to be, colonized by a set of assumptions we did not initially assume. Social inclusion could be one of these concepts unless we maintain a very keen eye on the background temperature and who is in control of the gauge.

And Just What Are We Including Them in?

This problematic of who benefits most by an emphasis on inclusion, rather than a critique of exclusion, becomes more apparent when we examine the different ways its advocates define its end. The first major policy shift based on the concept was in France, in 1988.

As with many of the economically advanced countries, France was faced with high unemployment, particularly among its traditional, semi-skilled manufacturing workers. This was due to capitalism's transformation to a digital economy and its liberalized ability to locate more labour-intensive production in low-wage countries. Fearing a loss in social cohesion, the centre-right government adopted a *revenue minimum d'insertion*, a guaranteed minimum income, but only if people "inserted" themselves into economic or civil life through training and work programs with the private sector, government, and voluntary associations (Guildford, 2000). A slightly more nuanced form of "workfare" programs, this was

not the first time France attempted a project of social reintegration necessitated by fundamental shifts in capitalist production. A century earlier, rural farmers and craftpersons, economically marginalized by another great shift in capitalism, the development of factory production, drank more and killed themselves quite regularly. This led French sociologist Emile Durkheim to coin the concept of *anomie*, a loss of personal meaning that arises with deep tears in the social fabric that normally binds people together. His policy recommendation: creation of "corporative organizations"—community betterment groups—whose purpose would be to change how people thought of themselves, essentially transforming their social identities to conform with how the economy had changed (Taylor & Ashworth, 1987). This is a gloss of Durkheim's sociological thought, but it makes my point: that social inclusion or social integration tends to adapt people to the needs of markets rather than regulate markets to the needs of people.

We see this even more sharply in the UK, where social inclusion has been truncated to labour market attachment (Lister, 2000). If you have a job, you're OK and more likely to display socially inclusive and nicely cohesive attitudes and behaviours. If you don't, you're more likely to be poor, a drain on social welfare, and prone to "anti-social" drug abuse, hooliganism, and crime. This isn't to minimize the importance of work to people's lives. Work satisfies far more dimensions of our being than simply the monthly wage packet. Rather than neighbourhoods, workplaces are where people form many of their enduring friendships (see Box 18.2). But we also know the bleaker side of work: its physical hazards, its psychosocial threats, and, subsequent to today's liberalized capital and episodic encounters with a crisis of overproduction, its increasingly non-standard form in which regular hours, living wages, extended benefits, and longer-term security are being swept away as uncompetitive relics of a bygone era, "labour market rigidities" that constrain our domestic productivity.

It is naive, then, to claim, as some have, "policies to combat social exclusion offer the hope of increasing employment opportunities and reducing poverty" (Guildford, 2000, p. 16). These poverty-reducing jobs will be created in one of three sectors: the public, the private, or the informal/underground. Informal sector work is highly insecure, private sector employment increasingly so, and the public sector has been under two

---

Box 18.2: Social inclusion the "A-way"

People with mental health disabilities often face social exclusion. In the mid-1980s, many psychiatric institutions began closing their wards and releasing psychiatric "consumer/survivors," as they began calling themselves, into communities, often without adequate support services. Key problems faced by many of these people were inadequate income, insufficient social support, and a lack of something to do.

A-Way Express, a Toronto community economic-development program for psychiatric consumer/survivors founded in 1987 by two agencies, offers a good example of both the possibility and the problematic of promoting health using a social inclusion approach.[4] A-Way Express is a courier service operating in Metropolitan Toronto run by people who have had some treatment for mental health difficulties. Couriers utilize public transit, especially the subway system, as their main source of transportation. All of its couriers work for welfare top-up. None of them are employed full-time, most working three five-hour shifts a week. Several professional staff manage, coordinate, and train couriers for the service. A-Way Express is proud of its ability to integrate economic-development activities with support services for psychiatric consumer/survivors. Income, a sense of meaningful social contribution, social support, and self-confidence are all part of the health-promoting, social inclusion "package" that A-Way, and many other consumer/survivor industries, are able to offer. Employment generally provides one sense of community to people. In enterprises such as A-Way, this sense of community is heightened due to employees' integrated participation in the formation and implementation of the organization's policies.

But the "social inclusion" offered by such community economic-development projects is not primarily about strengthening participants' labour market attachment, or making them wholly independent of state-funded support programs. Indeed, such projects are unlikely to become fully self-sufficient in the short, or even medium, term, owing partly to the historic social exclusion of many of the people for whom they create part-time employment. The economic dimension of social inclusion is merely one facet of a more holistic approach they are taking to the successful social integration of people with long-term psychiatric histories.

---

decades of right-wing attack to reduce its expenditures by trimming its labour force. Only "strong state" regulatory and redistributive policies might reallocate employment opportunities in some more durably inclusive way. Yet it is these very policy instruments that are being traded away in free trade negotiations, in such accords as the General Agreement on Trade in Services (which could further privatize public services, and under foreign ownership and even provision), the Agreement on Trade-Related Investment Measures (which prevents governments from putting equity-oriented "performance requirements" on foreign investment), and the Agreement on Government Procurement (which could bind government contracting-out to purely commercial criteria, including "national treatment" of foreign bidders) (Labonte, 2003).

Social Justice: Equality of Opportunity or Equality of Outcome?

What pulls these concepts of social inclusion/social exclusion in sometimes contrary directions, strange as it might first appear, is social justice. This is because

there are two broad norms of social justice defined by their emphases on equality of opportunity or equality of outcome. Both norms are ideal types. There can never be equality of opportunity because different individuals or groups have vastly differing resources or capacities that automatically disadvantage the less well endowed. There can never be equality of outcomes because there are differences between people that cannot be, or should not be, bludgeoned into similitude. But equality of opportunity, the mantra of neo-liberalism and, it seems, central to the UK and other countries' approach to social inclusion, is a grossly insufficient norm if some degree of distributive fairness is our goal.

A pithy illustration of the conflict between these two norms is a cartoon from a newspaper in Aotearoa, New Zealand, from 1991. This was the year that country began its radical dismantling of labour and welfare rights and entitlements as part of a program begun in 1984 of embracing free trade and neo-liberal economic policies. (It has since partially reversed this trend, which gave that country one of the highest growth rates in poverty—doubling between 1988 and 1996—and poorest records of economic growth among the wealthy nations making up the Organisation for Economic Co-operation and Development; Kelsey, 2002.) The cartoon showed a massive giant and a little pipsqueak in a wrestling ring. The match: rich and powerful vs. poor and powerless. As one of the ringside commentators enthused, "It should be a good match. They're playing on a level playing field." The "level playing field"—equality of opportunity—is exactly what is allowing our new global trade regime to ensure that the rich will get richer and the poor, even if they are successful in gaining ground materially, will fall further behind the rich in the economic power game. In strictly economic terms, the biggest winners of the past 20 years of increased global market integration have been the world's wealthiest nations, reversing the trend of the previous two decades (1960–1980) when economic growth in poor countries outpaced that in rich ones (Weisbrot et al., 2001; Milanovic, 2003). The biggest struggle in the World Trade Organization today is not between civil society protestors and trade negotiators. It is between poor and rich countries. Poor countries want stronger "special and differential" exemptions to trade rules so that they can grow their economies by expanding their exports while protecting their domestic markets from imports; by directing foreign investment to where it will do the most developmental good; and by copying technological innovations without threat of trade sanctions. Despite having "developed" their economies using precisely these strategies, rich countries now want the "level playing field" to deny poorer countries the same opportunity (Labonte, 2003).

Equality in outcome demands inequalities in opportunity. Full stop. "Inequalities in opportunity" does not mean targeted programs at the expense of universal programs. But universal programs without some targeting within them (some deference to greater disparity, greater need, greater historic *exclusion*) can heighten inequalities in outcome because of who is better able to avail of such programs.

The Need for a Global Lens

Consider, finally, that social inclusion/exclusion requires a global and not simply a national or local lens. Given the same or largely unchanged economic and political rules or structures that are *socially excluding*, does success in including one group come at the expense of

excluding another? Are we at risk, not of redistributing wealth and opportunity, but of redistributing poverty and marginalization?

Globally, for example, increasing numbers of women in developing countries are now being "included" in the economic wage-labour system, partly because capital has "excluded" from the same system the semi-skilled, blue-collar, primarily male, primarily White labour force in developed countries. For many women, this foreshadows a shift in their empowerment. Yet much of women's employment remains low-paid, unhealthy, and insecure in "free-trade" export zones that often prohibit any form of labour organization and employ only single women. Often, the income they earn still goes to male household members. Women are favoured in such employment because they can be paid less. Most developing countries lack pay-equity laws; the gender income gap in many countries is widening (Gyebi et al., 2002). Public caring supports for young children have been declining in many trade-opened countries, portending future health inequalities. There is also evidence of a global "hierarchy of care." Increasing numbers of women from developing nations are getting employment as domestic workers or other service providers in wealthy countries. They become "socially included," at least in an economic sense. They send much-valued currency back home to their families, which helps in their social inclusion back home. Some of this money is used to employ poorer rural women in their home countries to look after the children they have left behind. These rural women, in turn, leave their eldest daughter (often still quite young and ill-educated) to care for the family they left behind in the village (Hochschild, 2000). In the absence of changes in the rules by which we trade and govern, the process of including some will almost inevitably exclude others.

Conclusion

Our concern, then, should not be with the groups or conditions that are excluded, but with the socio-economic rules and political powers that create excluded groups and conditions and the social groups who benefit from this. Borrowing from similar cautions I made about last season's first blush with social capital (Labonte, 1999), I offer a focal question for practitioners, researchers, and policy-makers.

For practitioners, social inclusion/exclusion may be a useful idea in their ongoing struggles to keep some resources flowing into that part of their work that aims to see the less powerful become the more powerful, the disorganized more organized, the less capable more resourced and confident in their capacities. Like ideas of community empowerment and capacity before it, social exclusion should give practitioners pause to question: How has their work improved the situation for the least well-off within the ambit of their communities? And how has it avoided "excluding" others, perhaps almost as least well-off, from the support and resource access they might require?

For researchers, social inclusion/exclusion could represent a new opportunity for research funding grants, peer-reviewed publications, theoretical refinements, and invitations to health determinants conferences in nice places around the world. The problem is that the term becomes more a vehicle for career advancement than for social change. The question for those in the academy, then, is: How will theorizing and researching social inclusion/exclusion create differently new knowledge and argument useful for community workers and citizens, media sound-biters and policy-makers, in redirecting public governance toward the end of a "good life" for all, to which the market is necessarily subordinate? That is, does this idea prompt us to pose important questions for which we do not already have adequate answers?

For policy-makers, those unenviably straddling political discourses that have captured the noun by eroding the adjective, the question may be: How can the arguments elicited by social inclusion/exclusion convince the free market ideologues of the necessity of disciplining economic practices toward fairness in the distribution of wealth and sustainability in the use of natural resources? Can a social inclusion argument be extended to what we know are important health determinants residing in our economic practices (adequate income and its equitable distribution, access to universal and fairly financed public services), forcing the evidence-based policy conclusion that these conditions require a return to the strong, redistributive state policies we have seen eroded over the past 20 years? Can a social exclusion argument be used to challenge the orthodoxy of equal opportunity with the ideal of equal outcome?

I sow these questions in this chapter as seeds rather than transplanted agendas. I encourage debate upon them, since disagreement is usually more enlightening than prescription.

And I conclude this chapter by drawing attention to how I titled it: "dancing the dialectic." A dialectic is a form of reasoning or argument based on "a contradiction of ideas that serves as the determining factor in their interaction" (www.hyperdictionary.com). I don't want to discard the hopefulness that infuses the social inclusion/ social exclusion concept. The dialectic dances between seeking to include more people into social systems stratified by exclusion even while trying to transform these systems. It's an old dialectic, one that never fully resolves but remains at best a grapple-able task, one that straddles the imperatives of revolution with the pragmatics of reform. It would be hubris to deny that many excluded groups simply want the same chance to climb the ladders of wealth and power that others have before them. It would be unethical to criticize the existence of such ladders in the first place, or to join in struggles to shrink their height.

I also like the idea of dancing. I recently returned from Brazil, where I learned the samba and where every year during Carnival the social incohesion of that country's skewed wealth distribution—rivalling South Africa's as the worst on the planet—is momentarily obliterated in the world's biggest dance festival. Or, as Emma Goldman, the early 20th-century anarchist, feminist, and trade unionist, inspirationally aphorized: "If I can't dance, then it's not my revolution."

Notes

1. There is a long history of critique of the romanticized community. Good overviews are provided by Lyon (1989), who points out that every century produces its own laments for the lost halcyon community of earlier, simpler times; Hunter and Staggenborg (1988), who chide many community workers for failing to distinguish between "communities of limited liabilities" (our decentred opportunity networks) and "communities of enforced locality" (the ghettoes into which we would like to lock up the threatening poor); and Friedmann (1992), who urges a development paradigm in which state/civil society, globalism/localism, and many of the other dualities encountered in community theory and practice literature (such as inclusion/exclusion) are problematized rather than dichotomized.

2. Income inequalities per se may be less a direct threat to health than the more stubborn poverty and loss of social solidarity that such inequalities create.

3. I am sympathetic to the aim of many of today's social capital and health researchers, who should not take my critique of the construct as undermining the importance of understanding better, why, *ceteris paribus* (which they never are), some communities are healthier than others. But rather than working toward a better theorization and operationalization of social capital to study how or why it is a determinant of health, I would urge that studies examine the cultural history and political economy of nations and communities to understand better the determinants of social capital, i.e., to link social capital conceptually and analytically to the structured inequalities created by economic capital and capitalism.

4. The A-Way story is adapted from a report, *Equity in Action*, Ontario Premier's Council on Health, Well-being, and Social Justice (Labonte et al., 1994).

Critical Thinking Questions

1. Given the importance of work in many people's lives, is the emphasis of most social inclusion projects on "including" people in labour markets as unreasonable as this chapter argues?

2. How does approaching social exclusion as an effect of social power relations improve our understanding of exclusionary processes (and possible interventions) vs. listing groups of people who have been marginalized for whatever reasons?

3. From the vantage of social inclusion/exclusion, why are universal interventions preferred to those that target the most disadvantaged?

4. Can you identify other examples where wilful social exclusion is an act of empowerment, rather than of marginalization?

5. How do these two terms advance a more emancipator discourse on public policy? Or do they at all?

Recommended Readings

Clutterbuck, P. & Novick, M. (2002). *Building inclusive communities: Cross-Canada perspectives and strategies.* Draft Discussion Paper prepared for the Federation of Canadian Municipalities and the Laidlaw Foundation. Online at www.laidlawfdn.org/.

This report draws together findings from a cross-Canada series of "community soundings" that engaged 250 city leaders, agency professionals, and social advocates in 10 urban centres in 2002 to assess social vulnerabilities and civic capacities. It develops a vision of inclusive communities and cities, and outlines the institutions, strategies, and resources for successful implementation.

(The above description is taken from the CPRN *Nexus* Newsletter "Urban Nexus No. 4—Cities and Social Inclusion," January 2003.)

Craig, C. & Porter, D. (2005). "The third way and the third world: Poverty reduction and social inclusion strategies in the rise of 'inclusive' liberalism." *Review of International Political Economy, 12*(2) (May 2005), 226–263.

A theoretically dense and challenging essay, the authors are highly critical of the "facile" use of terms such as "inclusion," "exclusion," and "empowerment" that pepper contemporary policy discourse. The nub of their argument is that such terms, which emerged at the same time as modern globalization (liberalization, privatization, marketization) came to dominate political economy, attempt to defuse subsequent social protests arising from globalization's profound dislocations by emphasizing local "inclusion" projects.

Making the case for social and economic inclusion. Online at www.hc-sc.gc.ca/hppb/regions/atlantic/documents/e_abs1.html#14.

This report examines the development of policies and programs to combat social exclusion in Europe over the past decade, and the potential of social inclusion for contributing to the development of healthy social policy in the Atlantic region. It includes a 19-page annotated bibliography of articles, reports, and books relating to the concept of social inclusion.

(The above description is taken from the Health Canada Web site: www.hc-sc.gc.ca/hppb/phdd/ news2001/pdf/social_exclusion_en.pdf.)

Richmond, T. & Saloojee, A. (Eds.). (2005). *Social inclusion: Canadian perspectives.* Halifax: Fernwood Publishing.

This edited collection argues for policies and programs that increase social inclusion, generally taken to mean increasing the participation of those in society who are relatively deprived. While some authors specifically critique contemporary liberalism/neo-liberalism as the cause of social exclusion, most use the terms somewhat uncritically. Uzma Shakir's contribution offers a lone skeptical view.

Social Exclusion Knowledge Network, WHO Commission on Social Determinants of Health. (2007). *Understanding and tackling social exclusion.* Online at www.who.int/social_determinants/resources/latest_publications/en/.

This final report of the Social Exclusion Knowledge Network for the three-year WHO Commission on Social Determinants of Health (2005–2008) usefully identifies three ways in which the concept can be used: (1) a neo-liberal approach and its emphasis on labour market inclusion and welfare minimalism; (2) a relabelling of poverty approach that incorporates other exclusionary processes besides simply income; and (3) a transformational approach that focuses on exclusionary processes arising from socio-economic and institutional power relationships. The report argues the importance of state policies that are universal and fairly (progressively tax-) financed, noting that targeting programs or conditional transfers (such as workfare programs or income transfers based on parents taking their children to clinics or keeping them in schools, increasingly popular in international development work) can be stigmatizing (victim-blaming) and hence exclusionary.

Related Web Sites

Centre for Economic and Social Inclusion—www.cesi.org.uk

The UK-based Centre for Economic and Social Inclusion is an independent, not-for-profit organization working with government, the voluntary sector, business, and trade unions. The site contains several policy and research papers and a monthly journal, titled *Working Brief.*

European Union Community Action Programme to Combat Social Exclusion—www.ec.europa.eu/employment_social/spsi/poverty_social_exclusion_en.htm

The European Union adopted a program of community action to "eradicate poverty and social exclusion by 2010" by "sustained economic growth, more and better jobs and greater social cohesion." This site, titled "The Social

Inclusion Process," describes and contains documents, including reports, studies, and monitoring of national action plans, related to this 10-year goal.

Inclusive Cities Canada—www.inclusivecities.ca

A project of five municipal social planning councils and the Federation of Canadian Municipalities, with funding from Social Development Canada and the Laidlaw Foundation, the ICC project is attempting to "create a horizontal civic alliance on social inclusion across urban communities in Canada." Its Web site contains numerous documents and reports on social inclusion, including municipal reports from Saint John, Toronto, Burlington, Edmonton, and Vancouver.

Policy Research Initiative of Canada—www.policyresearch.gc.ca

The Policy Research Initiative of Canada, a branch of the federal government, has several policy programs involving research studies, conferences, and scholarly opinion pieces.

Social Exclusion Unit/Social Exclusion Task Force—www.cabinetoffice.gov.uk/social_exclusion_task_force.aspx

The UK Social Exclusion Unit, operating out of the office of the deputy prime minister, is a governmental body charged "by the Prime Minister to help improve Government action to reduce social exclusion by producing 'joined-up solutions to joined-up problems." Its original Web site offers this definition: "Social exclusion is a shorthand term for what can happen when people or areas suffer from a combination of linked problems such as unemployment, poor skills, low incomes, poor housing, high crime environments, bad health and family breakdown."

Chapter 19

——————◆——————

THE HEALTH OF ABORIGINAL PEOPLES

Janet Smylie

Introduction

At this point in the text, the classic socio-economic determinants of health (income security, employment, education, food, and shelter) have been covered in some detail. The immediately preceding chapters have highlighted societal processes and structures that result in differential access of social groups to critical resources. The focus has been on groups who have restricted resource access due to societal processes relating to race, ethnicity, gender, health status, and migration status. Restricted resource access has, in turn, been linked to poverty, exclusion from the labour market, poor housing, community disadvantage, and, ultimately, inequities in health status outcomes.

This chapter will focus on the social determinants of health of Aboriginal peoples living in Canada, from an Indigenous-specific and decolonizing perspective. The 1.2 million Aboriginal peoples living in Canada (Statistics Canada, 2008) are part of a larger global population of 370 million Indigenous peoples living in 70 countries around the world (Horton, 2006). In both developing and developed countries, Indigenous peoples face some of the heaviest burdens of ill health (Marmot, 2007; World Health Organization, 2007). Although all of the classic socio-economic determinants of health (such as income security, employment, education, food, and shelter) apply to Indigenous populations, there is evidence that

the societal processes of European colonization are a fundamental and underlying determinant of health (International Symposium on the Social Determinants of Indigenous Health, 2007). Our discussion of social determinants will therefore begin with an overview of the wide-reaching, devastating, diverse, and ongoing impacts of European colonization on First Nations, Inuit, and Métis people and their societies. This will provide the foundation for the discussion of other known social determinants of First Nations, Inuit, and Métis health, as well as an overview of First Nations, Inuit, and Métis health status. We will close the chapter with an introduction to current national and international policy efforts to redress the historic and ongoing injustices that are at the root of Indigenous health inequity.

Socio-demographics of Aboriginal Peoples Living in Canada

Aboriginal peoples living in Canada are part of the larger global population of Indigenous peoples. Prior to European colonization, the Indigenous populations of the Americas were extremely diverse linguistically and culturally. In what is now North America, there were approximately 300 distinct Indigenous languages, which have been grouped into over 50 distinct language families. This linguistic diversity was approximately ten-fold that of Europe at the time (Goddard, 1999).

Currently, at a national level in Canada, Aboriginal peoples represent themselves politically as belonging to one of three major groups: First Nations, Inuit, and Métis. These groupings are also reflected in Section 35 of Canada's Constitution Act, which also recognizes and reaffirms Aboriginal rights and treaty rights (Hurley, 1999). Culturally, Aboriginal peoples in Canada comprise over 50 distinct and diverse groups, each with its own distinct language and traditional land base. Each of these larger groups represents a complex network of communities and kinship systems, often with their own distinct language dialects. Table 19.1 presents the major linguistic groups and languages, and figures 19.1A and 19.1B show the traditional land bases of First Nations and Inuit (1A), as well as Métis (1B).

Aboriginal peoples may refer to themselves by their specific tribal affiliation (such as Mi'kmaq, Cree, Dene, Tsimshian), or identify as First Nations, Inuit, or Métis. First Nations peoples may also be referred to as Native or "Indian," although the latter term is a misnomer based on early European explorers' assumption that they had travelled to Asia; as a result, this term can be offensive to some First Nations peoples. For over 130 years, the federal government has been further classifying First Nations peoples according to whether or not they are registered under the federal Indian Act. People who are registered under the Act are referred to as "Status Indians" and those who are not registered as "non-Status Indians" (Smylie, 2000).

The Inuit traditionally lived above the treeline of what is now Canada and are part of a larger circumpolar Inuit population that includes Greenland, Alaska, and Russia (Smylie, 2000). There are now four Inuit regions in Canada, all with settled land claims: Nunavut, Inuvialuit, Nunavik, and Nunatsiavut.

The Métis are a grouping of Aboriginal peoples whose ancestry can be traced to the intermarriage of European (mainly French and Scottish) men and First Nations women in the western provinces during the 17th century. Over the next two centuries, the Métis became a sizable nation with a distinct language (Michif), culture, and economic role in the fur trade. Individuals of mixed First Nations and non-First Nations ancestry who are not directly connected to the Métis of the historic Northwest

may also self-identify as Métis. Métis are recognized in the Constitution Act, but have historically been excluded from treaty negotiations and the Indian Act (Smylie, 2000).

According to the 2006 national Census, just under 1.2 million people in Canada report Aboriginal identity (Statistics Canada, 2008). This represents 3.8 percent of the total Canadian population. Approximately 60 percent identified as North American "Indian",[1] 33 percent identified as Métis, 4 percent identified as Inuit, and the remaining 3 percent identified with more than one Aboriginal group and/or were registered Indians[2] or members of First Nations bands who didn't identify as Aboriginal (Statistics Canada, 2008). These numbers underestimate the actual Aboriginal population as there was significant non-participation in the Census by a number of First Nations on-reserve communities (Statistics Canada, 2008). Further, it is likely that a significant number of individuals chose not to self-identify Aboriginal ancestry to government workers. Figure 19.2 depicts the Aboriginal population distribution by ethnic group.

First Nations, Inuit, and Métis populations are all much younger than the rest of the Canadian population, with a collective median age of 27 years, compared to 40 years in the non-Aboriginal population. In 2006, children and youth under the age of 24 accounted for just under half (48 percent) of all Aboriginal peoples, compared to 31 percent of the non-Aboriginal population. Another important trend is the growing transition of First Nations, Inuit, and Métis peoples into urban areas. In 2006, over half (54 percent) of the Aboriginal population in Canada lived in urban centres (Statistics Canada, 2008).

Colonization and Its Subsequent Impacts as a Fundamental Determinant of First Nations, Inuit, and Métis Health

> Everyone agrees that there is one critical social determinant of health, the effect of colonization. (International Symposium on the Social Determinants of Indigenous Health, 2007)

In April 2007, as part of the ongoing deliberations of the World Health Organization's Commission on Social

Table 19.1: Linguistic groupings and languages of Aboriginal peoples in Canada

ALGONKIAN	Kaska	Onendaga	SIOUAN
Abenaki	Kutchin	Seneca	Dakota
Blackfoot	Sarcee	Tuscarora	
Cree	Sekani		TLINGIT
Delaware	Slave	KUTENAIAN	Inland Tlingit
Malecite	Tagish	Kutenai	
Mi'kmaq	Tahitan		TSIMSHIAN
Montagnaia	Tuchone	MICHIF	Coast Tsimshian
Ojibwa			Nass-Gitksan
Potawatomi	HAIDAN	SALISHAN	
Squamish	Haida	Bella Coola	WAKASHAN
		Comox	Haista
ATHAPASKAN	INUIT	Halkomeiem	Heiltshuk
Beaver	Inuktitut	Lilooet	Kwakiuti
Carrier		Oakanagan	Nootka
Chilcotin	IROQUOIAN	Sechelt	
Dogrib	Cayuga	Shuswap	
Han	Mohawk	Straits	
Hare	Oneida	Thompson	

Source: Adapted from Smylie, J. (2000). "A guide for health professionals working with Aboriginal peoples: The sociocultural context of Aboriginal peoples in Canada." *Journal of Society of Obstetricians and Gynaecologists of Canada, 22*(12), 1070–1081.

Determinants of Health, Indigenous representatives from the Americas, Asia, Australia, New Zealand, and the Philippines met to discuss the following three questions:

- What actions on the social determinants of Indigenous health would mitigate risk conditions and improve health outcomes for Indigenous peoples globally?
- What examples are there of successful action on the social determinants of health that have resulted in positive outcomes for the health and well-being of Indigenous peoples?
- What policies concerning the social determinants of health are most likely to be effective in improving the health of Indigenous peoples?

The colonization of Indigenous peoples emerged during the meeting and its follow-up as a fundamental underlying health determinant. Restitution of the right of Indigenous peoples to self-determination, including the

implementation of the standards in the UN Declaration on the Rights of Indigenous Peoples was identified as one key requirement for reversing colonization. The persistent and ongoing effects of colonization—including dislocation from traditional lands and lifestyles; policies of cultural or linguistic suppression and forced assimilation; industrial processes' degradation of traditional lands; the impacts of interpersonal and institutional racism—were identified as important determinants of Indigenous health. A recommendation was made that the Indigenous land rights necessary for sustaining Indigenous culture and livelihoods be restored as this and other forms of economic restitution were linked to Indigenous poverty and its subsequent health consequences (International Symposium on the Social Determinants of Indigenous Health, 2007). The summary of outcomes for the symposium is reproduced in Box 19.1 and the Articles of the UN Declaration on the Rights of Indigenous Peoples, which refer to health, are reproduced in Table 19.2.

Given the importance of colonization as a determinant of Indigenous health, it is critical for policy-makers,

Figure 19.1A: Traditional land base of Aboriginal peoples in Canada according to language/ethnic group

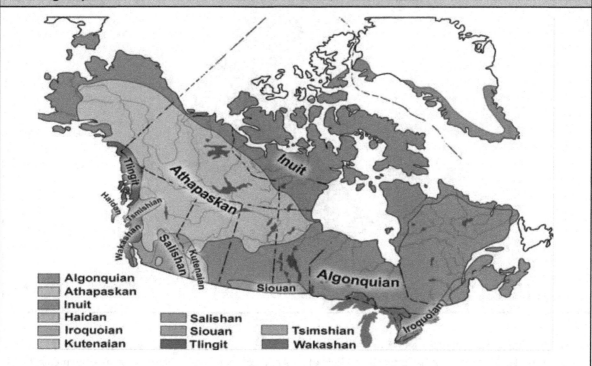

Source: Smylie, J. (2000). "A guide for health professionals working with Aboriginal peoples: The sociocultural context of Aboriginal peoples in Canada." *Journal of Society of Obstetricians and Gynaecologists of Canada, 22*(12), 1070–1081.

Figure 19.1B: Métis Homeland

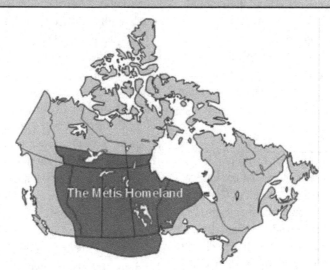

Source: Smylie, J. (2000). "A guide for health professionals working with Aboriginal peoples: The sociocultural context of Aboriginal peoples in Canada." *Journal of Society of Obstetricians and Gynaecologists of Canada, 22*(12), 1070–1081.

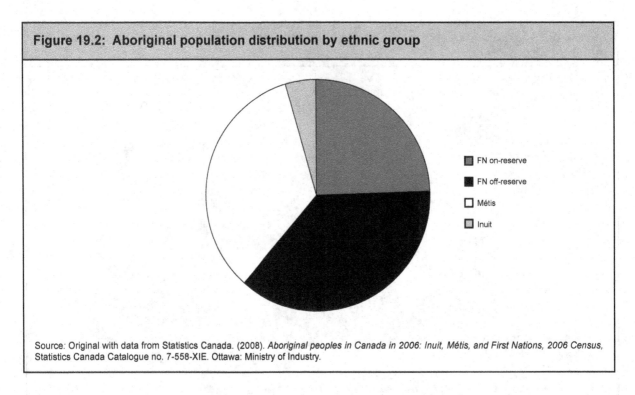

Figure 19.2: Aboriginal population distribution by ethnic group

- FN on-reserve
- FN off-reserve
- Métis
- Inuit

Source: Original with data from Statistics Canada. (2008). *Aboriginal peoples in Canada in 2006: Inuit, Métis, and First Nations, 2006 Census,* Statistics Canada Catalogue no. 7-558-XIE. Ottawa: Ministry of Industry.

service providers, and scholars working in the area of Aboriginal health to have a basic understanding of colonization processes and their effects on First Nations, Inuit, and Métis peoples living in Canada. This part of Canadian history is often ignored or oversimplified despite the reality that colonial processes in Canada have occurred over a 500-year period and are ongoing. These processes vary according to time, geographic location, and Aboriginal group. What follows are four specific examples of colonial policies and their links to First Nations, Inuit, and Métis health. For a more comprehensive coverage of colonial policy, please refer to the recommended reading list.

The Indian Act

The Indian Act is a body of federal legislation that was first enacted in 1876. It is a current statute of Canadian federal law, and despite significant amendments in 1951 and 1985, the original 1876 framework is essentially still intact (Hurley, 1999). The first Indian Act of 1876 reflects governmental policies of assimilation of Aboriginal populations in Canada and appropriation of Aboriginal lands. This Indian Act (and all subsequent Acts) clearly defines who is an "Indian" and who is not. The Indian Act also imposes a system for the management of First Nations lands, as well as the governance of First Nations communities. Box 19.2 includes an excerpt from the 1876 Indian Act, which defines an "Indian" as "Any male person of Indian blood reputed to belong to a particular band; any child of such a person; any woman who is or was lawfully married to such a person."

This definition clearly imposed European standards of male lineage and marriage upon First Nations communities, and meant that for over a century, if a First Nations woman married a person who did not meet this imposed definition of "Indian," she lost her status. It also restricted the definition of "Indian" to people who were registered under the Indian Act. Thus, if someone did not wish to register under the Indian Act or belonged to a First Nations community that refused to sign a treaty; was away when registration was taking place; was a mixed-blood person who chose to take half-breed scrip instead of registering; or was not included on the band lists that were being created by the imposed band council governance systems, then he or she was no longer considered "Indian." Although many First Nations women who had lost their "Indian status" by

---

Box 19.1: Social determinants and Indigenous health

The International Experience and Its Policy Implications
Report on specially prepared documents, presentations and discussion at the International Symposium on the Social Determinants of Indigenous Health Adelaide, 29–30 April 2007 for the Commission on Social Determinants of Health (CSDH).

Summary of Outcomes
Emerging from the proceedings of the International Symposium and associated material are a range of "key themes" and "areas for action." Through the forthcoming *Report of the Commission on the Social Determinants of Health*, these are meant to both inform globally oriented advocacy on Indigenous health and to prompt reflection by individual WHO Member States and, where appropriate, Member States at a regional level.

An understanding common to Symposium delegates and other contributors was that, despite very significant differences in the circumstances of Indigenous Peoples globally, numerous issues and problems are shared. So too are many policy implications.

The following is a selection from the range of other points over which there was wide agreement in the documents prepared for the Symposium and in the ensuing proceedings.

The colonization of Indigenous Peoples was seen as a fundamental underlying health determinant. This process continues to impact health and well-being and must be remedied if the health disadvantages of Indigenous Peoples are to be overcome. One requirement for reversing colonization is self-determination, to help restore to Indigenous Peoples control over their lives and destinies.

The failure to apply or implement various UN instruments, agreements and treaties directed at securing self-determination and other rights for Indigenous Peoples was a closely related matter of concern. Symposium participants and the papers canvassed issues suggesting that more specific standards, such as those enunciated in the draft UN Declaration on the Rights of Indigenous Peoples, were required. The Symposium heard examples of where the inability of Indigenous Peoples to enjoy fundamental freedoms impacted adversely on their health and well-being. Another fundamental health determinant stressed in the Symposium is the disruption or severance of ties of Indigenous Peoples to their land, weakening or destroying closely associated cultural practices and participation in the traditional economy essential for health and well-being. Rights to land necessary for sustaining Indigenous culture and livelihoods should be restored. Linked to land rights is the resolution of Indigenous poverty and economic inequality. Poor health was seen as the corollary of poverty and inequality. Economic redistribution was considered essential for moving towards equality in health outcomes.

Along with this, the Symposium and papers highlighted the impact of widespread and devastating land degradation and climate change as a determinant of Indigenous Peoples' health and well-being. This is through the limitations it imposes on Indigenous Peoples' cultural and economic opportunities and freedoms. A repeatedly mentioned means for tackling poverty and associated low socio-economic status is through much greater investment in education, more particularly that of children and for building Indigenous leadership.

Too often Indigenous Peoples and their social conditions are invisible. Much better data and quality research on Indigenous health needs to be generated, but this must be with the specific agreement of Indigenous Peoples. In this regard, cooperation across national borders is a particular challenge.

One of the strongest messages from the Symposium concerned the lack of understanding of Indigenous culture and world views. The papers and Symposium gave examples of instrumental and constitutive value attributed by Indigenous Peoples to culture and world views as a determinant of their health and well-being. The repeated implication is for increased respect for Indigenous Peoples and their cultures. This includes the need to take account of Indigenous Peoples' holistic approaches to, and understandings of, health and well-being. Such "difference blindness" compounded the impact of interpersonal and institutional racism that repeatedly emerged in the Symposium discourse as a determinant of health. Participants called for firm action on the part of Member States and civil society to urgently treat this danger to health and well-being.

Going beyond this was the call for broader reform of institutions and service arrangements. Reforms must extend from governmental structures, including systems of political representation; through legal and judicial arrangements, including securing practical equality before the law and the recognition of customary laws; to the extension of service delivery arrangements to ensure equitable access and accountability to

Indigenous People. Delegates referred frequently to the need for, and value of, properly funded primary health care services under Indigenous control. Finally, there was a strong belief amongst Indigenous delegates that international cooperation is an important ingredient in tackling common problems. This is sustained by a conviction that "we are all connected as Indigenous Peoples worldwide."

Source: International Symposium on the Social Determinants of Indigenous Health. (2007). *Social determinants and Indigenous health: The international experience and its policy implications: Report on specially prepared document, presentations and discussion at the International Symposium on the Social Determinants of Indigenous Health*.Adelaide: International Symposium on the Social Determinants of Indigenous Health. Online at www.who.int/social_determinants/resources/indigenous_health_adelaide_report_07.pdf

Table 19.2: Average individual incomes of the population by gender, Aboriginal identity, and area of residence, Canada, 2000

Gender	Total Aboriginal	Registered Indian			Métis	Inuit	Other Aboriginal	Non-Aboriginal
		Total	On Reserve	Off Reserve				
Women 15 +	16519	15365	13968	16483	18144	18721	16240	23065
Men 15+	21958	18724	14907	22849	26634	21103	23827	37265

Source: Hull, J. (2006). *Aboriginal women: A profile from the 2001 Census*. Prepared for Women's Issues and Gender Equality Directorate, Indian and Northern Affairs Canada. Online at www.ainc-inac.gc.ca/pr/pub/abw/index_e.html

marrying a "non-Indian" achieved a reinstatement of Indian status in the 1985 amendment to the Indian Act, these long-standing imposed definitions of "Indianness" have contributed to current divisions among and between First Nations and Métis peoples (Lawrence, 1999).

The Constitution Act of 1867 and subsequent Indian Acts legalized the removal of First Nations communities, which had signed treaties, from their homelands to "reserve lands" that were controlled by the Government of Canada on behalf of "Indians." The Indian Acts of 1876, 1880, and 1884 later outlawed First Nations ceremonies such as the sundance and potlatch and gave the Indian agent authority over the foods, goods, and travel available to on-reserve First Nations peoples. These policies also supported the abduction of Aboriginal children to residential schools, where language and culture were actively suppressed (Smylie, 2000). The dislocation of First Nations communities from their traditional territories to federal Indian reserves undermined the livelihood and local economies of these communities, which was strongly tied to traditional lands. Harvesting opportunities were often quite limited in the new reserve lands, and food-security issues were heightened on the Prairies as the buffalo population diminished.

At the same time, communities continued to struggle with infectious diseases such as influenza, measles, and smallpox. These diseases, imported into First Nations communities through contact with Europeans, had devastating impacts. Aboriginal communities had not been previously exposed prior to European contact and therefore had limited immunity. All of these changes had dramatic impacts on the health and well-being of First Nations and Métis people, and by the mid-1880s, 10 years after the first Indian legislation, starvation, violence, infectious disease, cultural suppression, imposed religious practice, as well as family and community disruption, were common realities for First Nations and Métis peoples. Many First Nations leaders resisted signing land treaties with the Canadian government and most fought for better treaty terms; however, these deteriorating conditions and policies, such as the withholding of food rations by Canadian authorities until the treaties were signed, eventually left them in a poor position to argue (Dickason, 1992).

Box 19.2: Excerpt from the Indian Act, 1876

CHAP. 18.
An Act to amend and consolidate the laws respecting Indians.
[Assented to 12th April 1876.]

TERMS
3.3 The term "Indian" means
First. Any male person of Indian blood reputed to belong to a particular band;
Secondly. Any child of such person;
Thirdly. Any woman who is or was lawfully married to such person:
(a) Provided that any illegitimate child, unless having shared with the consent of the band in the distribution moneys of such band for a period exceeding two years, may, at any time, be excluded from the membership thereof by the band, if such proceeding be sanctioned by the Superintendent-General:
(b) Provided that any Indian having for five years continuously resided in a foreign country shall with the sanction of the Superintendent-General, cease to be a member thereof and shall not be permitted to become again a member thereof, or of any other band, unless the consent of the band with the approval of the Superintendent-General or his agent, be first had and obtained; but this provision shall not apply to any professional man, mechanic, missionary, teacher or interpreter, while discharging his or her duty as such:
(c) Provided that any Indian woman marrying any other than an Indian or a non-treaty Indian shall cease to be an Indian in any respect within the meaning of this Act, except that she shall be entitled to share equally with the members of the band to which she formerly belonged, in the annual or semi-annual distribution of their annuities, interest moneys and rents; but this income may be commuted to her at any time at ten years' purchase with the consent of the band:
(d) Provided that any Indian woman marrying an Indian of any other band, or a non-treaty Indian shall cease to be a member of the band to which she formerly belonged, and become a member of the band or irregular band of which her husband is a member:
(e) Provided also that no half-breed in Manitoba who has shared in the distribution of half-breed lands shall be accounted an Indian; and that no half-breed head of a family (except the widow of an Indian, or a half-breed who has already been admitted into treaty), shall, unless under very special circumstances, to be determined by the Superintendent-General or his agent, be accounted an Indian, or entitled to be admitted into any Indian treaty.

Source: Parliament of Canada, Indian Act, 1876, *Report of the Royal Commission on Aboriginal Affairs*, Indian and Northern Affairs Canada. Online at www.ainc-inac.gc.ca/ch/rcap/sg/sg17_e.html

The Cree Chiefs negotiating Treaty #6 did manage to include a "medicine chest clause" in this treaty when it was signed in 1876, which reads: "In the event hereafter the Indians ... being overtaken by any pestilence, or by a general famine, the Queen ... will grant to the Indians assistance ... sufficient to relieve them from the calamity that shall have befallen them. A medicine chest shall be kept at the house of each Indian agent for the use and benefit of the Indians at the direction of such agent" (Morris, 1880, para. 18). This clause has been interpreted by many that the federal government's provision of health care services to First Nations peoples is a negotiated treaty right (Smylie, 2000).

Disregard for Métis Land Claims

In 1869, the Hudson Bay Company transferred its lands in Canada's Northwest and authority for these lands to the Government of Canada. These lands represented over one-third of the land base of what is now Canada, including the watershed of all rivers and streams flowing into Hudson Bay, and the watershed of the Arctic Ocean and Pacific Ocean. The Hudson Bay Company had previously been granted trading monopolies for these areas, and received £300,000 and one-twentieth of the fertile areas that were to be opened for settlement in return for the transfer (*Canadian Encyclopedia*, 2007).

At the time of the transfer, First Nations and Métis were by far the biggest populations living in these areas. For example, in 1871, according to the Census in the Red River area (now Winnipeg, Manitoba), there were 9,800 Métis and 1,600 Whites (the First Nations population was not counted). This transfer did not include any provision for the First Nations and Métis peoples who were living on these lands, and social unrest was therefore a predictable outcome.

Under the leadership of Louis Riel, Métis in the Red River resisted the transfer of governing authority and formed a provisional government. Eventually, representatives from this provisional government were able to meet with then Prime Minister Macdonald and ensured that the existing occupancies and titles of Métis and First Nations peoples were recognized in the creation of the province of Manitoba under the Manitoba Act. The Manitoba Act also reserved 1.4 million acres of Crown land for the unmarried children of Métis (Dickason, 1992).

Unfortunately, incoming settlers showed disregard for Métis land claims and the implementation of the land provisions for the Métis in the Manitoba Act was plagued by delays, speculation, and theft. For example, out of 93 Métis claims for their established river lots, 84 were rejected. In 1872, Métis asked then Lieutenant-Governor Archibald to let them know "what steps they should adopt to secure to themselves the right to prohibit people of other nationalities from settling in the lands occupied by them, without the consent of the Community." The Métis' proposals to have a block of land reserved for their collective use were refused, and they were forced to apply for their land grants as individuals. The government began offering these grants in the form of scrip to "half-breed" heads of families and their children. Scrip quickly became an item of speculation and could be taken in the form of money instead of land. Many Métis took the money ($160 for heads of families). In the end, the large majority of land set aside for Métis children in the Manitoba Act ended up being acquired by speculators for only a fraction of its value and less than a quarter was actually occupied by Métis. By 1880, it was clear that the implementation of the provisions in the Manitoba Act were to be of little benefit for the Métis (Dickason, 1992).

Frustrated and dispossessed of their lands and houses, many Métis groups left the Red River to establish independent settlements further west. In 1872, a large group of Métis, under the leadership of buffalo-hunt captain Gabriel Dumont, settled at the South Saskatchewan River north between what is currently Saskatoon and Prince Albert. The settlement became known as Batoche and a local governance system, complete with laws and taxes, was established in 1873. Unfortunately, over the next 10 years, this group's attempts to be recognized by the Government of Canada as a colony with special status acknowledging their Aboriginal rights were unsuccessful. Another provisional government was initiated by Riel, who had returned to Canada from the United States in 1884. Tensions escalated and there was a series of armed confrontations between the Métis and Canadian government forces. This culminated in a three-day battle at Batoche, which ended when the Métis ran out of ammunition. Following the battle, Canadian forces burned and pillaged the Batoche settlement, and Riel was hung as a traitor. The Métis once more were dispossessed of their land and homes. Fearful of further persecution, following the battle of Batoche, many Métis changed their names and others fled to the United States (Dickason, 1992).

The disruption of Métis families and communities resulting from federal governmental disregard for and appropriation of their lands has had a long-standing impact on Métis. It is important to note that prior to the Hudson Bay land transfer in Manitoba and the uprising in Batoche, many Métis families on the Prairies were economically prospering (Dickason, 1992, p. 295). Following these events, Métis struggled economically and commonly faced racial prejudice from European settlers, which, in turn, limited job prospects (Lutz, Hamilton & Heimbecker, 2005). As a result of not having their land claims officially recognized in the same way that First Nations claims were recognized through treaties, Métis have been, for the most part, excluded from federal Aboriginal health programming and service initiatives up until the current day. This exclusion contributes to health services access challenges for Métis, including challenges in accessing preventative health programming, purchasing prescription drugs, as well as obtaining medical transportation to tertiary services for Métis living in rural areas.

Relocation of Inuit Communities

Inuit experiences of colonization differed from those of First Nations and Métis, although the theme of dislocation from traditional lands is common among the three groups. Although Inuit communities in Canada's North had been in contact with Europeans since the 11th century, there was no official federal government presence until 1903, when the North West Mounted Police established posts at Herschel Island and Fort McPherson. During and after the Second World War, the federal government had a policy of "encouraging" Inuit to relocate into permanent villages in areas selected by the government (Dickason, 1992, pp. 396–397). Permanent villages did not exist among the Inuit prior to the arrival of Europeans. However, in order to receive family allowance, children were required to attend schools in these villages. In addition, family allowances and old-age pensions did not come in the form of cheques but as credit at Hudson Bay Company posts, which were located in these towns and villages. One of the first relocation attempts occurred in 1934. Twenty-two Inuit from Kinngait (Cape Dorset), 18 from Mittimatalk/Tununiq (Pond Inlet), and 12 from Pangnirtuuq (Pangnirtung) were transported to Dundas Harbour. During the 1950s and 1960s, many more Inuit families were moved from their traditional lands to permanent settlements (Dickason, 1992, pp. 396–397). The hunting conditions of the new sites were usually suboptimal, interfering with traditional food supply. The impact of these relocations upon the Inuit is described in the following excerpt from the Royal Commission on Aboriginal Peoples (RCAP) report:

"Although the intentions were to have Inuit gain better access to government services, this movement initiated a period of social, cultural, and economic upheaval for the Inuit. Within the space of a few years, many of us had left a life that was based on an intimate reliance on the resource of the land and sea and stepped into a different way of living" (Inuit Tapirisat of Canada, 2000). In addition to food insecurity, unemployment, and housing issues, the move to permanent settlements

was accompanied by outbreaks of tuberculosis. By 1964, more than 70 percent of Keewatin Inuit had been in TB sanatoria. Sometimes, children sent to sanatoria were adopted by southern families without their parents being informed (Dickason, 1992).

Residential Schools

Approximately 100 residential schools operated in Canada from 1849–1983. Indian Act legislation in 1920 made school attendance compulsory for all First Nations children between the ages of seven and 15. The residential school experience is described in the following excerpt from the *First Nations and Inuit Regional Health Survey*:

> In some areas as many as five separate generations of children were removed from their homes, families, culture, and language.... At the schools children's long hair was cut off and school uniforms issued ... many of the children endured long years of isolation and loneliness.... Children entered a strange new world in residential boarding schools.... Scores of children died from disease; others were emotionally and spiritually destroyed by the harsh discipline and living conditions. Children were referred to as "inmate." Survivors report being hungry all the time. In some cases, children were separated from their siblings, tortured for speaking their mother tongue, forbidden to honour their traditions. Grievous sexual abuse also occurred in some schools, but other outstanding issues include physical abuse and poor quality of education. (First Nations and Inuit Regional Health Survey, 1999)

Inuit children were not spared the residential school experience. Mary Carpenter summarizes her experience of residential school:

> After a lifetime of beating, going hungry, standing in a corridor on one leg, and walking in the snow with no shoes for speaking

Inuvialuktun, and having a heavy stinging paste rubbed on my face, which they did to stop us from expressing our Eskimo custom of raising our eyebrows for "yes" and wrinkling our nose for "no," I soon lost the ability to speak my mother tongue. When a language dies, the world it was generated from is broken down too. (Royal Commission on Aboriginal Peoples, 1996b)

The traumatic impact of residential schools on the individual is described in the same article:

Former students have expressed the pain and confusion of not fitting in either world, of being caught between two cultures—the white culture of the residential schools and their Inuit culture. This chasm within has caused various illnesses of the soul, leading to depres-sion, hopelessness and destructive behaviours such as alcoholism, drug addictions, sexual promiscuity or violence, all with their own tragic consequences. (Royal Commission on Aboriginal Peoples, 1996b)

Métis children and youth in some parts of the country also attended residential schools. In addition, they were also commonly excluded and/or barred from attending community schools set up for the children of European colonists.

Unfortunately, the impact of residential schools goes far beyond the impact on individual survivors. Dr. Cornelia Wieman highlights the enduring aftermath of the residential schools, asserting that:

In addition to the damage caused to the individual survivors who endured emotional, physical, and sexual abuse, we must consider the long-term, cumulative intergenerational effects on First Nations Communities ... including dislocation from one's community, loss of pride and self-respect, loss of identity, language, spirituality, culture, and ability to parent. The roots of this damage and these losses are reflected in the abysmal statistics

which reflect levels of family violence, suicide, alcohol and other substance abuse in Aboriginal communities today. (Wieman, 1999)

Additional Social Determinants of First Nations, Inuit, and Métis Health

Participants at the International Symposium on the Social Determinants of Indigenous Health made clear links between the failure to recognize Indigenous land rights, poverty, and inequality. First Nations, Inuit, and Métis communities in Canada have not recovered from the historic and ongoing social, cultural, and economic disruption brought about by colonial policies. In this section, the magnitude of this poverty and inequality is described in the areas of income, employment, education, food security, and housing. Additional determinants of Indigenous health detailed by symposium participants included: the marginalization of Indigenous peoples and perspectives from the planning and implementation of health policies, programs, and services; attitudinal and systemic racism; and geographical and jurisdictional barriers to health services access. None of these additional determinants are well measured in Canada at the current time; however, they represent important topics for future inquiry.

Income

According to the 2001 Census, the average annual income for Aboriginal men and women over the age of 15 was $21,958 and $16,519 respectively. These figures correspond to 58 percent of the average annual income for non-Aboriginal men and 72 percent of the average annual income for non-Aboriginal women (Hull, 2006). For First Nations men and women living on-reserve, their average annual incomes were 40 percent and 61 percent of the incomes for non-Aboriginal men and women respectively (Hull, 2006). These annual income ratios are slightly better for First Nations people living off-reserve, Inuit, and Métis, but still significantly below the annual incomes for non-Aboriginal Canadians (see Hull, 2006, Table 3).

These income disparities are all the more alarming when the household and demographic characteristics of Aboriginal families are taken into account. We know that

35 percent of Aboriginal children live with a lone parent, and that children and youth account for just under half of the Aboriginal population (Statistics Canada, 2008). Therefore, the reduced annual incomes of Aboriginal adults described above will often be providing for a larger group of dependants, compared to non-Aboriginal households. In keeping with this situation, it is not surprising that over one in four (26 percent) of Aboriginal households had an income below the low-income cut-off in 2001, compared to 12 percent of non-Aboriginal households (Statistics Canada, 2003a).

Employment

Participation in the labour force is lower and the unemployment rate is higher for Aboriginal peoples compared to non-Aboriginal Canadians. In 2001, the unemployment rate for Aboriginal peoples was 14 percent, compared to 7 percent for non-Aboriginal Canadians. For First Nations peoples living on-reserve, the rate of unemployment was 28 percent, compared to a rate of 14 percent for First Nations peoples living off-reserve. Unemployment rates were 20 percent for Inuit and 12 percent for Métis (Statistics Canada, 2003b).

Education

In 2001, 49 percent of Aboriginal men and 53 percent of Aboriginal women over the age of 15 who were not attending school full-time had at least completed high school, compared to 71 percent of non-Aboriginal men and 70 percent of non-Aboriginal women. In the same year, 40 percent of First Nations men living on reserve and 43 percent of First Nations women living on-reserve had at least high school education. For First Nations men and women living off-reserve, the rates of having at least high school education were 56 percent and 57 percent respectively. Forty-three percent of both Inuit men and women had achieved at least high school completion. For Métis men and women, the rates of at least high school completion were 65 percent and 63 percent respectively (Hull, 2006). Levels of post-secondary education have improved over the past 30 years. In 1968, approximately 800 Aboriginal peoples were known to have post-secondary education; this has increased to over 210,000 in 2001 (Statistics Canada, 2003c).

Food Security

Information regarding the rates of food security and insecurity among First Nations, Inuit, and Métis populations in Canada is patchy and inconsistent. This is of concern given the strong links between food security, income, and employment. Based on the income and employment statistics above, we know that Aboriginal peoples will be at risk of food insecurity. Data quality is further complicated by the use of different measurement instruments, most of which have not been validated in First Nations, Inuit, and Métis contexts. Information from the 1996 *National Longitudinal Survey of Children and Youth* (NLSCY) indicates that people of Aboriginal descent living off-reserve were four times more likely to report hunger than other respondents (McIntyre, Walsh & Connor, 2001). This finding is consistent with the results of the 2004 *Canadian Community Health Survey* (CCHS), which found that 33 percent of Aboriginal households surveyed experienced moderate and severe food insecurity compared to 8.8 percent of all of the non-Aboriginal households surveyed. The disparity is exacerbated when severe food security alone is examined—14.4 percent of Aboriginal households surveyed reported severe food security compared to 2.7 percent of non-Aboriginal households (Health Canada, 2007).

The CCHS excludes on-reserve First Nations populations and Inuit populations living in the territories. With respect to food insecurity for First Nations populations living on-reserve, reported rates vary from 21–83 percent (Power, 2007). For example, in the Cree community of Fort Severn, Ontario, a 2002 household study found total rates of food insecurity 67 percent. Food insecurity in this study had two categorizations: with hunger and without hunger. Twenty-four percent of all of the households with children surveyed reported child food insecurity with hunger (Lawn & Harvey, 2004). In a 1997 study of Inuit women in the northern communities of Qausuittuq (Repulse Bay) and Mittimatalk/Tunniq (Pond Inlet), 48 percent and 53 percent of women respectively reported not having enough to eat in the house over the past month. Remote and/or northern Aboriginal communities can face additional food security challenges as nutritious food can be difficult and costly to find. For example, in a 2001 study, a healthy food basket to feed a family of four was priced at $327 in a northern Inuit community, compared to $135–$155 in southern cities (Lawn & Harvey, 2001).

Housing

Aboriginal peoples living in Canada are four times more likely than non-Aboriginal people to live in a crowded dwelling. They are also close to four times more likely than non-Aboriginal people to live in a home that requires major repairs (Statistics Canada, 2008). This situation varies according to the Aboriginal group and where they are living. For example, 38 percent of Inuit living in Inuit Nunaat (northern Inuit territories) were challenged by crowded homes, compared to 11 percent of the total Aboriginal population and 3 percent of the non-Aboriginal population. As discussed in the preceding section, this overcrowding is linked to the relocation of Inuit from their traditional territories and impermanent, readily constructed dwellings to permanent housing in villages and cities. Not surprisingly, given these crowded conditions, Inuit children face some of the highest rates of severe lower respiratory tract infection in the world (Kovesi, Gilbert, Stocco, Fugler, Dales, Guay & Miller, 2007).

Of additional concern for many on-reserve First Nations communities is the lack of a safe household drinking water supply. In 2001, Indian and Northern Affairs Canada undertook an on-site assessment of water and wastewater systems on reserves and found that in about three-quarters of the water systems, there was a significant risk to the quality or the safety of community drinking water (Office of the Auditor General of Canada, 2005).

Health Status Inequities

Not surprisingly, given the inequities in health determinants described above, First Nations, Inuit, and Métis children and their families experience a disproportionate burden of illness and premature death compared to the rest of Canada (Health Council of Canada, 2005; First Nations Centre, National Aboriginal Health Organization, 2005; MacMillan, MacMillan, Offord & Dingle, 1996).

Although there are challenges in both the coverage and quality of health status measures (Smylie & Anderson, 2006), the information we do have indicates clear and inarguable health status disparities. The large majority of these health status disparities can be directly linked to the socio-economic determinants of health described in the preceding section, which, in turn, are linked to colonial processes and the resultant inequities in access to societal resources.

Life expectancies for First Nations peoples with status and Inuit people in Canada are five to 14 years less than those of the total Canadian population, with Inuit men and women experiencing the more extreme disparities (Statistics Canada, 2008; Canadian Institute for Health Information, 2004). Contributing to the shorter life expectancy are infant mortality rates that are 1.5 to four times the Canadian rates (Luo, Kierans, Wilkins, Liston, Uh & Kramer, 2004; Luo, Wilkins, Platt & Kramer, 2004; Wilkins et al., 2008), as well as high rates of premature death due to injury and suicide among First Nations with status (Health Canada, 2005). There is no life expectancy, infant mortality, or disease-specific mortality information for Métis and First Nations peoples without status even though they account for close to half of Canada's Aboriginal population. This exclusion from basic public health assessment typifies the current federal policies regarding Métis and First Nations peoples without status, which is still primarily guided by the Indian Act.

Rates of infectious diseases, including tuberculosis (Public Health Agency of Canada, 2007), pertussis, rubella, shigellosis, and chlamydia, are higher for Aboriginal peoples compared to other Canadians (Health Canada, 2005). While these rates vary according to Aboriginal group, children are particularly vulnerable and rates of hospitalization and/or death due to respiratory illness among young Inuit and First Nations children are elevated compared to non-Aboriginal Canadians (Kovesi et al., 2007; Orr, Mcdonald, Milley & Brown, 2001; Trovato, 2000). Despite the increased risk of infectious disease, coverage rates for routine immunizations among two-year-olds were lower among First Nations children for all antigens (Health Canada, 2005). Aboriginal peoples are overrepresented in the HIV epidemic in Canada. Of new HIV case reports between 1998 and 2006 that identified ethnicity, 22 percent reported Aboriginal ethnicity (Public Health Agency of Canada, 2006). The rates of tuberculosis among Aboriginal peoples in Canada is over five times the rate of the general Canadian population and has been linked to the effects of poverty, including crowded housing (Public Health Agency of Canada, 2007).

The prevalence of major chronic diseases, including arthritis/rheumatism, hypertension, asthma, and diabetes, is higher among First Nations and Métis populations compared to the total Canadian population (Statistics Canada, 2003d). Diabetes is of particular concern, with adult prevalence rates of up to 25 percent being reported in specific First Nations on-reserve communities (Young, Reading, Elias & O'Neil, 2000; Harris et al., 1997) and elevated rates were also reported among subpopulations of First Nations youth (Dean, 1998; Dean, Mundy & Moffatt, 1992; Harris, Perkins & Whalen-Brough, 1996). Obesity, which can lead to diabetes, has also emerged as a major problem in many First Nations communities and is linked to changes in diet and lifestyle (Young, 1996). High rates of obesity have also been reported for First Nations children living on-reserve (First Nations Centre, National Aboriginal Health Organization, 2005).

Aboriginal peoples in Canada also experience a disproportionate burden of mental health issues, which have been directly linked to colonial processes (Kirmayer, Brass & Tait, 2000). Suicide rates five to six times higher than non-Aboriginal rates have been reported among subpopulations of First Nations and Inuit youth (Chandler & Lalonde, 1998; Inuit Tapiriit Kanatami, 2007). An examination of First Nations youth suicide in British Columbia identified an inverse relationship between youth suicide and community systems that were community-controlled and/or facilitated cultural continuity (Chandler & Lalonde, 1998). With respect to other mental health issues, 18 percent of participants in the 1997 *First Nations and Inuit Regional Longitudinal Health Survey* met the criteria for major depression; 27 percent reported problems with alcohol; and 34 percent reported sexual abuse during childhood (First Nations and Inuit Regional Health Survey Steering Committee, 1999). Finally, Aboriginal families are more likely than non-Aboriginal families to experience violence (Adelson, 2005).

Concern regarding environmental exposures is also a commonly cited health priority for First Nations, Inuit, and Métis communities, particularly in communities where there is still significant consumption of hunted game and fish. Dozens of environmental contaminants have been identified in the food chains and living environments of Aboriginal peoples in Canada. For example, polychlorinated biphenyl (PCB) has been identified in Inuit traditional food sources (Hoekstra, Letcher, O'Hara, Backus, Solomon & Muir, 2003) and the breast milk of Inuit mothers living in Nunavik (Dewailly, Ryan, Laliberte, Bruneau, Weber, Gingras & Carrier, 1994) and mercury in the fish consumed by members of Grassy River First Nations (Kinghorn, Solomon & Chan, 2007). Such environmental exposures are clearly linked to environmental degradation through mostly non-Aboriginal commercial exploitation of traditional lands.

Despite the disruption of family and culture that has been experienced historically by First Nations, Inuit, and Métis peoples, there is evidence also of the resilience of extended kinship systems and the transmission of language and culture. For example, 63 percent of Inuit children indicated they could speak Inuktitut at least relatively well (Adelson, 2005) and 93 percent of *First Nations Regional Longitudinal Health Survey* (FNRLHS) respondents rated the learning of a First Nations language as important. FNRLHS respondents were also able to identify a wide range of people who helped children learn their culture (First Nations Centre, National Aboriginal Health Organization, 2005).

Regrettably, there have been many opportunities to document the devastating impacts of European colonization worldwide and the resultant patterns of illness and disease that have inevitably followed. Early health status impacts include famine, high rates of infectious disease, and high death rates, especially among infants and children. Subsequently there is a decline in infectious disease and rapid population growth. Finally, there is a rise in chronic and degenerative disease (Locust, 1999).

The health status information presented above clearly demonstrates that First Nations, Métis, and Inuit populations have and continue to experience the full range of health status consequences of colonization. Although rates of infectious disease and mortality, including infant mortality rates, improved over the course of the 20th century, persistent disparities continue and improvement appears to have levelled off over the past decade. Demographically, there is rapid population expansion, with a 45 percent increase in total Aboriginal population over the past 10 years (six times the growth rate of the non-Aboriginal population) (Statistics Canada, 2008). There is also a more recent rise in chronic and degenerative disease.

Health status disparities persist and chronic disease rates continue to rise despite federal/provincial/territorial governments' increased investment in health services and programs for on-reserve First Nations and northern Inuit communities. Although First Nations, Inuit, and Métis stakeholder groups tend to agree that these health services and program investments are inadequate, they are also keenly aware that the longer-term solution to addressing Aboriginal health status disparities needs to involve resolution of the gross inequities in underlying health determinants (Assembly of First Nations, 2006). For Indigenous peoples worldwide, this includes redressing the historic and ongoing injustices that are the root causes of Indigenous health inequity.

Policy Efforts

The federal government should begin the cycle of renewal with an act of national intention—a new Royal Proclamation.

The Commission is calling for a sharp break with past practices, mired as they are in fallacies about Aboriginal people and their rights, tarnished as they are with failed negotiations and broken promises. We propose a new Royal Proclamation, stating Canada's commitment to principles of mutual recognition, respect, responsibility and sharing in the relationship between original peoples and those who came later. (Royal Commission on Aboriginal Peoples, 1996a)

In 1996, following five years of consultations with Aboriginal and non-Aboriginal stakeholders from across Canada, the Royal Commission on Aboriginal Peoples (RCAP) released its report. The RCAP report recommended fundamental changes in the Government of Canada's approach to First Nations, Inuit, and Métis peoples. These included a call to recognize the inherent moral, historic, and legal rights of Aboriginal peoples to self-determination and hundreds of specific recommendations. Major recommendations included the following:

- legislation, including a new Royal Proclamation stating Canada's commitment to a new relationship and companion legislation setting out a treaty process and recognition of Aboriginal nations and governments
- recognition of an Aboriginal order of government, subject to the Charter of Rights and Freedoms, with authority over matters related to the good government and welfare of Aboriginal peoples and their territories
- replacement of the federal Department of Indian Affairs with two departments, one to implement the new relationship with Aboriginal nations and one to provide services for non-self-governing communities
- creation of an Aboriginal Parliament
- expansion of the Aboriginal land and resource base
- recognition of Métis self-government, provision of a land base, and recognition of Métis rights to hunt and fish on Crown land
- initiatives to address social, education, health, and housing needs, including the training of 10,000 health professionals over a 10-year period, the establishment of an Aboriginal peoples' university, and recognition of Aboriginal nations' authority over child welfare. (Hurley & Wherrett, 2000)

Additional RCAP recommendations specific to health included reorganizing the existing network of services for Aboriginal peoples into a system of health and healing centres under Aboriginal control, and adapting mainstream services "to accommodate Aboriginal people as clients and as full participants in decision making" (Royal Commission on Aboriginal Peoples, 1996b).

Since the release of the RCAP report, there has been some slow progress in the area of Aboriginal-controlled health services, as well as the identification of Aboriginal health human resources. However, more generally, the Canadian government's lack of implementation of the RCAP recommendations has been extensively criticized by national and international human rights bodies, including the Canadian Human Rights Commission, the United Nations Human Rights Committee, and the United Nations Committee on Economic, Social, and Cultural Rights (Hurley & Wherrett, 2000).

With respect to the development and implementation of Aboriginal-controlled health policies, programs, and services, initiatives vary with respect to the amount and type of Aboriginal input. The current federal government's response to its treaty promise to provide health care for Aboriginal peoples includes the Non-Insured Health Benefits Program, the Community Programs Directorate, and the Primary Care and Public Health Directorate, housed at First Nations and Inuit Health Branch (FNIHB), Health Canada. FNIHB limits their services to First Nations and Inuit peoples who are registered with the Department of Indian and Northern Affairs Canada (INAC) and many of their programs are restricted to people living on-reserve. As mentioned earlier, Métis and First Nations peoples without status are excluded from FNIHB health services, benefits, and programs.

FNIHB infrastructure is systemically geared toward producing centralized policies with respect to First Nations and Inuit health. Their national office generates national-level program and service strategies, which are then devolved in a hierarchical manner to their regional offices. This process limits the opportunities for substantive local input into policy development and too often there is little room for local First Nations and Inuit understandings of health. FNIHB has been working for over 10 years to implement a strategy that would transfer autonomy and control of health programs to First Nations and Inuit communities and, to date, 279 out of 609 communities have signed transfer agreements (First Nations and Inuit Health Branch, 2007a).

These agreements do allow communities the freedom to design new programs and redirect funding to high-priority areas as long as core services are maintained.

However, these agreements come with additional accountability requirements, limited or "enveloped" funds, and are usually restricted to health programs, with FNIHB maintaining control over other programs such as non-insured health benefits (First Nations and Inuit Health Branch, 2007b). The degree to which the FNIHB transfer program is aligned with the principles of self-determination is thus a subject that merits discussion. Some First Nations organizations have requested control for a greater scope of services, which would allow them to undertake a more holistic approach to health service delivery. New models are currently in development (First Nations and Inuit Health Branch, 2005).

Other ongoing challenges for First Nations, Inuit, and Métis health policies, programs, and services are the complexities and lack of clarity in the relationships among federal, provincial/territorial, and local health region jurisdictions. For the general Canadian population, health and public health services are primarily the responsibility of the provinces and territories. However, in the case of Aboriginal populations, provinces and territories often defer their responsibility for the provision of health and public health services to the federal government. But we have seen above that federal services have an on-reserve focus and are limited to First Nations and Inuit peoples registered with Indian and Northern Affairs Canada. Thus, Métis, non-status First Nations, off-reserve First Nations, and Inuit living in the South are caught between jurisdictions, and may receive little or no health and public health services. For example, there is no integrated system to track disease outbreaks among these populations. As the Aboriginal population becomes increasing urbanized, these jurisdictional issues are of escalating urgency. Nationally, First Nations peoples living on-reserve represent only 25 percent of the Aboriginal population. This leaves 75 percent of the Aboriginal population potentially caught between jurisdictions, with unclear accountabilities for their health and public health services.

Central to Indigenous self-determination of health services and programs is the incorporation of Indigenous beliefs, knowledge, and skills at the centre rather than at the margins of Indigenous health policy, programming, and service delivery (International Symposium on the

Figure 19.3: Policy framework, Aboriginal healing and wellness strategy

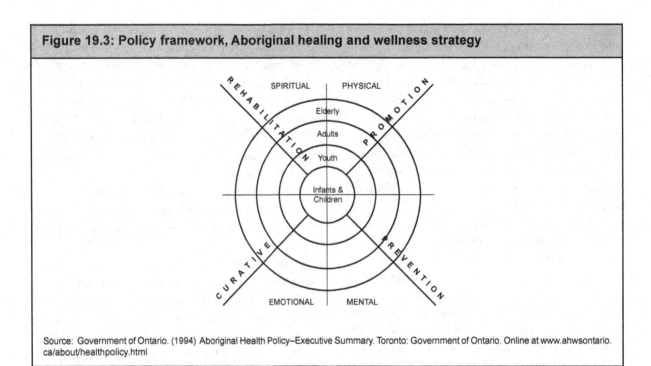

Source: Government of Ontario. (1994) Aboriginal Health Policy–Executive Summary. Toronto: Government of Ontario. Online at www.ahwsontario. ca/about/healthpolicy.html

Social Determinants of Indigenous Health, 2007; Royal Commission on Aboriginal Peoples, 1996a). Fortunately, First Nations, Inuit, and Métis communities have been creative in their responses to federal and provincial policies that, for the most part, continue to marginalize Indigenous perspectives regarding their health and well-being (Royal Commission on Aboriginal Peoples, 1996a; Smylie, Anderson, Ratima, Crengle & Anderson, 2006).

Figure 19.3 displays one of very few examples where such an Indigenous theoretical and mechanistic framework has been at the centre of a health policy, programming, and service-delivery planning and implementation process (Ontario Ministry of Health, 1994). This model clearly demonstrates a linkage between life stages; physical, mental, spiritual, and emotional health; as well as the continuum of health programs and services from health promotion to rehabilitation. This model is in active use by the Aboriginal Healing and Wellness Strategy (AHWS) in Ontario, Canada, which is governed by a joint board that includes representatives from Aboriginal organizations and governing bodies, as well as provincial government departments. The AHWS has been operational for over 12 years, involves 15 Aboriginal and

four provincial government partners, and delivers over $40 million of health programs and services annually to Indigenous peoples living in Ontario (Aboriginal Healing and Wellness Strategy, 2006). AHWS provides over 650 full-time equivalent health service positions. Evaluation of AHWS programming reveals that services meet or exceed expectations for 97.7 percent of participants, with 88 percent indicating that programming was useful and 61 percent reporting an improvement in their health status (Aboriginal Healing and Wellness Strategy, 2007).

Another key requirement in the redress of the historic and ongoing injustices that are at the root of First Nations, Inuit, and Métis health inequities is the resolution of poverty. Earlier in this chapter, we established that the roots of this poverty have clear links to the historic dislocation of First Nations, Inuit, and Métis peoples from their traditional lands. This direct connection between Aboriginal economic marginalization and the ongoing dispossession of Aboriginal peoples from their lands was also clearly recognized by the Royal Commission on Aboriginal Peoples. The RCAP recommended a redistribution of Canadian lands and resources in order to restore Aboriginal self-reliance and autonomy (Royal Commission on Aboriginal Peoples, 1996a). This included legislation to establish new processes and principles for recognized Aboriginal nations to renew their existing treaties or create new ones, with protections to ensure that such negotiations were conducted and financed fairly (Royal Commission on Aboriginal Peoples, 1996a). To date, as with most of the RCAP recommendations, there has been little progress in this area. The Inuit have successfully negotiated four land claims settlement areas: Nunatsiavut, Nunavik, Nunavut, and the Nunakput region (Inuit Tapiriit Kanatami & Inuit Circumpolar Council, 2007). First Nations face over 800 unresolved land claims, with an average of over 13 years to resolve a single land claim issue (Canadian Broadcasting Corporation, 2007).

Recent federal government attempts to improve the land claim process were criticized for not adequately involving First Nations leaders in the development of these policies (Assembly of First Nations, 2007). There has also been little movement forward on the RCAP recommendation regarding a Métis land base. A 25-year-old lawsuit that sought compensation for the lands promised, but for the most part not delivered to Métis under the Manitoba Act, was recently dismissed in court (CTV, 2007).

Given the very slow progress in the restitution of Aboriginal rights, lands, and resources on the domestic front, Aboriginal leaders from Canada have also been actively linking and advocating at an international level.

Box 19.3: List of Indigenous rights pertaining directly to health in the UN Declaration of the Rights of Indigenous Peoples

Article 21

1. Indigenous peoples have the right, without discrimination, to the improvement of their economic and social conditions, including, *inter alia*, in the areas of education, employment, vocational training and retraining, housing, sanitation, health and social security.
2. States shall take effective measures and, where appropriate, special measures to ensure continuing improvement of their economic and social conditions. Particular attention shall be paid to the rights and special needs of indigenous elders, women, youth, children and persons with disabilities.

Article 23

Indigenous peoples have the right to determine and develop priorities and strategies for exercising their right to development. In particular, indigenous peoples have the right to be actively involved in developing and determining health, housing and other economic and social programmes affecting them and, as far as possible, to administer such programmes through their own institutions.

Article 24

1. Indigenous peoples have the right to their traditional medicines and to maintain their health practices, including the conservation of their vital medicinal plants, animals and minerals. Indigenous individuals also have the right to access, without any discrimination, to all social and health services.
2. Indigenous individuals have an equal right to the enjoyment of the highest attainable standard of physical and mental health. States shall take the necessary steps with a view to achieving progressively the full realization of this right.

Article 29

1. Indigenous peoples have the right to the conservation and protection of the environment and the productive capacity of their lands or territories and resources. States shall establish and implement assistance programmes for indigenous peoples for such conservation and protection, without discrimination.
2. States shall take effective measures to ensure that no storage or disposal of hazardous materials shall take place in the lands or territories of indigenous peoples without their free, prior and informed consent.
3. States shall also take effective measures to ensure, as needed, that programmes for monitoring, maintaining and restoring the health of indigenous peoples, as developed and implemented by the peoples affected by such materials, are duly implemented.

Source: United Nations General Assembly. (2007). *United Nations Declaration on the Rights of Indigenous Peoples* (Geneva: United Nations. Online at www.iwgia.org/graphics/syndron-Library/Documents/InternationalProcesses/DraftDeclaration/07-09-13ResolutiontextDeclaration.pdf

Indigenous health stakeholders from Canada were important contributors at the International Symposium on the Social Determinants of Indigenous Health, which has already been described in some detail. Aboriginal organizations from Canada have also been actively involved with the United Nations Working Group on the Draft Declaration of the Rights of Indigenous Peoples (Office of the High Commissioner for Human Rights, 1995). After over a decade of work, this declaration was finalized and adapted by the United Nations General Assembly in September 2007. A listing of the key articles from the UN declaration that pertain to Indigenous health can be found in Box 19.3. Unfortunately, but perhaps not surprisingly, given the current domestic policy record, Canada was one of the four countries that voted against the adaptation of the declaration. Interestingly, Canada was accompanied by Australia, New Zealand, and the United States in its dissent, all relatively affluent countries that conceivably could easily address the underlying inequities facing their minority Indigenous populations.

Conclusion

The chapters in this section of the text highlight the health consequences of inequitable access to societal resources, particular for those population groups that are experiencing restricted access. In this chapter we have detailed how the inequitable and restricted access of First Nations, Inuit, and Métis peoples living in Canada is fundamentally linked to the historic and ongoing processes of colonization. The impacts of colonization have been identified internationally as unique and fundamental social determinants of Indigenous health to which all other Indigenous social and health status inequities are linked. It follows that any attempt to resolve Indigenous social and health status inequities will only be partially successful unless it includes the redress of historic and current colonial policies. In Canada, this would require a redistribution of lands and resources sufficient to restore First Nations, Inuit, and Métis autonomy and self-sufficiency. Each of these populations has unique histories, challenges, and health service needs. Because the majority of Aboriginal peoples in Canada currently live away from their traditional homelands (having been dislocated and/or needing to leave to pursue educational and employment opportunities), this restitution needs to occur in a way that would benefit all First Nations, Inuit, and Métis peoples regardless of their place of residence.

The RCAP report and the UN Declaration on the Rights of Indigenous Peoples set out clear policy frameworks that would enable Canada to attend to its social, moral, and legal obligations to First Nations, Inuit, and Métis peoples both nationally and internationally. As one of the richest countries in the world, Canada is well placed to right past wrongs and ensure that all Canadians, including Canada's First Peoples, are able to enjoy living conditions that promote health and well-being. The biggest barrier at this time appears to be the political will of those who are experiencing privileged access to societal resources, for in our current democratic system, it will be these populations who will have to choose equity and fairness over personal accumulation of wealth.

Notes

1.   This is the Census term used to identify people of First Nations ancestry. It is in quotations marks because the word "Indian" is recognized as a misnomer for Aboriginal peoples of First Nations ancestry.
2.   This term indicates that an individual of First Nations ancestry is federally recognized by the Indian Act.

Critical Thinking Questions

1.   On which Aboriginal groups' traditional land base do you currently live and work?
2.   Who are the First Nations, Inuit, and Métis peoples currently in the region where you live and work?

3. What are their perspectives and understandings of their health and how to improve it?
4. What are the Aboriginal/non-Aboriginal socio-economic and health status disparities in your region?
5. How does your day-to-day life and work impact on these disparities?

Recommended Readings

Anderson, K. & Lawrence, B. (2003). *Strong women stories: Native vision and community survival.* Toronto: Sumach Press.

This collection of 17 essays presents original and critical perspectives from writers, scholars, and activists on issues that are pertinent to Aboriginal women and their communities in rural and urban settings in Canada. Through topics such as the role of tradition, reclaiming identities, and protecting Native children and the environment, they identify the restraints that shape their actions and the inspirations that feed their visions.

Dickason, O.P. (1997). *Canada's First Nations.* Don Mills: Oxford University Press.

Canada's First Nations is an exploration of the experience of these peoples from their first appearance among the giant mammals that once roamed the land to their confrontations with contemporary Canada. Aboriginal peoples have displayed both ingenuity and flexibility in their survival techniques. While the history of Canada's Native peoples is also the history of the exploitation of the North American continent, it also reveals the recreation of the Native community in the fight for land claims, self-government, and recognition of Aboriginal rights.

First Nations Centre, National Aboriginal Health Organization. (2005). *First Nations Regional Longitudinal Health Survey (RHS) 2002/03: Results for adults, youth and children living in First Nations communities.* Ottawa: First Nations Centre. Online at www.rhs-ers.ca/english/pdf/rhs2002-03reports/rhs2002-03-technicalreport-afn.pdf.

The first *Regional Health Survey* took place in 1997 and involved First Nations from all provinces across Canada. The RHS provided, for the first time, a detailed picture of the health of First Nations peoples across Canada. As such, the RHS was established as an invaluable resource for First Nations health care workers; non-Aboriginal health care providers; and federal, provincial, and territorial policy-makers, among others. The RHS 2002–2003 is designed as a longitudinal survey and is considered the most comprehensive study of First Nations health and living conditions in Canada.

Royal Commission on Aboriginal Peoples Report—Highlight from the Report. (1996). Online at www.ainc-inac.gc.ca/ch/rcap/rpt/index_e.html.

This book introduces you to some of the main themes and conclusions in the final report of the Royal Commission on Aboriginal Peoples. That report is a complete statement of the commission's opinions on, and proposed solutions to, the many complex issues raised by the 16-point mandate set out by the Government of Canada in August 1991. Chapters are devoted to major topics such as treaties, economic development, health, housing, Métis perspectives, and the North.

United Nations General Assembly. (2007). *United Nations Declaration on the Rights of Indigenous Peoples.* Geneva: United Nations. Online at www.iwgia.org/sw248.asp.

With an overwhelming majority of 143 votes in favour, only four negative votes cast (Canada, Australia, New Zealand, and the US), and 11 abstentions, the United Nations General Assembly adopted the Declaration on the Rights of Indigenous Peoples on September 13, 2007. The Declaration has been negotiated through more than 20 years between nation-states and Indigenous peoples. Les Malezer, chair of the International Indigenous Peoples' Caucus, welcomed the adoption of the Declaration in a statement to the General Assembly: "The Declaration does not represent solely the viewpoint of the United Nations, nor does it represent solely the viewpoint of the Indigenous

Peoples. It is a Declaration which combines our views and interests and which sets the framework for the future. It is a tool for peace and justice, based upon mutual recognition and mutual respect."

Related Web Sites

Aboriginal Healing Foundation—www.ahf.ca
"Our mission is to encourage and support Aboriginal peoples in building and reinforcing sustainable healing processes that address the legacy of physical abuse and sexual abuse in the residential school system, including intergenerational impacts. We see our role as facilitators in the healing process by helping Aboriginal people help themselves, by providing resources for healing initiatives, by promoting awareness of healing issues and needs, and by nurturing a supportive public environment."

Aboriginal Portal—www.aboriginalcanada.gc.ca/acp/site.nsf/en/index.html
The Aboriginal Canada Portal (ACP) is your single window to First Nations, Inuit, and Métis online resources, contacts, information, and government programs and services in Canada. The Aboriginal Canada Portal is a partnership between government departments and the Aboriginal community, which allows better quality service and information delivery and, to the degree possible, ensures that the site continues to evolve in a user-friendly and useful manner.

Assembly of First Nations—www.afn.ca
The Assembly of First Nations (AFN) is the national organization representing First Nations citizens in Canada. The AFN represents all citizens regardless of age, gender, or place of residence.

Congress of Aboriginal Peoples (CAP)—www.abo-peoples.org
CAP is the national voice of off-reserve Aboriginal peoples throughout Canada. It is a grassroots-driven, national voice for our communities, advocating for the rights and interests of off-reserve and non-Status Indians and Métis peoples, living in urban, rural, and remote areas of Canada.

Inuit Tapiriit Kanatami—www.itk.ca
Inuit Tapiriit Kanatami is the national Inuit organization in Canada representing four Inuit regions—Nunatsiavut (Labrador), Nunavik (northern Quebec), Nunavut, and the Inuvialuit Settlement Region in the Northwest Territories. This site reflects their ancient and modern history and allows communication to the global community instantly, making the notion of a "global village" more real.

Métis National Council—www.metisnation.ca
This Web site is part of the Métis National Council's ongoing efforts to keep the citizens from throughout the Metis Nation Homeland informed on developments and initiatives being undertaken at the national and international level. Since 1983, the Métis National Council has represented the historic Métis nation in Canada at the national and international level.

National Aboriginal Health Organization—www.naho.ca
The National Aboriginal Health Organization (NAHO) is an Aboriginal-designed and -controlled body committed to influencing and advancing the health and well-being of Aboriginal peoples by carrying out knowledge-based strategies. Incorporated in 2000, NAHO is a unique, not-for-profit organization founded upon and committed to unity while respecting diversity. NAHO gathers, creates, interprets, disseminates, and uses both traditional Aboriginal and contemporary Western healing and wellness approaches.

Native Women's Association of Canada—www.nwac-hq.org

The Native Women's Association of Canada (NWAC) is founded on the collective goal to enhance, promote, and foster the social, economic, cultural, and political well-being of First Nations and Métis women within First Nation, Métis, and Canadian societies. NWAC is an aggregate of 13 Native women's organizations from across Canada and was incorporated as a non-profit organization in 1974.

Part Six

Public Policy

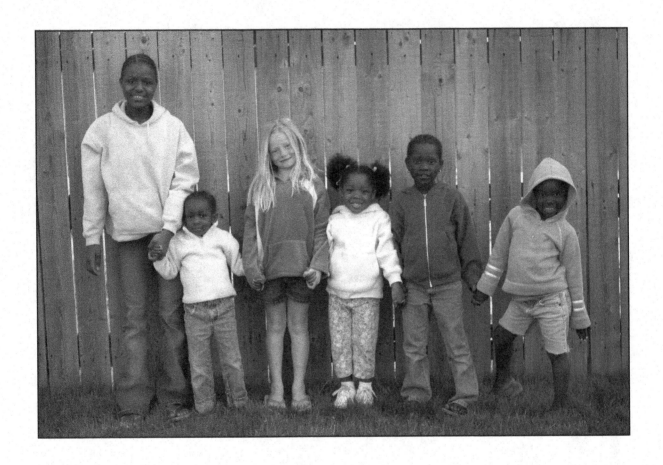

In all of the preceding sections, there has been a clear recognition that the quality of social determinants of health is profoundly influenced by governments' public policy decisions. In this section, specific focus is on public policy developments in Canada and how these influence the social determinants of health. Public policy is primarily concerned with the organization and distribution of economic, political, and social resources. States or governments have the power to intervene to influence the well-being of individuals and the communities in which they reside. These interventions affect the distribution of income, the available health and human services, and the extent of social exclusion. As noted by other contributors, increasing globalization profoundly affects how governments consider and implement public policy. Public policies, therefore, affect the quality of numerous social determinants of health and, by extension, the health of Canadians. And as documented in this volume, women and working, low-income, new, racialized, and Aboriginal Canadians are especially vulnerable to the effects of regressive social policy.

David Langille offers an analysis of the political forces influencing the social determinants of health. The erosion of many social determinants of health, verified by numerous indicators of social well-being in Canada, results from the shaping of Canadian public policy to business needs. The ideology of neo-liberalism, driven by owners and managers of major transnational enterprises, has wielded an enormous influence over public policy. Langille sees the main levers affecting policy related to the social determinants of health as being macroeconomic policy that sets constraints on the role and scope of government. While Canada has never been richer, and never had so many resources as it does now, Canadians have been led to believe that social and other programs are not affordable. The solution to this crisis is a better balance between equality and freedom. Equality must be reclaimed as a positive social value. The means by which this can occur are presented.

Elizabeth McGibbon examines the relevance of a human rights perspective for considering the intersection of the social determinants of health, various personal identities, and geography with access to health care issues. She notes that while there is active debate about whether health care is a social determinant of health, the

clear inequities in access to health care point to such a conclusion. A human rights-based approach to health care would consider how social inequities interact with socially produced health inequities to create profoundly unequal outcomes among various Canadian population groups. She is particularly critical of biomedical and lifestyle approaches for neglecting these important contextual issues and suggests that little progress will be made unless these contextual issues are addressed. McGibbon proposes a number of action strategies for implementing what she terms human rights stewardship in Canadian health care.

Lars Hallstrom provides an in-depth introduction to how political scientists think about public policy and policy analysis. He points out that the role of the state or government is evolving and, some argue, it is losing its ability to influence the lives of citizens. Much of this is due to the marketplace's increasing importance, which is enhanced by increasing economic globalization. These developments provide a backdrop for explaining three differing periods in Canadian public policy-making, culminating in the present neo-liberal period. He then provides a history of health policy in Canada, showing that medicare represents a social democratic approach to governance, which is somewhat inconsistent with the traditional liberal Canadian approach. Seriously addressing the social determinants of health will require policy-makers to intervene more forcibly in the workings of the marketplace and shift health policy from a curative to a preventive emphasis. Whether this is likely remains unclear.

Pat Armstrong discusses the importance of a gender-based perspective for research and public policy-making. The distinction of gender versus sex is explored, as is the relationship between the two. Developments that have facilitated attention to gender as a social determinants of health are reviewed and their implications for health-related research and public policy-making are explored. Examples of gender-based approaches adopted by the Canadian government and various research institutes are provided. Armstrong then goes on to explore how gender provides a lens through which various other social determinants of health can be analyzed for their impact upon women. The relationships among gender and these determinants are profound. She concludes that despite the importance of gender, little research and policy-making incorporates such an analysis. Such neglect results in bad science and bad policy-making.

Dennis Raphael and Ann Curry-Stevens consider the various barriers that work against having a social determinants approach direct public policy-making. These barriers become especially problematic within a political economy that places the marketplace as the primary institution of society. Canada is seen as having a relatively undeveloped welfare state that makes a social determinants perspective difficult to implement. They then direct attention to various models of the public policy-making process to help identify means of having governments address these issues. Finally, they provide an intensive analysis of some of the psychological and social forces that lead to the social determinants of health being so low on the policy agenda. How does the public view health and its determinants? Why are social determinants of health so neglected by health-related institutions and authorities? How can governmental reluctance to address social determinants of health issues be surmounted? Examples of social determinants of health-related activities are provided.

———————●———————

Chapter 20

FOLLOW THE MONEY:
HOW BUSINESS AND POLITICS DEFINE OUR HEALTH

David Langille

Introduction

It has been demonstrated that social factors play an enormous role in determining the health of Canadians. And it is also clear that many of the indicators of social well-being have eroded in recent years. Why has there been this erosion in our social fabric? How can we explain or understand this deterioration?

This chapter shows that Canadian public policy has been moulded to the needs of business over the last three decades. It shows how the ideology of neo-liberalism has been applied in the Canadian context, and how global competition has influenced politics and public policy.

The driving forces shaping our social determinants of health have been the owners and managers of major transnational enterprises—the men who have defined our corporate culture and wielded an enormous influence over public policy. Their main instrument has been macroeconomic policy, which they have used to set constraints on the role and scope of government. They have pushed for Canadian governments to adopt a free market or neo-liberal approach to macroeconomic policy.

The analysis shows that the corporate offensive to regain control over the state was a response to democratic pressure for regulation and redistribution. It shows that democratic politics might once again put the public interest ahead of corporate interests. By identifying the political actors behind what are often seen as impersonal market forces, citizens come to understand that progressive change is possible—and how they might improve the social determinants of health.

Explaining Recent Socio-economic Trends

Out of respect for the complexity and diversity of modern life, we often lose sight of the primary forces driving our society. Perhaps this is deliberate: "Although the knowledge that social and economic inequality produces inequities in health status has long been available, policy-makers avoid their root causes" (Hofrichter, 2003, p. xvii). Why do policy-makers shy away from the root causes of inequality? We need to examine a host of policy changes by federal and provincial governments, policies that not only took apart the social safety net erected by the welfare state in previous decades, but contributed to a fundamental reduction in the role and scope of the state.

There is a tendency to cite economic factors—e.g., lack of funding—as if the economy was some inexorable or omnipotent force that dictated social outcomes. There might be some merit to such an argument if our economy had collapsed, but our gross domestic product (GDP) has increased by 75 percent over the last two decades, from $733 billion in 1986 to $1,282 billion in 2006 (constant 2002 dollars). On a per capita basis, GDP increased 40 percent during this period (Centre for the Study of Living Standards, Tables on Aggregate Income and Productivity, June 22, 2007, Table 1, www.csls. ca/data/iptjune2007.pdf). The country is now far richer and could have sustained or increased expenditures on social programs.

Rather than keep pace with economic growth, overall program spending by all levels of governments fell during the period 1986–2006. At the federal level, total program expenditures fell by 31.5 percent, from 17.1 to 13 percent of GDP (Canada, Department of Finance, 2003, Fiscal Reference Tables, www.fin.gc.ca/frt/2007/ frt07_2e.html#8, Table 8). Provincial and territorial expenditures decreased by 15 percent, from 20.1 to 17.5 percent of GDP (Canada, Department of Finance, 2003, www.fin.gc.ca/frt/2007/frt07_5e.html#31, Table 31). Declining program expenditures cannot be blamed on the costs of servicing public debt.

Total spending (program expenditures plus public debt charges) followed a downward trend regardless of whether debt charges went up or down (Canada, Department of Finance, 2003, www.fin.gc.ca/frt/2007/ frt07_2e.html#8, Table 8; see Table 20.1). Given that our governments could have spent more on program spending but chose to spend less, we are more likely to find our explanation in the realm of politics than economics.

There is no doubt that changing ideology has had an enormous impact, as manifested in the triumph of neo-conservatism or neo-liberalism (Harvey, 2005; Klein, 2007; McBride, 2001; Navarro & Shi, 2003). Both these ideologies celebrate the merits of free enterprise, but the neo-conservatives are more likely to retain a strong state in order to defend religious values, national security, and domestic law and order. Classic examples of neo-conservatism include Ronald Reagan, Margaret Thatcher, and George W. Bush. While neo-liberalism allows more scope for individual rights, they are likely to be more fiscally conservative, keeping government spending and taxation to minimal levels and taking a conservative approach to monetary policy, with strict control over interest rates and the money supply to protect capital against inflation, even if it means slowing down growth and job creation. The ranks of the neo-liberals include Carter and Clinton in the US; Blair in Britain; and Mulroney, Chrétien, and Martin in Canada. Such changes in ideology are important, but we need to probe a little deeper to uncover what these ideologies have in common, where they originated, and how they are being

Table 20.1: Federal budgetary expenses and GDP, 1961–2006, Canada

	GDP per capita (2002 CAD$)	Total federal government spending (per cent of GDP)
1961	$14,512	18.2
1962	$15,238	16.9
1963	$15,751	17.4
1964	$16,459	16.5
1965	$17,189	15.7
1966	$17,998	16.1
1967	$18,189	17.2
1968	$18,774	17.1
1969	$19,435	17.4
1970	$19,749	18.2
1971	$20,127	19.2
1972	$20,802	19.8
1973	$21,987	19.5
1974	$22,480	20.9
1975	$22,562	22.3
1976	$23,419	21.1
1977	$23,943	21.0
1978	$24,638	20.9
1979	$25,327	19.8
1980	$25,557	21.5
1981	$26,117	23.0
1982	$25,069	25.4
1983	$25,493	23.7
1984	$26,721	24.3
1985	$27,742	22.9
1986	$28,136	22.7
1987	$28,965	22.6
1988	$30,002	21.9
1989	$30,262	22.1
1990	$29,861	22.6
1991	$28,872	23.1
1992	$28,783	23.3
1993	$29,118	22.3
1994	$30,190	21.7
1995	$30,715	21.0
1996	$30,888	19.0
1997	$31,872	17.9
1998	$32,894	17.5
1999	$34,435	16.5
2000	$35,905	16.2
2001	$36,164	15.9
2002	$36,807	16.0
2003	$37,132	15.6
2004	$37,896	16.3
2005	$38,681	15.2
2006	$39,354	15.4

Source: Canada, Department of Finance (2003). *Fiscal Reference Tables, October 2003.* Centre for the Study of Living Standards. Online at www.fin.gc.ca/frt/2003/frt03_e.pdf

transmitted—the carriers, bearers, or communicators who propagate the ideology of free markets and less government. For example, the words of academics may have political impact only when they are championed by a think tank and passed on to the mass media, prompting us to ask who sponsors the think tanks and who owns the media.

Public opinion has been manipulated by those who ascribe reduced social spending to a change in public priorities and a preference for tax cuts over public goods. Progressive critics of the welfare state acknowledge that governments failed to sustain the support of many who depended on its largesse (Albo, Langille & Panitch, 1993). But public opinion polls show Canadians routinely prefer public spending to tax cuts. Although some corporate spokespeople blame the public for changing their values or priorities (and do everything within their power to promote such changes), there is strong evidence that Canadians remain a compassionate, caring society that places a high value on public goods and services (Adams, 2003). Why, then, are they not getting policies to reflect their priorities? Perhaps the answer is not so much the corruption of our politicians as the corruption of our political process.

Let us exorcise another suspected culprit, globalization. Apologists for reduced social spending often invoke the need to be competitive and surrender to the dictates of the world economy (D'Aquino & Stewart-Patterson, 2001). As we will see, the same interests have also been working hard to remove whatever protected us from the vagaries of world markets and expose us to more competitive pressures (Clarkson, 2002; Dobbin, 2003a; Klein, 2007; McBride 2001). Globalization is increasingly understood as a political project or process that exploited new technologies of communication and transportation to weaken national barriers and create a world market for the transnational corporations.

An Historical Perspective

It helps to understand the current corporate offensive against the welfare state and the political role of the popular sector if we retrace some history. Although there has been an ongoing struggle between classes inspired by their conflicting interests, our story begins after the Industrial Revolution when the free enterprise of those

dark satanic mills was gradually regulated due to the slow extension of the franchise and the exercise of democratic or popular power. Reforms and concessions were made not only to foster capital accumulation but to maintain the legitimacy of capitalist rule. The welfare state rested on a tension between two systems of decision making: democratic government and the capitalist marketplace. When the conditions were right, the welfare state was a powerful mix and able to beat off challenges from fascism and communism.

Canada was to adopt a welfare state due to the powerful influence of business, which enjoyed a very close and influential relationship with the federal government no matter whether Conservative or Liberal parties were in power (McBride, 2001; Moscovitch & Albert, 1987; Teeple, 2000). Under the rubric of economic development, the state provided business with its infrastructure, its funding guarantees, bailouts, and subsidies. The state also helped to raise the qualifications and reduce the expectations of the labour force, as required. The Canadian political system was described as a confraternity of power, or a system of elite accommodation (Panitch & Leys, 2003). However, there was sufficient democratic pressure from the 1940s to the 1970s that the Canadian state gained greater autonomy from capital than it has enjoyed before or since. As we shall see, this pandering to the popular will sparked a reaction from the corporate community, which launched a political offensive to reassert their control over the state.

Comparisons with the United States often help to clarify what is distinct about Canadian politics. Despite the elaborate system of checks and balances that circumscribe the power of the American state, it has more often served as a tool of populist sentiment—witness the trust-busting era at the turn of the century, and Roosevelt's New Deal during the Dirty Thirties. Canadian business was never subjected to the sort of strict anti-combines legislation as found in the United States; perhaps we place less faith in the merits of free competition. The American state was also more supportive of organized labour, at least for a time in the 1930s and 1940s, and it adopted a stricter set of environmental controls in response to the public interest movement of the 1970s (McCann, 1986). Although Canadians have enjoyed a more extensive welfare state, the Canadian state has, at the same time, been more supportive of or beholden to business. This may be because the state has been dependent on the support of a very concentrated corporate community, which has been more closely tied to capital in London and New York than to their Canadian workers. Given our high dependence on foreign trade and investment, Canadian business leaders have always had a "global consciousness" and have used it to lever support from Canadian governments (McBride, 2001; McBride & Shields, 1997).

Clearly, the state was a terrain of political struggle. Corporate influence was being contested by social movements struggling to exert democratic control, a struggle in which artisans and craft unions, suffragettes, farmers, and industrial unions all played critical roles (Brodie & Jenson, 1988). In fact, the growing strength of the labour movement posed a challenge to business leaders. As labour institutionalized and developed its trade union bureaucracy, so too the business community created its trade associations and chambers of commerce.

We ended up with two systems of representation: political parties and interest groups. "Interest groups" was the term used by liberal-pluralist political theorists to legitimize the influence wielded by these new participants in the political process. It was obvious that individual citizens wielded less influence, and a plurality of groups was preferable in their eyes to a polarization between classes, so they redefined democratic politics as a struggle between competing groups. However, it was misleading to assume any sort of inherent equality or balance between these groups—e.g., between business associations and daycare supporters—and to assume that the state would play the role of a neutral arbiter between them, giving equal attention to all and rendering a balanced decision in the public interest. This was unlikely given that our liberal democracy exists within a capitalist economy, an economic and social system that is structurally imbalanced, dominated by powerful economic interests able to translate their economic power into political influence.

Democracy Delivered! We Won—for a While ...

Under these conditions, ordinary working people have to be mobilized and organized to act in a collective fashion if they are to have political power, i.e., if democracy is

to work. That is what happened—people mobilized and democracy delivered—for a while. There was an upsurge in democratic activity following the Great Depression and the Second World War. First, the labour movement was able to secure their rights to collective bargaining and enjoy a share of increasing productivity. (Unfortunately, the Canadian government's commitment to a Keynesian system of economic regulation began to falter soon after the war when pressure from the political left began to ease. Due in part to the open nature of the Canadian economy, the government was never able to maintain steady growth, full employment, and rising incomes. However, by the time stagflation hit in the mid-1970s and the Keynesian tools were finally abandoned, a social safety net had been erected that helped to protect workers from the worst effects of the economic crisis.)

Meanwhile, the civil rights struggle had erupted, followed by the anti-war movement, the environmental movement, and the struggle for women's rights. It was a time when businesspeople were vilified as polluters and corporate welfare bums, and citizen participation, via public interest groups, helped increase state regulation and redistribution.

Corporate leaders became concerned. A report to the Trilateral Commission in 1975 warned about "an excess of democracy" that was placing too many demands on government (Crozier, Huntington, & Watanuki, 1975). It complained about too much welfare, too much protection for workers, a top-heavy bureaucracy, and too many critics in academe and the media. The answer was to strengthen government's commitment to economic growth by centralizing authority and reducing its susceptibility to democratic inputs from citizens whose diverse demands undermined "efficient planning" (Marchak, 1991). This call was taken up by corporate leaders in all of the industrialized countries where state intervention and labour demands were threatening corporate profits. They organized a political counteroffensive to regain full control of the state (Frank, 2000; Montbiot, 2000; Phillips, 2002).

Capital Strikes Back: A New Era of Corporate Rule

The corporate offensive against the Canadian welfare state was led by the Business Council on National Issues (BCNI). Over the last 30 years, the BCNI, and their new incarnation as the Canadian Council of Chief Executives, has become well known to those familiar with Canadian politics. It was founded in 1976 by corporate leaders anxious to exert more influence over a state that they felt had grown too large and interventionist. They organized 150 chief executives from the major, transnational corporations so as to be able "to contribute personally to the development of public policy and the shaping of national priorities." As their Web site notes, these companies administer $3.5 trillion in assets; earn revenues of over $800 billion per year; and account for a significant majority of Canada's private sector investment, exports, research and development, and training. Although the Business Council on National Issues had always subordinated the national interest in the pursuit of world markets, they changed their name in 2001 to the Canadian Council of Chief Executives when

"it became clear that 'national issues' increasingly had global dimensions" (CCCE Web site, www.ceocouncil. ca/). Box 20.1 shows there are other actors involved in implementing the neo-liberal agenda, but the BCNI/ CCCE has exerted a greater impact on Canadian public policy than any other interest group, social movement, or non-governmental organization (Langille, 1987). Given that all but two or three of its 150 members are men, it is also the strongest institution of patriarchy in the country.

The Canadian Council of Chief Executives is an intersectoral business association that has become the senior voice of business within Canada. It is also a participant in the new right political offensive, which transnational corporations helped inspire throughout the industrialized countries. Discussions of such capitalist restructuring are often conducted at such a level of

---

Box 20.1: The institutions of neo-liberalism in Canada: How corporate priorities are realized

Business Associations

Canadian Bankers Association: The leading lobby group for the chartered and foreign banks. Nancy Hughes Anthony is president and CEO.

Canadian Chamber of Commerce: A coalition of local chambers of commerce representing the interests of many large and small businesses. Perrin Beatty is president and CEO.

Canadian Council of Chief Executives: The voice of big business, representing the 150 CEOs of the major transnational corporations, formerly known as the Business Council on National Issues. Tom D'Aquino is president and CEO.

Canadian Manufacturers and Exporters: Canada's oldest business lobby group represents large manufacturers and exporters. Jayson Myers is president.

Think Tanks

C.D. Howe Institute: The voice of the Bay Street business elite, led by president and CEO William B.P. Robson.

Fraser Institute: Founded in 1974 by Michael Walker to represent the "new right" devotion to free markets. Mark Mullins is the current executive director.

Institute for Research on Public Policy: A liberal response to the economic challenges of the 1970s, allowing more scope for government. Mel Cappe is president.

Citizens' Front Groups

Canadian Taxpayers Federation: A watchdog for the well-to-do against the "special interests" responsible for "runaway spending." John Williamson is the federal director.

National Citizens Coalition: Funded by business leaders to defend individual freedom against government intervention. Peter Coleman is president and CEO.

Lobbyists

"Government relations consultants" hired to help firms increase their influence and gain favours from government. A growth industry in recent years as dozens of firms enter the market. Examples include Earnscliffe, GCI, Hill and Knowlton, and Strategy Corp.

abstraction that we risk losing sight of the political actors. However, political theorists such as Antonio Gramsci, Robert Cox, Stephen Gill, Giovanni Arrighi, Immanuel Wallerstein, and Sidney Tarrow help us appreciate how such structures are socially constructed—to see how social forces make history. It is important to expose in this way what are otherwise seen as impersonal market forces—all-powerful forces that move inexorably and cannot be resisted. Once we appreciate how political actors emerge and trace their struggles over time, we gain a better sense of their vulnerabilities and of the possibilities for opposition forces.

Guided by their primary objective of curbing the role and size of the state, the Canadian Council of Chief Executives (and their former incarnation as the Business Council on National Issues) has helped maintain the fight against inflation, cut back public spending, and restore corporate profits. Their greatest success to date has been to engineer support for high-level agreements facilitating world trade and investment, beginning with CUFTA and NAFTA, agreements that do not guarantee free trade, but serve as a new economic constitution for the Americas, guaranteeing an investment climate conducive to the prosperity and expansion of transnational corporations. These agreements further undermine the sovereignty of the Canadian state and the policy capacity of our provincial governments, which find themselves forced to compete in a process of downward harmonization, offering less services to their citizens in an effort to sustain business confidence. The net effect has been a serious erosion of support for government and a loss of faith in democratic possibilities.

Taking Stock of the Political Dynamics and Assessing the Balance of Forces

As we have seen, Canada's social movements and citizens groups exerted pressure on the state to constrain the corporate sector and redistribute wealth. Threatened with a loss of control and the erosion of profits, the corporations launched a counteroffensive. Quite self-consciously, they have been waging a class struggle and winning. Economic trends, many of them politically inspired, have reinforced the power of capital while weakening the social movements: unemployment (often induced by technological change or other corporate restructuring

initiatives); the increase in part-time work; the erosion of social security; international competition; the mobility of capital and of production; and the deregulation of trade, financial, and labour markets. Consequently, the organizations of capital have not had this much political, economic, or social power in 50 years.

But the popular sector is certainly not powerless or ineffectual. If further evidence is required, one can look at the fluctuations in corporate political activity over the past few decades as they have been forced to respond to threats from below. Although the Council of Chief Executives prefers to maintain a rather low profile and not wield their weight in public, to avoid squandering their political capital or wasting other resources, they have been forced to take public stands on several issues over the past 20 years. In fact, their very origins stemmed from an outbreak of public concern over "corporate welfare bums," and their first action was to collaborate with organized labour in a quest to remove wage and price controls. The BCNI mobilized in the early 1980s in response to the outbreak of economic nationalism associated with the National Energy Program (NEP) and the Foreign Investment Review Agency (FIRA). The organization was then able to lie low during the first Mulroney years, confident that the Conservatives were doing their best to implement the BCNI's agenda. However, in the run-up to the federal election of 1988, they were galvanized to defend the Canada–US free trade agreement when it appeared that opposition forces might derail the deal. The Business Council had to organize the Canadian Alliance for Trade and Job Opportunities and raise many millions of dollars for its advertising campaign in order to win that battle. Also in that decade, the BCNI's Task Force on Defence and International Security responded to pressure from the peace movement, which called for Canada to "refuse the Cruise" and reduce military spending. Instead, they kept flogging the threat of the Soviet Union as an aggressive superpower in order that a few high-tech manufacturers could profit from the arms race. Similarly, the Business Council created its Task Force on the Environment to develop their own interpretation of "sustainable development," and subsequently came out as a leading opponent of the Kyoto Accord, the international effort to reduce the gas emissions that contribute to global warming. The CCCE began clamouring for action on climate change only when the pressure on governments became irresistible, intervening to advocate for market-based solutions rather than regulation (D'Aquino & Dillon, 2008).

Manufacturing the Debt and Deficit Mania

By focusing on the fiscal framework, the Canadian Council of Chief Executives has not dictated all aspects of public policy, but has set the boundaries or constraints on what governments can do. BCNI/CCCE President Tom D'Aquino used to consider the free trade fight to be his greatest victory, and the failure to reduce the deficit his greatest liability. But as soon as the 1988 election confirmed the Canada–US trade agreement, the BCNI launched its campaign to reduce the deficit by cutting government spending. Although the Ontario NDP government tried to use conventional Keynesian techniques to ride out the recession of the early 1990s, they eventually succumbed to the (business) pressure for restraint. The only serious threat to corporate priorities came from within the Liberal Party as it sought to be elected on a commitment to job creation. After the Liberal victory in 1993, there was a further period of uncertainty about which direction the new government would take, and the BCNI resurfaced as vocal champions of deficit reduction. Finance Minister Paul Martin's first budget confirmed the defeat of the reform liberals. Since then the combined efforts of business and government have had a considerable impact on public opinion, generating a deficit mania and a fixation with balanced budgets. Worse still, there have been ideological zealots in both Canada and the US so obsessed with reducing government and cutting taxes that they have been willing to induce a revenue crisis and manufacture a deficit, helping to delegitimate any collective response via public policy.

Paul Martin proved to be the ideal champion of the neo-liberals. The former CEO of Canada Steamship Lines obviously knew about and cared about social problems, yet consistently delivered what was best for business. The legend about Martin designing and delivering an amazing economic recovery in Canada while ridding the nation of chronic deficits was largely a myth. Murray Dobbin has shown that his enormous cuts to health and education did not eliminate the deficit, but rather it was the Bank of Canada's decision to dramatically lower interest rates that sparked a burst of economic growth and generated nearly $100 billion in surpluses from 1997–2003.

Canada's performance in the 1990s was the worst of any decade in the 20th century except the 1930s. By virtually every economic measure of importance—GDP growth, employment, new investment, productivity, standard of living, wages and salaries—the 1990s were a flat-out disaster…. The productivity gap with the U.S. is growing, not shrinking. GDP growth is still anemic, wages and salaries have increased only marginally, job growth is weak and we still have the second-highest number of low-wage jobs among all industrialized countries. We still attract less foreign investment per capita than the U.S., and most of it is used to buy up existing assets. (Dobbin, 2003b, p. B4)

Consistent with corporate priorities, Finance Minister Paul Martin was primarily committed to improving trade. He made cuts of 50 or 60 percent to the many departments that were long associated with nation-building—agriculture, fisheries, transportation, natural resources, regional and industrial development, and the environment. There was such faith that trade would drive the economy that the government abandoned its traditional tools of industrial and regional development, tools that had built the domestic economy. In fact, less than 20 percent of our real GDP is accounted for by trade. The policies designed to facilitate trade benefited a relatively small number of Canadian businesses. Just 4 percent of all exporting establishments accounted for 82 percent of the total value of merchandise exports, while 80 percent of Canadian enterprises do not export at all (Dobbin, 2003b). But those few large companies were there to support Martin when he wanted to lead the Liberal Party and become prime minister. As Professor Bob MacDermid has shown, "Corporations and corporate executives gave over 9 million dollars to Paul Martin's leadership campaign, often giving $100,000 or more" (MacDermid, 2005).

The Social Implications

Martin's legacy was rising inequality. Canada's 100 best-paid CEOs made an average of $8,528,304 in 2006—more than 218 times as much as a Canadian working full-time for a full year would earn on average

(Mackenzie, 2007). Since the BCNI was founded in 1976, disparities of income among Canadians have increased enormously—after-tax median income of the top 10 percent of families was 31 times higher than that of the bottom 10 percent in 1976—and it was 82 times higher by 2004 (Yalnizyan, 2007).

Although there is clear evidence that poverty and inequality reduce health outcomes (Raphael, 2007), there is good reason to question the corporate commitment to address the problem. The CCCE leaders have pledged to "ensure that the real disposable incomes of the worst-off 20 percent of Canadian families—their incomes after taxes, govt transfers and inflation—should grow over the next ten years at least as quickly as that of the average Canadian" (D'Aquino & Stewart-Patterson, 2001, p. 300). That would increase the incomes of poor people by one-third over the decade, which the authors suggest "would clearly represent real progress by any definition," but it would, in fact, mean that they fall further behind other Canadians and it would widen the gap between the rich and poor. While a one-third increase in an income of $9,000 would add $3,000, a one-third increase in an income of $90,000 amounts to $30,000. The corporate executives aren't calling for a substantial reduction in poverty, and they are not even offering to reduce inequality. It's just not on their agenda.

Instead, the CCCE is pushing for increased continental integration. "Canadian business leaders believe that the time has come for the next big step forward in the Canada–United States relationship" (CCCE Web site). The North American Security and Prosperity Initiative was launched in January 2003, and calls for action on five fronts:

- *Reinventing borders*—removing barriers to trade between Canada and the US, and harmonizing our immigration policies
- *Maximizing economic efficiencies*—harmonizing regulations
- *Negotiation of a comprehensive resource security pact*—ensuring free access
- *Reinvigorating the North American defence alliance*—putting more troops and weapons systems under US control
- *Creating a new institutional framework*—creating a stronger partnership

Integrating more closely with the United States could not fail to put further pressure on Canada's frail social safety net and further exacerbate inequalities in income, wealth, and power (Grinspun & Shamsie, 2007).

Corporate Power and Democratic Resistance

Citizens need to know why the corporate leaders have so much power and are able to exert so much influence if they are to challenge their hegemony. As Box 20.2 shows, the power of the Canadian Council of Chief Executives rests primarily on their control over enormous economic assets. But they have also demonstrated very effective political organization—recruiting their members into task forces that served as a virtual "shadow cabinet" for the government—covering the national economy, social policy, political reform, environmental policy, the international economy and foreign affairs, defence, and corporate governance. The council does not typically engage in lobbying and influence peddling to boost the profits of a particular company or sector, but makes an orchestrated effort to create a favourable climate for business—to privilege private, for-profit activity.

In promoting its agenda, the CCCE has been aided by a network of research institutes, including the C.D. Howe and the Fraser Institutes. Most of the corporations that fund and support these institutes are also members of the CCCE. Together, these corporate think tanks organize conferences, seminars, retreats, and briefings on major public policy concerns to which they invite politicians, journalists, academics, and other community leaders or elites. To maintain a common front in the business community, the chief executives consult the heads of the Canadian Chamber of Commerce, the Canadian Manufacturers and Exporters, and le Conseil du patronat in Quebec. While they do not have formal alliances with the National Citizens' Coalition or the Canadian Taxpayers Association, these right-wing networks helped spread their message to the general public.

Box 20.2 also shows how citizens can learn a great deal from the CCCE about how they might mobilize an effective resistance. If citizens are to reassert their power and restore democracy, they will first have to raise public awareness about the threat of corporate control. They will have to elect politicians ready to put citizens first, and that requires not only banning corporate contributions to candidates and parties, but eliminating tax deductions for lobbying or other political activities. We will have to reimpose stronger regulations at both domestic and international levels and withdraw from agreements that put corporate interests ahead of citizens.

What Is to Be Done to Improve the Social Determinants of Health

Based on the foregoing analysis, it appears that a key step to improving the social determinants of health is to curb corporate power and restore democratic control.

If you are a health professional, you have a special responsibility to act and you face special burdens. On the one hand, health professionals are better informed about how social factors affect health outcomes, and they have the capacity to educate for change. On the other hand, the health sciences have a conservative bias whereby health problems are individualized, localized, desocialized, and depoliticized (Hofrichter, 2003). Therefore, in order to be effective, committed health professionals have to become active in the wider community.

The following suggestions are addressed to citizens at large. Rather than look for a single quick-fix solution, action is required on several fronts:

1. Social Movements
This is often where change starts. Get together with people who share your values and lead the struggle for social change. Rather than try to build a movement in support of health, or persuade governments to adopt the social determinants of health framework, work directly to reduce inequality and strengthen our democracy. Tackling the other determinants of health—such as the lack of affordable housing, child care, or food security—is useful, but most of these problems have their roots in the corporate influence over public policy. However, you need not demonstrate in the streets, as most of this work involves educating and organizing. You can also be useful as a chequebook activist, supporting non-governmental organizations involved in research, education, and advocacy.

2. Community
Learn more about the problem and share the information with our families, friends, neighbours, and colleagues.

Box 20.2: Why the chief executives are so powerful—and how citizens can regain democratic control

1. POWER IN NUMBERS
Their power comes from 150 corporations with:
- Assets of $3.5 trillion (up from $440 billion in 1982)
- Earning revenues of over $800 billion/year (up from $170 billion in 1982)
- Employing less than 1.3 million Canadians (down from nearly 2 million in 1982)

What can citizens do?
HAVE POWER IN NUMBERS
- 33 million Canadian citizens
- 6 billion global citizens

2. GOOD POLITICAL ORGANIZATION
- They are pre-emptive and proactive. They have a long-term vision and seize the initiative. Citizens can do that.
- They focus on a few critical areas, and do good research. Citizens can do that.
- They speak everyday language in an effort to define common sense. Citizens can do that.
- They form task forces that shadow government departments and offer new policy initiatives. Citizens can form networks of academics and activists to shadow corporations and government—and offer their own citizens' agenda, alternative budgets, and legislation.
- They champion the national interest, pretending that what's good for the corporations is good for Canada. *But they're the real special interests.*

Such conversations are more persuasive than the mass media, most of which is in corporate hands.

Lessen our dependence on the transnational corporations by producing and consuming more local products. Bio-regionalism saves energy and reduces chemical preservatives. Stronger public services and social enterprises can help us decommodify our lives. Medicare offers a fine model—let's add pharmacare, child care, and home care. Our European trading partners offer free university, so why can't we? Offering free public transit would reduce automobile use and help save our planet.

3. Good Government
Get partisan and help elect progressive political leaders committed to improving the social determinants of health.

Push for more democracy so as to give more people more control over their lives. State power is the most powerful tool available to democrats. Use it to regulate in the public interest. Show how taxes are the best investment for social well-being (see Box 20.3).

Conclusion

This chapter has demonstrated how politics overdetermines the social determinants. It has put a human face on the abstract notions about capital, corporate power, and economic restructuring, so citizens can know in concrete terms who we are dealing with if we hope to regulate and redistribute in the public interest. Regulation and redistribution are key to improving the many social determinants of health. Although some gains can be achieved via local initiatives, it is clear that overall conditions are continuing to deteriorate because the federal and provincial governments are being run according to the needs, interests, and priorities of transnational corporations. Despite their rhetoric to the contrary, such corporate policies stand in fundamental and concrete opposition to the public interest—they are not conducive to improving the health of Canadians.

What are the prospects for the social determinants of health? The Canadian economy is benefiting from a resource boom that is sheltering us from the downturn in the US economy, where years of deficit-financed consumer spending are coming to a crashing end. As the American economy goes into recession, commodity prices will likely drop, and the Canadian dollar will

decline as well. Our economic situation is not based on solid fundamentals—it is more precarious than ever. As David Harvey warns, "when income and wealth inequalities reach a point—as they have today—close to that which preceded the crash of 1929, then the economic imbalances become so chronic as to be in danger of generating a structural crisis" (Harvey, 2005, p. 188).

In retrospect, neo-liberalism delivered wealth for a few, but economic insecurity for the rest. Even when it reached its peak under Clinton and Chrétien, wealth did not trickle down to the majority of working people. Although the rhetoric continues, the neo-liberal dream has lost it lustre and its legitimacy (Harvey, 2005). People want progressive policies that will mitigate their pain and reduce their insecurity, policies that the neo-liberals can't deliver. Progressive politicians seeking popular support have to offer a social democratic program, such as universal health care in the US or a poverty-reduction strategy in Canada.

Unfortunately, there is another route to power, as Naomi Klein (2007) describes in *The Shock Doctrine*. Neo-conservative politicians like Bush and Stephen Harper play on people's fears and prejudices. Their "war on terror" caters to those who sell weapons and oil, but leaves people everywhere feeling more fearful and insecure. Although the tactics of disaster capitalism were politically successful in countries around the world, they turned "the already wealthy into the super-rich and the organized working class into the disposable poor." Klein concludes that "the cost of that victory has been the widespread loss of faith in the core free-market promise—that increased wealth will be shared" (2007, pp. 534–535). There will be little improvement in the social determinants of health if Harper can continue selling our resources with so little concern for sustainability or climate change, or continue to bribe voters with their own tax dollars.

At a philosophical and personal level, the solution is to find a better balance between equality and freedom. We need to reclaim equality as a positive social value—it has gone out of fashion in recent decades, having been squelched in the pursuit of free enterprise. The values of the marketplace—individual greed, fear, insecurity—triumphed, and our rich legacy of social values—compassion, caring, sharing—were demeaned. The pertinent question is: What values should govern

Box 20.3: Impact of $60 billion in tax cuts on the social determinants of health

As Health Studies students, we have learned that social and economic factors have a large influence on our well-being—often more than doctors, drugs, and diagnostic machines. That's why we were concerned to hear the Federal Government announce $60 billion in tax cuts when there are so many pressing social needs in this country.

We were wondering if the Government couldn't have used that $60 billion to eliminate poverty and homelessness, reduce the danger of climate change, fix up our cities, and offer free childcare, homecare, pharmacare or university tuition. So we began investigating how much it would cost to achieve these worthwhile goals which would improve our health (and help create the Canada of our dreams.) Here is what we found:

Aboriginal Issues: It would cost about $5 billion to improve healthcare, education, economic opportunities and housing for First Nations peoples, as First Ministers and First Nations leaders agreed in the Kelowna accord of 2005. An additional $15 billion would settle every outstanding land claim.

Child Care: A universally accessible child care system for children ages 3–5 would cost $3.5 billion annually, and a complete national child care program including early childhood education would cost $10 billion.

Environment: Spending $2.5 billion to generate 12,000 MW of renewable energy would improve our air quality and help to meet our climate change responsibilities under the Kyoto protocol. The Coalition also call for $2 billion to improve energy efficiency in transportation and public housing, $800 million for the retrofit of existing buildings and houses, and $460 million to establish a solar roofs program for private homes. A total investment of $5.76 billion would reduce health service use by $24 billion over a period of 24 years.

Food Security: At $275 per child, it would cost $2.139 billion to provide approximately 8 million Canadian children below age 19 with a nourishing breakfast and lunch through a government-funded school nutrition program.

Health: $26.6 billion per year would cover the cost of prescription drugs for all Canadians. For $6.77 billion per year, Canadians could enjoy universal dental care.

Mental Health: It would cost $17 million to establish a mental health commission; $224 m for a mental health housing initiative; $215 m for a "basket" of community service initiatives; $50 m to implement a concurrent disorders program; $2.5 m to improve telemental health for distant and inaccessible communities, another $2.5 m to develop peer-support programs; and $25 m to continue and enhance research, totaling to $536 million annually or $5.5 billion over a ten-year implementation period.

Housing: Funding for affordable housing in Canada has declined sharply in the last twenty years. Canada is now the only developed country without a national housing strategy. At the same time, the gap between new affordable housing units and new market-rent units is growing. An annual investment of $2 billion would restore previous federal funding for social housing, ensuring an adequate supply of affordable, decent housing for low-income families.

Seniors: The $60 billion tax cut could have been used to double Old Age Security payments from a maximum of $500 per month to $1000 per month, and double the Guaranteed Income Supplement from $600 to $1150 per month maximum, That would mean 4 million seniors might receive $12,000 per year, and 500,000 low-income seniors receive $25,800.

University Education: About $4.4 billion annually would remove tuition costs for all students currently enrolled in Canadian universities. (Using data from the Canadian Information Centre on International Credentials.)

Obviously we cannot solve all of these problems at once, but accomplishing any one of them would have made Mr. Harper a great Canadian prime minister. Poll after poll reminds us that tax cuts are not the priority for Canadians. Given the choice, they would rather see our governments invest in health, education, the environment or other problems.

How we spend our money is a reflection of our priorities—it reflects our values as a nation. As citizens we need to ask, what values shall govern Canada?

Source: The Students of UNI 300: An Introduction to Health Care Policy in Canada, University of Toronto.

Canada?

Critical Thinking Questions

1. Why are governments and the medical establishment not taking faster action to improve the social determinants of health?
2. Based on what you have read in this chapter, how can citizens improve the social determinants of health? What should we expect of the health community?
3. If there was strong political support for improving the social determinants of health and a government committed to that goal was elected, what obstacles would the government face?
4. What can we learn from the Canadian Council of Chief Executives about how to influence the policy agenda and improve the social determinants of health?
5. Given all the evidence against delivery of health care for profit, who exactly is pushing for privatization and greater reliance on the market? Identify the individuals and organizations locally, provincially, and nationally.

Recommended Readings

Canadian Council of Chief Executives. (2004). *A Canadian agenda for progress and prosperity: Where Canada's business leaders stand.* Ottawa: Canadian Council of Chief Executives.

A comprehensive summary of the CCCE's positions across the full spectrum of economic and social policy, at home and abroad. It is organized along three key strategic themes: setting the fiscal framework, encouraging innovation and competitiveness, and fostering human and community development.

Clarkson, S. (2002). *Uncle Sam and us: Globalization, neoconservatism, and the Canadian state.* Toronto: University of Toronto Press.

While Clarkson focuses on how Canada has always been strongly influenced by its southern neighbour, he offers a good guide to understanding how public policy in this country is being affected by the corporate pressure for further continental integration.

Dobbin, M. (2003). *The myth of the good corporate citizen: Democracy under the rule of big business* (2nd ed.). Toronto: James Lorimer.

An account of how corporate globalization has affected Canadians by undermining our democracy and eroding our social and economic well-being.

Doern, B. (Ed.). (2007). *How Ottawa spends 2007–2008: The Harper Conservatives—climate of change.* Montreal & Kingston: McGill-Queen's University Press.

This annual series offers chapters analyzing the politics and public policy of particular sectors such as education, health care, housing, pensions, poverty, and deregulation.

Hofrichter, R. (Ed.). (2003). *Health and social justice: Politics, ideology, and inequity in the distribution of disease.* San Francisco: Jossey-Bass.

This collection offers a broader analysis of the politics of health inequalities, covering the effects of racism, social class, and gender discrimination. It also examines the political implications of various perspectives used to explain health inequities and explores alternative strategies for eliminating them.

McBride, S. (2001). *Paradigm shift: Globalization and the Canadian state.* Halifax: Fernwood.
    McBride reveals how the pressure to remove obstacles to global trade and investment has contributed to growing inequality and insecurity, as well as undermining Canadian sovereignty and democratic governance.

Related Web Sites

Canadian Centre for Policy Alternatives—www.policyalternatives.ca
    The CCPA conducts research on issues of social and economic justice and produces a range of publications, including a monthly digest of progressive research and opinion.

Canadian Council of Chief Executives—www.ceocouncil.ca
    Given how the most powerful pressure group in the country manages to set the agenda for government, watch this site in order to keep abreast of emerging trends in Canadian public policy.

Canadian Policy Research Network—www.cprn.com
    The CPRN's mission is to create knowledge and lead public debate on social and economic issues important to the well-being of Canadians.

Centre for Social Justice—www.socialjustice.org
    The CSJ undertakes research, education, and advocacy in an effort to narrow the gap in income, wealth, and power. It offers a range of materials covering the social determinants of health.

Institute for Research on Public Policy—www.irpp.org
    The IRPP seeks to improve public policy in Canada by generating research, providing insight, and sparking debate on public policy.

Chapter 21

———————⬤———————

HEALTH AND HEALTH CARE:
A HUMAN RIGHTS PERSPECTIVE

Elizabeth McGibbon

We take it as a basic fact that we all live and act in bodies that literally embody—biologically, across the lifecourse—our societal and ecological context. (Krieger, 2005, p. 8)

Introduction

In Canada, health care includes health care services, health promotion, public health, and prevention (Health Canada, 2008). It is now widely acknowledged that health is related to a broad range of goods and services beyond health care. There is continued debate regarding whether or not health care ought to be considered a social determinant of health (SDOH). Although it is sometimes included in lists of SDOH (*Ottawa Charter*, 1986; *Toronto Charter*, 2004), it is not included in important Canadian health system-based frameworks of the SDOH (Public Health Agency of Canada, 2006; Canadian Nurses Association, 2006), or in the World Health Organization's SDOH frameworks (Wilkinson & Marmot, 2003). The *Toronto Charter* SDOH include: early childhood development, employment and working conditions, income and its equitable distribution, food security, health care services, housing, education, social exclusion, and social safety nets. Since increases in health care expenditures have not resulted in improvements in population health, health care services are sometimes not viewed as a social determinant of health. However, analysis of the relationships among health care and health outcomes have largely focused on comparisons of health system expenditures, service availability, service-utilization rates, and population health statistics. Inequities in access are not considered in the equation.

If we assume that all Canadians enjoy equal access to health care, these analyses certainly indicate that increasing health care expenditures does not improve the health of a society. Yet there has been little sustained examination of how inequities in access to health care are linked to morbidity and mortality. Not surprisingly, inequities in access are intimately related to the social determinants of health. These inequities are broad in scope and include everyday, local barriers such as lack of money for transportation to health care appointments, and less concrete barriers such as health care providers' lack of cultural competence. Barriers related to inequities in health service access are linked to inequities in health outcomes and the systemic, policy-based obstacles that sustain them. Explicit attention to policy-sustained inequity requires a human rights approach to health system change. Health systems promote "health equity when their design and management specifically consider the circumstances and needs of socially disadvantaged and marginalized populations, including women and their children, the poor, and groups who experience stigma and discrimination, thus enabling social action by these groups and the civil society organizations supporting them" (Gilson, Doherty, Loewenson & Francis, 2007, p. v).

This chapter focuses on a human rights perspective to guide stewardship in Canada's health care system, and draws upon an intersectionality methodology. Health system change is discussed in terms of inequities in access to health care at the intersections of: (1) SDOH; (2) identity; and (3) geography. The social determinants of mental health are discussed in the context of the medicalization of oppression. Lifestyle approaches to primary health care are critiqued using an anti-oppressive participatory framework, and suggestions are made for an equities-competent health care system. Concern is raised regarding the increasingly influential role of multinational pharmaceutical corporations in shaping and directing Canada's health care system. The chapter concludes with a summary of action strategies for human rights stewardship in Canadian health care.

Health System Change through the Lens of Human Rights

The social movement to link health and human rights is relatively recent. The United Nations (UN) implemented the first worldwide public health and human rights strategy in the 1980s through its global program in AIDS. Further, the World Health Organization's (WHO) initiatives in the 1990s, based on the UN Charter of Rights and Freedoms, brought health and human rights together in international law (Gruskin, Mills & Tarantala, 2007). Decades earlier, in the challenge of the Jim Crow laws, which legalized the dehumanization of African-Americans, leaders in the civil rights movement in North America linked civil rights with the right to health care, based on the lack of access to basic health care for African-American people. The successful challenge of these laws led to the creation of a civil rights report card, which detailed the results of human rights violations in the United States health care system (Smith, 2005a). This direct link between human rights and health care remains one of the earliest strategies to address health inequities through legalization of equitable health care treatment. A human rights perspective on health care reframes healthy population outcomes as a legal entitlement rather than a desired, but not always achievable, goal. The movement toward defining health as a human right requires a social injustice-based analysis of the relationships among health and social policy decisions, health and social service

expenditures, population health outcomes, and the social determinants of health.

The Canadian Charter of Rights and Freedoms (1982), and a number of international human rights instruments that Canada has ratified, provide a legal and social policy basis for civil society pressure to remove barriers in access to health care. Relevant international documents include the United Nations Universal Declaration of Human Rights (1948), the International Covenant on Economic, Cultural, and Social Rights (1966), and the Convention on the Elimination of All Forms of Discrimination against Women (1979). For example, the latter convention obligates the state to uphold the right of rural women to "have access to adequate health care facilities, including information, counseling and services in family planning ... to enjoy living conditions, particularly in relation to housing, sanitation, electricity and water supply, transport and communications" (United Nations General Assembly, 1979). The Convention on the Rights of the Child (1989), Article 24, requires that states "recognize the right of the child to the enjoyment of the highest attainable standard of health and to facilities for the treatment of illness and rehabilitations of health ... and strive to ensure that no child is deprived of his or her right of access to such health care services" (1989). Under Canada's Charter of Rights, Section 15, inequitable access to health care is unconstitutional.

The sheer weight of evidence regarding inequities in health care treatment and health outcomes requires a systems-based and human rights perspective beyond individual biophysical status and genetic endowment. Systemic social structures influence the distribution of wealth and thus the distribution of physical and psychological wellness. A country's political, economic, and social structures and policy processes are a determinant of the health status of its citizens. When social democratic principles are used as a policy compass in nations, citizens have better health outcomes. Countries with social democracies tend to have the best health outcomes of all nations (Navarro, 2002). Canada, once a leader in progressive principles of equity and participation in approaches to public health, has fallen behind other nations due to its shift from community-based health promotion to other areas such as disease and infection control, and lifestyle approaches such as smoking cessation, exercise, and diet (Raphael & Bryant, 2006).

Government commitment to Tommy Douglas's vision for health care has gradually shifted from concerns about universal and equitable access to the development of an increasingly market-driven health care system. Douglas, known as the father of Canadian social medicine, successfully lobbied for a universally accessible health care system, which was nationally legislated in 1966. Douglas's vision for the health of Canadians focused squarely on designing and sustaining public policy to promote equity and dignity in the provision of health care. Privatization of health care is underway in Canada, reinforced by the Canadian Medical Association's Medicare Plus recommendations: "If, and only if, the public system fails to provide timely care, Canadians should have access to private insurance that can cover the cost of obtaining care in the private sector" (Canadian Medical Association, 2007, p. 685). A two-tier health care system, with private-pay clients, will create differential access based on ability to pay—the very problem that prompted Douglas to fight for social medicine in the 1960s. Inequitable access to health care, even in the publicly funded system, is not supported by Canadian law. Although the Canada Health Act (1984) legislated universality and accessibility in Canada's health care system, equitable access to health care is a human right that has not been realized for millions of Canadians.

Inequities in Health Outcomes and Access to Health Care

Inequities in access to health care have become an important benchmark of systemic inequities. In Canada "there is a strong 'pro-rich,' 'pro-educated,' 'anti-poor,' and 'anti-non-educated' bias in the probability of receiving any care from a specialist" (Curtis & MacMinn, 2007, p. 23). The debate about whether or not health services are a social determinant of health needs to shift to a sustained examination of the relationships among systemic barriers in access to health care, and the resulting devastating impact on the health of many Canadians who do not have equitable access to the goods and services of our health care system. These barriers have their genesis in economic inequity, social disenfranchisement, and systemic oppression that is reflected in the health care system. In other words, *it may not be so much that health service expansion is not influencing health outcomes,* *but rather that expansion of services, which do not explicitly address inequities in service access, show no positive impact on health outcomes.* Since increases in conventional medical services do not necessarily improve health outcomes, it is important to address barriers and poor health outcomes, which are created by providing non-participatory health care.

The health sector has been relatively slow in grasping the connections among human rights, social injustice, and how everyday life unfolds for patients. The quest for scientific objectivity has made it very difficult to come to grips with the lived experience of oppression, and the relationships among physical and mental health outcomes and oppression. Scientific objectivity, in the form of biomedicine, requires a social context-free analysis of health problems (McGibbon, 2000). This is, in part, why substantial advances in areas such as cardiac care and diagnostic and treatment practices may have only a marginal effect on the population health of marginalized and racialized people and groups. For example, population health database analyses have shown that people diagnosed with a mental illness in Nova Scotia have significantly increased mortality from cancer, diabetes, heart disease, and cerebrovascular disease. Limited access to services was cited as possible contributing factor (Kisley et al., 2005). First Nations peoples living on reserves have reported rates of heart diseases 16 percent higher than the overall Canadian rate (Statistics Canada, 2001), and First Nations women and men have life expectancies 5.3 and 7.4 years shorter, respectively, than overall Canadian rates (Health Canada, 2003). Chronic and infectious disease rates are higher in Indigenous (First Nations, Inuit, and Métis) peoples on- and off-reserve than in non-Indigenous Canadians: arthritis and rheumatism (26 percent for Indigenous peoples, 16 percent for non-Indigenous), high blood pressure (15 percent vs. 13 percent), and tuberculosis rate per 100,000/year (21 vs. 1.3) (Canadian Population Health Institute, 2004).

Studies have shown decreased access to services for African-Americans, even when insured and non-insured statuses are taken into account. Black women are statistically significantly less likely than White women to have received minimum expected therapy for breast cancer (Breen et al., 1999). In some studies, Black women have been shown to be 70 percent more likely to die of cervical cancer, more likely to be diagnosed at a later stage of the cancer, and less likely to receive treatment than white women (Brooks et al., 2000; Edwards & Buescher, 2002). African-Americans are significantly less likely to receive major colorectal treatment for their cancer, follow-up treatment, or chemotherapy (Ball & Elixhauser, 1996; Cooper, Yuan & Rimm, 2000; Schrag, Cramer, Bach & Begg, 2001). African-American lung and cancer patients are less likely to receive chemotherapy (Earle et al., 2000), and more likely to receive no treatment for prostate cancer (Mettlin, Murphy, Cunningham & Menck, 1997). Although most available statistics regarding the health of peoples in the African diaspora are United States-based, there is no reason to believe that rates in Canada are not similar. Population health statistics, such as these, direct attention to factors such as gender, race, and age as determinants of health care access and physical and mental health outcomes.

Further, to complicate any health system analyses regarding inequitable access to services, some of our *health*-related services are actually provided outside of the health system, as previously defined, especially for more vulnerable populations. Thoughtful health services and population health outcomes analyses need to acknowledge this issue. For example, early intervention services for children and families grappling with a variety of developmental delays and related issues are often delivered by community-based, not-for-profit agencies. In Atlantic Canada and other regions, these organizations typically lobby to garner non-core funding annually from a whole host of unpredictable and unsustainable funding sources, including provincial and federal governments, registered charities, and the communities at large. This is often the state of services for some of our most disenfranchised and marginalized citizens, including children with chronic health issues, pregnant teens, and homeless youth.

Intersectionality and Access to Health Care

At the core of a human rights perspective on health care is the concept of oppression. Intersectionality is a framework that recognizes the synergistic effects of various forms of oppression. The framework has been used to describe the interwoven influences of identities

such as gender, sexual orientation, race, ethnicity, (dis)ability, and age on experiences of injustice (James, 2003; Dei & Calliste, 2000). Some definitions of the SDOH have begun to include identities such as gender and race, which have been established as predictors of health outcomes. Evolving definitions notwithstanding, complexities in access to health care may usefully be considered within an intersectionality framework that includes SDOH, identity, and geography. Figure 21.1 depicts the intersections of the social determinants of health, identity, and geography. This section provides some current Canadian and international statistics to underscore the meaning of intersectionality in terms of health care access.

When individuals and families access health care, they arrive with more than their immediate physical and mental health concerns. The intersections of their identities (i.e., age, gender, race, social class) and intersections of their social determinants of health (i.e., early childhood development, employment) are inextricably linked to their health concerns. Statistics in the previous section provided evidence of the direct and often devastating relationship between these intersectionalities and inequities in access to health care. For example, the vast majority of health care in Canada is provided with the assumption that individuals and families can afford costs currently considered as peripheral: transportation, prescription medications, over-the-counter antibiotics and anti-inflammatory drugs, orthopaedic braces, time away from work, child care, and so on. Adequate employment and income thus become prerequisites for full health care access, particularly for rural, remote, and northern Canadians.

Health care then becomes a powerful determinant of health by virtue of its neutrality or presumptuousness regarding these hidden costs of full access, and its employment-neutral stance regarding which Canadians can or cannot afford access and health-maintenance costs. When individuals and families cannot afford to follow up on recommended treatments due to lack of money, they are at risk for being labelled "non-compliant" and thus having their health problems blamed on their lack of initiative. Lack of affordability is age-, gender-, race-, and social class-related. Canada now has 15.5 percent of children living in "relative poverty," defined as households with income below 50 percent of the national

Figure 21.1: Health care access and intersectionality lens

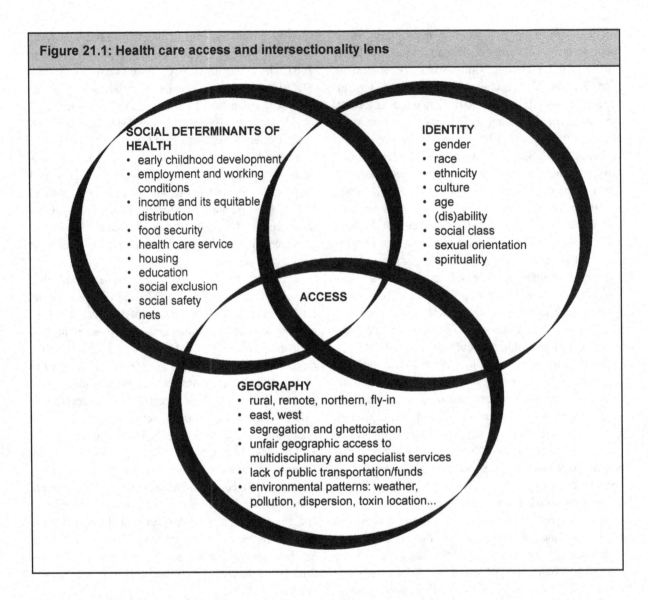

SOCIAL DETERMINANTS OF HEALTH
- early childhood development
- employment and working conditions
- income and its equitable distribution
- food security
- health care service
- housing
- education
- social exclusion
- social safety nets

IDENTITY
- gender
- race
- ethnicity
- culture
- age
- (dis)ability
- social class
- sexual orientation
- spirituality

ACCESS

GEOGRAPHY
- rural, remote, northern, fly-in
- east, west
- segregation and ghettoization
- unfair geographic access to multidisciplinary and specialist services
- lack of public transportation/funds
- environmental patterns: weather, pollution, dispersion, toxin location...

median, thus ranking 17th/23 in developed countries (UNICEF, 2005). Canadian women are less likely to be employed and they earn an average of only 62 percent of what men earn. The income of women aged 55–64 is barely over half that of men in their pre-retirement years (Statistics Canada, 2005).

Gender

Gender intersects with race to cause an even higher rate of unemployment among immigrant, Indigenous, and African-Canadian women (Galabuzi, 2006; Statistics Canada, 2006; Stout & Kipling, 1998). Poverty has been directly linked to decreased access to health care and

decreased health outcomes. Here the intersections of age, race, gender, and social determinants of health, such as employment and income, combine to limit health care access. Immigrant women of colour, who earn less than the Canadian average for women, face additional barriers related to geography, since their extended families are often far away and many immigrant individuals and families lack the resources to maintain connections with their country of origin. Senior Canadians are at particular risk, regardless of gender, race, or ethnicity, since home care or family care is becoming medical support "on the cheap." Family members, usually women, have taken on the additional burden of home care. "Canada's health care system is becoming de-institutionalized but no less medicalized" (McDaniel & Chappell, 1999, p. 129).

Women with disabilities are twice as likely to be unemployed when compared to the Canadian average for women. In 2000, women with disabilities aged 15 and over had an average income from all sources of $17,200, almost $5,000 less than women without disabilities, and $9,700 less than men with disabilities (Statistics Canada, 2005). Low income has particular consequences for people with disabilities, who have the additional burden of costs such as those associated with mobility enhancement, special diets, and rehabilitation. Men in the poorest income groups have the highest rates of ischemic heart disease in Canada (Canadian Population Health Institute, 2006). In 1996, 36.8 percent of women and 35 percent of men in racialized communities were low-income earners, compared to the Canadian average of 19.2 percent and 16 percent respectively. In 1995, the rate of children living in poverty in racialized communities was 45 percent—almost twice the overall Canadian rate of 26 percent (Galabuzi, 2006). For these children, age, race, social class, and family employment status intersect to create enormous barriers in access to health care. Family access to adequate full-time employment with benefits, and thus money, is a powerful indicator of their capacity to successfully navigate the health care system.

Geography

Geography is increasingly cited as a determinant of health. Rural, remote, "fly in", northern, and urban location all impact on health care access and health outcomes. Eastern Canadians experience the poorest health outcomes in Canada when compared to the health of the general population. The Maritime region has one of the highest percentages of rural populations in Canada (Canadian Population Health Institute, 2006). Degree of rurality contributes to health indicators above and beyond socio-economic factors, and living in areas with low population density is associated with special health risks. Macroeconomic changes, such as boom-and-bust economic cycles, which particularly impact rural communities, have an especially negative effect on the health of rural communities, particularly those with dependence on one industry for economic sustainability. Rural Canadians are more likely to report poorer socio-economic conditions and lower educational attainment, and to have higher overall mortality rates (Canadian Institute for Health Information, 2006).

Women living in the most rural areas form the highest proportion of people reporting fair/poor health (Canadian Institute for Health Information, 2006). In 1996, infant mortality rates in rural areas were 30 percent higher than the national average (Ministerial Advisory Council on Rural Health, 2002). In terms of rural, remote, and northern health care, there is a lack of diagnostic services, poor access to emergency and acute care services, lack of non-acute health services, and underservicing of special needs groups, such as seniors and people with disabilities. Health care restructuring has centralized or reduced acute care services without enhancing community-based services (Ministerial Advisory Council on Rural Health, 2002). Rural, remote, and northern geographic regions are home to over 50 percent of Canada's 1.4 million Indigenous peoples. The health status of rural Indigenous peoples follows the same pattern of decreased life expectancy and increased morbidity as Canada's Indigenous peoples as a whole.

The geography of segregation and its relationship to health care access and health outcomes has barely begun to be investigated in Canada. Current efforts to eliminate racial and ethnic disparities in health care treatment fail to address the effect of segregation—the physical separation of the races in residential contexts—on health disparities. Segregation causes racial disparities in health (Smith, 2005; Williams & Collins, 2001). Recent literature suggests a growing relationship between the clustering of certain visible minority groups in urban neighbourhoods and the spatial concentration of poverty in Canadian cities, raising the spectre of ghettoization (Galabuzi, 2006; Walks & Bourne, 2006). Since health care access is often dependent upon economic status (money for transportation, employment benefits, medications, etc.) and the cultural competence of service providers, segregation based on race has important implications for access to health care and the already evident racial disparities based on segregation. The unjust historical legacy of segregation of Canadian Indigenous peoples on reserves continues today.

Geography is relational: rural, remote, northern, eastern, western, urban, geographic segregation and ghettoization, weather patterns (especially in the North), and pollution dispersion patterns all contribute and intersect to shape the health status of Canadians and their access to health care and other services. People living in geographies with high pollution rates have an unfair toxic burden that is not necessarily reflected in increased access to cancer and respiratory health care. Hazardous waste facilities, landfill sites, and incinerators are all disproportionately located near communities of colour, regardless of country or region (Cole & Foster, 2000). Geography thus acts as a foundation that underscores health system inequities.

Health care design and delivery—which do not have the policy-driven capacity to accommodate intersections of SDOH, identity, and geography—will continue to create and sustain inequities in health care access and in health outcomes. When one considers the relationship between access and health outcomes, it is not surprising that increases in intersectionality-neutral or intersectionality-biased health care do not improve the overall health of Canadians. The following real-life case example (Box 21.1) illustrates the complex struggle for many Canadians when they attempt to navigate a health care system that does not yet have the capacity to accommodate and embrace intersectionality.

Recognizing that there are long-standing and complex problems with the publicly funded health and human services system for the child and youth population, innovative ways to coordinate interdepartmental and cross-sectoral policy development, priority setting, service planning, and service implementation have been piloted over the past decade in Canada. The interorganizational and interdepartmental Child and Health Network model, pioneered in eastern Nova Scotia and embraced by the Nova Scotia provincial government, has been shown to be particularly favourable, especially in terms of increasing system sensitivity and responsiveness to the population's needs. This model has also flourished in several other Canadian provinces, including British Columbia, Alberta, and Ontario (McPherson, Popp & Lindstrom, 2006). Cross-sectoral governmental teamwork is foundational to the success of countries such as Sweden in addressing population health inequities (Clancy, Adshead, Laurell & Carlson, 2005).

Human Rights and the Social Determinants of Mental Health

The rurality tax calculations and access costs in the above case example could readily be applied to access to mental health and addictions services. Intersections of the SDOH, identity, and geography create similar barriers in access to mental health care, and play an important role in mental health outcomes. For example, social determinants of health such as employment, working conditions, and housing have long been associated with an individual's mental health and resiliency. Similarly, gender, race, and age are markers of mental health (Ali, Massaquoi & Brown, 2003; Enang, 2001; McIntyre, Wien, Rudderham, Etter, Moore, MacDonald & Johnson, 2001). Depression serves as a case in point. Depression, predicted to be the second leading cause of global disability burden by 2020, is twice as common in women (World Health Organization, 2006a). In Canada, 9.2 percent of women are at probable risk of depression, compared to 5 percent for men (Hayward & Colman, 2003). Elderly women have the highest rates of depression, and being a woman is a significant predictor of being prescribed mood-altering psychotropic drugs. An estimated 80 percent of 50 million people affected by violent conflicts, civil wars, disasters, and displacement are women and children. The high prevalence of sexual violence to which women are subjected has been positively related to the fact that they are the largest single group of people who suffer from post-traumatic stress (World Health Organization, 2006a).

Not surprisingly, depression and post-traumatic stress are often experienced together. Depression in women and men has been linked to unemployment and adverse working conditions (Bonde, 2008), which are disproportionately experienced by people in the lower socio-economic gradients; people of colour; and people with disabilities, regardless of gender. Social class exploitation sets the stage for, and interacts with, racial discrimination to determine racial inequalities in physical and mental health (Oliver & Muntaner, 2005). Depression is a major risk factor for heart disease, cancer, and other chronic physical illnesses (Pratt, Fred, Crum, Armenan, Gallo & Eaton, 1999). Research has shown that racial discrimination is associated with depression, thus creating a double jeopardy for people of colour, and triple

Box 21.1: Case example

Health for some: Chronic illness, rurality, and Canada's working poor

Marya (pseudonym) is seven years old. She has recently been diagnosed with juvenile rheumatoid arthritis (JRA), an autoimmune condition that causes, among other problems, painful and possibly deforming swelling in her joints, particularly her ankles, her wrists, and her knees. Her family lives in a rural area where there are no clinicians with expertise in rheumatology, or its subspecialty, JRA. The nearest pediatric rheumatologist is a two-and-a-half hour drive away. Appointments are routinely booked without consultation regarding family availability, and cancelling an appointment results in delays of up to six months for another appointment, even if Marya's condition worsens. Mom works as a cashier at a large supermarket ($9/hour), and Dad works as a carpenter ($23/hour). His work is seasonal. Since the family must travel two-and-a-half hours to the city for an appointment, one of the parents must negotiate a full day off work, thus losing a day's pay (the average is $120 in lost wages). Marya also has other autoimmune conditions, and her long-term prognosis remains precarious and thus very worrisome for her parents. The family has a car, but it is used only for local travel due to its condition. They borrow a neighbour's car (gas and mileage = $210 return). Even though the neighbours will not charge mileage, the material cost is still incurred.

The appointment with the rheumatologist happens in tandem with other specialist appointments with an occupational therapist and a physiotherapist. At the occupational therapy appointment, the therapist fits Marya with special support braces for her wrists. After the fitting and moulding of the braces is complete, the parents are told that they must pay for the braces. They receive the bill two weeks later ($88). The occupational therapist recommends over-the-counter ankle supports for both ankles, which Marya finds very helpful in decreasing her pain ($50). Marya's wrist movements are increasingly painful, and the physiotherapist recommends regular warm-wax treatments at home. The device for warm-wax treatments costs $425. The family opts for a double boiler ($40) and buys the first batch of wax at the grocery store ($8); however, Mom and Dad worry about the safety of implementing the wax treatments at home.

The physician recommends methotrexate, an immune system suppressant. Neither of the parents has a drug plan through employment. The drug costs $38/month, and Marya requires three refills before her next appointment ($114). Between appointments, the family has access to the hospital's nurse clinician, who provides expertise via phone consultation as needed. Due to complications with medication, it has been necessary to consult the nurse clinician five times since Marya's last appointment ($70 long-distance charges). Marya develops movement-restricting deformities in some of her fingers. Her parents try to negotiate some adjustment with her school, and they are told that they will have to go through a process of having Marya declared disabled in order to obtain the laptop computer she needs to be able to write in class ($1,500). Dad works with his extended family to navigate the application process, but Marya must go without the computer, and is unable to take notes without a high level of pain, for at least her first term in grade two. Marya's parents strongly desire the expertise of a naturopathic physician who will work with their rheumatologist ($125 initial consultation). They have friends who have had very encouraging results with such an arrangement, and there is a highly respected naturopath with a rural practice near their home. They cannot afford the naturopath.

TOTAL COST: $700
Rurality tax/visit: $220 (return trip gas and mileage, phone charges between visits)
The family's minimum annual rurality tax (10 visits): $2,200

Marya's situation is not dissimilar to the expenses and constraints experienced by thousands of Canadian families with children who have chronic conditions. Her story illustrates the myth of universality in Canadian health care access. Marya's long-term prognosis will undoubtedly be heavily influenced by her family's socio-economic circumstances. Parental unemployment at any time in the course of Marya's illness will have a devastating effect on their ability to maintain contact with health services, and thus on Marya's health. Her family's rural location sets in motion an ongoing rurality tax that is inconsistent with her legal right to health care. Rurality tax is defined as the extra amount of money that rural and remote individuals and families must pay if they are to have the same possibilities of access to health care as urban people. If Marya's family is from a racialized group, she will experience additional and powerful barriers related to racism in the health care system.

jeopardy for women of colour (Brown, Keith, Jackson & Gary, 2003; Etowa, Keddy, Egbeyemi & Eghan, 2007). Barriers in access to mental health services for lesbian, gay, bisexual, and transgendered adolescents have also been linked to systemic discrimination. Lesbian, gay, and bisexual youth have higher depression and suicide rates than the overall rate for youth (Medeiros, Seehaus, Elliot & Melaney, 2004; Morrison & L'Heureux, 2001), and are more likely to be homeless than the general youth population (Shelby, 1999). Young Inuit men have the highest suicide rates in Canada (Isaacs, Keogh, Menard & Hockin, 2000). These examples depict the compounding effects of each oppression.

The intersecting relationships among the social determinants of health, identity, and mental health struggles such as depression have led to a growing critique of biomedical and, in particular, psychiatric approaches to assessment and intervention. An individualistic focus does not accommodate, and can actually mislead and confuse, attention to the social and economic conditions that cause or exacerbate mental health problems. Most publicly funded mental health services in Canada use the psychiatric diagnostic categories outlined in the *Diagnostic and Statistical Manual of Mental Disorders* (DSM-IV-TR) (American Psychiatric Association, 2004). Although the assessment system in the DSM-IV-TR includes a category entitled "psychosocial and environmental problems," its brief (one-and-a-half pages out of 900 pages) description *has remained exactly the same* in the 2004 edition as it was in the 1994 edition. Culture, gender, and age features are discussed in terms of epidemiological, rather than sociological, significance. This token and outdated attention to the influence of the SDOH and identity in the development of mental health and wellness is indicative of a much larger problem in the delivery of mental health services in Canada. Consistent historical reliance on the biomedical model of psychiatry, a framework that has limited capacity for incorporating spiritual, economic, and political origins of mental health struggles, has made it next to impossible to develop a mental health system that responds to social determinants of health-related stress.

In the widely used DSM-IV-TR (2004) classification system, depression is described as a psychiatric disorder, and the predominant mode of treatment is psychotropic medications. Since experiences of depression and stress are strongly influenced by the SDOH, those experiencing stress related to (un)employment and working conditions, racism, inadequate or no housing, and social exclusion are at risk for the medicalization of social problems. Medicalization has been defined as the rendering of life experiences as processes of health disorders, which can be discussed exclusively in medical terms and to which only medical solutions can be applied (Illich, 1976). Although many clinicians explore SDOH-related concerns, the Canadian diagnostic frame remains rooted in the individual-based DSM-IV-TR in most publicly funded health services. The resulting medicalization of oppression causes systemically created social problems to be reframed as individual psychiatric disorders. This, in turn, frequently results in the prescription of psychotropic drugs. The efficacy of psychotropic drugs for some individuals notwithstanding, the consistent overprescription of these drugs to women and elders, particularly elderly women, points to the medicalization of gender and age-based inequity (Stoppard, 2000). Elderly women have the highest rate of prescription of benzodiazepines, the Valium drug group. They are also the poorest people in Canada, with a 23.5 percent rate of poverty, compared to 10 percent for men in 1999 (Canadian Council on Social Development, 2007).

It is important to note that the fastest-rising health expenditure in Canada is in pharmaceuticals. Drug therapies accounted for 9 percent of total health expenditure in 1975 and, by 2005, expenditures nearly doubled to 18 percent, replacing payments to physicians as the second-largest expenditure, behind hospitals (Health Canada, 2005). At the current rate, the $10 million spent on pharmaceuticals in 1996 will reach $85 billion by 2017—one out of every $4 spent on health care will go to drugs (Morgan, 2006). This trend means that the multinational pharmaceutical industry now has an influential political role in shaping and directing Canada's vision of physical and mental health care. Since corporate profit is the goal of the pharmaceutical industry, these statistics should be cause for concern and action, particularly since numerous scholars have linked oppression with overmedication or mismedication of marginalized people and groups.

Critical questions need to be publicly asked and debated: Through what political and policy-based processes did the pharmaceutical industry gain such a massive share in Canadian health care expenditures? Who are the winners and who are the losers in the drive to make drugs a leading intervention in health care? These questions show that current health spending trends are at direct odds with social determinants of health knowledge about the health of Canadians.

Politicizing Primary Health Care

Poverty Is Not a Lifestyle

Primary health care (PHC) was affirmed unanimously by all WHO member countries in the Alma-Ata Declaration (1978), which affirmed that health care should be rooted in universal, community-based, preventive, and curative services with substantial community involvement, and inclusion of nurses and health extension officers who would be educated to work in community health centres. The money for these initiatives was to be secured from diversion of world resources from armaments and military conflicts. Policies of peace and détente would release funds for the promotion of health care services in the form of primary health care, which included social and economic development. PHC did not achieve its goals, chiefly due to: (1) the refusal of experts and politicians in developed countries to accept that communities should be in charge of the direction of their health care; and (2) changes in economic philosophy that led to the replacement of PHC by "health sector reform" based on market forces (Hall & Taylor, 2003).

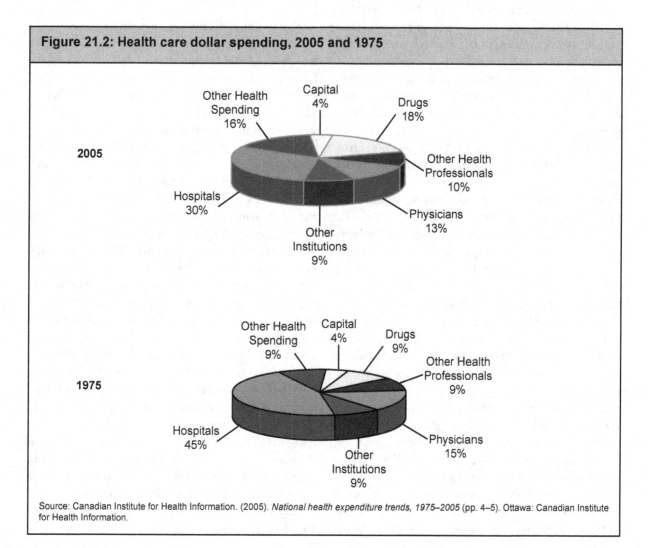

Figure 21.2: Health care dollar spending, 2005 and 1975

2005

Other Health Spending 16%
Capital 4%
Drugs 18%
Other Health Professionals 10%
Physicians 13%
Other Institutions 9%
Hospitals 30%

1975

Other Health Spending 9%
Capital 4%
Drugs 9%
Other Health Professionals 9%
Physicians 15%
Other Institutions 9%
Hospitals 45%

Source: Canadian Institute for Health Information. (2005). *National health expenditure trends, 1975–2005* (pp. 4–5). Ottawa: Canadian Institute for Health Information.

In Canada, primary health care has not achieved the participatory, community-driven, and community-based goals of PHC. Hospitals have been renamed "health centres," while the real work of bringing participatory health care to the neighbourhoods and streets of communities is undertaken largely by not-for-profit community agencies across the country. While hospitals are increasingly affiliated with these centres, the participatory goals of the Alma-Ata have been muted by an increasingly corporate model of health care delivery. PHC has shifted to a focus in "primary prevention." A focus on healthy lifestyles has been central to health-promotion strategies in Canada since the Lalonde Report (1974), strengthened, at least in principle, by the *Ottawa Charter* (1986). The lifestyles framework seems a natural fit for primary health care, including physical and mental health care, with its focus on prevention and early intervention. However, this approach is increasingly problematic because it hinges on the assumption of free choice. Smoking tobacco, eating cheap and fatty cuts of meat, and not making time for a walk become individual behavioural choices that produce self-induced ill health.

The logic of promoting healthy lifestyle choices rests on the belief that people have considerable control over their everyday activities, their grocery bill, and organizing the possibility of time for a safe place to walk. Since control over one's life circumstances rests heavily on one's economic circumstances, the logic and efficacy of lifestyle approaches to health promotion increasingly disintegrate as one descends the socio-economic gradient. Expectations that people living in poverty need to "try harder to overcome lack of money, be more organized, stop smoking, and be more creative in their combinations of high-protein legumes," trivialize the lived experience of poverty (Ocean, 2005). Moreover, when people in poverty do not follow such advice, they are blamed for their poor health.

Although lifestyle approaches may be important for some, the widening economic gap between the rich and the poor makes this approach ineffective and, some would argue, unethical for many Canadians. For example, the physical and mental health status of Indigenous peoples in Canada can best be traced to the oppression of colonialism rather than deficits in "lifestyle." While nutritious diets and exercise play a role in improving health status, these measures will ultimately not ameliorate the present-day health consequences of the brutal treatment of Indigenous peoples at the hands of White colonial power. Rather, systemic social change is imperative. Perhaps most importantly, the healthy lifestyle-choice approach shifts the locus of responsibility and intervention to the individual level rather than toward systemic social change to address health inequities related to the social determinants of health. Large and relatively expensive health-promotion campaigns regarding healthy lifestyles powerfully reinforce this apolitical approach to improving health. These campaigns divert attention away from the need for change in health systems and policy analysis, and the failure to honour the community ownership goals of the Alma-Ata Declaration.

Reclaiming the Meaning of Participation

Citizen participation is central to a human rights approach to health system change. Politicizing primary health care means that policy initiatives must start from a foundation of community development beyond its current conceptualization, which focuses on involving stakeholders in decision making, taking steps to provide communities with a greater say in how health care is delivered, and ensuring that there are community members on hospital and health boards. Although these approaches have provided clear avenues for citizen participation in health care design and delivery, they stop short of meaningfully embracing social action.

In contrast, an anti-oppressive community development model, which explicitly focuses on building capacity for social change and political action, has had encouraging success throughout Canada, mostly in non-profit community agencies that combine health care with a broad range of support, including housing, educational upgrading, food and job security, and legal aid services. The North End Community Health Centre (NECHC) model, in Halifax, Nova Scotia, could serve as a philosophical and practical template for broader health system change. Important gains could be realized if a meaningful portion of primary health care funds were dedicated to supporting local initiatives for increasing community wellness *while at the same time* building capacity for social and political action through civil society engagement. Although institutional, hospital-based health care, and the public health system in

Box 21.2: The North End Community Health Centre: The case for translating knowledge from community to conventional health services

The North End Community Health Centre (NECHC), Halifax, Nova Scotia, is an urban health service where nurses, nurse practitioners, social workers, dieticians, physicians, and support staff work in collaborative practice with community outreach and advocacy consistently and deliberatively integrated into everyday work. Support staff, often the first contact when individuals and families arrive at the centre, are pivotal in the centre's success. As one of Canada's oldest community-based health care services, the NECHC has demonstrated over 36 years of expertise in the application of community development principles to the health field. The centre practises within a well-developed and extensive repertoire of strategies for successful community and civil society engagement in health care and health outcome improvement. Notably, the centre's non-profit, independent status has meant that they operate at arm's length from government, and thus have been able to freely combine critical social scientific and community development ethics with health care delivery approaches. This may point to important areas for improvement in current conventional services. In an era where increasing numbers of health services and initiatives claim to practise community development, it is crucial that health services reclaim a social action-focused meaning of development, as evidenced and practised in NECHC's values:

- consensual decision making with the community
- inclusion and diversity
- transparency and open communication
- advocacy: the connection between social action and political action
- autonomy: the right to design and implement services for, and with, the community
- collaboration and partnership
- collegiality and teamwork
- respect and accountability
- a team culture
- continuous learning, development, and improvement

The following are some important directions for progressive health system change, which we can learn from the success of the NECHC:

1. *Back to the future:* Dedicate health dollars to social change-oriented, community development-based primary health care. Primary health care models largely do not follow community development principles of community ownership and active involvement in system change. Although an increasing number of Canadian cities and communities have services termed "community health centres," most of these services follow a biomedical approach to care delivery. Although the efficacy of approaches to care such as the NECHC has been demonstrated for several decades, policy-makers and politicians are slow to embrace health system change, which could promote community development-based primary health care. Research efforts should shift from proving the efficacy of community development to identifying and addressing points of resistance within the health system.
2. Actively transfer policy and clinical practice knowledge from NECHC kinds of approaches to primary health care and conventional, institution-based, tertiary health services. NECHC has successfully applied their principles and practices of addressing inequities in access to health services to their collaborative hospital-based services, which include prenatal programs and a shared care mental health model with two urban hospitals. This collaborative work with tertiary services recognizes and takes advantage of a well-recognized locus of expertise in social change-based community development. The shared care model, operating since 2000, has resulted in a dramatic increase in access to mental health services within the community, accompanied by a large reduction of mental health referrals to the tertiary-care hospitals. The template for system change is already flourishing in Canada. The genesis of community health centres such as NECHC lies in the inability of conventional health services to address barriers in access to the goods and services of the health care system.
3. Increase support for collaborative and interdisciplinary teamwork, which places the patient at the centre. Include an emphasis on collaborative team development in health human resources planning in Canada. Multidisciplinary and cross-community team work is foundational to increasing health system accessibility and civil society engagement.

Canada operate on a much larger scale than agencies such as NECHC, ethical and civil society principles, such as those embedded within the NECHC, could form a template for broader health system change. The NECHC exemplifies the primary health care philosophy of the Alma-Ata Declaration.

Civil society engagement is at the core of reclaiming participatory action for health system change. The World Health Organization's definition of civil society is "a social sphere separate from the state and market, made up of non-state, not-for-profit, voluntary organizations, ranging from formal organizations registered with authorities, to informal social movements coming together around a common cause" (World Health Organization, 2005, p. 5). A culture of capacity-building, and implementation of strategies for citizen involvement in the design and delivery of health care, are central to meaningful participation. The challenge of moving to equitable participation reflects the challenge of providing equitable health services themselves. When citizens are marginalized and racialized, their capacity for participation is inherently compromised. The same intersections of the social determinants of health, identity, and geography, described in Figure 21.1, which exclude people from access to health care, also exclude them from participation in civil society. Exclusion creates a diminished democracy, which encourages class- and race-biased health and public policy outcomes (Edwards, 2004; Skocpol, 2003). The exclusion of many Canadians in civil society participation is at odds with the principles of democracy.

In order for health care to make a difference in the health of Canadians, a cultural shift toward social action-based community development principles in the delivery of health care is necessary. This shift will not happen easily, since our health system is firmly entrenched in a hierarchical model with top-down decision making held by a few powerful actors. Shifting decision-making power closer to the community has broad implications for increasing political enfranchisement, and therefore influencing the subsequent choices citizens make regarding electoral preferences. Politicizing health care, through democratization of health system governance, will have important implications for Canada's increasingly for-profit health care system. Corporate culture is, by definition, hierarchical and market-driven. Privatization means that services are provided on a for-profit basis. Although the privatization debate is beyond the scope of this discussion, a few additional links are important to bring forward in the context of citizen participation.

The goals of privatization are efficient service production, satisfied health care consumers, and corporate profit. These goals are inconsistent with a civil society, participatory approach to improving health care, and the health of Canadians for at least two reasons. First, there is no mandate for participatory design. Consumer involvement, much beyond citizen recruitment for boards and committees, is inconsistent with corporate models of service delivery. Second, while privatization has been argued as a viable method to increase accessibility, as detailed earlier, it works only for people with sufficient financial resources. Globalization creates new and related challenges regarding profit, trade, and health. A globalization that is directed by large multinational corporations and by the governments that service the interests of multinationals is inconsistent with citizen-based movements toward human rights and social justice in health (Labonte, Schrecker & Gupta, 2005).

Toward an Equities-Competent Health Care System

National equities-competent health care systems would explicitly use a human rights and social justice framework. A human rights perspective would be meaningfully integrated into policy, practice, and service delivery. Professional associations would mandate competency in health-equities knowledge and strategies for knowledge translation into practice. Regarding the case example provided earlier, no matter how excellent Marya's clinical care is, significant determinants of the outcome of her arthritis are her family's social class position and their rurality. Best-practice models for chronic disease care must explicitly include the social determinants of health and measures for success in equities competence. Although health system mission statements and strategic plans are beginning to include the language of inclusion and equity, the translation into more effective and efficient equities-competent front-line health care is in its infancy.

A notable exception and a hopeful beginning is the Nova Scotia Department of Health's *Cultural Competence Guide for Primary Health Care Professionals* (2005), the first government-based initiative of its kind in the country. Racism, discrimination, and oppression are clearly defined and accompanied by action strategies. In an equities-competent system, protocols for diabetes management, in addition to directing insulin dose sliding-scale values, would include a detailed protocol regarding access to insulin, transportation, and food necessary for the diabetic diet. This is not to suggest that skilled clinicians do not already account for these aspects of diabetes care. Rather, there is no nationally developed protocol to which the health system must be held accountable. The following are possible strategies for equities competence, a set for the juncture where patient and provider meet, and another set for the overall health care system.

Strategies for equities competence where patient and provider meet:

1. Incorporate the explicit critical language of understanding oppression and working for social change as a mandate of practice in professional codes of ethics.

2. Build on already existing principles of reflexive practice to include the positioning of health care providers as also having a race, a gender, an ethnicity, a sexual orientation, and so on. Excellent tools already exist regarding White privilege (McIntosh, 2006) and heterosexism (Bella & Yetman, 2000). Tackle the myth of practitioner objectivity.

3. Require mandatory equities competency in education to ensure understanding of the links among human rights, oppression, injustice, and health outcomes. Educators in the health field often assume that human rights and social justice principles are already implicit in their teaching practice, and there is sometimes resistance to classroom incorporation of critical social scientific knowledge (see McGibbon & McPherson, 2006).

4. Require incorporation of cultural-competence theory and clinical practice standards in education and within institutional service delivery: race, ethnicity, sexual orientation, to name a few.

5. Support the providers. Health care workers are some of the unhealthiest workers in Canada. Fiscal instability creates cyclical unemployment in health workers, and the increasing casualization of nursing (Rachlis, 2004). Movement to democratization of health care cannot happen easily without the democratization of the workforce.

Strategies for equities competence in the health care system:

1. Numbers talk. Make health inequity visible through disaggregated health data: What is the self-reported health and wellness status of young men with disabilities? How does this rate compare with that of young men with disabilities whose families are living at the poverty line? How do race, social class, sexual orientation, and disability intersect with SDOH and geography to affect chronic illness outcomes? What is the relationship between these intersections and access to health care? The Canadian Institutes of Health Research (CIHR), and the Canadian Health Services Research Foundation (CHSRF) and its provincial counterparts should dedicate funds to develop methods and tools to disaggregate health and health system-utilization data. As an integral aspect of an equities-based system, disaggregated data would improve knowledge and visibility of the health of racialized and marginalized individuals and peoples.

2. Design and implement a Canada-wide, regionally specific Human Rights Health Report Card using disaggregated data wherever possible. Excellent templates and population health data analyses strategies for health inequities already exist (see Smith, 1998, 2005a; Williams & Doessel, 2006; Davies, Washington & Bindman, 2002). Include indicators such as infant mortality, Apgar scores (physical condition after delivery and any immediate need for extra medical or emergency care), immunization rates, perinatal

indicators such as percent low birth weight, percent term infants admitted to neonatal intensive care units within one day of delivery; oncology indicators such as use of tests critical to diagnosis, interdisciplinary treatment, and follow-up. Widely disseminate results annually across government, non-government, academic, and community venues with audience-tailored reports. Include in high school and post-secondary curricula. Provide data for citizen and policy action to improve health system accountability and provide evidence for change. Canadian provinces have developed a report card on child and family poverty (see New Brunswick Human Development Council, 2007), and they provide a clear and policy-based template.

3. Develop tools for social justice accountability in health policy documents such as the Canadian Nurses Association's Social Justice Gauge for measuring organizational success in achieving social justice (Canadian Nurses Association, 2006). Also see Vilshanskaya and Stride's (2003) *Four Steps towards Equity: A Tool for Health Promotion Practice.*

4. Require equities competence in health and public policy decision makers. Provide publicly funded workshops and equities-based policy seminars.

Conclusion: Action Strategies for Human Rights Stewardship in Canadian Health Care

A human rights perspective on health care would reorient health care system stewardship to actively pursue attainment of human rights for all Canadians. These are opportunities for systems change in many sectors and at various points of health care access and in the policy-making cycle. The following are summative suggestions for health system change.

- Expand analyses of health care as a social determinant of health. Direct sustained attention to inequities in access to health care.

- Democratize primary health care. Dedicate health dollars to social change-oriented, community development-based primary health care. Honour the principles of the Alma-Ata.

- Increase civil society engagement in the design and delivery of health services. Since the mid-1980s, the federal government has been transferring control of health services to First Nations peoples, under the federal First Nations and Inuit Health Branch (Ministerial Advisory Council on Rural Health, 2002). The resulting move toward integration of traditional medicine and First Nations' control of the design and delivery of health care serve as a model for culturally relevant, community-designed health services.

- Develop an equities-competent health care system. Create avenues for equities competence in service providers and in the system as a whole.

- Integrate critical social scientific knowledge across education, service delivery, and health systems policy-making. Make more energetic and explicit use of critical social science as a lens to inform primary health care, public health, health policy, and health systems policy analysis, creation, and evaluation (i.e., critical race theory, feminist theory, critical theory, queer theory). Globally, the language of human rights is the language of critical social science.

- Expand the applied health services and policy research agenda to systematically include qualitative, critical, and participatory methods. CIHR's gold standard of randomized controlled trials urgently needs to be augmented with the contextual perspective of lived experience and the social scientific exploration of how everyday life unfolds for Canadians. Critical social science health researchers have no clear home in tri-council (Canadian Institutes of Health Research, Canadian Health Services Research Foundation, Social Sciences and Humanities Research Council) fund allocation. Funding bodies could play a significant role in directing and enriching a health and human rights research agenda, and hence the policy agenda to address health inequity. Although qualitative, critical, and participatory methods have made some inroads, they are by far in the minority of provincially and nationally funded studies. Mixed-methods research, which could combine critical qualitative research with health geomatics, has barely begun in Canada, and there are excellent templates in the UK and the US (see Harvard Health Disparities Geocoding Project; Shaw, Dorling, Gordon & Smith, 1999).

• Increase cross-sectoral policy development, priority setting, service planning, and service implementation.

Figure 21.3 summarizes action strategies for a human rights stewardship to guide Canadian health system change. Democratizing health care in Canada would shift health care delivery toward equities competence and public debate and action about the health-for-some status of Canadian health care. Intersections of social determinants of health, identity, and geography create profound and avoidable systemic barriers in access to health care. Mental health care is at a crossroads in Canada. Our biomedical, psychiatric frame is at disturbing odds with the lived experience of marginalized and racialized individuals and families. Racism and poverty-created stress cannot be ameliorated with psychotropic drugs. Rather, social democratic policy initiatives must become a priority. Inherent in social democracy is the active participation of civil society. Increases in corporate dominance of health care delivery and the push toward privatization are inconsistent with social democracy. This dissonance will be the cornerstone of health care debates in the coming years. Fortunately, we have the visionary compass of Douglas's groundwork for social medicine in Canada.

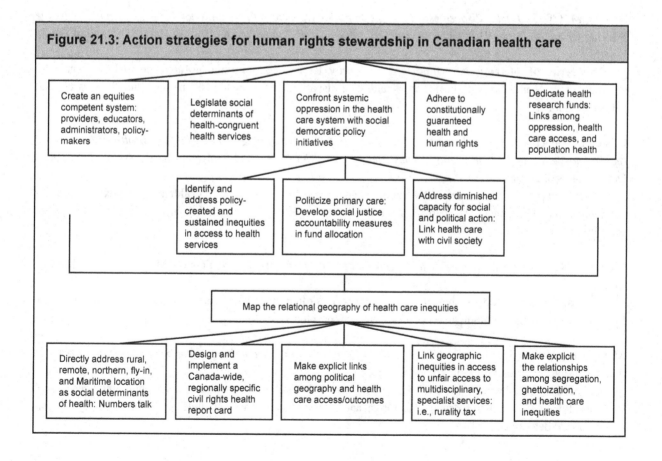

Figure 21.3: Action strategies for human rights stewardship in Canadian health care

Create an equities competent system: providers, educators, administrators, policy-makers

Legislate social determinants of health-congruent health services

Confront systemic oppression in the health care system with social democratic policy initiatives

Adhere to constitutionally guaranteed health and human rights

Dedicate health research funds: Links among oppression, health care access, and population health

Identify and address policy-created and sustained inequities in access to health services

Politicize primary care: Develop social justice accountability measures in fund allocation

Address diminished capacity for social and political action: Link health care with civil society

Map the relational geography of health care inequities

Directly address rural, remote, northern, fly-in, and Maritime location as social determinants of health: Numbers talk

Design and implement a Canada-wide, regionally specific civil rights health report card

Make explicit links among political geography and health care access/outcomes

Link geographic inequities in access to unfair access to multidisciplinary, specialist services: i.e., rurality tax

Make explicit the relationships among segregation, ghettoization, and health care inequities

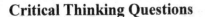

Critical Thinking Questions

1. What is the relevance of a human rights perspective on health care in Canada?
2. How do the social determinants of health, identity, and geography intersect to inform knowledge and action regarding inequities in access to health care?
3. Can a focus on the social determinants of mental health help to make the medicalization of oppression more visible?
4. How can involving civil society democratize Canada's health care system?
5. What are some action strategies for human rights stewardship in Canada's health care system?

Recommended Readings

Curtis, L.J. & MacMinn, W.J. (2007). *Health care utilization in Canada: 25 years of evidence*. Social and Economic Dimensions of an Aging Population (SEDAP) Research Paper no. 190. Hamilton: McMaster University.

   This paper focuses on inequity patterns in health care services (physicians, specialists, and hospitals). Detailed statistical evidence is presented regarding the complexities of analyzing health care access patterns, and the increasing socio-economic, status-based inequities in access to health care in Canada.

Drexler, M. (2005). *Health disparities and the body politic: A series of international symposia conducted by the Working Group on Health Disparities at the Harvard School of Public Health*. Boston: Harvard School of Public Health.

   This series of international symposia reports provides an economic and political perspective regarding governments' role in addressing health and health care disparities, new agendas for national health research, and paths to action.

Gilson, L., Doherty, J., Loewenson, R. & Francis, V. (2007). *Challenging inequity through health systems: Final report, knowledge network on health systems*. Geneva: The World Health Organization Commission on the Social Determinants of Health.

   This report presents the arguments for health systems as a social determinant of health in the context of inequities and civil society engagement. The paper concludes with the urgent need for initiating and sustaining health system transformation.

Illich, I. (1999). *Limits to medicine: Medical nemesis, the expropriation of health*. London: Marion Boyars Publishing Ltd.

   This book is a reprint of Illich's 1974 germinal text regarding the medicalization of human experience and the limited utility of applying biomedical solutions to social problems.

Morrow, M., Hankivsky, O. & Varcoe, C. (2007). *Women's health in Canada: Critical perspectives on theory and policy*. Toronto: University of Toronto Press.

   Gender is one of the most powerful determinants of health and health care access. This book includes critical analyses of women's health in a Canadian historical and current context. Topics include gender-based policy analysis and the social determinants of women's health.

Related Web Sites

Harvard Center for Society and Health (HCSH)—www.hsph.harvard.edu/centers-institutes/society-and-health/
The HCSH's work is focused on: researching the ways in which social and economic inequalities affect the public's health and well-being; formulating public- and private-sector policies that strive to improve people's health and quality of life; and communicating new findings on the social determinants of health to the general public.

International Development Research Center: Governance, Equity, and Health (IDRC-GEH)—www.idrc.ca/en/ev-11921-201-1-DO_TOPIC.html
The objectives of the IDRC-GEH are strengthening health systems, promoting civic engagement, and making research matter. The focus is the strengthening of Southern nations; however, the GEH's goals and research are very relevant to Canada's growing health and civil society participation gaps.

International Society for Equity in Health (ISEqH)—www.iseqh.org/journal_en.htm
The purpose of ISEqH is to promote equity in health and health services internationally through education, research, publication, communication, and charitable support. Goals include promoting equity and exposing inequity in health and in health care services internationally, and facilitating scientific interchange and research regarding equity in health and health care services.

International Union for Health Promotion and Education (IUHPE)—www.iuhpe.org
The mission of IUHPE is to promote global health and to contribute to the achievement of equity in health among and within countries of the world.

Pan American Health Organization Equidad Listserv Archive Web site—listserv.paho.org/archives/equidad.html
This global archive includes up-to-date resources, articles, and tool kits regarding equity and health, health economics, health legislation, gender, bioethics, ethnicity, human rights, health disparities, information technology, virtual libraries, and research and science concerns around the globe.

Chapter 22

PUBLIC POLICY
AND THE WELFARE STATE

Lars K. Hallstrom

Introduction

The political and policy-making context within which political scientists and policy analysts work has changed significantly in the past few decades. In addition to substantial challenges to the fundamental assumptions underlying the analysis of politics and political action (see, for example, Kuehls, 1996; Weber, 1995), factors such as the shift to neo-liberalism, environmental decline, and global pandemics such as avian influenza or SARS have increasingly made it apparent that: (1) states are no longer the primary unit of analysis for political science and international relations; (2) political authority is increasingly exercised not just within and between states, but also above and below the state (as characterized by the term "multilevel governance" (Harnisch, 2002; Peters & Pierre, 2002; Hooghe & Marks, 2001); and (3) markets now matter at least as much as states (and perhaps more) to political outcomes (Strange, 1996).

Despite the fact that the setting within which political authority rests is changing, there are a number of paradoxes in the domestic and international politics of today. While the state's political authority and power are declining, the degree of intervention in the daily lives of citizens by the state and state-based agencies has increased significantly. Additionally, even while the state's capacity and authority is in decline (particularly in the global North), there are increasing numbers of populations and regions that are demanding the elements of the sovereign nation-state: territory and sovereignty. Along with both comes the often implicit assumption that while the political state may be declining in both theoretical and practical or political importance, citizens regard the state's exercise of authority as important. However, this importance is attached not only to the activity of the state, but how that activity takes place—developed states such as Canada and Belgium[1] have both seen significant expressions of public dissatisfaction with elitist or top-down approaches to public policy and politics. More recently, the classic question of "who governs" (Dahl, 1961) has been complemented by "how do they govern," but a new dimension has been added—the question of what the effects of such patterns of governance are on issues such as justice, the distribution of resources, and the allocation of risks and costs to certain segments of the population.

Box 22.1: Key facts about Canada

Land mass: 9,984,670 sq. km
Population: 33,000,000
Political system: Bicameral Westminster model
Electoral system: Single-member plurality
Inception: 1867
Federalism: 10 provinces, 3 territories
National capital: Ottawa, Ontario
Head of state: Queen of Canada (Elizabeth II)
Head of government: Prime Minister

Given this rather amorphous environment, where states may be subservient to markets, multilateral treaties and large trans- or multinational corporations, the state still continues to affect the lives and activities of its citizens. In fact, the apparatus of the state, whether in Canada, the United States, or Bangladesh, while influenced or controlled by multiple factors, continues to move along a broad trajectory that began many decades ago with the emergence of the positive or welfare state. This trajectory, which seeks to reconcile the activities or inactivities of the state with the issues that society has identified as problematic, forms the backbone of the positive state: the idea that the state can and should play a role in either the provision of public goods[2] or the management of goods seen as necessary or beneficial to the lives of citizens (Brooks & Miljan, 2003).

As a result of both this role and citizens' expectations that the state will, in fact, be involved in some way in key parts of their lives, it has become increasingly difficult for citizens to understand public policy. At the same time, given the state's presence in almost every facet of citizens' lives, it is also important that citizens understand the state's interventions and the ways in which the emergence of the positive state has influenced their daily lives. Perhaps, even more importantly, a greater knowledge of the ways in which those actors and institutions interact, and the ways in which the welfare states functions, is a step away from apathy and uninformed cynicism toward greater awareness, involvement, and, ultimately, active citizenship and "strong" democracy.[3]

This is important for a number of reasons. First, as Pal (1997) pointed out, both the key problems that policy has sought to address, as well as the fundamental paradigm of the policy sciences—rationalism—have increasingly been in trouble. Critical areas of state-based action—such as unemployment insurance, poverty reduction or income assistance, and education—have actually declined or gotten worse in recent years despite significant expenditures and policies to the contrary. At the same time, the underlying idea that public policies can solve problems based on the rational, positivist application of the human intellect has been challenged since at least the early 1970s (see, for example, Ehrenfeld, 1981; Foucault, 1972, 1995), and particularly since the late 1980s (see, for example, Bobrow & Dryzek,

1987; Torgerson, 1986; Fisher, 1990, 1998; and Fisher & Forester, 1993). However, despite these challenges to both the efficacy and rationalism of late 20th- and early 21st-century public policy, the fact remains that public problems do exist; that states have some capacity to act upon these problems; and that citizens can and should judge the underlying values, methods, and objectives present in public policy (Barber, 1984; Pateman, 1980; Cook & Morgan, 1971).

This chapter outlines in broad strokes the nature of the positive state in Canada, with an eye on social policy and health policy more specifically. In doing so, it will map not only the historical patterns of social policy development and revision, but will place these patterns within the broader context of Canadian politics and public policy as part of Canada's development as a welfare state. Ultimately, the purpose of this chapter is to outline the basic concepts of public policy and policy analysis, and demonstrate not only where we are in terms of social and health policy, but also to place that location within a broader explanatory framework of institutions, ideologies, and globalization.

What Is Public Policy?

While numerous definitions of politics have been put forward, perhaps the most straightforward is: Who gets what, where, when, and how? Taking this distributive definition as a starting point, it then becomes possible to see public policy as the process by which this decision is made implemented (or not). In the words of Thomas Dye, public policy is "anything a government chooses to do or not to do" (Dye, 1972, p. 2). While perhaps overly simplistic as it treats every action of government as equal and provides no means of distinguishing important or meaningful actions from those of little consequence, this definition provides two key elements for better understanding what exactly public policy is: (1) the agent of public policy-making is a government (only the actions adopted or endorsed by the government constitute public policy); and (2) public policy involves a deliberate decision by governmental actors to pursue a specific course of action. While this action may actually involve doing nothing, it is still a deliberative choice to maintain the status quo (Howlett & Ramesh, 2003).

There are three central components of any public policy. The first is the identification or definition of a specific problem or issue area; the second is the identification of specific objectives and goals that are desired; and the third is the instruments or means by which the goals will be achieved and the problem resolved or at least somewhat alleviated. Of these three components, problem identification is perhaps the most critical in terms of generating policy activity, yet it is often the most contested, political, and complex of these components. Not only is there a large number of potential and real influences on the conception and causal nature of the problem from both lay and scientific standpoints (and even if a problem exists—see, for example, the ongoing debate on global climate change), but increasingly items that are recognized as problems cut across multiple dimensions, jurisdictions, and causal sources.

In addition to these complexities, and the increasing recognition that science does not necessarily present a unified or consistent perspective on the nature or causal relationships of policy problems, problem identification is further muddied by two additional factors: (1) that problems may appear as a result of perceived or substantial changes in a context or situation, rather than as new problems per se; and (2) that the question of causality (and therefore both the sources and potential solutions to a problem) can be not only multivariate (and indeed, may be neither linear nor direct), but also highly contested. This may occur not only on social, political, or ethical grounds, but also on the basis of different scientific paradigms, assumptions, discourses, and even political cultures (Buonanno, Zablotney & Keefer, 2001; ESRC Global Environmental Change Program, 1999; Caldwell, 1990; Fisher, 1990; Bernstein, 1983).

What emerges, therefore, is a complex image of contemporary public policy. Not only does it function within multiple locations of decision making, usually with multiple competing interests and actors, it can extend far beyond the realm of simple choices and action. In fact, public policy and, in turn, its analyses extend well into the domain of potential problems, potential effects, and potential choices both made and not made. Government decisions are not a reflection or indication of the free will of governmental decision makers. Rather, they are a recording of the interaction between that will and the various forces and constraints acting upon it at given points and contexts in time. Public policies, therefore, rarely deal with a single issue or problem. The reality of contemporary politics means that policies face "clusters" or "nodes" of entangled problems, many with contradictory or exclusive solutions and supporting actors. Policy problems, therefore, become far more than simple patterns of unilinear causation or connection where issues and policy determinants can be identified "upstream" or "downstream." Instead, they have been characterized as sets of interconnected problems with highly ambiguous boundaries or limits (Pal, 1997).

Due to the increasing recognition of the complexity of both problems and the public policies generated to resolve them, as well as the inherently political nature of public policy (Stone, 1997), public policy analysis emerged in the 20th century not only as a hypothesized necessary condition for effective and efficient governance in the positive state, but also as a potentially problematic activity that may have become overly specialized, methodologically driven, and "science-based" (Fisher, 1990). As countries such as the United States, Canada, the United Kingdom, and Germany began to provide high levels of public services and social policies, both as part of (in the case of the US) the New Deal and particularly after the Second World War, social scientists began to play a greater role in supporting the decision and policy-making process (Radin, 2000). The scope, scale, and imperatives of global war (and atomic weaponry) had brought new analytical methods to decision making based upon principles of rationality and scientific methodology. Found first in the natural sciences, both positivism (based upon laboratory-based experimental methods to discern true from false) and normative economic reasoning (based on market analogies and strict rationality) became increasingly present as mechanisms to guide the explanation of policy outcomes, and the prescription of desired public policies (Radin, 2000; Pal, 1997).

Since 1945, what has emerged in terms of both public policy analysis and the policy sciences is a desire to apply a highly specific set of skills and methodologies to the analysis of public policy processes (how decisions are arrived at and implemented), outputs, outcomes, and, of course, the underlying causes and problems. As a result, a range of terms and perspectives developed, including policy studies, policy evaluation, and policy sciences, and while there is a broad distinction to be made between those perspectives that sought to primarily descriptive and explanatory and those that were more applied and prescriptive, Harold Lasswell captured perfectly the need for both *knowledge of the policy process* and *knowledge in the policy process* in order to improve public policy (Lasswell, 1951).

One common thread links the different models and perspectives in policy analysis: Regardless of causal assumptions, the unit of analysis or the perceived constraints on policy-makers, the state is expected to play a role as either an active or reactive actor. Naturally, while different theoretical models present different expectations as to the characteristics and actions of the state, in each case the state is viewed not as some passive apolitical entity, but rather a collection of institutions, actors, agendas, and cultures that are both inherently political, and a significant factor in the design, provision, implementation, and analysis of public policies.[4]

This perspective is particularly relevant when the state's emergence as more than a simple guarantor of order and sovereignty is considered. As noted earlier, since the Great Depression, and particularly after the end of the Second World War, there has been a significant shift in the state's role and capacity in providing critical services to assist the welfare of citizens.[5] Without question, governments today "do" more than in the past, particularly when a longer-term historical lens is used. Particularly in systems such as Canada, the US, or the European states, not only do states now regulate or legislate over a much broader range of issues and topics than ever before (ranging from environmental emissions to minimum wages to tax rates to where an

individual can smoke), they do so using a larger share of national income, collect more taxes, and exert a greater influence on the day-to-day lives of citizens, and often even without citizens' awareness of that influence. As a result, not only is public policy (and social policy more specifically) a major component of contemporary politics, it is also significant in terms of the scope of modern public policy as it naturally constitutes a major portion of governmental expenditures. The contemporary state, therefore, has grown into an actor of major significance in "structuring life chances, in distributing wealth, privilege, information, and risks ... and providing the legal/regulatory framework for capitalism" (Eckersley, 2004).

As a developed Northern state, Canada has certainly participated in this trend, and over the past century has seen (in conjunction with independent statehood, decolonization, and globalization) both a massive increase in the scope and scale of state-based activity, as well as both a very real and publicly perceived shift away from state-based interventions. At the beginning of the 20th century, the Public Accounts for Canada consisted of only a few dozen departments and agencies of government. Nearly a century later, there were 120 (Brooks & Miljan, 2003). Similarly, total government expenditures in Canada, as in many other developed states, have grown almost ten-fold in Canada since Confederation. Rather than simply following the state's traditional functions concerned with social order, defence, and the creation of economic development, Canada's activities as a state have grown to encompass almost every aspect of social, political, cultural, and economic life, both as a

Table 22.1: Comparing the policy cycle and applied problem-solving	
Stages in the policy cycle	**Applied problem-solving**
1. Agenda setting	1. Problem recognition
2. Policy formulation	2. Proposal of solution(s)
3. Decision making	3. Selection of solution(s)
4. Implementation	4. Putting solution into effect
5. Policy evaluation	5. Monitoring results
6. Agenda/policy change	6. Identifying new problems

Source: Adapted from Howlett, M. & Ramesh, M. (2003). *Studying public policy: Policy cycles and policy subsystems* (p. 13). Oxford: Oxford University Press.

redistributive body and as a regulatory and decision-making body. For example, the Canadian state is now involved in the provision of education, health care, public health, income support, communications (including Canada Post), fiscal federalism (the redistribution of funds between subnational units), environmental protection and management, cultural and linguistic protection, unemployment insurance, pensions, natural resources protection, management and extraction, and infrastructure. As a result, not only is the state involved in many aspects of Canadian society, life, and economics, but this very involvement makes public policy and, in particular, the role of the Canadian state as a provider of transfer payments, a highly contested political domain.

Political debate of the past few decades has centred on these questions of redistribution. While the precise scope of governmental activities is typically a matter of personal preference and ideology, much of the content of Canadian politics and public policy has been concerned with attempting to find not only the right balance between intrusion and provision, but also with the right

mechanisms or methods by which to find that balance. However, while the debate is wide-ranging—particularly as neo-liberal discourses concerned with the extent of public sector deficits, national debt, and barriers to trade have become institutionalized since the late 1970s (see Langille, this text)—it is not quite accurate to state that the collectivist perspective, where individuals are seen to achieve dignity through communal associations and the collective is best suited to solving social and economic problems, has been defeated. Instead, while the precise nature, degree, and method of redistribution may be under contention, it is still apparent that the general premise of the collectivist perspective—that communally oriented goals such as promoting economic growth, protecting the weak and disadvantaged, and redistributing wealth—is accepted by most Canadians (Brooks & Miljan, 2003). That said, both the means of achieving these goals and the extent to which the state can or should be involved have continued to shift, due not only to changing national and regional political perspectives, but also to more general international pressures such as globalization, as well as more geographically specific arrangements such as the North American Free Trade Agreement.

Social Policy in Canada

The development of Canada as a welfare state and, in turn, its potential emergence as a regulatory state as well, is closely linked to its development as a federal system. In particular, as Banting and others have noted, the social programs that emerged in the second half of the 20th century in Canada came into being as different variants of federal-provincial relationships appeared. As a result, the Canadian welfare state and subsequent social policy have not developed evenly or uniformly. Instead, there are often striking inconsistencies—for example, as one of the liberal welfare states noted above, Canada's income security programs (such as pensions, unemployment insurance, and social assistance) tend to be oriented toward the principles of "self-help," 18th-century English liberalism, and faith in the superiority of markets, while the cores of the health care system reflect a much more social democratic approach. Naturally, not only are these differences derived from differing ideological and political traditions, but also from the use of social policy more generally as an instrument of statecraft to assist in

Table 22.2: Public expenditures as a percentage of total health expenditures, selected states (2000)

Country	Public expenditure (%)
Australia	72.4
Canada	71.2
Denmark	82.1
Finland	75.1
Germany	75.1
Iceland	84.4
Japan	76.7
Luxembourg	92.9 (1999 data)
Norway	82.8
Spain	69.9
Sweden	83.8
United Kingdom	81.0
United States	44.3

Source: Adapted from Brooks, S. & Miljan, L. (2003). *Public policy in Canada: An introduction* (4th ed.) (p. 186). Oxford: Oxford University Press.

the process of state-building, consolidation, and political integration.

In fact, the considerable variation between federal-provincial relations across social policy domains has led to the identification of three different models of federal-provincial relations embedded in the welfare state: (1) classical federalism, in which different levels of government act unilaterally with minimal interaction or coordination; (2) shared-cost federalism, where the federal government offers financial support to the provinces on specific terms; and (3) joint-decision federalism, where the formal agreement of both levels of government is required (Banting, 2005, p. 95). Depending on the specific area of social policy, the combination of ideology, political pragmatism, and the nature of federal relations has contributed to not only a mixed assortment of social policies, but also three distinct periods (consistent in part with the broader trends of both expenditure and withdrawal (see above). These are: (1) pre-1939 (characterized by the slow and limited development of social policy; (2) 1940–1970s, where social policy both developed and diversified; and (3) the 1980s onward, a period identified by Pierson as one of both resilience in the face of neo-liberalism as well as of "blame avoidance" (as cited in Obinger et al., 2005, p. 5).

Early Period (1867–1930s)

As might be expected in a relatively new country, the state's role in general was quite limited in Canada until the end of the First World War. Much like health care, welfare-type services were generally provided by private charities and religious organizations, and the predominantly agricultural structure of the economy (with accompanying conservative social and political ideologies) meant that there was little social basis or demand for the provision of welfare. Similarly, while the United States underwent significant social and economic change in the early 20th century due to the legalization of unions and the ability of both unions and other groups to challenge the status quo, Canada had limited capacity for alliances across labour and agriculture, and reform-oriented organizations such as women's and religious groups were located on the periphery of politics.

The decentralized federal structure of Canada has also served as an impediment to social policy provision.

Although some welfare initiatives did emerge in the early decades of the 20th century (Ontario, for example, introduced workers' compensation in 1914), these initiatives were neither universal, equitable, nor extensive. Poorer provinces, such as Prince Edward Island and New Brunswick, were not able to follow the lead of the Prairie provinces and Ontario in introducing the Mother's Allowance, and the benefits paid by such programs varied from $13.77 per month in Manitoba to $39.19 per month in British Columbia (Banting, 1987, 2005).

The Great Depression at the end of the 1920s brought the constraints and gaps of social policy into sharp relief. It resulted in both a fairly long-term debate as to the appropriate roles of provinces and federal government, as well as the economic implications of regional economic diversity and disparities. Much as the current economic boom in Alberta draws thousands of new Albertans every month in search of employment and riches, both federal and provincial concerns in the 1920s centred around the tendency for any province or city that appeared to resolve or at least mitigate the unemployment issue would naturally attract citizens from across the country, placing a massive further burden upon that solution. As a result, not only were there demands for consistency across the provinces, but as the implications for provincial competitiveness grew clearer, there were also demands and suggestions for federal jurisdiction.

Ultimately, the game of "jurisdictional hide-and-seek," with different levels of Canadian government attempting to both create and avoid social policies, lasted throughout much of the 1930s, but in 1927 federal action began to take place. Present in the form of old-age pensions for those aged 70 and older, but in the form of shared federal-provincial responsibility, this program marked a shift, but nothing along the scope or scale of the New Deal to the south. Uptake of the program was slow, but by 1936 a national system was in place, providing benefits at a comparable level across Canada, albeit not without problems. Many western provinces were nearly bankrupt, and federal contributions were often more than 50 percent of total expenditures.

Mid-Period (1945–1970s)

These tentative steps toward welfare reform (and initiation) were strengthened in the years after the Second

World War. The Canadian economy and demographic profile shifted significantly toward both urbanization and unionization following the Depression, and the combination of strong postwar economic performance, high tax revenues, and the perceived success of Keynesian-type fiscal policies all contributed toward increased support for a strong role for the state in resolving or at least mitigating social and economic problems. This was further supported by the evolution of Canadian party politics (particularly the shift of the Liberal Party toward social reform during the 1940s) and the relatively low profile of regional and linguistic tensions until the 1960s. As a result, the federal government was able to develop a significant regime centred around social policy, and while Quebec did at times complain about the federal profile over social policy,[6] other anglophone provinces did, in fact, push for even more federal involvement (Banting, 2005, p. 103).

Social policy in the years following the Second World War was, therefore, largely dominated by the federal footprint, but as time passed, the nature of the relationships between Ottawa and the provinces came to bear influence as well. By the 1960s, resistance in Quebec to federal dominance grew as a result of both Quebecois nationalism and the *révolution tranquille*, which included the modernization of government in Quebec. By 1965, Quebec had achieved an early form of asymmetrical federalism by winning the right to opt out of federal shared-cost programs (Banting, 2005). Other provinces followed suit (albeit not to the same degree) and while the first two decades following the war saw Ottawa taking the lead on social policies, the political and regional developments of the 1960s saw multiple approaches toward social programs, each reflecting a different reality of Canadian federal politics. In some cases, the federal government retained nearly total autonomy over social programs (such as income security), while others (such as pensions) are characterized by a complex process of joint federal-provincial decision making. Naturally, a third model also emerged, based on shared costs, in which both provinces and federal government are involved, but neither level maintains the power of veto. As a result, different policy domains have developed in different federal contexts, giving different levels of government, as well as different ideologies, greater or lesser influence over policy content. Thus, while health

care emerged under a shared-cost basis along with the accompanying federal-provincial dynamics, income security in Canada developed with a pronounced federal and liberal identity.

Neo-liberal Period (1975–Present)

Since the oil crises and recessions of the early 1970s and 1980s, there has been a pronounced shift in the policy "ideology" of many developed states. Relevant to both domestic and foreign policies, the term "neo-liberalism" has emerged to characterize a policy agenda based upon international comparative advantage, free trade and the reduction of trade and economic barriers, an increased reliance upon the efficiencies of free markets, and a broad withdrawal of the state from the provision of public goods in favour of privatization. Typically associated with politicians such as British PM Margaret Thatcher and US President Ronald Reagan, neo-liberalism has been heavily critiqued for: (1) its capacity to reinforce and even expand both the domestic and international disparities between the wealthy and those who are not; (2) its ideological reliance upon free markets and "the invisible hand"; and (3) the associated withdrawal of state intervention even as the economic and political gaps between the "haves" and the "have nots" increases (Castaneda, 1994; Overbeek & van der Pijl, 1993; Gill, 1993; Fernandez Kilberto, 1993; Baldwin, 1993; Fukuyama, 1992; Gamble, 1988).

From the Canadian perspective, neo-liberalism came into stark relief in the 1980s with the negotiation and signing of the North American Free Trade Agreement between Canada, the US, and Mexico. From the domestic perspective, this period marked the initiation of the Goods and Services Tax (GST), targeted directly at reducing Canada's international debt load in order to better attract international investors, and the initiation of many budgetary and programmatic cuts in order to limit the expenditures of both federal and provincial governments.

Framed largely in the language of economic rationalism, it has been argued in Canada and in other liberal welfare states that there is really "no choice" but to reduce the expenditures of government, given the high rates of public debt and interest rates. Based on the assumption that the expansion of the welfare state after the Second World War was the primary cause of this debt, the solution is seen to lie in smaller government, greater reliance on families and the private sector, and much more carefully targeted social programs. Since the mid-1980s and the Mulroney government, this has meant both an ideological and programmatic shifting of social policy toward individual responsibility, independence and employability, and individual characteristics as the most important reasons for not finding employment. However, as Baker pointed out in 1997, "What the Canadian programs overlook or downplay are the structural barriers to market income: the availability of work in the local economy, family responsibilities that might interfere with full-time employment, the availability of child care, and any idea of social responsibility for children" (1997, p. 3). In terms of health policy, as outlined in greater detail below, indirect changes to the state, typically in the form of modifications to the relationships of fiscal federalism, have been successful in diminishing the scope of the welfare state.

Health Policy in Canada

The system that has emerged to administer the health and health care needs of Canadians is a complex jumble of actors, organizations, and practices, each attempting to exercise influence over a largely provincial control over health care. While generally described as a public system,

Table 22.3: Total federal transfers for health care as a percentage of provincial health expenditures (1975–2000)	
Year	**Federal transfers (%)**
1975	41.3
1977	42.3
1980	43.7
1985	39.7
1990	33.9
1995	32.1
2000	29.3

Source: Banting, K. (2005). "Canada: Nation-building in a federal welfare state." In H. Obinger et al. (Eds.), *Federalism and the welfare state: New world and European experiences.* Cambridge: Cambridge University Press.

wherein the state takes on much of the responsibility for the provision of health care services, not all elements or services are covered by public health insurance.

Section 92, Subsection 7 of the Constitution assigns the responsibility for health policy in Canada to the provincial governments and, as noted above, the language of the Constitution reflects the early context of health policy and care provision in Canada. At the time of Confederation in 1867, the state's role in terms of health and health care was quite limited: Hospitals were typically created and administered by private organizations, while physicians billed patients directly. In fact, so limited was the state's role (at both federal and provincial levels) in health that provincial ministers of health did not exist until almost 20 years after Confederation, and the (federal) Dominion Department of Health did not emerge until after the First World War in 1919 (Brooks & Miljan, 2003).

Movement toward public health insurance was further slowed by Canadian federalism in the first half of the 20th century. The federal government's attempts to introduce health insurance via social insurance legislation and social policy more broadly in the "Green Books" were rejected by the courts and provinces respectively in 1937 and 1945, and it was not until 1947 that any movement toward universal insurance would emerge. In that year the Co-operative Commonwealth Federation (CCF) government of Saskatchewan implemented universal hospital insurance, and was followed by both British Columbia and Alberta. While this initiative would stall for almost 10 years, in 1957 a universal hospital insurance program was initiated, with Quebec joining in 1960.

Similarly, while different governments attempted to push through the social democratic approach toward health care, provinces such as Alberta and British Columbia preferred private coverage for all but the "hard to insure," i.e., the poor and the elderly. If not for the federal government's position following the recommendation of a Royal Commission, this model of health care probably would have prevailed. However, the popularity of a universal program with the Canadian electorate led to medicare programs in all provinces by 1971. This multilevel dynamic is continued today, with federalism creating both a space for negotiation, as well as for reform at the provincial level. In essence, federalism permitted a regional initiative to become the basis for a national-level policy based on social democratic norms, effectively displacing private health insurance in favour of provincially provided hospital, medical, and, later, public health services. That said, as the previous section demonstrated, Ottawa still plays a considerable role in health policy by setting rules, providing some funding, and even delivering health services to certain groups of the population. However, this dynamic has also led to a confusing mix, with the majority of health care costs covered by public expenditures, but with approximately one-third falling outside the public system.

There are two principal federal statutes for Canada's health care system: the Medical Care Act (1966) and the Canada Health Act (1984). The former set down for the first time the principles guiding cost-sharing health care for the provinces. These principles included: (1) non-profit operation by a public authority; (2) universal and equal access; (3) comprehensive health insurance plans; and (4) portable coverage.[7] Naturally, these principles provide considerable ambiguity in their interpretation and, as a result, the development and implementation of health policy in Canada has become increasingly political, with not only provincial and federal bureaucracies involved, but, more recently, the Supreme Court and the Charter of Rights and Freedoms. Brought into stark relief by the Chaoulli case in 2005 (see Box 22.2) issues

such as waiting times, the continuously growing costs of health care, emergency room and hospital closures, and even emergent pandemics such as SARS and avian influenza have made health policy a highly political item, with health care spending not only the largest public expenditure in provincial budgets, but also among the highest internationally (only the US, Switzerland, Germany, and France spend more as a percentage of GDP, and only Germany, France, Denmark, and Sweden spend more on public health) (Organisation for Economic Co-operation and Development, 2002). At the same time, public satisfaction with the health care system in Canada declined significantly during the 1990s (see Brooks & Miljan, 2003, p. 188), and Canadians are increasingly looking for reforms in that system in order to improve efficiency, efficacy, and access for both health care and public health.

Following the initiation of extra-billing in the 1970s, the Canada Health Act was developed to penalize provinces allowing extra-billing, a mechanism by which physicians could increase their revenues by charging patients a fee in addition to what they could claim from provincial insurance claims. The burden of these extra payments was, naturally, felt more by the poor and the unemployed, further exacerbating the inequalities

---

Box 22.2: Chaoulli v. Quebec (Attorney General) 2005, SCC 35

In June 2005, the Supreme Court of Canada decided that legislation in Quebec prohibiting private health insurance was in violation of Quebecers' rights. The Court found that the preservation of the public health insurance plan did not require prohibiting Quebecers from taking out insurance to obtain private sector services that were also available under the public plan.

Three of four judges found that the legislation in question violated the Canadian Charter of Rights and Freedoms, while one found that it violated only the Quebec Charter of Human Rights and Freedoms. Three judges dissented on the grounds that it was essentially a political question, and therefore beyond the remit of judges of constitutional law.

Based around the demands of an older man to be able to draw upon private sector services should wait times in Quebec prove too long, this decision essentially held that Quebecers who are willing to spend money to obtain services otherwise not available under the public plan due to the length of waiting times are allowed to do so. In essence, the state cannot restrict the pursuit of health care and services to just those provided by the state, particularly when the length of wait times may prove detrimental to the health of citizens. According to the first judgment in the case (provided by Deschamps J.), a prohibition on private health care would deny Quebecers a solution to long waiting lists, and thus was an infringement upon Quebecers' right to life and security. In the concurring judgment, McLachlin C.J., Major and Bastarache J.J. also noted that the legislation in question violated Section 7 of the Canadian Charter. The scheme put forward by the Quebec government, which essentially limited private health care to those so wealthy that they could afford to pay for treatments without needing insurance, would result in delays in treatment that adversely affect Quebecers' security of person.

between the "haves" and the "have nots." As a result, not only does the CHA reinforce the principles and spirit of the 1966 legislation, it also puts forward a strong role for the federal government in ensuring both the quality and consistency of health care as it is delivered by the provinces (Brooks & Miljan, 2003).

Despite this strong federal role created by the CHA, since the late 1970s the federal government has also increasingly moved away from sharing the costs of health care spending with the provinces, leading to a relative decline in Ottawa's ability to influence provincial health policy. In 1977, the government ceased matching provincial spending, and moved instead to the Established Programs Financing formula, where transfers for both health and post-secondary education were made on the basis of the previous year's spending, but adjusted to reflect any shifts in a province's gross provincial product. Over time, this has led to a steady decline in the proportion of cash transfers to the provinces, and while total per capita public spending on health care has increased significantly since the mid-1970s, the share of that spending undertaken by the provinces has increased. This has considerable implications for health care and services in Canada, particularly since 1995, when the Established Programs Financing was replaced by the Canada Health and Social Transfer (CHST).

Ottawa's primary contribution to the provinces until 2004, the CHST was a transfer to be divided between health care, post-secondary education, and social assistance. Although this transfer began at $26.9 billion, in 2004 this program was restructured into two different streams, the Canada Health Transfer (CHT) and the Canada Social Transfer (CST). The Canada Health Transfer allocated $25 billion for health costs, while the CST was significantly less. For the less prosperous provinces, the CHST is supplemented by equalization grants of almost $10 billion, part of which is usually spent by those provinces on health care and services. However, as the proportion of federal funds has diminished over the past 30 years, so too has Ottawa's ability to dictate or influence provincial policies. With the threat of withholding federal dollars in order to ensure compliance gradually diminishing (particularly for those provinces that do not rely upon equalization grants), the provinces' relative autonomy over health care and health policy has increased. This has taken place at the

same time that, as noted above, public satisfaction with health care and health policy more generally has declined, yet expectations of top-level technology, facilities, research, and care have increased. As a result, not only are provinces increasingly exerting influence over both what, and how much, is spent, they are doing so in an increasingly politicized environment in which demand for (often expensive) curative care, costs, and political attention are all increasing.

At the same time, despite initiatives such as the creation of the Public Health Agency of Canada (PHAC) in order to push population health, health promotion, and disease prevention, the Canadian health system and associated public policies continue to be largely curative in focus, with limited attention to public policies and interventions to address the social determinants of health. This is the result of a long-standing primacy of the curative and medicinal sciences in health, along with a significant media focus upon health care. However, there are also political reasons for this emphasis: Not only do the health professions and media play a significant role in shaping both public opinion and public policy (Page, 1996; Parenti, 1993), but the very political questions that lie at the heart of public health, health promotion, and the social determinants of health have made it difficult for health policy in Canada to move away toward a more preventative approach.

Conclusion

At its heart, both social and health policy in Canada have demonstrated not only how explicitly political the initiation, development, and implementation of such policies can be, but also how the structures and ideologies of Canadian politics have had a major effect in shaping health policy. As policy-makers, politicians, and those working in the applied health sciences have become more aware of the benefits of adopting a more preventative approach toward health policy, they are increasingly challenged by both the structural factors that have historically shaped policy, as well as the ideological and political realities of public policy-making. In particular, the rise of neo-liberalism, in combination with the federal structures of a "politics of blame," have led to a withering of the Canadian welfare state, and a marked shift in political rhetoric away from collective rights and welfare toward a politics of the individual.

Box 22.3: History of the Canada Health and Social Transfer

2007	Budget restructured the Canada Social Transfer (CST) to provide equal per capita cash support to provinces and territories, effective 2007–2008; similar changes to be made to the Canada Health Transfer (CHT) effective 2014–2015, when current legislation is renewed. The CST is extended to 2013–2014, and will grow by 3 percent annually as a result of an automatic escalator, effective 2009–2010.
2006	*September:* Budget provided $3.3 billion through five third-party trusts to help provinces and territories deal with immediate pressures in post-secondary education ($1 billion) and housing ($2.1 billion). *May:* Budget replaces the ELCC Initiative with the new Universal Child Care Benefit (UCCB).
2005	*March:* Budget introduced a new Early Learning and Child Care (ELCC) Initiative, providing $5 billion (2005–2006 to 2009–2010) to support development of a national ELCC framework outlining principles, objectives, and reporting requirements.
2004	*September:* First ministers signed the 10-Year Plan to Strengthen Health Care. The Government of Canada commits $41.3 billion in additional funding to provinces and territories for health. *April:* The CHST was restructured and two separate transfers were created, the Canada Health Transfer and the Canada Social Transfer.
2003	*March:* Budget announced $900 million over five years in increased federal support for ELCC. *February:* In support of the February 2003 First Ministers' Accord on Health Care Renewal, Budget confirmed: (1) a two-year extension of the five-year legislative framework with an additional $1.8 billion; (2) a $2.5 billion CHST supplement, giving provinces the flexibility to draw down funds as they required up to the end of 2005–2006; and (3) the restructuring of the CHST to create a separate Canada Health Transfer and a Canada Social Transfer effective April 1, 2004.
2000	*September:* First ministers agreed on an action plan for renewing health care and investing in early childhood development. The Government of Canada committed to investing $21.1 billion of additional CHST cash, including $2.2 billion for early childhood development over five years. *February:* Budget announced a $2.5 billion increase for the CHST to help provinces and territories fund post-secondary education and health care. This brought CHST cash to $15.5 billion for each of the years from 2000–2001 to 2003–2004.
1999	Budget announced increased CHST funding of $11.5 billion over five years, specifically for health care. Changes were made to the allocation formula to move to equal per capita CHST by 2001–2002.
1998	CHST legislation implemented with a cash floor of $12.5 billion.
1996	Budget announced a five-year CHST funding arrangement (1998–1999 to 2002–2003) and provided a cash floor of $11 billion per year. A new allocation formula to reflect changes in provincial population growth and to narrow existing funding disparities was introduced, moving halfway to equal per capita by 2002–2003.
1995	Starting in 1996, Established Programs Financing and Canada Assistance Plan programs would be replaced by a Canada Health and Social Transfer block fund. For 1995–1996, EPF growth was set at GNP-3, and CAP was frozen at 1994–1995 levels for all provinces. CHST was set at $26.9 billion for 1996–1997 and $25.1 billion for 1997–1998. CHST for 1996–1997 was allocated among provinces in the same proportion as combined EPF and CAP entitlements for 1995–1996.

There is no question that the policy and practitioner discourses on health in Canada have shifted toward a more socio-environmental conception of health that recognizes the social determinants of health since the Lalonde Report in 1974. Not only have the many authors critiqued the emphasis on the lifestyle approach to both improving and explaining health, but documents such as the *Ottawa Charter* (now 20 years old) and the Epp Report (known formally as the Health and Welfare Canada publication, *Achieving Health for All*), have been consistent with a more integrated and structural perspective on health. However, much of the more recent discourse on both health policy and health care has become tied not only to the economic perspectives of neo-liberalism (see, for example, Robertson, 1998), but have even provided a rationale for limiting the allocation of resources to health care.

At the same time that public policy, and public health in particular, have sought to become both more evidence-based or evidence-informed in order to be "objective" and apolitical, it has become increasingly apparent that all forms of policy, and health policy in particular, are not just explicitly political, but, as such, are an expression of multiple forms of power: epistemological, social, economic, and political. As a result, not only do the domestic and international contexts within which health policy takes place matter, so too do questions of political will, social values, and ideology.

As Robertson (1998) points out, the social determinants of health (and health promotion) are both explicitly and inherently political, making demands not on the allocation of resources to health care, but additionally on the fundamental inequities and disparities within Canadian society. In turn, the politics and policies of health in Canada are not only structurally and functionally complex and amorphous, but are also subject to the same discursive ambiguity and contests present in public policy more generally. Additionally, it may very well be that the political will and capacity to make a meaningful shift toward prevention is lacking.

As Brooks and Miljan (2003) note, a reformulation of Canadian health policy to actually address the social determinants of health will probably require greater government regulation, taxation, and involvement than citizens will permit. Ultimately, if Canadian citizens will not accept such a role, little more than a marginal shift in policy is likely to occur.

Notes

1. Both the Charlottetown Accord in Canada and the 1996 protests in Belgium.
2. Public goods may be either pure or partial. See Hampson, Daudelin, Hay, Martin & Reid (2002), for more.
3. See, for example, Nederveen Pieterse (2001); Barber (1984); Kramer (1982); Pateman (1980); Cook and Morgan (1971).
4. This is consistent with the political science literature of the 1980s and early 1990s concerned with "bringing the state back in." Following several years of dismissal or assumed impotence, authors drawing from sociology and other fields made a significant argument for the analysis of the state as a political actor itself. See, for example, Bremmer and Taras (1997); Barrow (1993); Mitchell (1991); Held (1989); Skocpol (1985, 1989); Laumann (1987).
5. As Hill correctly points out, social policy is often almost entirely absent in many of the developing countries of the world, despite the presence of severe social welfare problems and typically massive disparities between the "haves" and the "have nots" (Hill, 2006).
6. As had occurred in the 1930s, the differences between the political traditions of Quebec (oriented toward both conservatism and the Catholic Church) and the demands of the electorate meant that Quebec was vulnerable to federal social policy. Specifically, while the province opposed federal encroachment, Quebec was not in a position to initiate social policies at the provincial level. Additionally, social policies stemming from Ottawa were received positively by the Quebec electorate, placing further pressure on Quebec to accept such initiatives (Vaillancourt, 1988).
7. See the Commission on the Future of Health Care in Canada, *Interim Report* (February 2002), for greater detail.

Critical Thinking Questions

1. There are both domestic and international factors that have helped shape Canadian health policy. Is one level more important than the other? Why?

2. Federalism is easily identified as a key structural factor in Canadian social policy. What impact might other structures, such as the parliamentary or electoral systems, have upon this area of public policy?

3. Are there ways in which the effects of federalism on health policy in Canada can be viewed as positive?

4. Is there or has there been a common ideology attempting to shape social policy, and health policy specifically, in Canada? What is this ideology, and how does it seek to effect change?

5. What role has public opinion played in the development of health policy in Canada?

Recommended Readings

Banting, K. (1987). *The welfare state and Canadian federalism*, 2nd ed. Montreal: McGill-Queen's University Press.

In this text, Banting provides a critical overview of how the federal structures and resulting political tensions have contributed to the shape of the Canadian welfare state and social policy. Focusing on income security, Banting examines how political institutions directly contribute to policy outcomes.

Castles, F.G. (1999). *Comparative public policy: Patterns of post-war transformation*. Cheltenham: Edward Elgar.

This book provides a unique and systematic comparative perspective on the transformation of the post-Second World War welfare state. Based on comparisons of long-term members of the Organisation for Economic Co-operation and Development, Castles notes that no single variable explains the emergence or shape of welfare states.

Fisher, F. (1990). *Technocracy and the politics of expertise*. London: Sage Publications.

Fisher argues that a new model of governance and policy-making has emerged. One based on that has generally been built with an emphasis on a highly practical, utilitarian, and technocratic model of decision making: a "politics of expertise." This is where public policy is made by highly educated and informed bureaucratic elites and experts, with few opportunities for input from the general public.

Fisher, F., & Forester, J. (Eds.). (1993). *The argumentative turn in policy analysis and planning*. Durham & London: Duke University Press.

Fisher and Forester present a new perspective on the analysis of public policy by framing it within the context of the "linguistic turn." Drawing from authors such as Habermas and Foucault, this collection explores the ways in which conceptualizing public policy as being made of, and intimately affected by, language can help in its analyses.

Obinger, H., Leibfried, S., & Castles, F.G. (Eds.). (2005). *Federalism and the welfare state: New world and European experiences*. Cambridge: Cambridge University Press. This text provides a key set of comparative perspectives on the relationships between political institutions and public policy. Focusing on case studies of New and Old World federalism, countries such as Canada, the US, Switzerland, and Germany are used as case studies to assess a seemingly simple question with multiple and complicated answers: What effect does federalism have upon the emergence and form of social policy, and does federalism always inhibit the growth of social solidarity?

Torgerson, D. (1986). "Between knowledge and politics: Three faces of policy analysis." *Policy Sciences, 19*, 33–59.

Torgerson identifies various conceptual schemes that have been used to make sense of the diverse policy literature. Grounded in an attempt to understand policy analysis in terms of its political and historical significance, this essay points to three distinct faces, distinguished by differing relationships between knowledge and politics: (1) one where knowledge purports to replace politics; (2) one where politics masquerades as knowledge; and (3) one where knowledge and politics attain a measure of reconciliation.

Related Web Sites

Canadian Health and Social Transfers—www.fin.gc.ca/FEDPROV/hise.html

This government site provides a detailed history and explanation of the evolution of key social legislation and policies, as well as the key differences in funding allocation and budgetary growth/reduction.

Friends of Medicare—www.friendsofmedicare.ab.ca

The Friends of Medicare is a coalition of individuals, service organizations, social justice groups, unions, associations, churches, and organizations representing various sectors of our communities. Since 1979, it has called upon the federal and provincial governments to live up to the commitments they made in the original medicare legislation, the Canada Health Act.

Health Canada—www.hc-sc.gc.ca

Health Canada is the federal department charged with helping Canadians maintain and improve their health, while respecting individual choices and circumstances. Its goal is for Canada to be among the countries with the healthiest people in the world through the use of research, consultations, communications, and advocacy.

National Collaborating Centres for Public Health—www.nccph.ca

The six National Collaborating Centres are designed to provide knowledge syntheses and translation of the evidence base for different areas of public health. These are: Aboriginal Health, Environmental Health, Infectious Disease, Methods and Tools, Healthy Public Policy, and Determinants of Health.

Public Health Agency of Canada—www.phac-aspc.gc.ca

The Public Health Agency of Canada is a new agency charged with promoting and protecting the health of Canadians through leadership and action. Focused on more effective efforts to prevent chronic diseases, injuries, and respond to public health emergencies and infectious disease outbreaks, the Public Health Agency of Canada works closely with provinces and territories to keep Canadians healthy and to reduce the pressures on the health care system.

WHO Commission on the Social Determinants of Health—www.who.int/social_determinants

Initially commissioned in 2005, the WHO Commission on the Social Determinants of Health was created to bring together leading scientists and practitioners to provide evidence on policies that improve health by addressing the social conditions in which people live and work. It collaborates with countries to support policy change and monitor results. Its goals are to: (1) support policy change in countries by promoting models and practices that effectively address the social determinants of health; (2) support countries in placing health as a shared goal; and (3) help build a sustainable global movement for action on health equity and the social determinants.

Chapter 23

———◆———

PUBLIC POLICY, GENDER, AND HEALTH

Pat Armstrong

Introduction

Gender matters in health and care. The point may seem obvious, but it has only recently been acknowledged in health policy and research. Canada now recognizes gender as one of the dozen determinants of health. The 1995 federal government's plan for gender equality requires legislation and policy to include an analysis of the potential for differential impacts on women and men (Status of Women Canada, 1995). The Canadian Institutes of Health Research (CIHR), the main source of funding for research on health and care in this country, has just recently developed a policy on such gender-based analysis. According to the CIHR research guide, "implementing gender and sex-based analysis (GSBA) in health research is fundamental to achieving research excellence" (Canadian Institutes for Health Research, 2007, p. 2). The other major research funding body, the Social Sciences and Humanities Research Council of Canada, developed a policy on gender-based analysis several years earlier. In spite of these explicit and high-profile endorsements for gender-based analysis (GBA) in Canada, however, we are a long way from putting these policies into practice in research, health promotion, and care.

This chapter begins by examining what is meant by gender and gender-based analysis before outlining some of the research and pressures that led to the recognition of gender as a determinant of health. This sets the stage for a discussion of the role gender plays in the determinants of health and of our continued failure to integrate a gender-based analysis in policy and practices.

Gender-Based Analysis

In order to explain a gender-based analysis, it is first necessary to understand what is meant by gender. "Sex" is the term usually used to refer to biological differences between men and women, while "gender" most frequently refers to what is socially recognized as feminine and masculine (Greaves et al., 1999, p. 1). By differentiating between sex and gender, social scientists sought to stress the social construction of distinctions between women and men, boys and girls. They wanted to emphasize how many differences are created by us, and thus can be altered by us. But these terms raised their own problems. First, they implied that biological factors can be separated from social factors and that biological differences are firmly established. Second, they also implied that biology is unchanging, outside history and influence. Third, the distinction suggested that biology is irrelevant to an understanding of social distinctions between males and females.

It has long been recognized that sex differences play a role in health, especially when it comes to reproduction. Indeed, at times what were assumed to be biological differences between women and men were thought to create two distinct species and were used to justify both women's subordination to men and dramatically different treatment for women and men in all aspects of life. However, study after study has challenged the notion that biology determines behaviour and other differences in some direct manner and even the idea that we can describe two biologically distinct or universally distinct sexes (Fausto-Sterling, 2000; Lips, 2007; Rose et al., 1984). Research reveals an astonishing variety in gender relations that seems to deny biological determinism. Margaret Lock (1998), for example, found that the physical manifestations of menopause vary across cultures, while R.A. Anderson and colleagues (1999) showed that testosterone replacement had a different impact on male sexuality in Hong Kong than it did in North America. And claims that an extra Y-chromosome—the chromosome that must be present for the embryonic sex glands to develop in a male direction—leads to criminal behaviour has been rejected in US courts because the argument lacks scientific support (World Health Organization, 2008). Anne Fausto-Sterling has argued that it is impossible to determine which aspects of our behaviour are biologically determined because "an individual's capacities emerge from a web of interactions between the biological being and the social environment.... Biology may in some manner condition behaviour, but behaviour in turn can alter one's physiology. Furthermore, any particular behaviour may have many different causes" (1985, p. 8). This is why, as she has said more recently (Fausto-Sterling, 2000), that even with the latest techniques, scientists still disagree about differences and their impact. These debates are not surprising because people do not exist outside their social and economic environments. What are often called "biological processes" are influenced by those environments, as we see, for example, when our genes are altered by exposure to something like radiation.

The CIHR guide talks about gender and sex-based analysis. But the problem with using these two categories is that the labels may imply that sex and gender can be easily separated. There is a materiality to the body and there are significant differences related not only to reproductive and sexual organs but also to hormones, body size, and body processes. Only women get pregnant, menstruate, and lactate. And that matters. But, as those such as Michel Foucault (1978) argue, there are no bodies—or research—outside culture, history, space,

place, discourse, and social relations. The experiences, as well as the physical manifestations of pregnancy, menstruation, and lactation, vary significantly over time and with class, sexual orientation, and geographical location. Moreover, neither sex nor gender is one/two variables with clear lines between two sexes and two genders. Rather, they are continuums along which we can find multiple variations.

Gender-based analysis acknowledges that the biological always exists inside the social at the same time that it acknowledges that gender matters. Doing gender-based analysis means much more than analyzing data by sex, although it often begins with data collected on the basis of sex categories. It does not mean that sex is never used as a category, nor that dichotomies such as male/female, and feminine/masculine are never used. Rather, gender-based analysis means being constantly aware of the social shaping and evaluation of sex that makes it a gendered construct and of the variability in sex that challenges the notion of it as a dichotomous one. Lumping people into two categories may be the only way to use the data available; it may be the best way to develop a general picture of pattern and processes. But it is important to be aware of the complexity and variability hidden by those dichotomies and categories.

Gender-based analysis begins with the recognition that all populations are gendered, and that people experience their worlds and are treated in their worlds on the basis of gender. Of course, other social locations linked to age, culture, income, disability, and racialization—to name only some—also matter. But these, too, are divided by gender.

Gender-based analysis means recognizing how gender shapes and is shaped by conditions, practices, and relations, including relations of markets, power, and inequality. A gendered analysis in health and health care requires the assessment of causes, processes, and consequences by gender, "taking into account the context of individuals' lives" (DesMeules et al., 2003, p. 2). The impact of these may be contradictory for women, simultaneously or alternatively improving and challenging their health and capacity to provide care.

Gender-based analysis is an approach rather than a formula for assessing research, policy, and practices. It is a way of seeing and doing research rather than a set of standard methods. It requires beginning with the assumption that there are gender differences in how we live, work, and play, as well as in our power and resources. These differences have consequences for our health, our care and care work, our symptoms, our treatments and our outcomes. This assumption must play a role in our research questions, in our data collection and analysis, in the conclusions we draw and the strategies we develop to address what we find. It means asking how women and men, boys and girls differ in terms of causes, processes, consequences, alternatives, and power, and how such differences influence their health and care. It also means asking which women and which men, so that we can explore the ways other social and physical locations intersect with gender.

Gender-Based Analysis and Women's Health

Not surprisingly, much of the gender-sensitive research and policy in Canada has focused on women. It is not surprising because it was the women's movement that began demonstrating how gender and assumptions about gender permeate policy and practice, and do so in ways that assume male norms, standards, and subjects. They showed, for example, that almost all randomized clinical trails were done on young males and that research not only focused on men but generalized on the basis of this research to the entire population (Greaves et al., 1999, p. 7). They demonstrated that the consequences of what Karen Messing (1998, p. 3) has called "One-Eyed Science," a science that focused on men and biological processes, have been particularly harmful for women. As the authors of *The Politics of Women's Health* put it, medicine has played "an active role in perpetuating some aspects of women's oppression while helping to reduce other dimensions" (Sherwin et al., 1998, p. 3).

Women pushed to have research that both included them and considered differences. They demanded space and specificity. We are only beginning to see the results, results that bear out their contention that gender matters in everything from heart attacks to Aspirin consumption, from wait times to care work (Jackson, Pederson & Boscoe, 2006). But gender-based analysis is not exclusively about women. Gender is understood as a relationship. It thus requires paying attention to the relations among the genders. And it requires

recognizing that women have often been, and continue to be, subordinate in those relationships. Indeed, much of the research intended to demonstrate the importance of gender required comparative data on women and men. Moreover, a great deal of health behaviour, health care, and other health processes involves relations between women and men, a fact not lost on those beginning from a women's perspective. Power relations in particular have played a major role in the analysis, with an emphasis on the subordination shared by most women. It should be noted, however, that gender-sensitive research is not necessarily comparative. It can study women or men without searching for comparisons or emphasizing gender relations. Yet even those who have been most concerned with women's issues and who see women as subordinate in terms of both health and care recognize that strategies for change cannot be developed in many areas without understanding what is happening with men. Perhaps more critically, this women's research developed many of the tools of analysis that allow us to see gendered causes, consequences, processes, and contexts. What works for women does not necessarily work for men, just as what works for men does not necessarily work for women. In fact, that is a major point of gender-sensitive research.

This does not mean ignoring men's health. Indeed, it is a required aspect of GBA. But it does mean recognizing that male health has been considered the norm and that men often have more power. In other words, the causes, processes, and consequences of health care are not only different for women and men. They also contribute to inequality both between women and men and among women. Stephen Lewis's (2005) arguments about the role that gender plays in the spread of AIDS in Africa is just one example of how critical it is to understand women's health and the relationships between women and men. Moreover, what benefits women frequently benefits men as well. One example is the pressure to limit hours of work for doctors, which is often blamed on women moving into medical jobs. With more restrictions on demands for their time, male physicians, too, can now see their children.

In short, health and health care have clearly emerged as women's issues, and women have played an active role in revealing how gender matters. Women have shown that, although there is little that is universal about gender, it is universally relevant. Gender-based analysis is thus

Box 23.1: Health Canada and gender analysis

Health Canada's role is to foster good health by promoting health and protecting Canadians from harmful products, practices, and disease. Gender equality is a broad societal human rights, social justice, and health issue. As such, Health Canada will implement a gender-based analysis to ensure that policies and programs are responsive to sex and gender differences and to women's health needs, which results in remedies to inequality.

Gender-based analysis (GBA) is a method of evaluation and interpretation that takes into account social and economic differences between women and men, whether applied to policy and program development, or general life activities such as work/family roles.

The application of GBA is governed by a number of fundamental principles including:
- gender equality can be achieved only by recognizing the different impact of norms or measures on women and men according to their diverse life situations
- gender-based analysis is an integral part of the substantive analytical process and must be applied at each stage of this process
- gender-based analysis focuses not only on results but also on concepts, arguments, and language used in the work process
- gender-based analysis must lead to remedies to inequality

GBA and Women's Health

When GBA is applied to health policy and program development, gender stereotypes are eliminated and socio-economic factors affecting women's health are acknowledged. When equitable policies are applied to the health system, this sets the stage for the provision of services appropriate to women's needs.

GBA recognizes that the health needs of women and girls, and men and boys are different. It does this by ensuring that an analysis of the determinants of health is undertaken. This accounts for social factors that affect everyone's lives, such as issues of diversity including socio-economic status, ability, ethnicity, and sexual orientation.

Health Canada Initiatives

Health Canada's implementation of a gender-based analysis fully integrates gender into its day-to-day operations. It represents Health Canada's commitment to doing business in a way that is sensitive to women's health needs and concerns.

This federal government commitment is articulated in the Federal Plan for Gender Equality approved by Cabinet in 1995, which states that departments will put forward "a systematic process to inform and guide future legislation and policies at the federal level by assessing any potential differential impact on women and men."

Health Canada will ensure that:
- employees are given professional development seminars to learn the steps involved in GBA
- employees are given a guide on how to apply GBA to the substantive work of the department
- a network of gender equality specialists serve as resource persons for policy/program development and implementation, research, funding, data collection, surveillance, regulatory activities, health promotion, disease prevention, services to First Nations and Inuit, corporate management activities/ policies/consultations/communication plans
- managers will dedicate staff time for GBA training, analysis, committee work, etc.
- managers incorporate women's health plans in the development of the annual branch plans and business lines to ensure that gender equality is given priority as an integral part of the strategic planning process

The Women's Health Bureau has prepared a guiding document, *Women's Health Strategy*, which situates gender issues in the context of health, and will be the basis for Health Canada's GBA implementation.

The overall goal is to improve the health of women in Canada by making the health system more responsive to women and women's health.

Sources:
- *Women's Health Strategy*, Women's Health Bureau, Health Canada, 1999.
- *Health Canada's Implementation on Gender-Based Analysis*, Women's Health Bureau, Health Canada, 1999.
- *Exploring Concepts of Gender and Health*, Health Canada, Women's Health Bureau, 2003.
- *Gender-Based Analysis Backgrounder*, Human Resources Development Canada, Cat. no. SP-100-01-97E, 1997.
- *Gender-Based Analysis Guide*, Human Resources Development Canada, Cat. no. SP-101-01-97E, 1997.
- *Diversity and Justice: Gender Perspectives, a Guide to Gender Equality Analysis*, Department of Justice Canada, 1998.
- *Women's Health in the Context of Women's Lives*, Minister of Supply and Services, Cat. no. H39-324/1995E, 1995.
- *Working Together for Women's Health: A Framework for the Development of Policies and Programs*, Federal/Provincial/Territorial Working Group on Women's Health, April 1990.

Source: Women's Health Bureau of Health Canada, 2004. Available on-line at www.hc-sc.gc.ca/english/women/.

necessary for good science, effective policy, and efficient practices. There are ethical and moral reasons for gender-based analysis as well. If we are interested in promoting equity, we need to do GBA. Without a knowledge base that takes gender into account, we cannot determine and address inequity. It was evidence and pressure from the women's movement that led Canada to adopt the federal plan for gender equality mentioned in the introduction to this chapter. Also as a result of this pressure and evidence, Canada established a Women's Health Bureau within Health Canada, a Centres of Excellence Programme for Women's Health and a Canadian Women's Health Network.[1]

All these initiatives were based on the recognition that gender differences are critical in health and care, and that women were often excluded from research and treated inappropriately in practice. All of them include gender-sensitive research, policy, and practice in their mandate. Women worked equally hard to ensure that one of the federally funded Canadian Institutes of Health Research focused on gender, with a mandate "to support research to address how sex and gender interact with other factors that influence health to create conditions and problems that are unique, more prevalent, more serious or different with respect to risk factors or effective interventions for women and men" (Health Canada, 2003, p. 7). It is, in other words, devoted to research that focuses on either women or men, or each in relation to the other. The Institute of Gender and Health has funded

research on men's issues such as hormone treatment for prostrate cancer, the service needs of elderly gay men, and Black men's experience of violence, as well as many comparative projects such as the role of women and men in unpaid caregiving (Neufeld, Harrison, Hughes & Stewart, 2007).

This struggle to have gender taken into account in ways that serve women has not been an easy process, however, and it is one that is far from complete. Gender-based analysis is a work in progress and, as we shall see in the next sections that outline how gender pervades the determinants of health, we still have a long way to go.

Gender and the Determinants of Health

Largely as a result of pressure and evidence developed at home and abroad, Health Canada expanded the list of health determinants to include gender. Even the traditional focus on reproductive health is shifting. The range of sex issues is understood to be much broader and biology is increasingly understood as influenced by social contexts while gender is used to draw particular attention to the social construction of female/male differences. The inclusion of gender as a health determinant marks a major advance. However, it is equally important to examine how gender pervades all the other determinants as this section does.

It seems logical to begin a discussion of health determinants with biology and genetic endowments, given that they clearly play a role in gender and are often assumed to be the critical factors in health and illness. In general, women and men have different bodies and these bodies help create differences in risks and outcomes. Although most of the attention has focused on women's reproductive capacities, we are just beginning to learn about the ways in which biology and genetics influence other aspects of women and men's health. For example, women are two to three times more likely than men to develop lung cancer, even when they don't smoke, and this difference may be related to gene expression (Greaves & Richardson, 2007, p. 6).

However, biology is profoundly influenced by social and economic contexts, and influenced in ways that can shape the way bodies develop and experience. These contexts are unequally structured for women and men as well as for different groups of women and men and for different individuals. Age of puberty, for example, varies significantly among economic groups, and women employed in some jobs cease to menstruate as a result of the conditions in which they work (Messing, Lippel, Demers & Mergler, 2000). Even our genes are influenced by the physical, social, and economic environment (Fausto-Sterling, 2000), as are our definitions of what is genetic (Basen, Eichler & Lippman, 1993). Equally important, the meaning and the consequences of biological and genetic endowments are structured by such environments. In other words, while it is important to ask about male and female differences in genes and biology, it is also important to remember that all bodies are located in history and social relations.

Gender, understood as a term emphasizing the social construction of differences linked to sex, is separated from sex on the Health Canada list of determinants and does mean that social relations are recognized. This identification of gender as a determinant has the advantage of emphasizing that women in general share not only reproductive capacities but also an unequal position in relation to men. Lesley Doyal nicely sums up the argument for recognizing gender as a determinant in her groundbreaking book, *What Makes Women Sick* (1995, p. 7): "Though this subordination is linked in complex ways with divisions of race, class and nationality, women do have common experiences as objects of sexist practices." And these practices have a critical impact on health for both women and men. As Richard Wilkinson (2005, p. 217) shows, in "societies where women's status is closer to men's, both men and women had better health."

The Fourth World Conference on Women (United Nations, 1995) agreed that "Women's health involves women's emotional, social, cultural, spiritual and physical well-being and is determined by the social, political and economic contexts of women's lives as well as by biology." A gendered approach thus means understanding differences among women as well as differences related to their various social, cultural, sexual, physical, and economic locations and abilities. The claim is not that gender is primary, but that it always must be taken into account, considering the ways it intersects with other factors. Equally important, the claim is that gender is not only one of a list of factors, but one that pervades all the others, as we shall see as we look at the other 10 determinants recognized by Health Canada.

Racialization

Health Canada does not identify racialization as a determinant of health, but does identify culture as one, suggesting some differences related to the social relations of racialization. However, as Richard Wilkinson (2005, p. 229) explains, it is easier to remove cultural markers than it is to remove those linked to racialization, and racism may well be a more important factor in health. The absence of racialization from Health Canada's list could be understood as a failure to recognize the importance of racism, although it may also be meant to emphasize how other differences may be linked to discrimination, stigmatization, and exclusion that result in poor health. Nevertheless, research in Canada and elsewhere has highlighted the importance of racialization as a health determinant for women and men, although we need much more research on racism that provides a gender lens (Das Gupta, 1996; Doyal, Payne & Cameron, 2003; Guruge, Donner & Morrison, 2000). Moreover, research also suggests that government policy, such as those linked to immigration and social services, often fails to counteract racism or gender inequalities linked to racism and may even support it in ways that undermine health (Cohen, 2000; Creese, Dyck & McLaren, 2006). Equally important, we are only beginning to develop policies and practices that are intended to make health services more culturally sensitive and accessible in ways that understand gender relations (Laroche, 2000; Mulvihill, Mailloux & Atkin, 2002).

The federal and some provincial governments do have some policies on employment equity that acknowledge inequities resulting from racism and cultural discrimination. And the Canadian Charter of Rights and Freedoms can be understood to acknowledge racism. Some organizations have been able to use the Charter of Rights and Freedoms to help reduce harmful discrimination against some groups, such as gays and lesbians. However, the cancellation of the government program that provided funding for groups seeking to use the Charter in this way may mean little progress in the future. There is still a long way to go before a determinants approach makes racism central and recognizes the ways in which it interacts with gender in shaping health.

Income and Social Status

Income and social status also have a critical impact on health in ways that are profoundly gendered. The poor live shorter lives than the rich, and their lives are marked by more frequent bouts of ill health and disability (Wilkinson, 1992). It is not only absolute income that matters to health, however. Relative income is also very important. Indeed, overall inequality in a society is a critical indicator of overall health, with greater inequality leading to poorer health (Wilkinson, 2005). Not only is inequality increasing globally and nationally (Hennessy, 2006), but women are making little progress in relation to men. Women continue to be paid less than men and receive less in benefits from paid employment (Statistics Canada, 2006, Chapter 6). Women are more likely than men to parent alone and be poor when they do so. Senior women have, however, made important progress in terms of income, largely as a result of our universal pensions scheme (Statistics Canada, 2006, p. 144).

Income inequality and relative income are not the only factors, though. The "quality of social relations and low social status are among the most powerful influences on health" (Wilkinson, 2005, p. 101). Low social status is often linked to income, although it is also linked to jobs such as cleaning and doing laundry, which mainly women do, regardless of pay. There are clearly gendered patterns to employment and although women have made some gains in terms of access to more prestigious, male-dominated jobs, the labour force remains highly

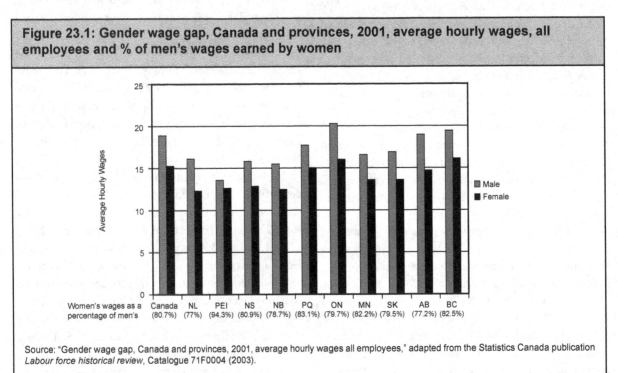

Figure 23.1: Gender wage gap, Canada and provinces, 2001, average hourly wages, all employees and % of men's wages earned by women

Source: "Gender wage gap, Canada and provinces, 2001, average hourly wages all employees," adapted from the Statistics Canada publication *Labour force historical review*, Catalogue 71F0004 (2003).

segregated, with women concentrated in jobs with the lowest status and pay (Statistics Canada, 2006, chapters 5 and 6).

Many of these social relations and much of this social status are related to employment. Paid work can promote health, by providing material and psychological rewards as well as social contacts (Carver & Ponée, 1995). And unemployment can destroy health (Avison, 1998). For many, however, the formal workplace is dangerous to their health in ways that are profoundly gendered (Stellman & Daum, 1973; Stellman, 1977). And the risk does not come only from obvious dangers such as chemicals and guns, falls and fumes. Research in the United Kingdom shows that there is a strong relationship between health and location in the hierarchy at the workplace, with mortality rates near the bottom three times higher than the rates for those near the top (Marmot, 1986). Lack of control over tasks and the ordering of tasks can produce more dangerous stress than does running the plant (Karesek, 1979; Karasek & Theorell, 1990), and few women run the plant. Low co-worker support can undermine mental health as well, as can sexual harassment. A summary prepared for the National Forum on Health (1998), a group appointed a decade ago by the prime minister to look at the future of health care, sets out a range of factors, starting with the global, national,

and sectoral contexts, through to organizational structure and environment, task requirements, and individual practices that shape health at paid work and that need to be addressed in promoting health. What the forum did not do, however, was bring a gender lens to bear on the workplace health issues even though we know gender shapes workplace health in quite distinct ways (European Agency for Safety and Health at Work, 2003).

Nor did the forum look at unpaid work in the household, where women account for the majority of the workforce. Households, too, can be workplaces that promote health or undermine it. Both violence and accidents are common consequences of relations and conditions in the household, especially for women (Lakeman, 2006; Rosenberg, 1990). Moreover, stress caused by the conflicting demands of paid and unpaid work can be a particular health hazard for women (Shields, 2006).

Paid workplaces and households often constitute our most important physical and social environments, as well as other determinants of health. Like the work that goes on within them, they can either promote or undermine health, or even do both at the same time. The 19th-century public health movement was built on the evidence demonstrating the importance of clean air and water, on the critical nature of housing and crowding,

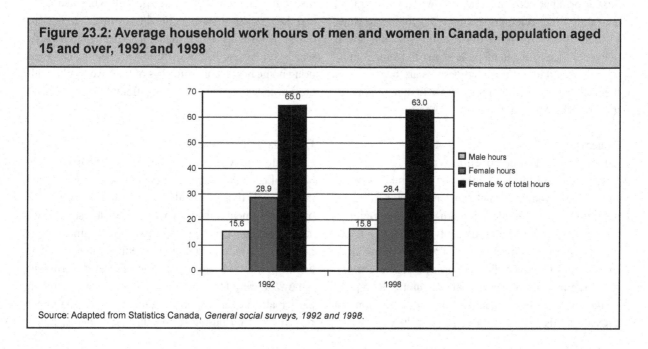

Figure 23.2: Average household work hours of men and women in Canada, population aged 15 and over, 1992 and 1998

Source: Adapted from Statistics Canada, *General social surveys, 1992 and 1998.*

and on the significance of safe, nutritious food. The identification of bacteria emphasized the importance of washed hands, clean surfaces, and sterile equipment while, more recently, Legionnaire's disease made us recognize that ventilation systems play an important role. And we have all become increasingly aware of air, water, and soil pollution. Health services constitute the physical and social environments not only for workers, but for patients and residents as well. The international magazine *Women and Environments* clearly shows that women have both a specific interest in environments and are influenced in particular ways by environments.

Employment

Employment, in turn, can provide us with the sort of social networks that promote good health or do the reverse by undermining our ability to form social networks. Although we most often associate social networks with households and communities, workplaces may not only be where we meet people but also where our health is influenced in ways that threaten social relations at home. As Jeanette Cochrane (1995, p. 131) succinctly put it, the "stressors we encounter in one area of our lives are certain to have an impact on other areas of our lives." And women especially feel stress from juggling their paid and unpaid work in ways that sustain relationships. Sexual or other harassment at paid work, for example, can undermine relations at home. At the same time, women often have more dense and rewarding social networks than men and often have more regular contact with their children. Such relationships are beneficial in themselves, and they promote access to other resources that contribute to health.

Education

Education is linked to employment and gender, influencing the kinds of jobs and income available. Increasingly women are matching or even outnumbering men in many higher education programs, although this has not paid off in terms of equivalent employment. Education can also mean that we know about the kinds of personal practices, like eating our vegetables and cooking them appropriately, that can contribute to good health (Breen, 1998). Equally important, education can provide skills that allow people to gain satisfaction

in both their paid and unpaid work. Doing a job well can promote health. It is an ongoing process, requiring continual attention to new learning from and with others. While formal education is the most obvious form, the informal acquisition of skills and knowledge that happens through work can be as important as the ones recognized through certification. The possibilities for learning on the job, however, are shaped by the organization of work as well as by the nature of the workplace relations and, of course, by gender. Women more often find themselves in precarious employment that fails to recognize or reward their skills and education or allow for this kind of learning (Vosko, 2006).

Healthy Child Development

The National Forum on Health (1998), devoted an entire volume to another of Health Canada's determinants; namely, healthy child development. It seems obvious that our early years have a profound impact not only on children's health, but also on our adult health. What may be less obvious are the ways the work of adults, and especially of mothers, influence the environments in which children grow up. Mothers who are stressed at their paid jobs take home their stress, and may take that stress out on their children. Every group we interviewed for one long-term care project talked about yelling at their children more as the pace of their work increased and the number of staff declined (Armstrong & Jansen, 2006). Women can also bring home other health hazards from work, as we learned with SARS, and so can men bring home health consequences of their work, although the hazards they face may be different from those of women.

Lifestyle Behaviours

Lifestyle behaviours, or what Health Canada calls personal health practices and coping skills, are perhaps the most talked-about health determinant. It is difficult to pick up a women's magazine without seeing a story about eating your spinach or joining a gym. Governments, too, have made fitness and eating a central theme in their health-promotion strategies. The federal government is now offering tax credits for parents whose children participate in certain sports that the revenue department regards as contributing to health. Undoubtedly, doing yoga and eating spinach can improve health. However, in order to participate in such activities, people have to have the time, energy, and resources. The will is often not good enough. With multiple paid jobs, for example, a long commute, and no access to child care, it is difficult for a woman to find the time for yoga. And in any case, yoga may not be sufficient to overcome the stress caused by such work demands. Moreover, workers may know about workplace health and safety strategies, but be unable to follow them because the equipment and/or the pace of their work are unsafe. Similarly, workers may have the money to buy spinach and even to cook it, but if the available spinach carries harmful bacteria, health is not promoted by the practice. Workplaces shape the possibilities for coping and for staying healthy, as does gender.

Health Services

Finally, health services are recognized as a determinant of health. This, too, seems obvious. Indeed, a determinants of health approach emphasizes how health is determined by more than medical interventions, assuming that health services play a critical role. The interaction with other factors tends to be less obvious, however. For example, recent research (Fowler et al., 2007) found that older women were less likely than men of a similar age to be admitted to the intensive-care unit for treatment of heart conditions and were more likely to die from their heart conditions. Earlier research suggests that Aboriginal women face multiple barriers in getting health services and encounter considerable discrimination within those services they do manage to get (Dion Stout, Kipling & Stout, 2001). In other words, gender is related to power over and relations within health services as well as to racialization. Similarly, conditions for work and pay of workers not only influence those providing care, but also the care they provide. Most of this paid and unpaid health care is provided by women.

In short, a determinants of health approach tells us that health is created in classed, racialized, and gendered ways. The determinants listed by Health Canada help us see the multiple factors at play. While it is important to recognize gender as a determinant, it is equally important to remember that gender pervades all the determinants of health.

Conclusion

Efforts by the women's health movement, as well as the evidence they have amassed, led Canada to recognize gender as a determinant of health and to policy that promotes a gender-based analysis. In spite of the evidence that gender matters, however, a great deal of research and policy fails to incorporate such an analysis. The result is poor science and often worse policy and practices, as well as continuing inequalities.

Note

1. Materials produced by these agencies and groups can be found at www.cewh-cesf.ca or www.cwhn.ca. To find the publications of the Coordinating Group on Health Care Reform and Women, click on "Health Reform."

Critical Thinking Questions

1. Should we always include a gender-based analysis when we do research on health?
2. Should we have separate health services for women and men?
3. How can we do research that takes women and men's multiple social locations into account?
4. What kinds of social policy are required to reduce gender-related inequalities?

Recommended Readings

Armstrong, Pat et al. (2002). *Reading Romanow.* Online at www. CWHN.ca.

The Romanow Report on the Future of Health Care in Canada was the outcome of a Royal Commission that not only conducted extensive research, but also held wider-ranging public hearings. It offered recommendations on how to construct a public health care system that is sustainable and that reflects Canadian values. In spite of submissions that called for a gender-sensitive analysis, and in spite of federal government policy requiring such analysis, the report was gender-blind. This document provides an example of gender-sensitive analysis in practice.

Grant, Karen et al. (Eds.). (2004). *Caring for/caring about: Women, home care, and unpaid caregiving.* Aurora: Garamond.

Women account for four out of five caregivers. Women also do the overwhelming majority of unpaid care work. This collection of articles offers a conceptual guide to caregiving as well as an assessment of existing research on gender and caregiving. One article focuses specifically on women with disabilities, while another focuses on Aboriginal women. Additional articles develop portraits of women who give and receive care in Quebec and Ontario.

Jackson, Beth, Pederson, Ann & Boscoe, Madeline. (2006). *Gender-based analysis and wait times: New questions, new knowledge.* Online at www.cwhn.ca

This article, published as an appendix to a federal government report on wait times, provides an excellent example of gender-based analysis applied to practices, showing why gender matters in health services.

Lorber, Judith. (2000). *Gender and the social construction of illness.* Oxford: Rowman and Littlefield.

The author explores the interaction between gender and medicine, focusing on how both are social constructions that are understood within a context of power and politics.

Messing, Karen. (1998). *One-eyed science: Occupational health and women workers.* Philadelphia: University of Philadelphia Press.

Internationally recognized as a definitive work on the importance of gender in occupational health, this book provides a comprehensive assessment of theory and research in this critical field.

Van Esterik, Penny (Ed.). (2003). *Head, heart, and hands partnerships for women's health in Canadian environments,* vol. 1. Toronto: National Network on Environments and Women's Health.

This volume brings together papers written under the auspices of the National Network for Environments and Women's Health, a federally funded Centre of Excellence for Women's Health. Beginning with conceptual frameworks and methodological approaches, the collection moves on to consider conditions of work in care, health, and locality, and perceptions of risk. The articles cover a wide range of perspectives, issues, methods, and topics, making it an excellent source for those interested in acquiring an understanding of the breadth of women's health issues.

Related Web Sites

Canadian Centre for Policy Alternatives—www.policyalternatives.ca

The CCPA is a research organization that covers multiple topics directly related to health.

Canadian Health Coalition—www.healthcoalition.ca

This site offers analysis of current critical issues in health care and the social determinants of health. The coalition brings together brings together community, religious, and union organizations dedicated to protecting and promoting public care.

Canadian Institutes of Health Research, Institute of Gender and Health—www.cihr-irsc.gc.ca

The institute funds research on gender and health. It also publishes material on integrating gender-sensitive research.

Canadian Women's Health Network—www.cwhn.ca

This Web site not only provides access to publications from the Centres of Excellence for Women's Health, it also links directly to sources around the world on a broad range of issues related to women's health.

Department of Gender, Women, and Health—www.who.int/gender/en

This agency of the World Health Organization is a particularly good source for comparative information on research from countries around the world.

Chapter 24

SURMOUNTING THE BARRIERS:
MAKING ACTION ON THE SOCIAL DETERMINANTS
OF HEALTH A PUBLIC POLICY PRIORITY

Dennis Raphael and Ann Curry-Stevens

Introduction

The current state of affairs concerning the social determinants of health and their effects upon the health of Canadians has been presented. Each contributor has carefully presented evidence concerning the social determinants of health and their effects upon health. They have also provided various policy options to improve their quality, which would improve the health of Canadians. Clearly, concerted action is needed to raise Canadians' awareness of the importance of the social determinants of health and press policy-makers to undertake actions to improve their quality. The key issues addressed in this concluding chapter are:

1. Considering what is known about these social determinants of health and their importance for promoting the health of Canadians, why does there seem to be so little action being undertaken to improve them?
2. What are the means by which such action can be brought about?

Our analysis requires consideration of issues that are only sporadically discussed in the health sciences literature but appear especially important to implementing a social determinants of health agenda. The first issue considers the role that professional and societal discourses—ways that health professionals,

the public, and policy-makers understand and consider an issue—play in having a concept such as the social determinants of health taken seriously. What are the ideas about health and illness—the ideologies—held by health professionals, the public, and policy-makers concerning the sources of health and causes of disease? How do these ideas influence receptivity to a social determinants of health approach to promoting health?

This analysis is important as there are numerous aspects of a social determinants of health approach that are foreign to traditional ways of thinking about health issues. Some of these aspects include: (1) how issues in the health sciences in general, and in epidemiology in particular, are generally conceived and acted upon; (2) the role that the beliefs in individualism and individual responsibility play in Canadian society; and (3) the increasing market orientation of Canadian society and how this emphasis weakens support for a social determinants of health approach to promoting health.

The second issue is concerned with what is known about the policy change process in Canada and other developed nations. There are varying approaches to understanding the policy change process (Brooks & Miljan, 2003). The pluralist approach sees policy development as driven primarily by the quality of ideas in the public policy arena so that those judged as beneficial and useful will be translated into policies by governing authorities. The materialist approach is that policy development is driven primarily by powerful interests who assure their concerns will receive rather more attention than those not so situated. In Canadian society, these powerful interests are usually based in the economic market sector and have powerful partners in the political arena. The public choice view of policy-making tries to get into the heads of policy-makers to understand why they act on some issues and not others. Each approach provides differing explanations for understanding the present situation and each proposes different means of moving a social determinants of health agenda forward.

The pluralist approach suggests the need for further research, knowledge dissemination, and public policy advocacy with the aim of *convincing* policy-makers to enact health-supporting public policy (Wright, 1994). The materialist model suggests the need for developing strong social and political movements with the aim of *forcing* policy-makers to enact health-supporting public policy. The public choice model has little to say about raising these issues, but can be drawn upon to develop ways of understanding and influencing policy-makers' decision processes. The exploration of these two key issues constitutes much of the content of this chapter.

Finally, we provide an analysis of some of the psychological and social—in additional to the political and economic—forces that account for why the social determinants of health concept is so low on the public policy agenda. How does the public view health and its determinants? Why are social determinants of health so neglected by health-related professionals such as the health care, public health, and health research communities? Are governments reluctant to raise the issues of the social determinants of health because of the role they themselves play in weakening these health determinants through faulty public policy-making?

Ideology, Health Discourses, and the Social Determinants of Health

Most Canadians believe that academic disciplines, such as the health sciences and their applied expressions, public health agencies, and governmental health ministries, carry out their activities based on objective facts drawn from empirical research studies. Within this framework we would understand the health field's current preoccupation with biomedical advances and with what sociologist Sarah Nettleton (Nettleton, 1997) calls the "holy trinity of risk" of tobacco, diet, and physical activity as reflecting the accumulated evidence that these domains are the primary determinants of citizens' health status in developed nations. We would also understand the profound neglect by the health sciences, public health, and governmental health authorities of the social determinants of health examined in this volume as reflecting a lack of evidence that these issues play an important role in determining the health status of Canadians.

Clearly, the accumulating evidence concerning the importance of the social determinants of health does not support this argument. There must be more to this neglect of the social determinants of health than meets the eye and indeed, numerous hypotheses are available to inform this analysis. The first concerns the nature—that is the focus and the analytical tools available—of research and action in the health sciences in general and epidemiology in particular.

Traditional Approaches to the Health Sciences

Raphael and Bryant (2002) have identified some of the characteristics of traditional health sciences and epidemiological approaches that are problematic. These include: (1) a reliance on quantitative and statistical approaches to understanding health and its determinants; (2) a tendency toward viewing the sources of health and illness as emanating from individual dispositions and actions rather than resulting from the influence of societal structures; (3) a professed commitment to objectivity or what is termed a non-normative approach to health issues; and (d) a profound depoliticizing of health issues. All of these reflect an adherence to positivist science as the preferred means of understanding health and its determinants (Wilson, 1983). These categories will be used to inform our discussion of the disjuncture between traditional health sciences and the social determinants of health approach.

The health sciences in general, and epidemiology in particular, are a reflection of what has been termed "positivist science" (Wilson, 1983). Positivist science is based on a natural sciences approach associated with the rise of physics, chemistry, and biology as areas of study. It is focused on the concrete and observable. It has also been called a reductionist approach whereby effort is expended to identify specific variables that can be placed into statistical equations in order to identify putative causes and effects. While positivist science has led to impressive advances in the natural sciences, its application to the fields of the health sciences and other areas of social inquiry has been problematic.

When applied to the health and social sciences, positivist science generally avoids dealing with aspects of broader environments (Lincoln & Guba, 1985). In the medical field it leads to a focus upon cells, body organs, and bodily systems by biomedical researchers and a focus on behavioural risk factors by public health authorities (Bezruchka, 2006). The study of environments—i.e., the social determinants of health—and the public policies and political, economic, and social forces that shape the quality of these environments is generally neglected (Raphael & Bryant, 2006). Positivist health and social science also avoids analysis of the abstract, implying the study of the underlying economic, political, and social structures of society are beyond its analytical and methodological grasp. The role of politics and political ideology in shaping these environments is even more uncommon.

Another important aspect of positivist science is its professed commitment to objectivity. This leads to researchers and workers being unwilling to make what are termed "normative" judgments as to what "should be" as opposed to describing "what is." This professed commitment to objectivity and avoidance of normative judgments is a pretense as all health science researchers and public health workers identify their clear commitments to promoting treatment regimens to improve biomedical markers and to reduce so-called risk behaviours such as smoking, excessive consumption of alcohol, physical inactivity, and diets lacking in fruits and vegetables. These commitments to the importance of—and need to influence—biomedical markers and behavioural risk factors to the neglect of broader issues are so strong as to constitute in itself a normative ideology of what is a health issue and what is not (Tesh, 1990). This is—by any analysis—not an "objective" approach to understanding and promoting health.

The professed commitment to objectivity, therefore, serves as a means to avoid consideration of broader issues

concerned with political, economic, and social issues. Also unlikely to be discussed is how the class biases of health researchers and workers come to influence what is conceived as being either within—or outside—the realm of health sciences inquiry (Muntaner, 1999). A perceived threat to career prospects that may arise by raising broader issues associated with the social determinants of health is also not to be dismissed (Raphael, 2003). Extensive discussions of how these issues shape the health sciences and public health sectors' apparent unwillingness to consider a social determinants of health approach are available (Raphael, 1998, 2002, 2003).

Within the traditional health sciences approach, health problems remain individualized, localized, desocialized, and depoliticized (Hofrichter, 2003). It is important to note that such an approach is congruent with conservative and neo-liberal political ideology, whereby social problems such as unemployment, poverty, and racism are framed as individual rather than societal issues (Coburn, 2004). Policy solutions under conservative and neo-liberal ideologies are residual (dealing with problems as a last resort) and desocialized (focused on individual rather than communal aspects of society). Government responses to the effects of social problems are eroded as exemplified by the increasing ineligibility of many Canadians to access unemployment insurance or students experiencing increasing difficulty in financing their education (Black & Shillington, 2005).

Frequently, these public policy developments are explicit, such as outright cancellation of progressive programs or are done by stealth through clawbacks, de-indexation, or incremental cuts to programs (Stanford, 2004). While traditional health science approaches may not be overtly conservative in orientation, they are congruent with such an ideology and justify the retreat of governments around the world from investing in our collective health and well-being (Raphael & Bryant, 2006a, 2006b).

Individualism and the Social Determinants of Health

The second barrier to having a social determinants of health approach taken seriously by professionals, the public, and governmental policy-makers is the societal commitment to the ideologies of individualism and individual responsibility as opposed to communal responsibility (Hofrichter, 2003). Individualism is the belief that one's place in the social hierarchy—one's occupational class, income and wealth, and power and prestige, as well as the effects of such placement such as health and disease status—comes about through one's own efforts (Travers, 1997). At the very minimum, it places the locus of responsibility for one's health status within the individual's motivations and behaviours rather than recognizing that health status is a result of how a society organizes its distribution of a variety of resources.

The importance of individualism to understanding how the determinants of health are conceptualized has been thoughtfully explored by Hofrichter:

> Individualism, a powerful philosophy and practice in North American, limits the public space for social movement activism. By transforming public issues into private matters of lifestyle, self-empowerment, and assertiveness, individualism precludes organized efforts to spur social change. It fits perfectly with a declining welfare state and also influences responses to health inequities. From this perspective, each person is self-interested and possessed of a fixed, competitive human nature. Everyone has choice and the potential for upward mobility through hard work—ignoring how we develop through the process of living in society. Individualism presumes that individuals exist in parallel with society instead of being formed by society. (Hofrichter, 2003, p. 28)

Individualism in health has numerous effects in relation to the social determinants of health. First, it leads to a strong bias toward understanding health problems as individual problems rather than societal ones. Second, it specifies the cause of the health problem as residing within faulty biomedical markers, specific individual motivations, and risk behaviours that are somehow under individual control. Third, it specifies that improving health will result from modifying these markers, motivations, and behaviours. Fourth, it says little about society and its structures and its effects upon health. Fifth, it says even less about how such societal structures could be modified.

An alternative paradigm for understanding health and its mainsprings is available. Sociologists and social epidemiologists working in the historical materialist tradition have long attempted to illuminate how various modes of production, especially in capitalist societies, influence the distribution of economic, social, and political resources within the population, thereby influencing health (see Raphael, 2006). Despite this long-standing tradition, these analyses concerning the structural determinants of health—and their clear impacts on health—remain outside the mainstream of current discourse on determinants of health among policy-makers and health researchers in Canada. It is unclear whether the efforts associated with the International Commission on the Social Determinants of Health can reverse this tendency.

Increasing Market Orientation of Canadian Society and the Social Determinants of Health

Finally, the increasing market orientation of Canadian society weakens support for a social determinants of health approach to promoting health. The rise of capitalism and the market economy grew in tandem with a strong belief in individualism and the ability of the individual to control his or her destiny (Esping-Andersen, 1990). The uncritical belief in this ideology was associated with the rise of market-oriented societies that saw little role for governmental or state intervention in the marketplace and in the provision of various forms of security for its citizens. At its heyday, such a belief saw the rise of tremendous inequalities in wealth and health in Victorian England, for example, and, more recently, during the 1930s and since the 1970s in many developed nations (Alesina & Glaeser, 2004).

The rise of differing forms of welfare states in Europe during the 19th century was a response to these excesses of *laissez-faire* capitalism (Esping-Andersen, 1990). In continental Europe a conservative form of the welfare state arose whose main concern was with reducing unrest and promoting a modicum of security for citizens. The dominant ideological inspiration of this type of welfare state has been identified as *solidarity*, achieved through social stability, wage stability, and social integration (Saint-Arnaud & Bernard, 2003) (see Figure 24.1).

In Scandinavia the social democratic welfare state arose, which saw active promotion of equality and human rights and the provision of citizen security across the lifespan (Esping-Andersen, 1985). There, the dominant ideological inspiration is *equality,* achieved through the reduction of poverty, inequality, and unemployment (Saint-Arnaud & Bernard, 2003). The third form of the welfare state—the liberal—is the weakest of all and Canada falls within this group. In the liberal welfare state, the dominant ideological inspiration is *liberty,* achieved through minimizing governmental interventions, and minimizing so-called "disincentives to work," such as social programs and supports.

The liberal welfare state and its associated ideology provide barren soil for a serious social determinants of health approach (Raphael & Bryant, 2006a). Within liberal welfare states, liberty and its close neighbour, self-determination, become available only to a narrow band of the population—those who have sufficient financial resources and cultural capital to define their own living conditions (Coburn, 2006). Liberty and self-determination are out of reach for much of the population.

Scholarship has specified the mechanisms by which these differing forms of the welfare states developed and how their trajectories shape the making of public policy (Esping-Andersen, 1990). Importantly, these differing forms of the welfare state have been shown to be related to clear differences in the quality of numerous social health determinants of health and population health outcomes (Esping-Andersen, 1999; Navarro et al., 2004).

Even so, the end of the Second World War saw a clear desire by all nation-states to avoid the economic and social conditions that gave rise to totalitarianism (Teeple, 2000). Attention to promoting citizen security was increased across all developed nations so that by the 1970s, the ideology of the Canadian welfare state was seen by some as rivalling that of Sweden at the time (Myles & Pierson, 1997).

Yet the rise of what has been termed "neo-liberalism," or a retreat from government intervention in the marketplace, has threatened these social reforms (Coburn, 2004; Teeple, 2000). This has especially been the case in the liberal political economies such as Canada. Neo-liberalism refers to the dominance of markets and the market model. According to Coburn, the

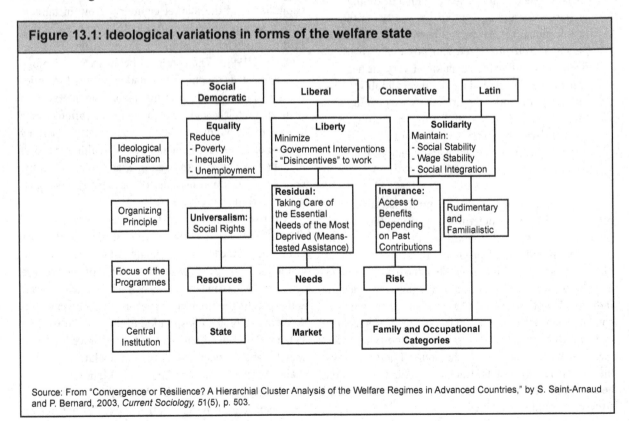

Figure 13.1: Ideological variations in forms of the welfare state

Source: From "Convergence or Resilience? A Hierarchial Cluster Analysis of the Welfare Regimes in Advanced Countries," by S. Saint-Arnaud and P. Bernard, 2003, *Current Sociology,* 51(5), p. 503.

primary tenets of neo-liberalism are: (1) markets are the best and most efficient allocators of resources in production and distribution; (2) societies are composed of autonomous individuals (producers and consumers) motivated chiefly or entirely by material or economic considerations; and (3) competition is the major market vehicle for innovations (Coburn, 2000). The essence of neo-liberalism, in its pure form, is a more-or-less thoroughgoing adherence, in rhetoric if not in practice, to the virtues of a market economy and, by extension, a market-oriented society (Coburn, 2000). Such ideology sees little space for governmental action in strengthening the social determinants of health.

Conservative and social democratic political economies have been more able to resist neo-liberal forces than liberal political economies (Vandenbroucke, 2002). Consistent with this view, it has been argued that Canadian society is moving more and more toward that of the most extreme liberal welfare state, the United States (Scarth, 2004). It should therefore not be surprising that implementation of a social determinants of health approach has been lacking in Canada (Canadian Population Health Initiative, 2002). Those attempting to raise these issues through the provision of evidence and policy options run smack into resistance driven by ideological beliefs concerning the nature of society, as well as concrete pressures to resist such an agenda. Some of these concrete forces become clearer in the following examination of how public policy is made in nations such as Canada.

Understanding Policy Change

Another key issue is the policy change process in Canada and other developed nations. The pluralist approach sees policy development as driven primarily by the quality of ideas in the public policy arena. An alternative materialist approach is that policy development is driven primarily by powerful interests. The public choice model gets into the heads of policy-makers and focuses on the process by which they develop and implement policies (Brooks & Miljan, 2003).

Each approach provides differing explanations for understanding the present situation and each proposes different means of moving such an agenda forward. As noted the social determinants of health appear to be underdeveloped in Canada as compared to most other developed nations. Much of this has to do with public policies that determine how the resources of the nation are to be distributed among the population.

Pluralist View

The pluralist view is that public policy decisions result from governments and other policy-makers choosing public policy directions based on the competition of ideas in the public arena (Brooks & Miljan, 2003). This competition of ideas, according to this view, is facilitated by various interest groups that lobby governments to accept their position. Pluralists recognized that there may not be a level playing field in these lobbying attempts, with political, economic, and social elites having an upper hand. Nevertheless, the pluralist approach assumes that the governmental policy-making process is generally open and that those with the better ideas will come to see governments adopt their views.

Additionally, pluralists assume that Canadian policy-making is a democratic process. Policy-making is a rational process whereby the best ideas are put into practice. Individuals, communities, agencies, organized groups, labour, and business all have a place at the policy-making table. Canadian governments are not seen as being the handmaiden of the elites. Rather, they strive to implement the Canadian constitutional principles of peace, order, and good government by implementing reasonable public policy. If Canada lags behind in social determinants of health-supportive policy, it requires education of policy-makers and lobbying of these same policy-makers with the expectation that with the right knowledge dissemination, translation, or exchange, these health-supportive policies will come to pass. The pluralist view argues, therefore, that advocates of the social determinants of health view need to get organized and have their voices heard by policy-makers. Ongoing consciousness-raising, advocacy and lobbying, and building coalitions will achieve policy change.

Taking this view at face value, we would expect that all of the policy recommendations presented in this volume would be of interest to policy-makers. The only problem is that these policy options have been presented numerous times over the past decade to policy-makers, their benefits have been outlined repeatedly, yet no action seems forthcoming. For example, in the 1st edition of this volume, we presented the following options:

Policies to Reduce the Incidence of Low Income
The following steps would reduce the number of Canadians living with low incomes, reduce economic inequality, and improve population health:

- Raise the minimum wage to a living wage.
- Improve pay equity.
- Restore and improve income supports for those unable to gain employment.
- Provide a guaranteed minimum income.

Policies to Reduce Social Exclusion
Numerous analyses have considered how social exclusion occurs and the role it plays in threatening population health (Atlantic Centre of Excellence for Women's Health, 2000; Shaw et al., 1999). The following steps—in addition to reducing low income—would reduce social exclusion in Canada:

- Enforce legislation that protects the rights of minority groups, particularly concerning employment rights and anti-discrimination.
- Ensure that families have sufficient income to provide their children with the means of attaining healthy development.
- Reduce inequalities in income and wealth within the population through progressive taxation of income and inherited wealth.
- Assure access to educational, training, and employment opportunities, especially for those such as the long-term unemployed.
- Remove barriers to health and social services, which will involve understanding where and why such barriers exist.
- Provide adequate follow-up support for those leaving institutional care.
- Create housing policies that provide enough affordable housing of reasonable standard.
- Institute employment policies that preserve and create jobs.
- Direct attention to the health needs of immigrants and to the unfavourable socio-economic position of many groups, including the particular difficulties many new Canadians face in accessing health and other care services.

Policies to Restore and Enhance Canada's Social Infrastructure
Canadian federal program spending as a percentage of gross domestic product has been decreasing since 1987 so that current federal spending is at 1950 levels (Hulchanski, 2002). Indeed, these data indicate that many aspects of program spending in Canada are now lower than that seen in the US!

These decreases have occurred in tandem with decreases in tax revenues resulting from modifications to the tax structure that favour the well-off (McQuaig, 1987, 1993). The concept of universality is an important cornerstone of policies designed to promote social inclusion. Programs that apply to all are more likely to engender political support from the public. The federal and provincial governments should:

- Restore health and service program spending to the average level of OECD nations.
- Develop a national housing strategy and allocate an additional 1 percent of federal spending for affordable housing.
- Provide a national daycare program.
- Provide a national pharmacare program.
- Restore eligibility and level of employment benefits to previous levels.
- Require that provincial social assistance programs be accessible and funded at levels to assure health.
- Assure that supports are available to support Canadians through critical life transitions.

Yet, there is little evidence that any of these recommendations have been taken seriously. Why is this the case? Perhaps we need an alternate model of policy change to explain the current situation and point the way forward. The materialist model provides such an alternative.

The Materialist View of Public Policy-making
The materialist view is that governments in capitalist societies such as Canada enact policies that serve the interests of economic elites (Brooks & Miljan, 2003). These elites are the owners and managers of large corporations whose primary goals are to maximize profits, provide growing profits to shareholders, and institute public policies that keep business costs down.

These interests are also likely to lobby for minimal governmental intervention in business practices and to resist business regulation and progressive labour legislation (see Langille, this volume). Lowering corporate and income taxes is also an important policy objective. Since taxes are required to fund governmental services, economic interests frequently call for reduction in program spending to allow tax decreases. Business interests generally oppose moves that enable workers to form unions that would see the realization of collective bargaining. Collective bargaining is related to the receipt of higher wages, stronger benefits, and increased employment security for union members. We have come through a generation of governments retreating from their role in supporting its most vulnerable citizens, and even much of the middle class.

We have seen a dramatic set of cuts to progressive taxes such as income tax and corporate taxes, and a correlated rise in regressive taxes such as the GST. We have also seen massive cuts to income-support programs such as social assistance (in most provinces) and unemployment insurance. On the program side, extensive cuts have been made to public housing, education, mental health, and violence against women services (Scarth, 2004). Failed promises in child care and supports for the homeless reveal that even when gains are made through social movements, governments can undo them through an array of means. Labour legislation has been rolled back in many provinces, undoing gains made in the postwar era.

Economic interests are able to influence governments through a variety of processes. First, they are able to influence government through their ability to shift investment capital from location to location (Brooks & Miljan, 2003). A government that institutes non-business friendly policies could see business and investment leaving the jurisdiction. Second, lending agencies whose interests are consistent with business can raise borrowing rates for debt-ridden jurisdictions that institute what they see as problematic policies. Third, the people who have the financial resources to consider running for the dominant political parties may either come from the business class and/or hold similar values. These individuals cannot only expect to receive financial support for their runs at political office, but can also be assured of employment opportunities within these same

sectors if they fail to be re-elected or upon their retirement from public office (Raphael, 2007b).

Increasing income and wealth inequality, and the weakening of social infrastructure, result from the concentration of wealth and power within a nation with attendant weakening of civil society (Raphael, 2007a). What is to be done? The materialist model suggests organizing the population to oppose and defeat the powerful interests that influence governments to maintain poverty (Wright, 1994). These defeats can occur in the workplace through greater union organization and the promotion of class solidarity. These defeats can also occur in the electoral and parliamentary arena by the ascendance of working-class power.

This would come about by achieving greater equity in political power (Zweig, 2000). This can be achieved by restoring programs and services and reintroducing more progressive income tax rates. Independent unions are a necessity, as is legislation that strengthens workers' ability to organize. Re-regulating many industries would reverse current trends toward the concentration of power and wealth. Internationally, the development and enforcement of agreements to provide adequate working and living standards that would support and promote health and well-being across national barriers is essential.

The provision of a social wage—government-provided services that people need to live and develop their ability to work—is a way to restore the social infrastructure that has been so weakened in nations such as Canada and the US. Resistance to the privatization of public services is essential.

Public Choice Model

The public choice model focuses on the individual policy-maker and the process by which he or she develops and implements policies that maximize the benefits to society (Brooks & Miljan, 2003). In this model, the policy-maker is said to look out for societal interests as well as his or her own interests by balancing the interests of a wide range of stakeholders: interest groups including business, labour, the needs of elected officials and senior civil servants, and the media, among others.

The public choice model would suggest that it is not in the overall interests of Canadian policy-makers to address the social determinants of health. People who experience poor-quality determinants have little influence with policy-makers since their concerns are not seen as being the concerns of most Canadians and, in any event, these people are less likely to vote.

In contrast, those interests who experience weak social determinants are highly organized, and are able to exert influence upon policy-makers, thereby controlling the public policy agenda. Put simply, raising and addressing social determinants of health issues provides little benefit for governing parties. The public choice model argues that policy dynamics must change so that policy-makers who do not address poverty will suffer consequences and their political masters will experience electoral consequences.

Understanding Professional and Citizen Priorities

Moving beyond these models of the political process, we need to understand the means by which health and other service workers as well as the public come to accept this current state of affairs. There are pragmatic reasons for the image of health policy-makers, authorities, and advocates as ostriches digging their collective heads in the sand. Consider the everyday situation of those either responsible for formulating health policy or those working directly with vulnerable populations. In both cases, health assessments and solutions need to be offered. To appreciate fully the policy implications of the health issues identified in this volume is to come face to face with problems of vast proportions—poverty, inequality, poor access to food, workplace stress, inadequate housing, racism, and inadequate child care, among others (Raphael & Bryant, 2006a).

What would it take to solve these monumental social and economic ills? In the Canada of 2008, it would require a profound reordering of political priorities and reinvestment in social infrastructure and program spending. Such a reordering would not be revolutionary. It would simply represent adopting health policy directions consistent with many European nations and directions that, until recently, made Canada a world leader in developing and implementing healthy public policy (O'Neill, Pederson, Dupere & Rootman, 2007). Without such commitment, it is unlikely that any health-promotion activities will make a dent in addressing

emerging Canadian health issues by addressing the social determinants of health (Raphael & Bryant, 2006b).

Health and Service Workers
Faced with such formidable policy options, many turn to community development as a means of improving health and well-being. Working on small-scale projects, frequently with limited resources, offers some workers enough hope for change. While this might resonate for some as a liberal model of change (Curry-Stevens, 2003), it is a location from which good work can be done. On a day-to-day basis, do you as a health or other worker choose to work directly with a community of people struggling for a better life, or spend your days divorced from the vulnerable attempting to effect policy change by those who may never heed your call? For many, the choice of moving upstream to prevention looks less attractive, and perhaps futile.

The General Public
We can appreciate why health and other workers turn away from health paradigms based on the social determinants of health. Why, then, do vulnerable communities and individuals—those most affected by the conditions described in this volume—appear complacent in accepting the economic and social conditions under which they are required to live? Why are workers not pressing for fairer tax systems? Better wages? Fleeing low-income jobs? Demanding better minimum-wage protection from their governments? Or insisting on expanding regulated child care or assisted housing programs? In other words, where is the public outrage? A number of reasons may be responsible for this.

On Income and Inequality Issues, Masked by Debt
As incomes erode for a significant portion of the population, and they slide lower down the income ladder, why is there not greater outrage over declining standards of living, especially as this is the case for numbers of Canadians that approach the majority?

Canadians are borrowing to compensate for this loss, with credit easier to secure and more abundantly provided. A study by the Vanier Institute of the Family explored the most recent data on the wealth of Canadians (Sauve, 2002). Revealed are two trends on debt—one is that 30 percent of all households were now uncomfortable with their debt load and the second is that more families are failing to save for their retirement.

A study by Statistics Canada itself compared debt levels between 1984 and 1999 (Statistics Canada, 2001). The findings confirm that Canadians are living with greater levels of debt, and are most likely to compensate for shortfalls in income. The debt figures are available as a percentage of assets. For every $100 of assets, Canadians now carry $18 of debt, rising from $14 in 1984. The highest burden is carried by those aged 25–34 years, and it is $40, more than double the debt load of others, and in comparison with 1984, up from $30. The most compelling available data on this topic is that from the Canadian Labour Congress, which indicates that "the personal savings rate in the first half of 2003 was just 2.3%, well down from the already low level of 4.2% in 2002" (Canadian Labour Congress, 2003, p. 2). It is now negative, with the average Canadian spending more than he or she earns each and every year (Tal & Preston, 2005). Rising debts and stalling incomes mean increasing economic vulnerability is stretching into Canada's middle class at an alarming pace (Curry-Stevens, in press).

Hidden from View

The evidence provided by the various contributors to this volume is sometimes, but certainly not always, consistent with common sense, or at least not the common sense being forwarded by our leading political parties, most of whom want the news about the economy to be seen as good news. This perception is important as our economy—the value of the Canadian dollar, the bond rating that foreign debtors place on the debts we owe, our interest rates and access to credit, the value of the stock market—is vulnerable to what can loosely be called "confidence." No mainstream political leader wants to reveal how the market is failing the majority of its citizens and advancing the interests of a small proportion of the population. They would much rather hide this failing behind glowing reports of the rise in GDP or the increases in "average" incomes.

Pointed in the Wrong Direction

It serves the economic elite for low- and middle-income earners to point the blame for their social ills at other marginalized groups. These groups include immigrants, "who steal our jobs"; the welfare poor, "who are just a

drain on our resources"; the beneficiaries of employment equity, "who take the jobs we should have got"; and even the unionized workers, "who get much more that they deserve." One explaining factor is that competition increases as resources dry up, and that this competition generates hostility, particularly between those most alike. Any objective analysis of the current state of Canadian society quickly recognizes the role that uncaring corporations and those who wish to preserve their excessive income and wealth levels are playing in weakening the social determinants of health.

Replaced by Self-Blame

Dominant culture in Western civilization emphasizes individual achievement and personal agency. Embedded within our social and cultural norms is the myth of personal success, framing the individual as the author of his or her own life. Such a notion of where agency originates redirects anger at the structural aspects of society that create unhappiness toward the self. Those who do not achieve "view such failure in terms of personal inadequacy or the 'luck of the draw'" (McLaren, 2003, p. 77).

Through this process, we become agents in our own marginalization, a process identified by Gramsci as hegemony. Drawing from McLaren (2003), the prevailing image for our political system is a benevolent one, whereby the interests of the political and economic elite "supposedly represent the interests of all groups" (McLaren, 2003, p. 78). Canadians rarely confront their governments as to why they are not being firm with corporate giants or more generous to its citizens. While we are not coerced into such an analysis, we are conditioned to view the cause of our social ills as residing within ourselves. The power of such analysis rests with the "common sense" of such beliefs, and it even seems to have been generated by that common sense.

Such beliefs manifest themselves in voting preferences and profoundly disturbs progressive Canadians as many struggling Canadians vote for right-wing political parties. While noting such a process in the US, Gore Vidal observes: "the genius of our system is that ordinary people go out and vote against their interests. The way our ruling class keeps out of sight is one of the greatest stunts in the political history of any country" (McLaren, 2003, p. 79). And, apparently so, too, in Canada.

Stuck in Real Human Dilemmas

The mobility of workers stalls as one gets poorer. Lacking money for first and last months' rent, a car to drive to distant locations, or even enough for public transit keep many in dire poverty. Even information about wages is the privilege of higher-income groups. The "money taboo" (Ehrenreich, 2001) keeps workers from sharing information that might fruitfully be used to even know where better-paying jobs exist. All these dynamics limit access to decent work.

Also at fault is the real drain that high housing costs place on our ability to make ends meet. The disappearance of cheap housing (safe or otherwise) leaves families in shelters, motels, trailers, and even cars. The withdrawal of the federal government and most provincial governments from public and co-operative housing (although signalled to reverse) deepens this crisis. If ever there was a market failure for the supply of a commodity in response to high demand, housing is truly that failure.

Minimum wages fail to keep working families and most individuals out of poverty. When costs for housing are high, and benefit programs meagre (and prescription drugs out of reach, employment insurance likely unavailable, and pension savings non-existent), low-wage workers are poor and increasingly vulnerable to economic shocks such as job loss, old age, and ill health. When coupled with the ideological strain that individualism places on one's psyche (that "these problems are mine, and it is my responsibility to dig myself out of this hole"), low-wage workers suffer psychologically and materially.

Feeling Futile and Disempowered ... Distanced from Our Political Leadership

Consider the political landscape today. Trust in government has been shrinking over the last 35 years (since such polling began). The EKOS survey, *Canadian and American national election studies*, uncovered the answer to the following question: "How much do you trust the government in Ottawa to do what is right?" The answer was resoundingly poor, falling from a high of 57 percent (answering "just about always/most of the time") in 1968 to a level of just 27 percent in May 2002 (EKOS Research Associates, 2002). And the ever-popular Ipsos-Reid *Canada Trust Survey* (*Readers Digest Canada*, 2003) was repeated in 2003, revealing that the trust[1]

Canadians place in the federal politicians ranks last of a list of 26 professions—even car salespeople rank one position higher at 25th. Local politicians score no better, as they take the 24th spot. Those who score higher include pharmacists (1st), doctors (2nd), teachers (4th), the police (5th), charitable organizations (9th), religious institutions (14th), lawyers (18th), journalists (19th), trade unions (21st), and CEOs (22nd). Emerging is a growing crisis in the reputation of our political leadership.

Further evidence of this dramatic change is revealed in the EKOS survey, as it articulates the shrinking importance of the public interest. The following question was posed: "When the federal government makes decisions, whose interests do you think are given the greatest importance?" From 1998–2002, the public interest shrank from 18 percent of the population to 16 percent, while the combined importance of "the interest of politicians and their friends" and "the interest of big business" rose from 60 percent to 67 percent in just four years.

There is clear evidence of growing distrust in politicians and rising concern with the interests and activities of big business. In tandem, these trends displace the importance of the public interest. As a decision-making body, today's political leaders show themselves to be seriously out of step with the majority of the population. To explore the causes of this destabilizing dynamic, we need to turn to theory drawn from the study of privilege. Hobgood asserts that there is a natural process in play for the privileged whereby their separation (socially and economically) from the majority population leads to an ignorance that stems from their lack of contact with the lived realities of the average and more vulnerable citizens (Hobgood, 2000). This ignorance, in time, leads to an arrogance that stems from assuming that the world works for the majority in much the same way that it works for the privileged.

Asserting this to be a natural process of alienation, Hobgood thus calls on us to problematize the world of privilege. It is they who are out of touch and suffering the effects of social exclusion, not the majority world that lies below them (Curry-Stevens, 2004). The gravely serious arrogance that is bred unfolds as follows: The privileged person looks at the lived reality of the less privileged and assumes that the world works for others the way it works for themselves. The reality is, in fact, contrary to this logic. They assume that if they lived their lives as a poor, blue-collar, racialized immigrant or as a woman, they would achieve largely the same accomplishments as they have as White, male, and upper class. What they do not realize is that nothing would be the same. They would not have gotten off home plate. As encapsulated by Hatfield, when discussing George Bush Junior, "He's one of those guys who was born on third base and thinks he hit a triple" (Hatfield, 2002, p. 53).

And Finally, Duped by the Hope (and Sometimes the Promise) That We, Too, Can Be Rich

Let's start at the beginning. Our statistics reveal that only 15 percent of Canadian families earn more than $100,000/year (Murphy, Roberts & Wolfson, 2007). The same study reveals that only 5 percent of individuals have incomes of $89,000 and up, yet the myth of income mobility is held out in front of us like a carrot, intertwined by the promise that hard work will get us ahead. Social commentators such as Michael Moore claim that in the United States, citizens are afraid to hold corporations accountable as they bought the lie "that we too could some day become rich. So we don't want to do anything that could harm us on that day we end up millionaires" (Moore, 2003, p. 140). In calculations done for Moore's book, he asserts that the chance of the average American at middle-income levels becoming rich is about one in a million. Similarly, too, we imagine this statistic for Canadians.

Having scanned these various social and economic impediments to change, there remains the need to debunk the rhetoric of the status quo as well as political projects that aim to lower labour costs, lower taxes, shrink governments, and expand the role of corporate voices in the governing decisions of the country. These pressures have reconfigured social policy as we know it, but, from our view, their position is weak, becoming exposed as self-interested, with cracks beginning to show.

Challenging the Assertion: "We Can't Afford This"

The costs of resolving all our social ills may appear to be prohibitive. One answer would be "We cannot afford not to effect such spending" as the costs of attending later to the problems of poverty and homelessness as two

examples escalate later down the line as more lives are damaged. Yet time frames in politics do not stretch far. They are limited to five-year time horizons or less if the next election looms.

So what arguments exist today in defence of enhanced social spending? Beginning with the basics of economic growth, we can illustrate that enhanced spending is not simply an expenditure item. Any spending that employs someone has a ripple effect. First, employment returns income taxes to the government, reducing the net outlay of the expenditure. Second, employment removes someone from the rolls of unemployment insurance or social assistance and puts him or her into the workforce. Thirdly, that income in turn is spent on goods and services that generate economic activity and the cycle of earnings and spending. It is only when those dollars are removed from the system through expenditures outside of the country or through savings that the ripple effects stop.

Consider whether government spending creates more ripple effects if placed in the hands of the rich or the poor. When placed in the hands of the rich, it is more likely to end up as savings or spent outside of the country, and it is also more likely to be saved, limiting its multiplier effect in the economy. This is the reason that deductions in capital gains taxes or reduced income taxes do not serve our economy. Yet direct social spending strongly serves economic growth, particularly if it is placed in the pockets of those who spend it locally. Hundreds of businesses went bankrupt in the Toronto area when social assistance rates were cut and purchase of goods and services were reduced. Cuts in employment insurance serve the same function, reducing the quality of life in our neighbourhoods as the spending power of Canadians shrinks.

Linking Individuals to Ideologies

The various forms of analysis we bring to understanding the failure to take action on the social determinants of health informs our understanding of solutions. The public choice model suggests that agreement might be possible or, at the very least, a decision-making process would be in place to ensure that democratic resolution is adhered to. In this approach, values such as consensus, fairness, and democracy would feature prominently. When we try to understand the failure to act on the social determinants of health, we would look to advance strategies that would ensure collection of research, dissemination of information, decision-making tables that allowed all perspectives to surface, and transparency and accountability in the decision-making process itself.

If, on the other end of the spectrum, we embrace a materialist perspective, we would work from the assumption that failure to advance action on the social determinants of health is simply a matter of power and influence. Quite simply, this failure is the result of sufficient power resting with the majority of the population, who would be likely to demand changes when faced with social movement campaigns that build awareness about how issues like housing, income, and job security shrink their health outcomes. Many readers would likely (and rightly) identify that many Canadians know the problem is not one of awareness, but one of power. Poor Canadians, particularly, know the toll that their perpetual disadvantage takes on them. In this situation, campaigns are needed to ensure that power is coalesced in strategic ways to force political decision makers to reject the voices of the powerful and accept those of the marginalized.

The choice of strategy depends on one's ideology and analytical lens. The authors of this chapter are reluctant to reject certain ideologies, with the exception of those that lead to residual social policies, a deepening concentration of capital, inequitable tax cuts that leave more money in the hands of those who need it least, and non-democratic decision-making processes. Within the pluralist, public choice, and materialist models, we advocate for continued efforts to enact policies that will improve health outcomes for all. Can we inform the public policy arena so as to change the terms in which health policy is considered? Yes, although it is frequently an uphill battle. Is there a chance that some policy-makers will voluntarily give priority to the social determinants of health? Yes, and we (as a community of allies and potential allies) hold the responsibility to find and support these leaders in the field. We also are pragmatists, and realize that placing responsibility for change in the hands of the economic and political elite is precarious—we support social movements that create more enduring alternatives (such as proportional representation, progressive media outlets, political reform), and citizen education that yields an engaged citizenry willing to get involved in the political process.

Conclusion

Developments in Europe indicate that concerted public health and community efforts can profoundly influence the development of policies that determine the extent of health inequalities and the overall state of population health within a nation (Mackenbach & Bakker, 2002, 2003). The policy directions being undertaken by nations such as Sweden and Finland are two such examples (Finnish Ministry of Social Affairs and Health, 1999, 2001, 2002; Government of Sweden, 2005; Swedish National Institute for Public Health, 2003). Similarly, the success of the WHO European Office Healthy Cities initiative is another example of the power of cities and communities to influence health policy (World Health Organization Regional Office for Europe, 1997, 2003). Canada has a rich history of concerted public pressure that can lead to positive policy change.

And there have been significant efforts in Canada to have a social determinants of health perspective taken seriously. Innovative and bold efforts have been undertaken by health units, municipalities, health and service provider associations, and various non-governmental associations to shine a spotlight on the social determinants of health and promote public policy in the support of health. Examples of these efforts are provided in Table 24.1.

The Toronto Charter on the Social Determinants of Health (see Appendix) is based on the content of this volume (Raphael, Bryant & Curry-Stevens, 2004). Toronto and Ottawa city councils have endorsed the *Charter* and it has gone before additional municipal councils across Canada for endorsement. This *Charter* itself is a tool for promoting health and social justice, both within and outside of Canada. It can be an impetus for change, notably by municipal council endorsement, followed by political action.

The social determinants of health concept can help make the links between government policy, the market, and the health and well-being of Canadians. For those working in the health sector, it can serve as motivation for working for change. The interests of their clients, patients, or consumers are served by speaking out against poverty, social exclusion, inequality, and inadequate services. There are potent barriers, however, to such actions. We hope that this volume will assist in these efforts.

Table 24.1: Examples of Canadian developments in addressing the social determinants of health
Alberta Public Health Association 2007 summer school addresses the social determinants of health
Alberta Public Health Units collaborate to create a Health Equity Network
Canadian Population Health Initiative publishes numerous reports addressing social determinants of health
City of Regina undertakes a social determinants of health approach to municipal public policy
Conference Board of Canada establishes roundtable on socio-economic determinants of health

Health-related organizations address the social determinants of health
    Association of Ontario Health Centres
    Canadian Nurses Association
    Chronic Disease Alliance of Ontario
    Registered Nurses Association of Ontario

"Ideas" program on CBC devotes a two-hour series to the social determinants of health
International Commission on the Social Determinants of Health places two learning hubs—early childhood and globalization—in Canada
National Collaborating Centre for Determinants of Health established at St. Francis Xavier University in Antigonish, Nova Scotia

Non-governmental organizations address social determinants of health
    United Nations Association of Canada
    Edmonton Social Planning Council
    Peterborough YMCA address the social determinants of health

Public health units address social determinants of health
    Interior Health (BC)
    Chinook (Alberta)
    Waterloo, Peterborough, Sudbury, Perth (Ontario)
    Montreal (Quebec)

Senate Sub-committee on Population Health addresses the social determinants of health
Sudbury Health Unit publishes a framework to incorporate social and economic determinants of health into the Ontario public health mandate

Note

1. This survey also inquired about the behaviours and attitudes that are most valued components of trust. These include honesty, integrity, and reliability.

Recommended Readings

Mackenbach, J. & Bakker, M. (Eds.). (2002). *Reducing inequalities in health: A European perspective.* London: Routledge.

    Social determinants of health approaches to health policy are much more prevalent in Europe than North America. This volume provides numerous case studies of efforts to address social determinants of health that provides examples for Canadian policy-makers to follow.

Navarro, V. (Ed.). (2002). *The political economy of social inequalities: Consequences for health and quality of life.* Amityville: Baywood Press.
Navarro, V. (Ed.). (2007). *Neoliberalism, globalization, and inequalities: Consequences for health and quality of life.* Amityville: Baywood Press.
Navarro, V. & Muntaner, C. (Eds.). (2004). *Political and economic determinants of population health and well-being: Controversies and developments.* Amityville: Baywood Press.

    These three collections of papers explicitly consider how ideology and politics influence the social determinants of health. The importance of the welfare state for health is clearly demonstrated.

Raphael, D. (2007). *Poverty and policy in Canada: Implications for health and quality of life.* Toronto: Canadian Scholars' Press Inc.

    This volume considers the political, economic, and social forces that lead to Canada's having poverty levels that are among the highest of developed nations. Poverty is seen as representing the situation where there is a clustering of negative experiences associated with a number of social determinants of health of low quality.

Raphael, D. (2003). "Towards the future: Policy and community actions to promote population health." In R. Hofrichter (Ed.), *Health and social justice: A reader on politics, ideology, and inequity in the distribution of disease* (pp. 453–468). San Francisco: Jossey Bass/Wiley.

    This chapter provides the means by which health public policy can be developed to influence the social determinants of health. Examples of successful initiatives are provided from Canada and elsewhere.

Rebick, J. (2000). *Imagine democracy.* Toronto: Stoddart.

    When considering change, very quickly our analysis turns to our system of democracy, with its associated faults of corporate influence, first-past-the-post electoral decisions, representative instead of participatory democracy, and the trust deficit that these (and other) factors engender. Rebick assesses our Canadian system and develops an argument for her model of effective citizenship.

Related Web Sites

Canadian Health Coalition—www.healthcoalition.ca
    This is the site of the Canadian Health Coalition, the major activist-oriented site on health issues. It has an excellent list of resources in their archives of current issues within health care. Although focused on medical care, it also provides information about food and food safety, genetically modified foods, privatization of health care, and the pharmaceutical industry. It positions itself as a watchdog on the Canadian health system.

National Institute of Public Health. (2004). Sweden's New Public-Health Policy—www.fhi.se/upload/PDF/2004/English/roll_eng.pdf
    This document provides an excellent example of a social determinants of health approach to national health policy. The Web site www.sweden.gov.se/sb/d/2942 provides links to other examples of Swedish health policy.

Rabble.ca—www.rabble.ca

Any set of resources is incomplete without a site that is dedicated to keeping us up-to-date on what is happening in Canada and around the world. Rabble.ca is an online news source that draws from Canada's best progressive journalists (both well known and lesser known) and provides commentary on current political issues.

Social Determinants of Health Listserv at York University, Canada

To subscribe, send the message "subscribe SDOH *yourfirstname yoursecondname*" in the text area to listserv@yorku.ca

This international listserv was established to: (1) provide the latest information on scholarship on social determinants of health; (2) explore the implications of these conditions for the health of citizens; and (3) provide support for those attempting to strengthen these social determinants of health in their local jurisdictions. It has over 1,200 members from around the world.

World Health Organization, European Office. (2003). *Healthy cities and urban governance*—www.euro.who.int/healthy-cities

This Web site provides resources for developing healthy cities based on 15 years of European experience. The Healthy Cities movement originated in Toronto, but has seen its successful implementation in Europe.

Appendix

———————

STRENGTHENING THE SOCIAL DETERMINANTS OF HEALTH: THE TORONTO CHARTER FOR A HEALTHY CANADA

From November 29 to December 1, 2002, a conference of over 400 Canadian social and health policy experts, community representatives, and health researchers met at York University in Toronto, Canada to: (1) consider the state of 10 key social or societal determinants of health across Canada; (2) explore the implications of these conditions for the health of Canadians; and (3) outline policy directions to improve the health of Canadians by influencing the quality of these determinants of health. The conference took place at a time when Canadian social and health policies were undergoing profound changes related to shifting political, economic, and social conditions.

Ten social determinants of health—early life, education, employment and working conditions, food security, health services, housing, income and income distribution, social exclusion, the social safety net, and unemployment and job insecurity were chosen on the basis of their prominence in Health Canada and World Health Organization policy statements and documents.

The conference was a response to accumulating evidence that growing social and economic inequalities among Canadians are contributing to higher health care costs and other social burdens. Indeed, the Kirby Report on the *Federal Role in Health Care* points out that 75 percent of our health is determined by physical, social, and economic environments. Evidence was also accumulating that a high level of poverty—an outcome of the growing gap between the rich and poor—has

profound societal effects as poor children are at higher risk for health and learning problems in childhood, adolescence, and later life, and are less likely to achieve their full potential as contributors to Canadian society.

The "Social Determinants of Health across the Lifespan" conference coincided with the release of the Romanow Report on the *Future of Health Care in Canada*, which called for strengthening the Canadian health care system by expanding its coverage, resisting privatization, and increasing financial investment. The report also discusses the importance of economic and social determinants of health. The evidence heard at the conference reinforced the view that immediate and long-term improvements in the health of Canadians depend upon investments that address the sources of health and disease.

The participants at the "Social Determinants of Health across the Lifespan" conference therefore resolve:

Whereas the evidence is overwhelming that the health of Canadians is profoundly affected by the social and economic determinants of health, including—but not restricted to—early life, education, employment and working conditions, food security, health care services, housing, income and its distribution, social exclusion, the social safety net, and unemployment and employment security; and

Whereas the evidence presented at the conference clearly indicates that the state and quality of these key determinants of health are linked to Canada's political, economic, and social environments and that many governments across Canada have not responded adequately to the growing threats to the health of Canadians in general, and the most vulnerable in particular; and

Whereas these social determinants of health are also human rights as defined in the *Universal Declaration of Human Rights* and the *International Covenant on Economic, Social, and Cultural Rights*, which Canada is obliged to protect and promote; and

Whereas the evidence presented indicates that investments in the basic social determinants of health will profoundly improve the health of Canadians most exposed to health-threatening conditions—the poor, the marginalized, and those Canadians excluded from participation in aspects of Canadian society by virtue of their living conditions—therefore providing health benefits for all Canadians; and

Whereas the evidence presented to us has indicated the following to be the case:

1. Early childhood development is threatened by the lack of affordable licensed child care and continuing high levels of family poverty. It has been demonstrated that licensed quality child care improves developmental and health outcomes of Canadian children in general, and children-at-risk in particular. Yet, while a national childcare program has been promised, 90% of Canadian families with children lack access to such care.

2. Education as delivered through public education systems has helped to make Canada a world leader in educational outcomes but our education systems are now at risk due to funding instability and poorly developed curriculum in many provinces. These conditions may weaken the trend toward greater number of students graduating despite evidence that those who do so show significantly better health and family functioning than non-graduates.

3. Employment and working conditions are deteriorating for some groups—especially young families—with potential attendant health risks. One in three adult jobs are now either peripheral or precarious as a result of increasing contracting out of core jobs and privatization of public employment. These jobs are often temporary, with low pay and high stress. Precarious working situations are directly related to the weakening of labour legislation in many jurisdictions. These changes threaten the gains made by workers in the past, jeopardizing their health and well-being.

4. Food security among Canadians and their families is declining as a result of policies that reduce income and other resources available to low-income Canadians. In Canada, food insecurity exists among 10.2% of Canadian households representing 3 million people. Monthly food bank use is 747,665 or 2.4% of the total Canadian population, which is double the 1989 figure; 41% of the food bank users or 305,000 are children under the age of 18.

5. Health care services can become a social determinant of health by being reorganized to support health. Many examples of effective—but all-too-rarely implemented—means of preventing deterioration among the ill through chronic disease management and rehabilitation are available. Screening that has been carefully assessed for its effectiveness can support health. Preventing disease in the first place by promoting the social and living conditions that support healthy lifestyles has also been neglected. While the Romanow Report reaffirmed the principles of the Canada Health Act, missing were strong statements about the important roles public health, health promotion, and long-term care play in supporting health.

6. Housing shortages are creating a crisis of homelessness and housing insecurity in Canada. Lack of affordable housing is weakening other social determinants of health as many Canadians are spending more of their income on shelter. More than 18% of Canadians live in unacceptable housing situations and one in every five renter households spent 50% or more of their income on housing in 1996, an increase of 43% since 1991.

7. Income and its equitable distribution have deteriorated during the past decade. Despite a 7-year stretch of unprecedented economic growth, almost half of Canadian families have seen little benefit as their wages have stagnated. Governments at all levels have let the after-tax-and-transfer income gap between rich and poor grow from 4.8:1 in 1989 to 5.3:1 in 2000. The growing vulnerability of lower-income Canadians threatens early childhood, education, food security, housing, social inclusion, and ultimately, health. Low-income Canadians are twice as likely to report poor health as compared to high-income Canadians.

8. Social exclusion is becoming increasingly common among many Canadians. Social exclusion is the process by which Canadians are denied opportunities to participate in many aspects of cultural, economic, social, and political life. It is especially prevalent among those who are poor, Aboriginal people, New Canadians, and members of racialized—or non-white—groups. As our racialized composition grows, it is unacceptable that these groups earn 30% less than whites and are twice as likely to be poor. These trends contribute to social and political instability in our society.

9. Social safety nets are changing in character as a result of shifting federal and provincial priorities. The 1990s have seen a weakening of these nets that constitute threats to both the health and well-being of the vulnerable. The social economy may provide opportunities for community organizations to provide services in more democratic, transparent, and community-sensitive ways. It may be, however, unable to meet emerging needs without further burdening caregivers in the community, many of whom are women, or inadequately compensating them.

10. Unemployment continues at high levels and **employment security** is weakening due to the growth of precarious, unstable, and non-advancing jobs. Higher stress, increasing

hours of work, and increasing numbers of low-income jobs are the mechanisms that link employment insecurity and unemployment to poor health outcomes. Unionized jobs are the most likely to help avoid these health-threatening conditions.

11. Canadian women, Aboriginal people, Canadians of colour, and New Canadians are especially vulnerable to the health-threatening effects of these deteriorating conditions. This is most clear regarding income and its distribution, employment and working conditions, housing affordability, and the state of the social safety net.

It is therefore resolved that:

Governments at all levels should review their current economic, social, and service policies to consider the impacts of their policies upon these social determinants of health. Areas of special importance are the provision of adequate income and social assistance levels, provision of affordable housing, development of quality childcare arrangements, and enforcement of anti-discrimination laws and human rights codes. It is also important to increase support for the social infrastructure including public education, social and health services, and improvement of job security and working conditions;

Public health and health care associations and agencies should educate their members and staff about the impacts of governmental decisions upon the social determinants of health and advocate for the creation of positive health promoting conditions. Particularly important is these associations and agencies joining current debates about Canadian health and social policy decisions and their impacts upon population health;

The media should begin to seriously cover the rapidly expanding findings concerning the importance of the social determinants of health and their impacts upon the health of Canadians. This would strike a balance between the predominant coverage of health from a biomedical and lifestyle perspective. It would also help educate the Canadian public about the potential health impacts of various governmental decisions and improve the potential for public involvement in public policymaking; and that

Immediate Action
As a means of moving this agenda forward, the conference recommends that Canada's federal and provincial/territorial governments immediately address the sources of health and the root causes of illness by matching the $1.5 billion targeted for diagnostic services in the Romanow *Report on the Future of Health Care in Canada* and allocating this amount towards two essential determinants of health for children and families: (1) affordable, safe housing; and (2) a universal system of high quality educational childcare; and

Long-Term Action
Similar to governmental actions in response to the *Acheson Inquiry into Health Inequalities in the United Kingdom*, the federal government should establish a *Social Determinants of Health Task Force* to consider these findings and work to address the issues raised at this conference. The *Task Force* would operate to identify and advocate for policies by all levels of government to support population health. The federal and provincial governments would respond to these recommendations in a formal manner through annual reports on the status of these social determinants of health.

So Resolved, this December 1, 2002, in Toronto, Canada, and Ratified, February 10, 2003.

REFERENCES

Chapter 1

Acheson, D. (1998). *Independent inquiry into inequalities in health.* Online at www.archive.official-documents. co.uk/document/doh/ih/ih.htm.

Bambra, C. (2004). "The worlds of welfare: Illusory and gender blind?" *Social Policy and Society, 3*(3), 201–211.

Barker, D.J., Osmond, C. & Simmonds, M. (1989). "Weight in infancy and death from ischemic heart disease." *The Lancet, 2,* 577–580.

Bartley, M. (2003). *Understanding health inequalities.* Oxford: Polity Press.

Benzeval, M., Judge, K. & Whitehead, M. (1995). *Tackling inequalities in health: An agenda for action.* London: Kings Fund.

Blane, D. (1999). "The life course, the social gradiant, and health." In M.G. Marmot & R.G. Wilkinson (Eds.), *Social determinants of health* (pp. 64–80). Oxford: Oxford University Press.

Blane, D., Brunner, E. & Wilkinson, R. (Eds.). (1996). *Health and social organization.* London: Routledge.

Bryant, T., Brown, I., Cogan, T., Dallaire, C., LaForest, S., McGowan, P., et al. (2004). "What do Canadian seniors say supports their quality of life?: Findings from a national participatory study." *Canadian Journal of Public Health, 95,* 299–303.

Burstrom, B., Diderichsen, F., Ostlin, P. & Ostergren, P.O. (2002). "Sweden." In J. Mackenbach & M. Bakker (Eds.), *Reducing inequalities in health: A European perspective* (pp. 274–283). London: Routledge.

Canadian Institute on Children's Health. (2000). *The health of Canada's children: A CICH Profile* (3rd ed.). Ottawa: Canadian Institute on Children's Health (CICH).

Canadian Population Health Initiative. (2002). *Canadian Population Health Initiative brief to the Commission on the future of health care in Canada.* Online at secure.cihi.ca/cihiweb/en/downloads/cphi_policy_romanowbrief_ e.pdf.

Canadian Population Health Initiative. (2004). *Select highlights on public views of the determinants of health.* Ottawa: CPHI.

Canadian Public Health Association. (1996). *Action statement for health promotion in Canada.* Online at www. cpha/cpha.docs/ActionStatement.eng.html.

Canadian Public Health Association. (2000). *Reducing poverty and its negative effects on health: Resolution passed at the 2000 CPHA Annual Meeting.* Online at www.cpha.ca/english/policy/resolu/2000s/2000/page2.htm.

Canadian Public Health Association. (2001). *CPHA policy statements.* Online at www.cpha.ca/english/policy/pstatem/ polstate.htm.

Canadian Senate. (2007). *Sub-committee on population health.* Online at tinyurl.com/ypwhhq.

Center for Disease Control and Prevention. (2006). *Social determinants of health.* Online at www.cdc.gov/sdoh/.

Chronic Disease Prevention Alliance of Canada. (2003). *Who we are.* Online at www.chronicdiseaseprevention. ca/content/about_cdpac/mission.asp.

Dahlgren, G. & Whitehead, M. (1992). *Policies and strategies to promote equity in health.* Copenhagen: World Health Organization, Regional Office for Europe.

Davey Smith, G. (Ed.). (2003). *Inequalities in health: Life course perspectives.* Bristol: Policy Press.

Davey Smith, G. & Ebrahim, S. (2001). "Epidemiology—is it time to call it a day?" *International Journal of Epidemiology, 30*(1), 1–11.

Davey Smith, G. & Hart, C. (2002). "Life-course approaches to socio-economic and behavioural influences on cardiovascular disease mortality." *American Journal of Public Health, 92*(8), 1295–1298.

Diderichsen, F., Whitehead, M., Burstrom, B. & Aberg, M. (2001). "Sweden and Britain: The impact of policy context on inequities in health." In T. Evans, M. Whitehead, F. Diderichsen, A. Bhuya & M. Wirth (Eds.), *Challenging inequities in health: From ethics to action* (pp. 241–255). New York: Oxford University Press.

Diez-Roux, A.V., Link, B.G. & Northridge, M.E. (2000). "A multi-level analysis of income inequality and cardiovascular disease risk factors." *Social Science & Medicine, 50*(5), 673–687.

Engels, F. (1845/1987). *The condition of the working class in England.* New York: Penguin Classics.

Epp, J. (1986). *Achieving health for all: A framework for health promotion.* Ottawa: Health and Welfare Canada.

Eriksson, J., Forsen, T., Tuomilehto, J., Winter, P., Osmond, C. & Barker, D. (1999). "Catch-up growth in childhood and death from coronary heart disease: Longitudinal study." *British Medical Journal—Clinical Research, 318*(7181), 427–431.

Esping-Andersen, G. (1990). *The three worlds of welfare capitalism.* Princeton: Princeton University Press.

Esping-Andersen, G. (1999). *Social foundations of post-industrial economies.* New York: Oxford University Press.

Esping-Andersen, G. (2002). "A child-centred social investment strategy." In G. Esping-Andersen (Ed.), *Why we need a new welfare state* (pp. 26–67). Oxford: Oxford University Press.

Evans, R.G., Barer, M.L. & Marmor, T.R. (Eds.). (1994). *Why are some people healthy and others not? The determinants of health of populations.* Hawthorne: Aldine DeGruyter.

Eyles, J., Brimacombe, M., Chaulk, P., Stoddart, G., Pranger, T. & Moase, O. (2001). "What determines health? To where should we shift resources? Attitudes towards the determinants of health among multiple stakeholder groups in Prince Edward Island, Canada." *Social Science & Medicine, 53*(12), 1611–1619.

Federation of Canadian Municipalities. (1999). *Quality of life reporting system: Quality of life in Canadian communities.* Ottawa: Federation of Canadian Municipalities.

Federation of Canadian Municipalities. (2001). *Second report: Quality of life in Canadian communities.* Ottawa: Federation of Canadian Municipalities.

Federation of Canadian Municipalities. (2003). *Falling behind: Our growing income gap.* Ottawa: Federation of Canadian Municipalities.

Federation of Canadian Municipalities. (2004a). *Highlights report 2004: Quality of life in Canadian municipalities.* Ottawa: Federation of Canadian Municipalities.

Federation of Canadian Municipalities. (2004b). *Income, shelter, and necessities.* Ottawa: Federation of Canadian Municipalities.

Gasher, M., Hayes, M., Ross, I., Hackett, R., Gutstein, D. & Dunn, J. (2007). "Spreading the news: Social determinants of health reportage in Canadian daily newspapers." *Canadian Journal of Communication, 32*(3), 557–574.

Gordon, D. (2000). "Inequalities in income, wealth, and standard of living in Britain." In C. Pantazis & D. Gordon (Eds.), *Tackling inequalities: Where are we now and what can be done?* (pp. 25–58). Bristol: Policy Press.

Gordon, D., Shaw, M., Dorling, D. & Davey Smith, G. (1999). *Inequalities in health: The evidence presented to the Independent Inquiry into Inequalities in Health.* Bristol: The Policy Press.

Gordon, D. & Townsend, P. (Eds.). (2000). *Breadline Europe: The measurement of poverty.* Bristol: The Policy Press.

Graham, H. (2004a). "Social determinants and their unequal distribution: Clarifying policy understandings." *Milbank Quarterly, 82*(1), 101–124.

Graham, H. (2004b). "Tackling health inequalities in health in England: Remedying health disadvantages, narrowing health gaps, or reducing health gradients?" *Journal of Social Policy, 33,* 115–131.

Hayes, M., Ross, I.E., Gasherc, M., Gutstein, D., Dunn, J.R. & Hackett, R.A. (2007). "Telling stories: News media, health literacy, and public policy in Canada." *Social Science & Medicine, 64*(9), 1842–1852.

Health Canada. (1998). *Taking action on population health: A position paper for health promotion and programs branch staff.* Ottawa: Health Canada.

Health Canada. (1999). *Statistical report on the health of Canadians.* Online at www.hc-sc.gc.ca/hppb/phdd/report/stat/pdf/english/all_english.pdf.

Health Canada. (2003). *Healthy living strategy.* Online at www.hc-sc.gc.ca/english/media/releases/2003/2003_14.htm.

Irwin, A. & Scali, E. (2007). "Action on the social determinants of health: An historical perspective." *Global Public Health, 2*(3), 235–256.

Kuh, D. & Ben-Shilmo, Y. (Eds.). (1997). *A life course approach to chronic disease epidemiology.* Oxford: Oxford University Press.

Lalonde, M. (1974). *A new perspective on the health of Canadians: A working document.* Online at www.hc-sc.gc.ca/main/hppb/phdd/resource.htm.

Lantz, P.M., House, J.S., Lepkowski, J.M., Williams, D.R., Mero, R.P. & Chen, J.J. (1998). "Socioeconomic factors, health behaviors, and mortality." *Journal of the American Medical Association, 279*(21), 1703–1708.

Mackenbach, J. & Bakker, M. (Eds.). (2002). *Reducing inequalities in health: A European perspective.* London: Routledge.

McKeown, T. (1976). *The role of medicine: Dream, mirage, or nemesis.* London: Neufeld Provincial Hospitals Trust.

McKeown, T. & Record, R.G. (1975). "An interpretation of the decline in mortality in England and Wales during the twentieth century." *Population Studies, 29,* 391–422.

McKinlay, J. & McKinlay, S.M. (1987). "Medical measures and the decline of mortality." In H.D. Schwartz (Ed.), *Dominant issues in medical sociology* (2nd ed.) (pp. 7–19). New York: Random House.

Navarro, V. (Ed.). (2004). *The political and social contexts of health.* Amityville: Baywood Press.

Navarro, V., Borrell, C., Benach, J., Muntaner, C., Quiroga, A., Rodrigues-Sanz, M., et al. (2004). "The importance of the political and the social in explaining mortality differentials among the countries of the OECD, 1950–1998." In V. Navarro (Ed.), *The political and social contexts of health* (pp. 11–86). Amityville: Baywood Press.

Navarro, V. & Shi, L. (2002). "The political context of social inequalities and health." In V. Navarro (Ed.), *The political economy of social inequalities: Consequences for health and quality of life* (pp. 403–418). Amityville: Baywood.

Nettleton, S. (1997). "Surveillance, health promotion, and the formation of a risk identity." In M. Sidell, L. Jones, J. Katz & A. Peberdy (Eds.), *Debates and dilemmas in promoting health* (pp. 314–324). London: Open University Press.

O'Neill, M., Pederson, A., Dupéré, S. & Rootman, I. (Eds.). (2007). *Health promotion in Canada: Critical perspectives* (2nd ed.). Toronto: Canadian Scholars' Press Inc.

Paisley, J., Midgett, C., Brunetti, G. & Tomasik, H. (2001). "Heart health Hamilton-Wentworth survey: Programming implications." *Canadian Journal of Public Policy, 92,* 443–447.

Pantazis, C. & Gordon, D. (Eds.). (2000). *Tackling inequalities: Where are we now and what can be done?* Bristol: Policy Press.

Pantazis, C., Gordon, D. & Levitas, R. (Eds.). (2006). *Poverty and social exclusion in Britain.* Bristol: Policy Press.

Raphael, D. (2000). "Health inequities in the United States: Prospects and solutions." *Journal of Public Health Policy, 21*(4), 392–425.

Raphael, D. (2001a). "Canadian policy statements on income and health: Sound and fury—signifying nothing." *Canadian Review of Social Policy, 48*, 121–127.

Raphael, D. (2001b). "From increasing poverty to societal disintegration: How economic inequality affects the health of individuals and communities." In H. Armstrong, P. Armstrong & D. Coburn (Eds.), *Unhealthy times: The political economy of health and care in Canada* (pp. 224–246). Toronto: Oxford University Press.

Raphael, D. (2001c). *Inequality is bad for our hearts: Why low income and social exclusion are major causes of heart disease in Canada.* Online at depts.washington.edu/eqhlth/pages/academic_resources/paperA15.html.

Raphael, D. (2001d). "Letter from Canada: An end of the millennium update from the birthplace of the Healthy Cities Movement." *Health Promotion International, 16*, 99–101.

Raphael, D. (2002). *Social justice is good for our hearts: Why societal factors—not lifestyles—are major causes of heart disease in Canada and elsewhere.* Online at tinyurl.com/2vou8c.

Raphael, D. (Ed.). (2004). *Social determinants of health: Canadian perspectives.* Toronto: Canadian Scholars' Press Inc.

Raphael, D. (2006). "Social determinants of health: Present status, unresolved questions, and future directions." *International Journal of Health Services, 36*, 651–677.

Raphael, D. (2007a). "Addressing health inequalities in Canada: Little attention, inadequate action, limited success." In M. O'Neill, A. Pederson, S. Dupéré & I. Rootman (Eds.), *Health promotion in Canada: Critical perspectives* (2nd ed.) (pp. 106–122). Toronto: Canadian Scholars' Press Inc.

Raphael, D. (2007b). "Canadian public policy and poverty in international perspective." In D. Raphael (Ed.), *Poverty and policy in Canada: Implications for health and quality of life* (pp. 335–364). Toronto: Canadian Scholars' Press Inc.

Raphael, D. (2007c). "Interactions with the health and service sector." In D. Raphael (Ed.), *Poverty and policy in Canada: Implications for health and quality of life* (pp. 173–204). Toronto: Canadian Scholars' Press Inc.

Raphael, D. (2007d). *Poverty and policy in Canada: Implications for health and quality of life.* Toronto: Canadian Scholars' Press Inc.

Raphael, D. (2007e). "Who is poor in Canada?" In D. Raphael (Ed.), *Poverty and policy in Canada: Implications for health and quality of life* (pp. 59–84). Toronto: Canadian Scholars' Press Inc.

Raphael, D., Anstice, S. & Raine, K. (2003). "The social determinants of the incidence and management of type 2 diabetes mellitus: Are we prepared to rethink our questions and redirect our research activities?" *Leadership in Health Services, 16*, 10–20.

Raphael, D. & Bryant, T. (2002). "The limitations of population health as a model for a new public health." *Health Promotion International, 17*, 189–199.

Raphael, D. & Bryant, T. (2006a). "Maintaining population health in a period of welfare state decline: Political economy as the missing dimension in health promotion theory and practice." *Promotion and Education, 13*, 236–242.

Raphael, D. & Bryant, T. (2006b). "The state's role in promoting population health: Public health concerns in Canada, USA, UK, and Sweden." *Health Policy, 78*, 39–55.

Raphael, D., Bryant, T. & Curry-Stevens, A. (2004). "Toronto Charter outlines future health policy directions for Canada and elsewhere." *Health Promotion International, 19*, 269–273.

Raphael, D. & Farrell, E.S. (2002). "Beyond medicine and lifestyle: Addressing the societal determinants of cardiovascular disease in North America." *Leadership in Health Services, 15*, 1–5.

Raphael, D., Macdonald, J., Labonte, R., Colman, R., Hayward, K. & Torgerson, R. (2004). "Researching income and income distribution as a determinant of health in Canada: Gaps between theoretical knowledge, research practice, and policy implementation." *Health Policy, 72*, 217–232.

Ross, D.P. & Roberts, P. (1999). *Income and child well-being: A new perspective on the poverty debate.* Ottawa: Canadian Council on Social Development.

Ross, D.P., Roberts, P. & Scott, K. (2000). "Family income and child well-being." *ISUMA, 1*(2), 51–54.

Roux, A., Merkin, S. & Arnett, D. (2001). "Neighbourhood of residence and incidence of coronary heart disease." *New England Journal of Medicine, 345*, 99–106.

Shaw, M., Dorling, D., Gordon, D. & Smith, G.D. (1999). *The widening gap: Health inequalities and policy in Britain*. Bristol: The Policy Press.

Shields, M. & Tremblay, S. (2002). "The health of Canada's communities." *Health Reports*, Supplement 13(July), 1–25.

Siddiqi, A. & Hertzman, C. (2007). "Towards an epidemiological understanding of the effects of long-term institutional changes on population health: A case study of Canada versus the USA." *Social Science & Medicine, 64*(3), 589–603.

Tarlov, A. (1996). "Social determinants of health: The sociobiological translation." In D. Blane, E. Brunner & R. Wilkinson (Eds.), *Health and social organization: Towards a health policy for the 21st century* (pp. 71–93). London: Routledge.

Teeple, G. (2000). *Globalization and the decline of social reform: Into the twenty-first century*. Aurora: Garamond Press.

Tesh, S. (1990). *Hidden arguments: Political ideology and disease prevention policy*. New Brunswick: Rutgers University Press.

Townsend, P., Davidson, N. & Whitehead, M. (Eds.). (1992). *Inequalities in health: The Black report and the health divide*. New York: Penguin.

United Way of Greater Toronto & Canadian Council on Social Development. (2002). *A decade of decline: Poverty and income inequality in the City of Toronto in the 1990s*. Toronto: Canadian Council on Social Development and United Way of Greater Toronto.

United Way of Ottawa. (2003). *Environmental scan*. Ottawa: United Way of Ottawa.

United Way of Winnipeg. (2003). *2003 environmental scan and Winnipeg census data*. Winnipeg: United Way of Winnipeg.

Virchow, R. (1848/1985). *Collected essays on public health and epidemiology*. Cambridge: Science History Publications.

Wilkins, R., Berthelot, J.-M. & Ng, E. (2002). "Trends in mortality by neighbourhood income in urban Canada from 1971 to 1996." *Health Reports, 13*(Supplement), 1–28.

Wilkinson, R. & Marmot, M. (2003). *Social determinants of health: The solid facts*. Online at www.euro.who.int/document/e81384.pdf.

World Health Organization. (1986). *Ottawa Charter for health promotion*. Online at www.who.int/hpr/NPH/docs/ottawa_charter_hp.pdf.

World Health Organization. (2004). *WHO to establish commission on social determinants of health*. Online at www.who.int/social_determinants/en/.

Chapter 2

Allison, K., Adlaf, E., Ialomiteanu, A. & Rehm, J. (1999). "Predictors of health risk behaviours among young adults: Analysis of the national population health survey." *Canadian Journal of Public Health, 90*(2), 85–89.

Armstrong, P. (1996). "Unravelling the safety net: Transformations in health care and their impact on women." In J. Brodie (Ed.), *Women and Canadian public policy* (pp. 129–150). Toronto: Harcourt Brace.

Armstrong, P. (2004). "Health, social policy, social economies, and the voluntary sector." In D. Raphael (Ed.), *Social determinants of health: Canadian perspectives* (pp. 331–344). Toronto: Canadian Scholars' Press Inc.

Armstrong, P., Lippman, A. & Sky, L. (1997). *Women's health, social change, and policy development, Synthesis paper*. Paper presented at the Fifth National Health Promotion Research Conference on "Gender and Health: From Research to Policy," Halifax, NS, July 5.

Avison, W. (1997). "Single motherhood and mental health: Implications for primary prevention." *Canadian Medical Association Journal, 156*(5), 661–663.

Barker, D., Forsen, T., Uutela, A., Osmond, C. & Eriksson, J. (2001). "Size at birth and resilience to effects of poor living conditions in adult life: Longitudinal study." *British Medical Journal—Clinical Research, 323*(7324), 1273–1276.

Bartley, M. (2003). *Understanding health inequalities.* Oxford: Polity Press.

Bartley, M., Power, C., Blane, D., Davey Smith, G. & Shipley, M. (1994). "Birthweight and later socioeconomic disadvantages: Evidence from the 1958 British cohort study." *British Medical Journal, 309(6967),* 1475–1478.

Bédard, M. (1998). *The economic and social costs of unemployment.* Applied Research Branch, Human Resources Development Canada. Online at www.hrdc-drhc.gc.ca/sp-ps/arb-dgra/publications/research/r-96-12e.pdf.

Benzeval, M., Dilnot, A., Judge, K. & Taylor, J. (2001). "Income and health over the lifecourse: Evidence and policy implications." In H. Graham (Ed.), *Understanding health inequalities* (pp. 96–112). Buckingham: Open University Press.

Benzeval, M., Judge, K. & Whitehead, M. (1995). *Tackling inequalities in health: An agenda for action.* London: Kings' Fund.

Brooks-Gunn, J., Duncan, G.J. & Britto, P.R. (1998). "Are SES gradients for children similar to those for adults? Achievement and health of children in the United States." In D.P. Keating & C. Hertzman (Eds.), *Developmental health and the wealth of nations: Social, biological, and educational dynamics* (pp. 94–124). New York: Guilford Press.

Brunner, E. & Marmot, M.G. (2006). "Social organization, stress, and health." In M.G. Marmot & R.G. Wilkinson (Eds.), *Social determinants of health* (2nd ed.) (pp. 17–43). Oxford: Oxford University Press.

Bryant, T. (2004). "Housing and health." In D. Raphael (Ed.), *Social determinants of health: Canadian perspectives* (pp. 217–232). Toronto: Canadian Scholars' Press Inc.

Canadian Population Health Initiative. (2004). *Select highlights on public views of the determinants of health.* Ottawa: CPHI.

Coburn, D. (2000). "Income inequality, social cohesion, and the health status of populations: The role of neo-liberalism." *Social Science and Medicine, 51*(1), 135–146.

Coburn, D. (2004). "Beyond the income inequality hypothesis: Globalization, neo-liberalism, and health inequalities." *Social Science and Medicine, 58,* 41–56.

Cohen, S., Kaplan, G. & Salonen, J. (1999). "The role of psychological characteristics in the relation between socioeconomic status and perceived health." *Journal of Applied Social Psychology, 29*(3), 445–468.

Davey Smith, G. (Ed.). (2003). *Inequalities in health: Life course perspectives.* Bristol: Policy Press.

Davey Smith, G., Ben-Shlomo, Y. & Lynch, J. (2002). "Life course approaches to inequalities in coronary heart disease risk." In S.A. Stansfeld and M. Marmot (Eds.), *Stress and the heart: Psychosocial pathways to coronary heart disease* (pp. 20–49). London: BMJ Books.

Davey Smith, G. & Gordon, D. (2000). "Poverty across the life-course and health." In C. Pantazis & D. Gordon (Eds.), *Tackling inequalities: Where are we now and what can be done?* (pp. 141–158). Bristol: Policy Press.

Davey Smith, G., Hart, C., Blane, D., Gillis, C. & Hawthorne, V. (1997). "Lifetime socioeconomic position and mortality: Prospective observational study." *British Medical Journal, 314*(7080), 547–552.

Davies, L., McMullin, J.A., Avison, W. & Cassidy, G. (2001). *Social policy, gender inequality, and poverty.* Ottawa: Status of Women Canada.

Dooley, M. & Curtis, L. (1998). *Child health and family socioeconomic status in the Canadian national longitudinal survey of children and youth.* Hamilton & Halifax: McMaster University Canadian International Labour Network, and Dalhousie University.

Fawcett, G. (2000). *Bringing down the barriers: The labour market and woman with disabilities in Ontario.* Ottawa: Canadian Council on Social Development.

Fitzpatrick, M. (2001). *The tyranny of health: Doctors and the regulation of lifestyle.* London: Routledge.

Forsen, T., Eriksson, J.G., Tuomilehto, J., Osmond, C. & Barker, D.J.P. (1999). "Growth *in utero* and during childhood among women who develop coronary heart disease: Longitudinal study." *British Medical Journal—Clinical Research, 319*(7222), 1403–1407.

Forssas, E., Gissler, M., Sihvonen, M. & Hemminki, E. (1999). "Maternal predictors of perinatal mortality: The role of birthweight." *International Journal of Epidemiology, 28*(3), 475–478.

Galabuzi, G.E. (2005). *Canada's economic apartheid: The social exclusion of racialized groups in the new century.* Toronto: Canadian Scholars' Press Inc.

Graham, E., MacLeod, M., Johnston, D., Dibben, C., Morgan, I. & Briscoe, S. (2000). "Individual deprivation, neighbourhood, and recovery from illness." In H. Graham (Ed.), *Understanding health inequalities* (pp. 170–185). Buckingham: Open University Press.

Graham, H. (Ed.). (2001). *Understanding health inequalities.* Buckingham: Open University Press.

Hadley, K. (2001). *And we still ain't satisfied: Gender inequality in Canada, A status report for 2001.* Toronto: Centre for Social Justice, Foundation for Research and Education and National Action Committee on the Status of Women. Online at www.socialjustice.org/pubs/womequal.pdf.

Hatfield, M. (1997). *Concentrations of poverty and distressed neighbourhoods in Canada.* Applied Research Branch, Human Resources Development Canada. Online at www.hrdc-drhc.gc.ca/sp-ps/arb-dgra/publications/research/w-97-1e.pdf.

Health Canada. (1999). *Toward a healthy future: Second report on the health of Canadians.* Health Canada, Statistics Canada, Canadian Institute for Health Information. Online at www.hc-sc.gc.ca/hppb/phdd/report/toward/pdf/english/toward_a_healthy_english.PDF.

Hertzman, C. (1998). "The case for child development as a determinant of health." *Canadian Journal of Public Health, 89*(Supplement 1), S14–S19.

Hertzman, C. (1999a). "The biological embedding of early experience and its effects on health in adulthood." *Annals of the New York Academy of Sciences, 896*, 85–95.

Hertzman, C. (1999b). "Population health and human development." In D.P. Keating & C. Hertzman (Eds.), *Developmental health and the wealth of nations: Social, biological, and educational dynamics* (pp. 21–40). New York: Guilford Press.

Hertzman, C. (2000a). "The case for an early childhood development strategy." *Isuma, 1*(2), 11–18.

Hertzman, C. (2000b). "The socioeconomic, psychosocial, and developmental environment." In J. Sussex (Ed.), *Improving population health in industrialized nations* (pp. 87–104). London: Office of Health Economics.

Hou, F. & Picot, G. (2003). *Visible minority neighbourhood enclaves and labour market outcomes of immigrants.* Ottawa: Analytic Studies Branch, Statistics Canada.

Innocenti Research Centre. (2000). *A league table of child poverty in rich nations.* Florence: Innocenti Research Centre.

Innocenti Research Centre. (2001). *A league table of child deaths by injury in rich nations.* Florence: Innocenti Research Centre.

International Labour Organization. (1999). *Country studies on the social impact of globalization: Final report.* Geneva: International Labour Organization.

Jackson, A. (2002). "Canada beats USA—but loses gold to Sweden." *Canadian Council on Social Development.* Online at www.ccsd.ca/pubs/2002/olympic/indicators.htm.

Jackson, A. (2004). "The unhealthy Canadian workplace." In D. Raphael (Ed.), *Social determinants of health: Canadian perspectives* (pp. 79–94). Toronto: Canadian Scholars' Press Inc.

Jackson, A. (2005). *Work and labour in Canada: Critical issues.* Toronto: Canadian Scholars' Press Inc.

James, P.T., Nelson, M., Ralph, A. & Leather, S. (1997). "Socioeconomic determinants of health: The contribution of nutrition to inequalities in health." *British Medical Journal, 314*(7093), 1545–1548.

Jarvis, M.J. & Wardle, J. (1999). "Social patterning of individual health behaviours: The case of cigarette smoking." In M.G. Marmot & R.G. Wilkinson (Eds.), *Social determinants of health* (pp. 224–237). Oxford: Oxford University Press.

Johnson, A.A., El-Khorazaty, M.N., Hatcher, B.J., Wingrove, B.K., Milligan, R., Harris, C. & Richards, L. (2003). "Determinants of late prenatal care initiation by African-American women in Washington, DC." *Maternal and Child Health Journal, 7*(2), 103–114.

Kawachi, I. & Kennedy, B. (2002). *The health of nations: Why inequality is harmful to your health.* New York: New Press.

Labonte, R. (1993). *Health promotion and empowerment: Practice frameworks.* Toronto: Centre for Health Promotion and ParticipAction.

Lawlor, D., Ebrahim, S. & Davey Smith, G. (2002). "Socioeconomic position in childhood and adulthood and insulin resistance: Cross-sectional survey using data from British women's heart and health study." *British Medical Journal, 325*(12), 805–807.

Lee, K. (2000). "Urban poverty in Canada: A statistical profile." *Canadian Council on Social Development.* Online at www.ccsd.ca/pubs/2000/up/.

Lochhead, C. & Scott, K. (2000). "The dynamics of women's poverty in Canada." *Status of Women Canada.* Online at www.swc-cfc.gc.ca/pubs/0662281594/200003_0662281594_1_e.html.

Lupien, S., King, E., Meaney, M. & McEwan, B. (2001). "Can poverty get under your skin? Basal cortisol levels and cognitive function in children from low and high socioeconomic status." *Development and Psychopathology, 13,* 653–676.

Lynch, J. (2000). "Income inequality and health: Expanding the debate." *Social Science and Medicine, 51,* 1001–1005.

Lynch, J.W., Davey Smith, G., Kaplan, G.A. & House, J.S. (2000). "Income inequality and mortality: Importance to health of individual income, psychosocial environment, or material conditions." *British Medical Journal, 320,* 1220–1224.

Lynch, J. & Kaplan, G.A. (2000). "Socioeconomic position." In L.F. Berkman & I. Kawachi (Eds.), *Social epidemiology* (pp. 13–35). New York: Oxford University Press.

Lynch, J., Kaplan, G. & Salonen, J. (1997). "Why do poor people behave poorly? Variation in adult health behaviours and psychosocial characteristics by stages of the socioeconomic lifecourse." *Social Science and Medicine, 44*(6), 809–819.

MacMillan, H.L., MacMillan, A.B., Offord, D.R.D. & Dingle, J.L. (1996). "Aboriginal health." *Canadian Medical Association Journal, 155*(11), 1569–1578.

Marmot, M. (2004). *Status syndrome: How your social standing directly affects your health and life expectancy.* London: Bloomsbury.

Marmot, M. & Wilkinson, R. (Eds.). (2006). *Social determinants of health* (2nd ed.). Oxford: Oxford University Press.

Muntaner, C. (2004). "Commentary: Social capital, social class, and the slow progress of psychosocial epidemiology." *International Journal of Epidemiology, 33*(4), 1–7.

Nettleton, S. (1997). "Surveillance, health promotion, and the formation of a risk identity." In M. Sidell, L. Jones, J. Katz & A. Peberdy (Eds.), *Debates and dilemmas in promoting health* (pp. 314–324). London: Open University Press.

Newbold, K.B. & Danforth, J. (2003). "Health status and Canada's immigrant population." *Social Science and Medicine, 57,* 1981–1995.

Ng, E., Wilkins, R., Gendron, F. & Berthelot, J.M. (2004). *Dynamics of immigrants' health in Canada: Evidence from the national population health survey.* Ottawa: Statistics Canada.

O'Loughlin, J.L., Paradis, G., Gray-Donald, K. & Renaud, L. (1999). "The impact of a community-based heart disease prevention program in a low-income, inner city neighbourhood." *American Journal of Public Health, 89*(12), 1819–1826.

Organisation for Economic Co-operation and Development. (2005a). *Health at a glance: OECD indicators 2005.* Paris: OECD.

Organisation for Economic Co-operation and Development. (2005b). *Society at a glance: OECD social indicators* (2005 ed.). Paris: OECD.

Pahlke, A., Lord, S. & Christiansen-Ruffman, L. (2001). "Women's health and well-being in six Nova Scotia fishing communities." *Maritime Centre of Excellence for Women's Health.* Online at www.medicine.dal.ca/mcewh/Publications/Fishnet%20Finalreport.pdf.

Picot, G. (2004). *The deteriorating economic welfare of immigrants and possible causes.* Ottawa: Statistics Canada.

Pomerleau, J., Pederson, L.L., Østbye, T., Speechley, M. & Speechley, K.N. (1997). "Health behaviours and socio-economic status in Ontario, Canada." *European Journal of Epidemiology, 13*(6), 613–622.

Potvin, L., Richard, L. & Edwards, A. (2000). "Knowledge of cardiovascular disease risk factors among the Canadian population: Relationships with indicators of socioeconomic status." *Canadian Medical Association Journal, 162*, S5–S12.

Power, C., Bartley, M., Davey Smith, G. & Blane, D. (1996). "Transmission of social and biological risk across the lifecourse." In D. Blane, E. Brunner & R. Wilkinson (Eds.), *Health and social organization* (pp. 188–203). London: Routledge.

Raphael, D. (2000). "Health inequalities in Canada: Current discourses and implications for public health action." *Critical Public Health, 10*(2), 193–216.

Raphael, D. (2003). "A society in decline: The social, economic, and political determinants of health inequalities in the USA." In R. Hofrichter (Ed.), *Health and social justice: A reader on politics, ideology, and inequity in the distribution of disease* (pp. 59–88). San Francisco: Jossey Bass.

Raphael, D. (2004). "Introduction to the social determinants of health." In D. Raphael (Ed.), *Social determinants of health: Canadian perspectives* (pp. 1–18). Toronto: Canadian Scholars' Press Inc.

Raphael, D. (2007). *Poverty and policy in Canada: Implications for health and quality of life.* Toronto: Canadian Scholars' Press Inc.

Raphael, D., Anstice, S. & Raine, K. (2003). "The social determinants of the incidence and management of type II diabetes mellitus: Are we prepared to rethink our questions and redirect our research activities?" *Leadership in Health Services, 16*, 10–20.

Raphael, D. & Farrell, E.S. (2002). "Addressing cardiovascular disease in North America: Shifting the paradigm." *Harvard Health Policy Review, 3*(2), 18–28.

Raphael, D., Macdonald, J., Labonte, R., Colman, R., Hayward, K. & Torgerson, R. (2005). "Researching income and income distribution as a determinant of health in Canada: Gaps between theoretical knowledge, research practice, and policy implementation." *Health Policy, 72*, 217–232.

Roberts, P., Smith, P. & Nason, H. (2001). *Children and familial economic welfare: The effect of income on child development.* Applied Research Branch, Human Resources Development Canada. Online at www.hrdc-drhc.gc.ca/sp-ps/arb-dgra/publications/research/2001docs/W-01-1-11/IW-01-1-11e.pdf.

Ronson, B. & Rootman, I. (2004). "Literacy and health." In D. Raphael (Ed.), *Social determinants of health: Canadian perspectives* (pp. 155–170). Toronto: Canadian Scholars' Press Inc.

Rosenberg, M.W. & Wilson, K. (2000). "Gender, poverty, and location: How much difference do they make in the geography of health inequalities?" *Social Science & Medicine, 51*(2), 275–287.

Ross, D.P. & Roberts, P. (1999). *Income and child well-being: A new perspective on the poverty debate.* Ottawa: Canadian Council on Social Development.

Ross, D.P., Roberts, P.A. & Scott, K. (1998). *Variations in child development outcomes among children living in lone-parent families.* Applied Research Branch, Human Resources Development Canada. Online at www.hrdc-drhc.gc.ca/sp-ps/arb-dgra/publications/research/w-98-7e.pdf.

Ross, N., Wolfson, M., Dunn, J., Berthelot, J.M., Kaplan, G. & Lynch, J. (2000). "Relation between income inequality and mortality in Canada and in the United States: Cross-sectional assessment using census data and vital statistics." *British Medical Journal, 320*(7239), 898–902.

Sapolsky, R.M. (1992). *Stress, the aging brain, and mechanisms of neuron death.* Cambridge: MIT Press.

Sarlio-Lahteenkorva, S. & Lahelma, E. (2001). "Food insecurity is associated with past and present economic disadvantage and body mass index." *The Journal of Nutrition, 131*(11), 2880–2884.

Shah, C. (2004). "Aboriginal health." In D. Raphael (Ed.), *Social determinants of health: Canadian perspectives* (pp. 267–280). Toronto: Canadian Scholars' Press Inc.

Shaw, M. (2001). "Health and housing: A lasting relationship." *Journal of Epidemiology and Community Health, 55*, 291–296.

Shaw, M., Dorling, D. & Davey Smith, G. (2006). "Poverty, social exclusion, and minorities." In M.G. Marmot & R.G. Wilkinson (Eds.), *Social determinants of health* (pp. 196–223). Oxford: Oxford University Press.

Shaw, M., Dorling, D., Gordon, D. & Davey Smith, G. (1999). *The widening gap: Health inequalities and policy in Britain.* Bristol: The Policy Press.

Stewart, M., Brosky, G., Gillis, A., Jackson, S., Johnston, G., Kirkland, S., Leigh, G., Pawliw-Fry, B., Persaud, V. & Rootman, I. (1996). "Disadvantaged women and smoking." *Canadian Journal of Public Health, 87*(4), 257–260.

Tarlov, A. (1996). "Social determinants of health: The sociobiological translation." In D. Blane, E. Brunner & R. Wilkinson (Eds.), *Health and social organization: Towards a health policy for the 21st century* (pp. 71–93). London: Routledge.

Townson, M. (2000). *A report card on women and poverty.* Ottawa: Canadian Centre for Policy Alternatives.

Travers, K.D. (1996). "The social organization of nutritional inequities." *Social Science and Medicine, 43*(4), 543–553.

Tremblay, D.G. (2004). "Unemployment and the labour market." In D. Raphael (Ed.), *Social determinants of health: Canadian perspectives* (pp. 53–66). Toronto: Canadian Scholars' Press Inc.

United Way of Greater Toronto. (2004). *Poverty by postal code: The geography of neighbourhood poverty, 1981–2001.* Toronto: United Way of Greater Toronto.

van de Mheen, H., Stronks, K. & Mackenbach, J. (1998). "A lifecourse perspective on socioeconomic inequalities in health." In M. Bartley, D. Blane & G. Davey Smith (Eds.), *The sociology of health inequalities* (pp. 193–216). Oxford: Blackwell Publishers.

Wamala, S., Lynch, J. & Horsten, M. (1999). "Education and the metabolic syndrome in women." *Diabetes Care, 22*(12), 1999–2003.

Wilkinson, R. (2001). *Mind the gap: Hierarchies, health, and human evolution.* London: Weidenfeld and Nicolson.

Wilkinson, R.G. (1996). *Unhealthy societies: The afflictions of inequality.* New York: Routledge.

Williamson, D. (2000). "Health behaviours and health: Evidence that the relationship is not conditional on income adequacy." *Social Science & Medicine, 51*(12), 1741–1754.

Willms, J.D. (1997). "Literacy skills and social class gradients." *Policy Options, 18*(6), 22–26.

Willms, J.D. (1999). "Quality and inequality in children's literacy: The effects of families, schools, and communities." In D.P. Keating & C. Hertzman (Eds.), *Developmental health and the wealth of nations: Social, biological, and educational dynamics* (pp. 72–93). New York: Guilford Press.

Willms, J.D. (2001). "Three hypotheses about community effects on social outcomes." *Isuma, 2*(1), 53–62.

Willms, J.D. (Ed.). (2002). *Vulnerable children: Findings from Canada's national longitudinal survey.* Edmonton: University of Alberta Press.

Chapter 3

Abella, R. (1984). *Equality in employment: The report of the Commission on Equality in Employment*. Ottawa: Supply and Services Canada.

Canada Employment and Immigration Advisory Council. (1992). *Last in, first out: Racism in employment*. Ottawa: Government of Canada.

Canadian Council for Refugees. (2000). *Report on systemic racism and discrimination in Canadian refugee and immigration policies*. Montreal: Canadian Council for Refugees.

Canadian Race Relations Foundation. (1999). *Unequal access: A Canadian profile of racial differences in education, employment, and income*. Toronto: Canadian Race Relations Foundation.

Commission on Systemic Racism in the Ontario Criminal Justice System. (1994). *Report of the Commission on Systemic Racism in the Ontario Criminal Justice System*. Toronto: Queen's Printer for Ontario.

Curry-Stevens, A. (2001). *When markets fail people: Exploring the widening gap between rich and poor in Canada*. Toronto: CSJ Foundation for Research and Education.

Curry-Stevens, A. (2004). Arrogant capitalism: Changing futures, changing lives. *Canadian Review of Social Policy, 52*: 158–164.

Curry-Stevens, A. (2008). "Building the case for the study of the middle class: Shifting our gaze from margins to centre." *International Journal of Social Welfare* [forthcoming].

Ehrenreich, B. (2001). *Nickel and dimed: On (not) getting by in America*. New York: Metropolitan.

Frenette, M. & Morisette, R. (2003). *Will they ever converge? Earnings of immigrant and Canadian-born workers over the last two decades*. Ottawa: Statistics Canada.

Galabuzi, G.E. (2001). *Canada's creeping economic apartheid*. Toronto: CSJ Foundation for Research and Education.

Lewis, S. (1992). *Stephen Lewis report on race relations in Ontario*. Submitted to Premier Bob Rae. Online at www.geocities.com/CapitolHill/6174/lewis.html.

Lindsay, C. & Almey, M. (2006). "Income and earnings." In *Women in Canada: A gender-based statistical report* (pp. 133–158). Ottawa: Statistics Canada.

Michalski, J.H. (2001). *Asking citizens what matters for quality of life in Canada: Results of CPRN's public dialogue process*. Ottawa: Canadian Policy Research Networks.

Morissette, R. & Zhang, X. (2006). "Revisiting wealth inequality." *Perspectives on Labour and Income, 7*(12), 5–16.

Murphy, B., Roberts, R. & Wolfson, M. (2007). "High-income Canadians." *Perspectives on Labour and Income, 8*(9), 5–17.

National Council of Welfare. (2006). *Poverty profile, 2002 & 2003*. Ottawa: Government of Canada.

Noël, A. (2002). *A law against poverty: Quebec's new approach to combating poverty and social exclusion*. Ottawa: Canadian Policy Research Networks–Family Network.

Ornstein, M. (1994). *Income and rent: Equality-seeking groups and access to rental accommodation restricted by income criteria*. Toronto: Institute for Social Research.

Ornstein, M. (1999). *The differential effect of income criteria on access to rental accommodation on the basis of age and race: 1996 census results*. Toronto: Centre for Equality Rights in Accommodation.

Sauve, R. (2002). *The dreams and the reality: Assets, debts, and net worth of Canadian households*. Ottawa: The Vanier Institute on the Family.

Scott, K. (2002). *A lost decade: Income inequality and the health of Canadians*. Presentation to the Social Determinants of Health across the Lifespan Conference, Toronto, November 2002.

Statistics Canada. (2001a). *The assets and debts of Canadians: An overview of the results of the Survey of Financial Security*. Ottawa: Statistics Canada.

Statistics Canada. (2001b). *2001 census of Canada.* Ottawa: Statistics Canada.

Task Force on the Participation of Visible Minorities in the Federal Public Service. (2000). *Embracing change in the federal public service.* Ottawa: Treasury Board of Canada.

Yalnizyan, A. (1998). *The growing gap: A report on growing inequality between the rich and poor in Canada.* Toronto: Centre for Social Justice.

Yalnizyan, A. (2000). *Canada's great divide: The politics of the growing gap between rich and poor in the 1990s.* Toronto: Centre for Social Justice.

Yalnizyan, A. (2007). *The rich and the rest of us: The changing face of Canada's growing gap.* Ottawa: Canadian Centre for Policy Alternatives.

Chapter 4

Aubin, J. & Traoré, I. (2007). *L'excès de poids en France et au Québec en 2003: Un regard sur les caractéristiques socioéconomiques associées.* Quebec: Zoom Santé, Institut de la statistique du Québec.

Barrett, C., Bussière, L., Darby, P., Lafleur, B., MacDuff, D. & Vail, S. (2003). *Performance and potential 2003–04: Defining the Canadian advantage.* Online at www.conferenceboard.ca.

Bill 112. (2002) *An Act to combat poverty and social exclusion* (Chapter 61). National Assembly, second session, 36th legislature. Quebec: Quebec Official Publisher.

Bordeleau, M. & Traoré, I. (2007). *Santé générale, santé mentale et stress au Québec: Regard sur les liens avec l'âge le sexe, la scolarité et le revenu.* Quebec: Zoom Santé, Institut de la statistique du Québec.

Ferland, M. (2003). *Variation des écarts de l'état de santé en fonction du revenue au Québec de 1987 à 1998.* Quebec: Institut de la statistique du Québec.

Hou, F. & Chen, J. (2003). "Neighborhood low income, income inequality, and health in Toronto." *Health Reports (Statistics Canada), 14*(2), 21–34.

Human Resources Development Canada. (2003). *Understanding the 2000 low income statistics based on the market basket measure* (Applied Research Bulletin, Strategic Policy). Online at www.hrdcdrhc.gc.ca/sp-ps/arb-dgra/ publications/research/2003docs/SP-569-03/e/SP-569-03_E_toc.shtml.

Institut de la statistique du Québec. (2006). *Recueil statistique sur la pauvreté et les inégalités socioéconomiques au Québec.* Ministère de l'Emploi et de la Solidarité sociale, Québec. Online at www.stat.gouv.qc.ca.

Institut national de santé publique du Québec et ministère de la Santé et des Services sociaux du Québec en collaboration avec l'Institut de la statistique du Québec. *Portrait de santé du Québec et de ses régions: Les analyses—Deuxième rapport national sur l'état de santé de la population du Québec,* gouvernement du Québec, 2006. Online at www.inspq.qc.ca/pdf/publications/546-PortraitSante2006_Analyses.pdf.

Kawachi, I. (2000). "Income inequality and health." In L. Berkman & I. Kawachi (Eds.), *Social epidemiology* (pp. 76–94). Oxford: Oxford University Press.

Kawachi, I. & Kennedy, B. (1997). "The relationship of income inequality to mortality: Does the choice of indicator matter?" *Social Science & Medicine, 45*(7), 1121–1128.

Kidder, K., Stein, J. & Fraser, J. (2000). *The health of Canada's children: A CICH profile* (3rd ed.). Ottawa: Canadian Institute on Children's Health.

Kozyrskyj, A.L., Dahl, M.E., Chateau, D.G., Mazowita, G.B., Klassen, T.P. & Law, B. (2004). "Evidence-based prescribing of antibiotics for children: Role of socioeconomic status and physician characteristics." *Canadian Medical Association Journal, 171*(2), 139–145.

Lemstra, M., Neudorf, C. & Opondo, J. (2006). "Health disparity by neighbourhood income." *Canadian Journal of Public Health, 97*(6), 435–439.

Lessard, R., Roy, D., Choinière, R., Bujold, R. et al. (1998). *Social inequalities in health: Annual report of the health of the population.* Montreal: Direction de la Santé Publique. Online at www. santepub–mtl.qc.ca/Publication/ autres/rapport1998.html#english.

Lessard, R., Roy, D., Choinière, R., Lévesque, J.F. & Perron, S. (2002). *Urban health: A vital factor in Montreal's development*. Montreal: Direction de Santé Publique. Online at www.santepub–mtl. qc.ca/Publication/autres/annualreport2002.html.

Lethbridge L.N. & Phipps, S.A. (2005). "Chronic poverty and childhood asthma in the Maritimes versus the rest of Canada." *Canadian Journal of Public Health, 96*(1), 18–23.

Lynch, J.W., Smith, G.D., Kaplan, G.A. & House, J.S. (2000). "Income inequality and mortality: Importance to health of individual income, psychosocial environment, or material conditions." *British Medical Journal, 320*, 1200–1204.

Massé, R. & Gilbert, L. (2003). *Programme national de santé publique 2003—2012*. Québec: Ministère de la Santé et des Services Sociaux.

McLeod, C.B., Lavis, J.N., Mustard, C.A. & Stoddart, G.L. (2003). "Income inequality, household income, and health status in Canada: A prospective cohort study." *American Journal of Public Health, 93*(8), 1287–1293.

Ministère de la Santé et des Services Sociaux. (1992). *La politique de la santé et du bien-être*. Quebec: Ministère de la Santé et des Services Sociaux.

NAPO. (2006). *The face of poverty in Canada: An overview.* National Anti-Poverty Organization. Online at www.napo-onap.ca/en/issues/2006POVERTYinCANADA.pdf.

Noël, A. (2002). *A law against poverty: Quebec's new approach to combating poverty and social exclusion* (Background Paper: Family Network). Canadian Policy Research Networks. Online at www.cpds.umontreal.ca/fichier/cahiercpds03–01.pdf.

Noël, A. (2004). *A focus on income support: Implementing Quebec's law against poverty and social exclusion.* Canadian Policy Research Networks. Online at www.cprn.org/documents/29659_en.pdf.

Pampalon, R. & Raymond, G. (2000). "A deprivation index for health and welfare planning in Quebec." *Chronic Diseases in Canada, 21*(3), 104–113.

Phipps, S. (2003). *The impact of poverty on health: A scan of research literature*. Canadian Institute for Health Information. Online at cihi.ca.

Phipps, S.A., Burton, P.S., Osberg, L.S. & Lethbridge, L.N. (2006). "Poverty and the extent of child obesity in Canada, Norway and the United States." *Obesity Reviews, 7*, 5–12.

Ross, D. & Roberts, P. (1999). *Income and child well-being: A new perspective on the poverty debate*. Ottawa: Canadian Council on Social Development.

Ross, N., Wolfson, M., Dunn, J., Berthelot, J.M., Kaplan, G. & Lynch, J. (2000). "Relation between income inequality and mortality in Canada and in the United States: Cross-sectional assessment using census data and vital statistics." *British Medical Journal, 320*, 898–902.

Séguin, L., Nikiéma, B., Gauvin, L., Zunzunegui, M.-V. & Xu, Q. (2007). "Duration of poverty and child health in the Quebec Longitudinal Study of Child Development: Longitudinal analysis of a birth cohort." *Pediatrics, 119*(5): e1060–1070.

Séguin, L., Xu, Q., Gauvin, L., Zunzunegui, M.-V., Potvin, L. & Frohlich, K.L. (2005). "Understanding the dimensions of socioeconomic status that influence toddlers' health: Unique impact of lack of money for basic needs in Quebec's birth cohort." *Journal of Epidemiology and Community Health, 59*, 42–48.

United Nations Human Development Report. (1999). "Globalization with a human face: Human development indicators, Part 1." Oxford: United Nations Development Programme, Oxford University Press. Online at hdr.undp.org/reports/global/1999/en/pdf/hdr_1999_back1.pdf.

United Nations Human Development Report. (2006). "Beyond scarcity: Power, poverty, and the global water crisis." Oxford: United Nations Development Programme, Oxford University Press. Online at hdr.undp.org/hdr2006/.

Webber, M. (1998). *Measuring low income and poverty in Canada: An update*. Income and labour dynamic working paper series. Ottawa: Statistics Canada.

Wilkins, R. (2006). *PCCF+ Version 4G, automated geographic coding based on the Statistics Canada postal codes to October 2005*. Health Analysis and Measurement Group, Statistics Canada.

Wilkins, R., Berthelot, J.-M. & Ng, E. (2002). "Trends in mortality by neighbourhood income in urban Canada from 1971 to 1996." *Health reports (Stats Can)*, Supplement 13, 1–28.

Xi, G., McDowell, I., Nair, R. & Spasoff, R. (2005). "Income inequality and health in Ontario: A multilevel analysis." *Canadian Journal of Public Health, 96*(3), 206–211.

Chapter 5

Arthur, M.B. & Rousseau, D.M. (Eds.). (1996). *The boundaryless career: A new employment principle for a new organizational era.* New York: Oxford University Press.

Cadin, L., Bender, A.F., Saint-Giniez, V. & Pringle, J. (2000). *Carrières nomades et contextes nationaux. Revue de gestion des ressources humaines.* Paris: AGRH.

Cette, G., Méda, D., Sylvain, A. & Tremblay, D.-G. (2007). "Activité d'emploi et difficultés de conciliation emploi-famille: Une comparaison fine des taux d'activité en France et au Canada." *Loisir et société/Leisure and Society, 29*(1), 117–154.

Chapon, S. & Euzéby, C. (2002). "Vers une convergence des modèles sociaux européens?" *Revue internationale de sécurité sociale, 55*(2), 49–71.

Dasgupta, S. (2001). *Employment security: Conceptual and statistical issues.* Geneva: International Labour Organization. Online at www.ilo.org/public/english/protection/ses/info/publ/employment.htm.

Doucet, A. & Tremblay, D.-G. (2006). "Leave policies in Canada, 2006." In P. Moss & M. O'Brien (Eds.), *International review of leave policies and related research, 2006* (pp. 78–88). Employment Relations Research Series no. 57. Department of Trade and Industry, United Kingdom.

Esping-Andersen, G. (1985). *Politics against markets: The social democratic road to power.* Princeton: Princeton University Press.

Fontan, J.-M., Klein, J.-L. & Tremblay, D.-G. (2005a). "Collective action in local development: The case of Angus Technopole in Montreal." *Canadian Journal of Urban Research, 13*(2), 317–336.

Fontan, J.-M., Klein, J.-L. & Tremblay, D.-G. (2005b). *Innovation sociale et reconversion économique. Le cas de Montréal.* Paris: L'Harmattan.

Freyssinet, J. (2003). "Les trois inflexions des politiques de l'emploi." *Alternatives économiques*, 210(January), 38–45.

Kapsalis, Costa & Tourigny, Pierre. (2004). "La durée de l'emploi atypique." *L'emploi et le revenu en perspective*, (December), 5–14.

Le Boterf, G. (1998). *L'ingénierie des compétences.* Paris: Les Editions d'Organisation.

Lowe, G., Schellenberg, G. & Davidman, Katie. (1999). *Re-thinking employment relationships.* CPRN Discussion Paper no. W-5.

OECD (Organisation for Economic Co-operation and Development). (1996). *L'économie fondée sur le savoir.* Paris: OECD.

Paugam, S. (1998). *Le revenu minimum d'insertion en France après six ans; un bilan contrasté.* Montreal: Interventions économiques. Online at www.teluq.uquebec.ca/interventionseconomiques.

Standing, G. (1999). *Global labour flexibility: Seeking distributive justice.* London: Palgrave.

Statistics Canada. (2005a). "Le marché du travail en 2004." *L'emploi et le revenu en perspective* (February), 1–15.

Statistics Canada. (2005b). *Regard sur le marché du travail.* Online at www41.statcan.ca/2621/ceb2621_000_f.htm.

Statistics Canada. (2005c). *Enquête sur la population active.* Special calculations of the Statistical Institute of Quebec (Institut de la statistique du Québec).

Thomsin, L. & Tremblay, D.-G. (2006). "Le 'mobile working': De nouvelles perspectives sur les lieux et les formes du télétravail." *Interventions économiques, 34.* Online at www.teluq.uqam.ca/interventionseconomiques.

Tremblay, D.-G. (2002a). "Les économistes institutionnalistes: les apports des institutionnalistes à la pensée économique hétérodoxe." *Interventions économiques journal*. Online at www.teluq.uquebec.ca/interventions economiques.

Tremblay, D.-G. (2002b). *Informal learning communities in the knowledge economy*. Proceedings of the 2002 World Computer Congress. Montreal: Elsevier Press, International Federation for Information Processing. Tremblay, D.-G. (2002c). "Balancing work and family with telework? Organizational issues and challenges for women and managers." *Women in Management, 17*(3/4), 157–170.

Tremblay, D.-G. (2003a). "New types of careers in the knowledge economy? Networks and boundaryless jobs as a career strategy in the ICT and multimedia sector." In *Communications & Strategies* (pp. 81–106). Montpellier-Manchester: IDATE.

Tremblay, D.-G. (2003b). "Telework: A new mode of gendered segmentation? Results from a study in Canada." *Canadian Journal of Communication, 28*(4), 461–478.

Tremblay, D.-G. (2003c). "Youth employment situation and employment policies in Canada." In Laurence Roulleau-Berger (Ed.), *Youth and work in the post-industrial city of North America and Europe* (pp. 175–189). Boston: Leiden.

Tremblay, D.-G. (2004a). *Économie du travail: Les réalités et les approches théoriques*. Montreal: Editions St-Martin.

Tremblay, D.-G. (2004b). *Conciliation emploi-famille et temps sociaux*. Quebec-Toulouse: Presses de l'Université du Québec et Octares.

Tremblay, D.-G. (2006). "L'évolution des politiques familiales et de conciliation emploi-famille au Québec et au Canada." In C. Bourreau-Dubois & B. Jeandidier (Eds.), *Économie sociale et droit*, vol. 2, *Famille et éducation* (241–255). Paris: L'Harmattan.

Tremblay, D.-G. (2007a). L'éclatement de l'emploi. Quebec: Presses de l'université du Québec.

Tremblay, D.-G. (2007b). Formes de travail et politiques d'emploi; les enjeux. Quebec: Presses de l'université du Québec.

Tremblay, D.-G. (2007c). Vers une articulation des temps sociaux tout au long de la vie; l'aménagement et la réduction du temps de travail. Quebec: Presses de l'université du Québec.

Tremblay, D.-G. (2007d). L'innovation continue. Les multiples dimensions du phénomène de l'innovation. Quebec: Télé-université.

Tremblay, D.-G., Chevrier, C. & Di Loreto, M. (2006). "Le télétravail à domicile: Meilleure conciliation emploi-famille ou source d'envahissement de la vie privée?" Interventions économiques, 34. Online at www.teluq.uqam.ca/interventionseconomiques.

Tremblay, D.-G., Chevrier, C. & Di Loreto, M. (2007). "Le travail autonome: Une meilleure conciliation entre vie personnelle et vie professionnelle … ou une plus grande interpénétration des temps sociaux?" *Loisir et société/ Leisure and Society, 29*(1), 191–214.

Tremblay, D.-G. & Fontan, J.-M. (1994). *Le développement économique local: La théorie, les pratique, les expériences*. Quebec City: Presses de l'Université du Quebec.

Tremblay, D.-G., Najem, E. & Paquet, R. (2006). "Articulation emploi-famille et temps de travail: De quelles mesures disposent les travailleurs canadiens et à quoi aspirent-ils?" *Enfance, Famille, et générations, 4*. Online at www.erudit.org/revue/efg/.

Tremblay, D.-G., Paquet, R. & Najem, E. (2006). "Telework: A way to balance work and family or an increase in work-family conflict?" *Canadian Journal of Communication, 31*(2), 715–731.

Tremblay, D.-G. & Rolland, D. (1998). *Modèles de gestion de main-d'oeuvre: Typologies et comparaisons internationales*. Quebec City: Presses de l'université du Québec.

Tremblay, D.-G. & Rolland, D. (2000). "Labour regime and industrialisation in the knowledge economy: The Japanese model and its possible hybridisation in other countries." *Labour and Management in Development Journal*, 7, 2–16. Online at www.ncdsnet.anu.edu.au.

Vosko, L., Zukewich, N. & Cranford, C. (2003). "Le travail précaire: Une nouvelle typologie de l'emploi." *L'emploi et le revenu en perspective* (pp. 40–51). Ottawa: Statistique Canada.

Chapter 6

Ackerman, B. & Alstott, A. (1999). *The stakeholder democracy*. New Haven: Yale University Press.

Ala-Mursula, L., Vahtera, J., et al. (2002). "Employee control over working time: Associations with subjective health and sickness absences." *Journal of Epidemiology and Community Health, 56*, 272–278.

Ali, J. & Avison, W.R. (1997). "Employment transitions and psychological distress: The contrasting experiences of single and married mothers." *Journal of Health and Social Behavior, 38*, 345–362.

Aneshensel, C.S. (1992). "Social stress: Theory and research." *Annual Review of Sociology, 18*, 15–38.

Appelbaum, E., Bailey, T., Berg, P. & Kalleberg, A. (2000). *Manufacturing advantage: Why high-performance work systems pay off*. Ithaca: ILR.

Appelbaum, S., Lavigne-Schmidt, S., Peytchev, M. & Shapiro, B. (1999). "Downsizing: Measuring the costs of failure." *Journal of Management Development, 18*(5), 436–463.

Beach, C., Finnie, R., et al. (2002). "Earnings over time." *Perspectives on Labour and Income, 3*(11), 13–14.

Belanger, J. (2000). *The influence of employee involvement on productivity: A review of research*. Applied Research Branch Discussion Paper R-00-4E. Ottawa: Human Resource Development Canada.

Benach, J., Muntaner, C., Benavides, F.G., Amable, M. & Jodar, P. (2002). "A new occupational health agenda for a new work environment." *Scandinavian Journal of Work, Environment, and Health, 28*, 191–196.

Betcherman, G. & Chaykowski, R. (1996). *The changing workplace: Challenges for public policy*. Applied Research Branch Discussion Paper, R-96-13E. Ottawa: Human Resources Development Canada.

Betcherman, G. & Lowe, G.S. (1997). *The future of work in Canada: A synthesis report*. Ottawa: Canadian Policy Research Network.

Bjarnason, T. & Sigurdardottir, T. (2003). "Psychological distress during unemployment and beyond: Social support and material deprivation among youth in six northern European countries." *Social Science & Medicine, 56*, 973–985.

Bobak, M., Pikhart, H. & Rose, R. (2000). "Socioeconomic factors, material inequalities, and perceived control in self-rated health: Cross-sectional data from seven post-communist countries." *Social Science & Medicine, 51*, 1343–1350.

Borrell, C., Muntaner, C., Benach, J. & Artazcoz, L. (2004). "Social class and self-reported health status among men and women: What is the role of work organisation, household material standards and household labour?" *Social Science & Medicine, 58*, 1869–1887.

Bosma, H., Peter, R., Siegrist, J. & Marmot, M.G. (1998). "Two alternative job stress models and the risk of coronary heart disease." *American Journal of Public Health, 88*, 68–74.

Broad, D. (2000). *Hollow work, hollow society? Globalization and the casual labour problem in Canada*. Halifax: Fernwood.

Burchell, B., Ladipo, D. & Wilkinson, F. (2002). *Job insecurity and work intensification*. London: Routledge.

Burke, M. & Shields, J. (1999). *The job-poor recovery: Social cohesion and the Canadian labour market*. Toronto: Ryerson Polytechnic University.

Burrell, D. (2001). "Weekend woes: Working hard can be hazardous to your holidays." *Psychology Today, 34*(20), 20.

Carter, T. (1999). *The aftermath of reengineering: Downsizing and corporate performance*. New York: Haworth.

CFO Forum. (1995). "Downsizing downsized." *Institutional Investor, 29*(12), 28.

Cohen, M. (1997). "Downsizing and disability go together." *Business and Health, 15*(1), 10.

Cranford, C.J., Vosko, L.F., et al. (2003). "Precarious employment in the Canadian labour market: A statistical portrait." *Just Labour, 3*(Fall), 6–22.

Davis-Blake, A., Broschak, J. & George, E. (2003). "Happy together? How using nonstandard workers affects exit, voice, and loyalty among standard employees." *The Academy of Management Journal, 46*(4), 475–485.

Dooley, D. (2003). "Unemployment, underemployment and mental health: Conceptualizing employment status as a continuum." *American Journal of Community Psychology, 32,* 9–20.

Duxbury, L. & Higgins, C. (2001). *Work-life balance in the new millennium: Where are we? Where do we go from here?* Ottawa: Canadian Policy Research Networks.

Duxbury, L. & Higgins, C. (2003). *Work-life conflict in Canada in the new millennium: A status report: A final report.* Ottawa: Human Research and Development Canada. Online at www.phac-aspc.ca/publicat/work-travail/report2/index.html.

Duxbury, L.E., Higgins, C.A. & Lee, C. (1994). "Work–family conflict: A comparison by gender, family type, and perceived control." *Journal of Family Issues, 15*(3), 449–466.

Elmuti, D. & Kathawala, Y. (2000). "Business reengineering: Revolutionary management tool, or fading fraud?" *Business Forum, 25*(1/2), 29–36.

Ertel, M., Pech, E. & Ullsperger, P. (2000). "Telework in perspective: New challenges to occupational health and safety." In K. Isaksson, C. Hogstedt, C. Eriksson, & T. Theorell (Eds.), *Health effects of the new labour market* (pp. 169–182). New York: Kluwer Academic.

European Foundation for the Improvement of Living and Working Conditions. (2002). *Quality of work and employment in Europe: Issues and challenges.* Foundation Paper. Dublin: EFILWC. Online at www.eurofound.eu.int/publications/files/EF0212EN.pdf.

Fagan, C. (2003). *Working-time preferences and work–life balance in the EU: Some policy considerations for enhancing quality of life.* Dublin: European Foundation for the Improvement of Working and Living Conditions.

Fagan, C. & Burchell, B. (2002). *Gender, jobs, and working conditions in the European Union.* Dublin: European Foundation for the Improvement of Working and Living Conditions.

Fairris, D. & Tohyama, H. (2002). "Productive efficiency and the lean production system in Japan and the United States." *Economic and Industrial Democracy, 23*(4), 529–554.

Farias, G. & Varma, A. (1998). "Research update: High-performance work systems: What we know and what we need to know." *HR Human Resource Planning, 21*(2), 50–54.

Ferber, M.A. & O'Farrell, B. (1991). *Work and family: Policies for a changing workforce.* Washington: National Academy Press.

Ferrie, J.E. (2001). "Is job insecurity harmful to health?" *Journal of the Royal Society of Medicine, 94,* 71–76.

Franks, S. (1999). *Having none of it: Women, men, and the future of work.* London: Granta Books.

Frone, M., Russell, M. & Cooper, L. (1997). "Relation of work–family conflict to health outcomes: A four-year longitudinal study of employed parents." *Journal of Occupational and Organizational Psychology, 70*(4), 325–335.

Gore, S. (1978). "The effect of social support in moderating the health consequences of unemployment." *Journal of Health and Social Behaviour, 19*(June), 157–165.

Green, F. (2002). *Work intensification, discretion, and the decline of well-being at work.* Paris: Conference on Work Intensification.

Hammer, M. & Champy, J. (1993). *Reengineering the corporation: A manifesto for business revolution.* New York: HarperCollins.

Heery, E. & Salmon, J. (2000). "The insecurity thesis." In E. Heery & J. Salmon (Eds.), *The insecure workforce* (pp. 1–24). London: Routledge.

Heisz, A., Jackson, A., et al. (2002). *Winners and losers in the labour market of the 1990s.* Ottawa: Statistics Canada.

Herzenberg, S.A., Alic, J.A., et al. (1998). *New rules for a new economy: Employment and opportunity in post-industrial America.* Ithaca & London: ILR.

International Labour Organization. (2007). *Working time around the world: Trends in working hours, laws, and policies in a global comparative perspective.* Geneva: International Labour Organization.

Jahoda, M. (1982). *Employment and unemployment: A social psychological analysis.* Cambridge: Cambridge University Press.

Johnson, J.V. (1991). "Collective control: Strategies for survival in the workplace." In J. Johnson & G. Johnson (Eds.), *The psychosocial work environment: Work organization, democratization, and health* (pp. 121–132). Amityville: Baywood Publishing.

Kasl, S.V. (1998). "Measuring job stressors and studying the health impact of the work environment: An epidemiologic commentary." *Journal of Occupational Health Psychology, 3*(4), 390–401.

Kasl, S.V., Rodriguez, E. & Lasch, K. (1998). "The impact of unemployment on health and well-being." In B.P. Dohrenwend (Ed.), *Adversity, stress, and psychopathology* (pp. 111–131). Oxford: Oxford University Press.

Kivimaki, M., Vahtera, J., Pentti, J. & Ferrie, J. (2000). "Factors underlying the effect of organisational downsizing on health of employees: Longitudinal cohort study." *British Medical Journal, 320*(7240), 971–985.

Landsbergis, P.A. (2003). "The changing organization of work and the safety and health of working people: A commentary." *Journal of Occupational and Environmental Medicine, 45*(1), 61–72.

Lewchuk, W., de Wolff, A., King, A. & Polanyi, M.F. (2003). "From job strain to employment strain: Health effects of precarious employment." *Just Labour, 3*(Fall), 23–35.

Lewchuk, W., de Wolff, A., King, A. & Polanyi, M. (2005). *Beyond job strain: Employment strain and the health effects of precarious employment.* Work in a Global Society Working Paper Series 2005-1. Hamilton: Labour Studies Programme, McMaster University.

Marshall, K. (1996). "A job to die for." *Perspectives on Labour and Income* (Summer), 26–31.

Martens, M.F.J., Nijhuis, F.J.N., et al. (1999). "Flexible work schedules and mental and physical health: A study of a working population with non-traditional hours." *Journal of Organizational Behavior, 20,* 35–46.

Mattiasson, I., Lindgarde, F., Nilsson, J.A. & Theorell, T. (1990). "Threat of unemployment and cardiovascular risk factors: Longitudinal study of quality of sleep and serum cholesterol concentration in men threatened with redundancy." *British Journal of Medicine, 301,* 461–466.

Maxwell, J. (2002). *Smart social policy: "Making work pay."* Ottawa: Canadian Policy Research Networks.

Mehmet, O., Mendes, E., et al. (1999). *Towards a fair global labour market: Avoiding a new slave trade.* London: Routledge.

Mohr, G.B. (2000). "The changing significance of different stressors after the announcement of bankruptcy: A longitudinal investigation with special emphasis on job insecurity." *Journal of Organizational Behavior, 2,* 337–359.

Morris, J.K., Cook, D.G. & Shaper, A.G. (1992). "Non-employment and changes in smoking, drinking, and body weight." *British Medical Journal, 304,* 536–541.

Morissette, R. & Rosa, J. (2003). *Alternative work practices and quit rates: Methodological issues and empirical evidence for Canada.* Statistics Canada Research Paper no. 11F0019 no. 199.

Mustard, C.A., Cole, D.C., Shannon, H.S., Pole, J., Sullivan, T.J., Allingham, R. & Sinclar, S.J. (2001). *Does the decline in workers' compensation claims (1990–1999) in Ontario correspond to a decline in workplace injuries?* Working Paper no. 168. Toronto: Institute for Work and Health.

Nolan, J. (2002). "The intensification of everyday life." In B. Burchell & F. Wilkinson (Eds.), *Job insecurity and work intensification* (pp. 112–137). London: Routledge.

Osberg, L. & Sharpe, A. (2003). *An index of labour market well-being for OECD countries.* CSLS research report 2003–05, 1–37. Ottawa: Centre for the Study of Living Standards.

Polanyi, M.F. & Tompa, E. (2002). *Rethinking the health implications of work in the new global economy.* Working Paper, Comparative Program on Health and Society. Toronto: Munk Centre for International Studies, University of Toronto. Online at www.utoronto.ca/mcis.

Price, R.H., Choi, J.N., et al. (2002). "Links in the chain of adversity following job loss: How financial strain and loss of personal control lead to depression, impaired functioning, and poor health." *Journal of Occupational Health Psychology, 7*(4), 302–312.

Probst, T.M. & Brubaker, T.L. (2001). "The effects of job insecurity on employee safety outcomes: Cross-sectional and longitudinal explorations." *Journal of Occupational Health Psychology, 6*(2), 139–159.

Quinlan, M., Mayhew, C. & Bohle, P. (2001). "The global expansion of precarious employment, work disorganization, and consequences for occupational health: A review of recent research. *International Journal of Health Services, 31,* 335–414.

Ramsay, H., Scholarios, D. & Harley, B. (2000). "Employees and high-performance work systems: Testing inside the black box." *British Journal of Industrial Relations, 18*(4), 501–531.

Raphael, D. (2001). "From increasing poverty to social disintegration: How economic inequality affects the health of individuals and communities." In P. Armstrong, H. Armstrong & D. Coburn (Eds.), *Unhealthy times: The political economy of health and care in Canada* (pp. 224–246). Toronto: Oxford University Press.

Saunders, R. (2006). *Risk and opportunity: Creating options for vulnerable workers.* Vulnerable Workers Series no. 7. Ottawa: Canadian Policy Research Network.

Schor, J.B. (2002). *The overworked American: The unexpected decline of leisure.* New York: Basic Books.

Scott-Marshall, H., Tompa, E. & Trevithick, S. 2007. "The social patterning of underemployment and its health consequences." *International Journal of Cotemporary Sociology, 44*(1), 7–34.

Sharpe, A. & Hardt, J. (2006). *Five deaths a day: Workplace fatalities in Canada, 1993–2005.* Centre for the Study of Living Standards Research Paper 2006-04. Ottawa: Centre for the Study of Living Standards.

Shields, M. (1999). "Long working hours and health." *Health Reports, 11*(2), 33–48.

Smith, V. (1997). "New forms of work organization." *Annual Review of Sociology, 23,* 315–339.

Sparks, K., Cooper, C., Fried, Y. & Shirom, A. (1997). "The effects of hours of work on health: A metaanalytic review." *Journal of Occupational and Organizational Psychology, 70*(4), 391–408.

Sparks, K., Faragher, B., et al. (2001). "Well-being and occupational health in the 21st-century workplace." *Journal of Occupational and Organizational Psychology, 74*(4), 489–509.

Sverke, M., Hellgren, J., et al. (2002). "No security: A meta-analysis and review of job insecurity and its consequences." *Journal of Occupational Health Psychology, 7*(3), 242–264.

Tompa, E., Dolinschi, R., Trevithick, S. Scott-Marshall, H. & Bhattacharyya, S. (2005). *Work-related precariousness: Canadian trends and policy implications.* Institute for Work & Health Working Paper no. 218. Toronto: Institute for Work & Health.

Tompa, E., Scott-Marshall, H., Dolinschi, R., Trevithick, S. & Bhattcharyya, S. (2007). "Precarious employment experiences and their health consequences: Towards a theoretical framework." *Work: A Journal of Prevention, Assessment, and Rehabilitation, 28*(7), 209–224.

Townson, M. (2003). *Women in non-standard jobs: The public policy challenge.* Ottawa: Status of Women Canada.

Tremblay, D.-G. (2002). "New ways of working and new types of work? What developments lie ahead?" *Report for the Futures Forum: "Places of Work."* Ottawa: Policy Research Initiative.

Tremblay, D.-G. (2003a). *New types of careers in the knowledge economy: Networks and boundaryless jobs as a career strategy in the ICT and multimedia sector.* Research Note of the Canada Research Chair on the Knowledge Economy no. 2003-12A. Online at www.teluq.uquebec.ca/chaireecosavoir.

Tremblay, D.-G. (2003b). *The new division of labour and women's jobs: Results from a study conducted in Canada from a gendered perspective.* Research Note of the Canada Research Chair on the Knowledge Economy no. 2003-19A. Online at www.teluq.uquebec.ca/chaireecosavoir.

Tremblay, D.-G. (2003c). *Working time and work-family balancing: A Canadian perspective.* Research Note of the Canada Research Chair on the Knowledge Economy no. 2003-18. Online at www.teluq.uquebec.ca/chaireecosavoir.

Tremblay, D.-G., Davel, E. & Rolland, D. (2003). *New management forms for the knowledge economy: HRM in the context of teamwork and participaton.* Research Note of the Canada Research Chair on the Knowledge Economy no. 2003-14A. Online at www.teluq.uquebec.ca/chaireecosavoir.

Tremblay, D.-G. & Rolland, D. (2003). *The Japanese model and its possible hybridization in other countries.* Research Note of the Canada Research Chair on the Knowledge Economy no. 2003-20A. Online at www.teluq.uquebec.ca/chaireecosavoir.

Turner, J.B. (1995). "Economic context and the health effects of unemployment." *Journal of Health and Social Behaviour, 36*(3), 213–229.

Varma, A., Beatty, R., Schneier, C. & Ulrich, D. (1999). "High-performance work systems: Exciting discovery or passing fad?" *Human Resource Planning, 22*(1), 26–37.

Vosko, L.F., Zukewich N. & Cranford, C. (2003). "Precarious jobs: A new typology of employment." *Perspectives on Labour and Income, 4*(10). Online at www.statcan.ca/english/freepub/75-001-XIE/0100375-001-XIE.html.

Wagar, T. (1998). "Exploring the consequences of workforce reduction." *Canadian Journal of Administrative Sciences, 15*(4), 300–309.

Warr, P.B. (1987). *Work, unemployment, and mental health.* Oxford: Clarendon Press.

Wilkinson, R.G. (1996). *Unhealthy societies: The afflictions of inequality.* London: Routledge.

Wood, S. (1999). "Human resource management and performance." *International Journal of Management Reviews, 1*(4), 367–413.

Yates, C., Lewchuk, W. & Stewart, P. (2001). "Empowerment as a Trojan horse: New systems of work organization in the North American automobile industry." *Economic and Industrial Democracy, 22*, 517–541.

Chapter 7

Advisory Group on Working Time and the Distribution of Work (1994). *Report on working time and the distribution of work.* Ottawa: Human Resources Development Canada.

Breslin, F., Curtis, Pete Smith, Koehoorn, Mike & Lee, Hyunmi. (2006). *Is the workplace becoming safer?"* Statistics Canada Cat. no. 75-001-XIE. Perspectives on Labour and Income, December.

Brisbois, Richard. (2003). *How Canada stacks up: The quality of work—an international perspective.* Ottawa: Canadian Policy Research Networks.

Dunn, James R. (2002). *A population health approach to housing.* Ottawa: Canadian Mortgage and Housing Corporation.

Duxbury, Linda & Higgins, Chris. (2002). *The 2001 national work-life conflict study.* Ottawa: Health Canada. Online at www.hc-sc.gc.ca.

Duxbury, Linda, Higgins, Chris & Lyons, Sean. (2007). *Reducing work-life conflict: What works? What doesn't?* Ottawa: Health Canada.Online at www.hc-sc.gc.ca/ewh-semt/alt_formats/hecs-sesc/pdf/pubs/occup-travail/work-travail/balancing-equilibre/report-rapport_e.pdf.

European Foundation for the Improvement of Living and Working Conditions. (2000, 2007). *European working conditions survey.* Online at www.eurofound.europa.eu.

European Industrial Relations Observatory (EIRO). (2006). *Working time developments: Annual update 2.* Online at www.eiro.eurofound.eu.int.

Higgins, Chris, Duxbury, Linda & Johnson, Karen. (2004). *Exploring the link between work-life conflict and demands on Canada's health care system.* Ottawa: Health Canada. Online at www.phac-aspc.gc.ca/publicat/work-travail/report3/index.html.

Jencks, C., Perlman, L. & Rainwater, L. (1988). "What is a good job? A new measure of labour market success." *American Journal of Sociology, 93*, 1322–1357.

Karasek, R. & Theorell, T. (1990). *Healthy work: Stress, productivity, and the reconstruction of working life.* New York: Basic Books.

Lewchuk , W., de Wolff, A., King, A. & Polanyi, M. (2006). "The hidden costs of precarious employment: Health and the employment relationship." In L. Vosko (Ed.), *Precarious employment: Understanding labour market insecurity in Canada* (pp. 141–162). Montreal & Kingston: McGill-Queen's University Press.

Lewchuk, W. & Robertson, D. (1996). "Working conditions under lean production: A worker-based benchmarking study." *Asia Pacific Business Review,* 2, 60–81.

Lippel, K. (2006). "Precarious employment and occupational health and safety legislation in Quebec." In L. Vosko (Ed.), Precarious employment: Understanding labour market insecurity in Canada (pp. 241–255). Montreal & Kingston: McGill-Queen's University Press.

Livingstone, D.W. (2002). *Working and learning in the information age: A profile of Canadians.* Ottawa: Canadian Policy Research Networks.

Lowe, G. (2000). *The quality of work: A people-centred agenda.* Oxford: Oxford University Press.

Lowe, G. (2007). *21st-century job quality: Achieving what Canadians want.* Ottawa: Canadian Policy Research Networks.

Marshall, K. (2003). *Benefits of the job.* Statistics Canada Cat. no. 75-001-XIE. Perspectives on Labour and Income. Ottawa: Statistics Canada.

Organisation for Economic Cooperation and Development (2006). *OECD employment outlook, 2006 Edition: Boosting jobs and incomes.* Paris: Organisation for Economic Co-operation and Development.

Park, J. (2007). *Work stress and job performance.* Statistics Canada Cat. no. 75-001-XIE. Perspectives on Labour and Income. Ottawa: Statistics Canada.

Raphael, D. (Ed.). (2004). *Social determinants of health: Canadian perspectives.* Toronto: Canadian Scholars' Press Inc.

Shainblum, E., Sullivan, T. & Frank, J.W. (2000). "Multicausality, non-traditional injury, and the future of workers' compensation." In M. Gunderson & D. Hyatt (Eds.), Workers' compensation: Foundations for reform (pp. 58–95). Toronto: University of Toronto Press.

Shields, M. (2006). "Stress and depression in the employed population." *Health Reports. Statistics Canada 17*(4), 11–29.

Statistics Canada (2001). *Learning a living: A report on adult education and training in Canada.* Cat. 81-586-XIE.

Sullivan, Terrence (Ed.). (2000). *Injury and the new world of work.* Vancouver & Toronto: UBC Press.

Wilkins, Kathryn & Beaudet, Marie P. (1998). "Work stress and health." *Health Reports, 10*(3), 47–62.

World Health Organization. (1999). *Labour market changes and job insecurity.* Regional Publications/European Series no. 81. Copenhagen: World Health Organization.

Chapter 8

Advisory Committee on the Changing Workplace (1997). *Collective reflection on the changing workplace: Report of the Advisory Committee on the Changing Workplace.* Ottawa: Public Works and Government Services Canada.

Amick, B.C., McDonough, P., Chang, H., Rogers, W.H., Pieper, C.F. & Duncan, G. (2002). "Relationship between all-cause mortality and cumulative working life course psychosocial and physical exposures in the United States labour market from 1968 to 1992." *Psychosomatic Medicine, 64,* 370–381.

Aronowitz, S., Esposito, D., DiFazio, W. & Yard, M. (1998). "The post-work manifesto." In S. Aronowitz & J. Cutler (Eds.), *Post-work: The wages of cybernation* (pp. 31–80). New York: Routledge.

Arthurs, H.W. (2006). *Fairness at work: Federal labour standards for the 21st century.* Ottawa: Human Resource and Skills Development Canada.

Australian Institute of Family Studies. (2005). *Growing up in Australia: The longitudinal study of Australian Children.* Melbourne: Commonwealth of Australia.

Baum, F. (2007). "Cracking the nut of health equity: Top down and bottom up pressure for action on the social determinants of health." *Promotion & Education, 14*(2), 90–95.

Belkic, K., Landsbergis, P.A., Schnall, P.L. & Baker, D. (2004). "Is job strain a major source of cardiovascular disease risk?" *Scandinavian Journal of Work, Environment, and Health, 30*(2), 85–128.

Benoit-Smullyan, E. (1944). "Status, status types, and status interrelations." *American Sociological Review, 9*(2), 151–161.

Bluestone, B. & Harrison, B. (1999). *Growing prosperity: The battle for growth with equity in the twenty-first century.* New York: Houghton Mifflin.

Borg, V. & Kristensen, T.S. (2000). "Social class and self-rated health: Can the gradient be explained by differences in life style or work environment?" *Social Science & Medicine, 51,* 1019–1030.

Brown, P. & Lauder, H. (2001). *Capitalism and social progress: The future of society in a global economy.* London: Palgrave Macmillan.

Brunner, E. (1997). "Socioeconomic determinants of health: Stress and the biology of inequality." *British Medical Journal, 314,* 1472–1476.

Cheung, L. (2005). *Racial status and employment outcomes.* Ottawa: Canadian Labour Congress.

Chung, L. (2004). "Low-paid workers: How many live in low-income families?" *Perspectives on Labour & Income, 5*(10), 5–14.

Cooperrider, D.L. & Srivastva, S. (1987). "Appreciative inquiry in organizational life." In W. Pasmore & R. Woodman (Eds.), *Research in organizational change and development,* vol. 1 (pp. 129–169). Greenwich: JAI Press.

Cornwall, A. & Jewkes, R. (1995). "What is participatory research?" *Social Science & Medicine, 41*(12), 1667–1676.

Crompton, S. (2002). "I still feel overqualified in my job." *Canadian Social Trends,* Winter, 23–26.

de Lange, A.H., Taris, T.W., Kompier, M.A., Houtman, I. & Bongers, P. (2003). "The very best of the millennium: Longitudinal research and the demand-control-(support) model." *Journal of Occupational Health Psychology, 8*(4), 282–305.

De Vogli, R., Ferrie, J.E., Chandola, T., Kivimaki, M. & Marmot, M.G. (2007). "Unfairness and health: Evidence from the Whitehall II Study." *Journal of Epidemiology and Community Health, 61*(6), 513–518.

Dressler, W.W. (1988). "Social consistency and psychological distress." *Journal of Health and Social Behavior, 29*(1), 79–91.

Drolet, M. (2002). *The persistent gap: New evidence on the Canadian gender gap.* Ottawa: Statistics Canada.

Duxbury, L. & Higgins, C. (1998). *Work-life balance in Saskatchewan: Realities and challenges.* Regina: Saskatchewan Labour, Government of Saskatchewan.

Duxbury, L. & Higgins, C. (2001). *Work-life balance in the new millennium. Where are we? Where do we need to go?* Ottawa: Canadian Policy Research Network.

Duxbury, L., Higgins, C. & Johnson, K.L. (1999). *An examination of the implications and costs of work-life conflict in Canada.* Ottawa: Health Canada.

Eaker, E.D., Sullivan, L.M., Kelly-Hayes, M., D'Agostino, R.B. & Benjamin, E.J. (2004). "Does job strain increase the risk for coronary heart disease of death in men and women? The Framingham offspring study." *American Journal of Epidemiology, 159*(10), 950–958.

Eakin, J.M. (2000). "Commentary." In B.D. Poland, L.W. Green & I. Rootman (Eds.), *Settings for health promotion: Linking theory to practice* (pp. 166–174). Thousand Oaks: Sage Publications.

European Commission. (1997). *Green paper: Partnership for a new organization of work.* Luxembourg City: European Commission.

European Foundation for the Improvement of Living and Working Conditions. (2002). *Quality of work and employment in Europe: Issues and challenges*. Dublin: European Foundation for the Improvement of Living and Working Conditions.

Ferrie, J.E., Head, J., Shipley, M.J., Vahtera, J., Marmot, M.G. & Kivimaki, M. (2006). "Injustice at work and incidence of psychiatric morbidity: The Whitehall II study." *Occupational and Environmental Medicine, 63*(7), 443–450.

Fried, M. (1998). *Taking time: Parental leave policy and corporate culture*. Philadephia: Temple University Press.

Gortz, A. (1999). *Reclaiming work: Beyond the wage-based society*. Malden: Blackwell Publishers Inc.

Hammar, N., Alfredsson, L. & Johnson, J.V. (1998). "Job strain, social support at work, and incidence of myocardial infarction." *Occupational and Environmental Medicine, 55*, 548–553.

Head, J., Kivimaki, M., Martikainen, P., Vahtera, J., Ferrie, J.E. & Marmot, M.G. (2006). "Influence of change in psychosocial work characteristics on sickness absence: The Whitehall II study." *Journal of Epidemiology and Community Health, 60*(1), 55–61.

Herzenberg, S.A., Alic, J.A. & Wial, H. (1998). *New rules for a new economy: Employment and opportunity in postindustrial America*. Ithaca: Cornell University Press.

Hill, A.B. (1965). "The environment and disease: Association or causation?" *Proceedings of the Royal Society of Medicine, 58*, 295–300.

Israel, B.A., Schurman, S.J. & House, J.S. (1989). "Action research on occupational stress: Involving workers as researchers." *International Journal of Health Services, 19*(1), 135–155.

Jacobs, J.A. & Gerson, K. (2001). "Overworked individuals or overworked families?" *Work and Occupations, 28*(1), 40–63.

Johnson, J.V. (2005). "The growing imbalance: Class inequalities in work and health in an era of flexibilization." Presentation at the 4th International Conference on Work, Environment, and Cardiovascular Disease, Newport Beach, California.

Johnson, J.V. & Hall, E.M. (1995). "Class, work, and health." In B.C. Amick, S. Levine, A.R. Tarlov & D. Chapman Walsh (Eds.), *Society and health* (pp. 247–271). New York: Oxford University Press.

Johnson, J.V., Stewart, W., Hall, E.M., Fredlund, P. & Theorell, T. (1996). "Long-term psychosocial work environment and cardiovascular mortality among Swedish men." *American Journal of Public Health, 86*(3), 324–331.

Karasek, R.A. (1979). "Job demands, job decision latitude, and mental strain: Implications for job re-design." *Administration Science Quarterly, 24*, 285–308.

Karasek, R. & Theorell, T. (1990). *Healthy work: Stress productivity and the reconstruction of working life*. New York: Basic Books Inc.

King, C., McPherson, R. & Long, D. (2000). "Public labor market policies for the 21st century." In R. Marshall (Ed.), *Back to shared prosperity: The growing inequality of wealth and income in America* (pp. 275–286). Armonk: M.E. Sharpe.

Kivimaki, M., Elovainio, M., Vahtera, J. & Ferrie, J. (2003). "Organisational justice and health of employees: Prospective cohort study." *Occupational and Environmental Medicine, 60*, 27–34.

Kivimaki, M., Elovainio, M., Vahtera, J. & Ferrie, J. (2004). "Organisational justice and change in justice as predictors of employee health: The Whitehall II study." *Journal of Epidemiology and Community Health, 58*, 931–937.

Kuper, H. & Marmot, M. (2003). "Job strain, job demands, decision latitude, and risk of coronary heart disease within the Whitehall II study." *Journal of Epidemiology and Community Health, 57*, 147–153.

Landsbergis, P. (2003). "The changing organization of work and the safety and health of working people: A commentary." *Journal of Occupational & Environmental Medicine, 45*(1), 61–72.

Landsbergis, P., Schnall, P., Pickering, T., Warren, K. & Schwartz, J. (2003). "Life course exposure to job strain and ambulatory blood pressure in men." *American Journal of Epidemiology, 157*(11), 998–1006.

Landsbergis, P., Schnall, P., Warren, K., Pickering, T. & Schwartz, J. (1999). "The effect of job strain on ambulatory blood pressure in men: Does it vary by socioeconomic status." *Annals of the New York Academy of Sciences, 896*, 414–416.

Lee, S., Colditz, G., Berkman, L.F. & Kawachi, I. (2003). "A prospective study of job strain and coronary heart disease in US women." *International Journal of Epidemiology, 31*, 1147–1153.

Lerner, S., Clark, C.M.A. & Needham, W.R. (1999). *Basic income: Economic security for all Canadians.* Toronto: Between the Lines.

Lowe, G.S. (2000). *The quality of work: A people-centred agenda.* Don Mills: Oxford University Press.

Lowe, G.S. (2007). *21st-century job quality: Achieving what Canadians want.* Ottawa: Canadian Policy Research Networks.

MacIntyre, S. (2003). "Evidence-based policy making." *British Medical Journal, 326*, 5–6.

Macleod, J., Davey Smith, G., Heslop, P., Metcalfe, C., Carroll, D. & Hart, C. (2001). "Are the effects of psychosocial exposures attributable to confounding? Evidence from a prospective observational study on psychological stress and mortality." *Journal of Epidemiology and Community Health, 55*, 878–884.

Malinauskiene, V., Theorell, T., Grazuleviciene, R., Azaraviciene, A., Obelenis, V. & Azelis, V. (2005). "Psychosocial factors at work and myocardial infarction among men in Kanus, Lithuania." *Scandinavian Journal of Work, Environment, and Health, 31*(3), 218–223.

Marmot, M.G. (2006). "Health in an unequal world." *Lancet, 67*(36), 2081–2094.

Marmot, M.G., Bosma, H., Hemingway, H., Brunner, E. & Stansfeld, S. (1997). "Contribution of job control and other risk factors to social variations in coronary heart disease incidence." *The Lancet, 350*(9073), 235–239.

Marshall, K. (2001). "Part-time by choice." *Perspectives on Labour & Income* (Spring), 20–27.

Maume Jr., D.J. & Houston, P. (2001). "Job segregation and gender differences in work-family spillover among white-collar workers." *Journal of Family and Economic Issues, 22*(2), 171–189.

Maxwell, J. (2002). *Smart social policy—making work pay.* Ottawa: Canadian Policy Research Networks.

McEwen, B. (1998). "Protective and damaging effects of stress mediators." *New England Journal of Medicine, 338*(3), 171–179.

Mergler, D. (1987). "Worker participation in occupational health research: Theory and practice." *International Journal of Health Services, 17*(1), 151–167.

Morissette, R. & Picot, G. (2005). *Low-paid work and economically vulnerable families over the last two decades.* Ottawa: Business and Labour Market Analysis Division, Statistics Canada.

Murray, S. & Mackenzie, H. (2007). *Bringing minimum wages above the poverty line.* Ottawa: Canadian Centre for Policy Alternatives.

Niedhammer, I. & Chea, M. (2003). "Psychosocial factors at work and self reported health: Comparative results of cross-sectional and prospective analyses of the French GAZEL cohort." *Occupational and Environmental Medicine, 60*, 509–515.

Nutbeam, D. (2003). "How does evidence influence public health policy? Tackling health inequalities in England." *Health Promotion Journal of Australia, 14*(3), 154–158.

Palameta, B. (2004). "Low income among immigrants and visible minorities." *Perspectives on Labour and Income, 16*(2), 32–37.

Peter, R., Gassler, H. & Geyer, S. (2007). "Socioeconomic status, status inconsistency, and risk of ischaemic heart disease: A prospective study among members of a statutory health insurance company." *Journal of Epidemiology and Community Health, 61*, 605–611.

Polanyi, M.F. & Cole, D.C. (2003). "Stakeholder engagement in the control of repetitive strain injury." In T.J. Sullivan & J.W. Frank (Eds.), *Preventing and managing disabling injury at work* (pp. 125–141). New York: Taylor & Francis.

Polanyi, M., Frank, J.W., Shannon, H.S., Sullivan, T.J. & Lavis, J.N. (2000). "Promoting the determinants of good health in the workplace." In B. Poland, L. Green & I. Rootman (Eds.), *Settings for health promotion: Linking theory to practice* (pp. 138–166). Thousand Oaks: Sage Publications.

Polanyi, M.F. & Tompa, E. (2002). *Rethinking the health implications of work in the new global economy.* Toronto: Munk Centre for International Studies, Comparative Program on Health and Society, University of Toronto.

Reskin, B. & Padavic, I. (1994). *Women and men at work.* Thousand Oaks: Sage.

Riese, H., Van Doornen, L.J.P., Houtman, I.L.D. & De Geus, E.J.C. (2004). "Job strain in relation to ambulatory blood pressure, heart rate, and heart rate variability among female nurses." *Scandinavian Journal of Work, Environment, and Health, 30*(6), 477–485.

Saunders, R. (2005). *Does a rising tide lift all boats? Low-paid workers in Canada.* Ottawa: Canadian Policy Research Network.

Saunders, R. (2006). *Risk and opportunity: Creating options for vulnerable workers.* Ottawa: Canadian Policy Research Network.

Schnall, P.L., Landsbergis, P.A. & Baker, D. (1994). "Job strain and cardiovascular disease." *Annual Review of Public Health, 15,* 381–411.

Scott, H.K. (2004). "Reconceptualizing the nature and health consequences of work-related insecurity for the new economy: The decline of workers' power in the flexibility regime." *International Journal of Health Services, 34*(1), 143–153.

Shields, M. (1999). "Long working hours and health." *Health Reports, 11*(2), 33–48.

Siegrist, J. (1996). "Adverse health effects of high-effort/low-reward conditions." *Journal of Occupational Health Psychology, 1*(1), 27–41.

Siegrist, J. & Marmot, M. (2004). "Health inequalities and the psychosocial environment—two scientific challenges." *Social Science & Medicine, 58,* 1463–1473.

Siegrist, J. & Peter, R. (1996). *Measuring effort-reward imbalance at work: Guidelines.* Dusseldorf: Heinrich Heine University.

Skocpol, T. (2000). *The missing middle: Working families and the future of American social policy.* New York: W.W. Norton & Company Inc.

Smith, G.S., Wellman, H.M., Sorock, G.S., Warner, M., Courtney, T.K., Pransky, G.S. & Fingerhut, L.A. (2005). "Injuries at work in the US adult population: Contributions to the total injury burden." *American Journal of Public Health, 95*(7), 1213–1219.

Smith, P.M. (2007). "A transdisciplinary approach to research on work and health: What is it, what could it contribute, and what are the challenges?" *Critical Public Health, 17*(2), 159–169.

Smith, P.M. & Frank, J.W. (2005). "When aspirations and achievements don't meet: A longitudinal examination of the differential effect of education and occupational attainment on declines in self-rated health among Canadian labour force participants." *International Journal of Epidemiology, 34*(4), 827–834.

Spurgeon, A., Harrington, J.M. & Cooper, C.L. (1997). "Health and safety problems associated with long working hours: A review of the current position." *Occupational and Environmental Medicine, 54,* 367–375.

Steptoe, A. & Marmot, M. (2002). "The role of psychobiological pathways in socio-economic inequalities in cardiovascular disease risk." *European Heart Journal, 23*(1), 13–25.

Sverke, M., Hellgren, J. & Naswall, K. (2002). "No security: A meta-analysis and review of job insecurity and its consequences." *Journal of Occupational Health Psychology, 7*(3), 242–264.

Tompa, E., Scott-Marshall, H., Dolinschi, R., Trevithick, S. & Bhattacharyya, S. (2007). "Precarious employment experiences and their health consequences: Towards a theoretical framework." [Review] *Work, 28*(3), 209–224.

Vahtera, J., Kivimaki, M., Pentti, J. & Theorell, T. (2000). "Effect of change in the psychosocial work environment on sickness absence: A seven-year follow-up of initially healthy employees." *Journal of Epidemiology and Community Health, 54,* 484–493.

Vail, J., Wheelock, J. & Hill, M. (1999). *Insecure times: Living with insecurity in contemporary society.* London: Routledge.

van Vegchel, N., de Jonge, J., Bosma, H. & Schaufeli, W. (2005). "Reviewing the effort-reward imbalance model: Drawing up the balance of 45 empirical studies." *Social Science & Medicine, 60,* 1117–1131.

Weisbord, M.R. & Janoff, S. (1995). *Future search: An action guide to finding common ground in organizations and communities.* San Francisco: Berrett-Koehler.

Chapter 9

Andersson, B.E. (1992). "Effects of day care on cognitive and socioemotional competence of thirteen-year-old Swedish school children." *Child Development, 63,* 20–36.

Beach, J., Bertrand, J., Forer, B., Michal, D. & Tougas, J. (2004). *Working for change: Canada's child care workforce.* Ottawa: Child Care Human Resources Sector Council.

Beach, J, & Flanagan, K. (2006). *People, programs and practices: A training strategy for the early childhood education and care sector in Canada.* Ottawa: Child Care Human Resources. Sector Council.

Cleveland, G., Colley, S., Friendly, M. & Lero, D. (2003). *The state of Canadian ECEC data.* Toronto: Childcare Resource and Research Unit, University of Toronto.

Doherty, G., Friendly, M. & Beach, J. (2003). *Canada background report.* Thematic Review of Early Childhood Education and Care. Ottawa: Government of Canada.

Doherty, G., Friendly, M. & Forer, B. (2002). *By default or design? An analysis of quality in for profit and non-profit child care centres using the You Bet I Care! data sets.* Occasional paper no. 18. Toronto: Childcare Resource and Research Unit, University of Toronto.

Doherty, G., Lero, D., Goelman, H., LaGrange, A. & Tougas, J. (2000). *You bet I care! A Canada-wide study on wages, working conditions, and practices in child care centers.* Guelph: Centre for Families, Work, and Well-Being, University of Guelph.

Federal, Provincial and Territorial Advisory Committee on Population Health. (1996). *Report on the health of Canadians: Technical appendix.* Catalogue No. H39-385/1-1996E. Ottawa: Health Canada.

Federal/Provincial/Territorial Ministers Responsible for Social Services. (2003). "Supporting Canada's children and families." Press release, March 13. Toronto: Multilateral Framework on Early Learning and Child Care.

Fournier, C. & Drouin, D. (2004). *Grandir en qualité 2003: Educational quality in child care centre daycares (installations de CPE)—Highlights.* Quebec City: Institute de la Statistique du Quebec.

Friendly, M. (2000). *Child care and Canadian federalism in the 1990s: Canary in a coal mine.* In G. Cleveland & M. Krashinsky (Eds.), *Our children's future* (pp. 347–351). Toronto: University of Toronto Press.

Friendly, M. (2001). *Is this as good as it gets? Child care as a test case for assessing the Social Union Framework Agreement.* Ottawa: Canadian Review of Social Policy. Online at www.childcarecanada. org/pubs/ bn/ isthisasgoodasitgets.html.

Friendly, M. (2006). *Early learning and child care: How does Canada measure up? International comparisons using data from Starting Strong 2.* Briefing Note. Toronto: Childcare Resource and Research Unit.

Friendly, M., Beach, J. & Doherty, G. (2005). *Quality in early learning and child care: What we know and what we think.* Working documents for Quality by Design. Toronto: Childcare Resource and Research Unit.

Friendly, M., Beach, J., Ferns, C. & Turiano, M. (2007). *Early childhood education and care in Canada 2006.* Toronto: Childcare Resource and Research Unit.

Friendly, M. & White, L. (2007). "From multilateralism to bilateralism to unilateralism in three short years: Early learning and child care and Canadian federalism." In H. Bakvis & G. Skogsted (Eds.), *Canadian federalism: Performance, effectiveness, and legitimacy* (2nd ed.) (pp. 182–204). Toronto: Oxford University Press.

Gallagher, J.J., Rooney, R. & Campbell, S. (1999). "Child care licensing regulations and child care quality in four states." *Early Childhood Research Quarterly, 14*(3), 313–333.

Goelman, H., Doherty, G., Lero, D., LaGrange, A. & Tougas, J. (2000). *You bet I care! Caring and learning environments: Quality in child care centres across Canada.* Guelph: Centre for Families, Work and Well-Being, University of Guelph.

Helburn, S. et al. (1995) *Cost, quality, and child outcomes in child care centers: Public Report* Denver, CO: University of Colorado.

Japel, C., Tremblay, R. & Côté, S. (2005). "Quality counts! Assessing the quality of daycare services based on the Quebec longitudinal study of child development." *Choices, 11*(5), 1–44. Montreal: Institute for Research on Public Policy.

Masse, L.N. & Barnett, S. (2002*). Benefit-cost analysis of the Abecedarian early childhood intervention.* New Brunswick: National Institute for Early Education Research, Rutgers University.

Meyers, M.K. & Gornick, J.C. (2000). *Early childhood education and care (ECEC): Cross-national variation in service organization.* New York: Institute for Child and Family Policy, Columbia University School of Social Work. Organization for Economic Co-operation and Development.

Mocan, H. (2001). *Can consumers detect lemons? Information asymmetry in the market for child care.* NBER Working Paper. Washington DC: National Bureau of Economic Research, Inc. Online at ideas.repec.org/p/nbr/ nberwo/8291.html.

Moss, P., Penn, H. & Mestres, B. (2004). *Quality in early learning and child care services: Papers from the European Commission Childcare Network.* Toronto: Childcare Resource and Research Unit, University of Toronto.

Organisation for Economic Co-operation and Development (OECD). (2001). *Starting strong: Early childhood education and care.* Education Division. Paris: OECD.

Organisation for Economic Co-operation and Development (OECD). (2004). *Canada country note.* Thematic Review of Early Childhood Education and Care.Education Division. Paris: OECD.

Organisation for Economic Co-operation and Development (OECD). (2006). *Starting strong 2: Early childhood education and care.* Thematic Review of Early Childhood Education and Care.Education Division. Paris: OECD.

Schweinhart, L.J. & Weikart, D.P. (1993). "Changed lives, significant benefits: The High Scope Perry Preschool Project to date." *High Scope Resource, 1*(Summer), 10–14. Ypsilanti: High Scope Press.

Shonkoff, J. & Phillips, D. (2000). *From neurons to neighbourhoods: The science of early childhood development.* Washington: National Academies Press.

United Nations Children's Fund. (2001). *The state of the world's children 2001.* New York: United Nations.

Whitebook, M., Howes, C. & Phillips, D. (1990). *Who cares? Child care teachers and the quality of care in America: Final report of the national staffing study.* Oakland: Child Care Employee Project.

Chapter 10

Bailey, D. (2002), "Are critical periods critical for early childhood education? The role of timing in early childhood pedagogy." *Early Childhood Research Quarterly, 17*, 281–294.

Bauer, A.M. & Boyce, W.T. (2004). "Prophecies of childhood: How children's social environments and biological propensities affect the health of populations. *International Journal of Behavioral Medicine, 11*(3), 164–175.

Berk, L.E. & Shanker, S. (2006). *Child development* (2nd Canadian ed.). Toronto: Pearson Education Canada Inc.

Black, J.E. (1998). "How a child builds its brain: Some lessons from animal studies of neural plasticity. *Preventive Medicine, 27*, 168–171.

Bruer, J. T. (1999). *The myth of the first three years: A new understanding of early brain development and lifelong learning.* New York: Free Press.

Canadian Council on Social Development (2006). *The progress of Canada's children and youth.* Ottawa: Canadian Council on Social Development.

Currie, J. (2001). "Early childhood education programs." *Journal of Economic Perspectives, 15*(2), 213–238.

Dennis, C. (2004). "The most important sexual organ." *Nature, 427*, 390–392. Online at www.nature.com/nature.

Eikeseth, S. (2001). "Recent critiques of the UCLA Young Autism Project." *Behavioral Interventions, 16*, 249–264.

Gagne, L.G. (2003). *Parental work, child-care use, and young children's cognitive outcomes.* Statistics Canada Catalogue no. 89-594-XIE. Ottawa: Statistics Canada.

Galobardes, B., Lynch, J.W. & Smith, G.D. (2004). "Childhood socioeconomic circumstances and cause-specific mortality in adulthood: Systematic review and interpretation." *Epidemiologic Reviews, 26*, 7–21.

Gottesman, I.I. (1963). "Genetic aspects of intelligent behaviour." In N.R. Ellis (Ed.), *Handbook of mental deficiency* (pp. 253–296). New York: McGraw-Hill.

Government of Canada. (2006). *The well-being of Canada's young children.* Statistics Canada Catalogue no.: HS1-7/2006E-PDF. Ottawa: Statistics Canada.

Harris, S.L. & Handleman, J.S. (2000). "Age and IQ at intake as predictors of placement for young children with autism: A four- to six-year follow-up." *Journal of Autism and Developmental Disorders, 30*(2), 137–142.

Heckman, J.J. & Masterov, D.V. (2005). *The productivity argument for investing in young children.* Chicago: American Bar Foundation and University College London.

Janowsky, J.S. & Finlay, B.L. (1986). "The outcome of perinatal brain damage: The role of normal neuron loss and axon retraction." *Developmental Medicine and Child Neurology, 28*, 375–389.

Kafer, K. (2004). "A head start to nowhere?" *USA Today.* Online at findarticles.com/p/articles/mi_m1272/is_2710_133/ai_n6113085/print.

Kolb, B. & Whishaw, I.Q. (2003). *Fundamentals of human neuropsychology* (5th ed.). New York: Worth Publishers.

Kuhl, P. (2004). "Early language acquisition: Cracking the speech code." *Nature Reviews: Neuroscience, 5*(11), 831–843.

Lefebvre, P. & Merrigan P. (2002). "The effect of childcare and early education arrangements on developmental outcomes of young children." *Canadian Public Policy, 28*(2), 160–186.

Lovaas, O.I. (1987). "Behavioral treatment and normal education and intellectual functioning in young autistic children." *Journal of Consulting and Clinical Psychology, 55*(1), 3–9.

Magnuson, K.A., Ruhm, C. & Waldfogel, J. (2005). "Does prekindergarten improve school preparation and performance?" *Economics of Education Review, 26*, 33–51.

Magnuson, K., Ruhm, C. & Waldfogel, J. (2007). "The persistence of preschool effects: Do subsequent classroom experiences matter?" *Early Childhood Research Quarterly, 22*(1), 18–38.

McCain, M.N. & Mustard, J.F. (1999). *Early years study: Reversing the real brain drain.* Toronto: Ontario Children's Secretariat; www.childsec.gov.on.ca.

Media-Awareness Network. (2007). *Statistics on TV viewing habits (1994–2000).* Online at www.media-awareness.ca/english/resources/research_documents/statistics/television/tv_viewing_habits.cfm.

Nelson, G., Westhues, A. & MacLeod, J. (2003). "A meta-analysis of longitudinal research on preschool prevention programs for children." *Prevention & Treatment 6*(31), 1–67.

Ramey, C.T. & Landesman-Ramey, S. (1998). "Early intervention and early experience." *American Psychologist, 53*(2), 109–120.

Roberts, P. & Gowan, R. (2007). *Workplace literacy: Canadian literature review and bibliography.* Ottawa: Canadian Council on Social Development.

Rutter, M. (2002). "Nature, nurture, and development: From evangelism through science toward policy and practice." *Child Development, 73*(1), 1–21.

Shea, V. (2004). "A perspective on the research literature related to early intensive behavioral intervention (Lovaas) for young children with autism." *Autism, 8*(4), 346–367.

Shields, M. (2005). *Measured obesity: Overweight Canadian children and adolescents.* Component of Statistics Canada Catalogue no. 82-620-MWE2005001. Ottawa: Statistics Canada.

Siegler, R.S. (1996). *Emerging minds: The process of change in children's thinking.* New York: Oxford University Press.

Skeels, H.M. (1966). "Adult status of children with contrasting early life experiences." *Monographs of the Society for Research in Child Development, 31,* Serial No. 105.

Slater, A. (2001). "Visual perception." In G. Bremner & A. Fogel (Eds.), *Blackwell handbook of infant development* (pp. 5–34). Malden: Blackwell.

Statistics Canada. (2007, February). "Child care." *The Daily.* Online at www.statcan.ca/Daily/English/050207/d050207b.htm.

Thatcher, R.W., Lyon, G.R., Rumsey, J. & Krasnegor, J. (1996). *Developmental neuroimaging.* San Diego: Academic Press.

Thompson, R. & Nelson, C. (2001). "Developmental science and the media." *American Psychologist, 56*(1), 5–15.

US Department of Health and Human Services, Administration for Children and Families. (2005). *Head Start impact study: First year findings.* Washington: US Department of Health and Human Services.

Zimmerman, F.J. (2007). "Television and DVD/video viewing in children younger than 2 years." *The Archives of Pediatrics Adolescents, 161,* 473–479.

Zimmerman, F.J., Christakis, D.A. & Meltzoff, A.N. (2007). "Associations between media viewing and language development in children under age 2 years." *Journal of Pediatrics, 151,* 364–368.

Chapter 11

Aikenhead, G.S. (2001). "Integrating Western and Aboriginal sciences: Cross-cultural science teaching." *Research in Science Education, 31,* 337–355.

Behnia, B. & Duclos, E. (2003). *2001 participation and activity limitation survey: Children with disabilities and their families.* Statistics Canada Catalogue no. 89-585-XIE. Ottawa: Statistics Canada.

Bohatyretz, S. & Lipps, G. (1999). "Diversity in the classroom: Characteristics of elementary students receiving special education." *Education Quarterly Review, 6*(2), 7–19.

Bowlby, J.W. & McMullen, K. (2002). *At a crossroads: First results for the 18- to 20-year-old cohort of the youth in transition survey.* Human Resources Development Canada. Online at www.hrdc-drhc.gc.ca/sp-ps/arb-dgra/publications/research/2002docs/YITS/yits-encov.pdf.

Bussière, P., Knighton, T. & Pennock, D. (2007). *Measuring up: Canadian results of the OECD PISA study: The performance of Canada's youth in science, reading, and mathematics—2006 first results for Canadians aged 15.* Ottawa: Minister of Industry.

Canadian Council on Learning. (2005). *Good news: Canada's high school dropout rates are falling.* Lessons in Learning. Online at www.ccl-cca.ca/CCL/Reports/LessonsInLearning/LiL-16Dec2005.htm.

Canadian Council on Learning. (2006a). *Survey of Canadian attitudes toward learning: Early childhood learning.* Online at www.ccl-cca.ca/NR/rdonlyres/866439A5-2715-42AA-B4A5-99731702BECF/0/FactSheetChildENGmtg.pdf.

Canadian Council on Learning. (2006b). *Survey of Canadian attitudes toward learning: Structured learning.* Online at www.ccl-cca.ca/NR/rdonlyres/D6B130CA-E00F-4AA2-AB08-6AF5C2E58F30/0/FactSheetStructureENGmtg.pdf.

Canadian Council on Learning. (2007). *The cultural divide in science education for Aboriginal learners.* Lessons in Learning. Online at www.ccl-cca.ca/CCL/Reports/LessonsInLearning/LinL20070116_Ab_sci_edu.htm.

Canadian Education Statistics Council. (2000). *Education indicators in Canada: Report of the Pan Canadian education indicators program 1999.* Ottawa: Statistics Canada. Online at www.statcan.ca/english/freepub/81-582-XIE/81-582-XIE.pdf.

Chandler, M. & Lalonde, C. (1998). "Cultural continuity as a hedge against suicide in Canada's First Nations." *Transcultural Psychology, 35*(2), 191–219.

Corak, M. (1999). Death and divorce: The long-term consequences of parental loss on adolescents. Family and Labour Studies, Statistics Canada. Online at www.statcan.ca/english/research/11F0019MIE/11F0019MIE1999135.pdf.

Delors, J., Al Mufti, I., Amagi, A., Carneiro, R., Chung, F., et al. (1996). *Learning: The treasure within: Report to UNESCO of the International Commission on Education for the Twenty-first Century.* Paris: UNESCO.

Garnett, B. (2006). "An introductory look at the academic trajectories of ESL students." A paper presented at the Immigration, Integration, and Language Conference, University of Calgary.

Department of Indian Affairs and Northern Development. (2002). *Basic departmental data.* Ottawa: Minister of Public Works and Government Services. Online at www.ainc-inac.gc.ca/pr/sts/bdd02/bdd02_e.html.

Drolet, M. (2005) *Participation in post-secondary education in Canada: Has the role of parental income changed over the 1990s?* Research Paper, Statistics Canada. Online at www.statcan.ca/english/research/11F0019MIE/11F0019MIE2005243.pdf.

Garnett, B. & Ungerleider, C. (2008). *An introductory look at the academic trajectories of ESL students.* Working Paper Series No. 08 – 02. Vancouver: Metropolis British Columbia. Online at riim.metropolis.net/Virtual%20Library/2008/WP08-02.pdf.

Heisz, A. (2007). *Income inequality and redistribution in Canada: 1976 to 2004.* Ottawa: Statistics Canada.

Kerr, D. & Beaujot, R. (2001). *Family relations, low income, and child outcomes: A comparison of children in intact, lone, and step families.* London, ON: University of Western Ontario, Population Studies Centre. Discussion paper 01-8. Online at www.ssc.uwo.ca/sociology/popstudies/dp/dp01-8.pdf.

Lipps, G. & Yiptong-Avila, J. (1999). *From home to school: How Canadian children cope: Initial analyses using data from the second cycle of the school component of the National Longitudinal Survey of Children and Youth.* Ottawa: Culture, Tourism, and the Centre for Education Statistics. Online at www.statcan.ca/english/indepth/81-003/feature/eqar1999006002s4a04.pdf.

McCall, D. (1998). *Transitions within elementary and secondary levels third national forum on education.* Council of Ministers of Education Canada. St. Johns, Newfoundland. Online at www.cmec.ca/nafored/english/cap.pdf.

Ontario. (2007). *6 Ways to reach every student: Student success-learning to 18.* Online at www.edu.gov.on.ca/eng/6ways/welcome.html.

Organisation for Economic Co-operation and Development. (2000a). Health data. Online at www.library.mun.ca/hsl/guides/oecd.php.

Organisation for Economic Co-operation and Development. (2000b). *Messages from PISA 2000.* Paris: Programme for International Student Assessment Organisation for Economic Co-operation and Development.

Organisation for Economic Co-operation and Development. (2003). *Learning for tomorrow's world: First results from PISA 2003.* Paris: Programme for International Student Assessment Organisation for Economic Co-operation and Development.

Organisation for Economic Co-operation and Development. (2006). *PISA 2006 science competencies for tomorrow's world.* Paris: Programme for International Student Assessment Organisation for Economic Co-operation and Development.

Organisation for Economic Co-operation and Development. (2007a). *Education at a glance 2007.* Paris: Organisation for Economic Co-operation and Development. Online at www.oecd.org/document/30/0,3343,en_2649_39263294_39251550_1_1_1_1,00.html.

Organisation for Economic Co-operation and Development. (2007b). *Equity in education: Students with disabilities, learning difficulties, and disadvantages.* Paris: Organisation for Economic Co-operation and Development.

Pepler, D.J. & Craig, W.M. (1997). "Bullying: Research and interventions." *Youth update.* Toronto: Institute for the Study of Antisocial Youth.

Phipps, S. & Lethbridge, L. (2006). *Income and the outcomes of children*. Ottawa: Statistics Canada.

Ravanera, Z.R. (2000). *Family tranformation and social cohesion: Project overview and integrative framework*. A revised version of Z.R. Ravanera & F. Rajulton, *Multiple levels of analysis: Prospects and challenges for the family transformation and social cohesion project*, a paper presented at the annual meeting of the Canadian Population Society in Edmonton, Alberta, May 28–30, 2000.

Ross, D., Roberts, P. & Scott, K. (2000) "Family income and child well-being." *ISUMA*, *1*(2), 51–54. See also Ross, D. & Roberts, P. (1999). *Income and child well-being: New perspectives on the poverty debate*. Canadian Council on social Development. Online at www.ccsd.ca/pubs/inckids/index.htm.

Ryan, B.A. & Adams, G.R. (1999). "How do families affect children's success in school?" *Education Quarterly Review, 6*(1), 30–43.

Sprott, J.B., Doob, A.N. & Jenkins, J.M. (2001, May). *Problem behavior and delinquency in children and youth*. Statistics Canada Catalogue Number 85-002-XPE 21(45). Ottawa: Juristat, Canadian Centre for Justice Statistics, Statistics Canada. Online at dsp-psd.tpsgc.gc.ca/Collection-R/Statcan/85-002-XIE/0040185-002-XIE.pdf.

Statistics Canada. (1998, April 14). "1996 Census: Education, mobility, and migration." *The Daily*. Online at www.statcan.ca/Daily/English/980414/d980414.htm#1996%20Census.

Statistics Canada. (2000, February 21). "Education indicators in Canada: Report of the Pan-Canadian Education Indicators Program 1999." *The Daily*. Online at www.statcan.ca/english/freepub/81-582-XIE/free.htm.

Statistics Canada. (2000, September 4). "Rural youth: Stayers, leavers, and return migrants." *The Daily*. Online at www.statcan.ca/Daily/English/000905/d000905b.htm.

Statistics Canada. (2001, December 7). "Participation in postsecondary education and family income: 1998." *The Daily*. Online at www.statcan.ca/Daily/English/011207/d011207c.htm.

Statistics Canada. (2002, January 23). "Youth in Transition Survey, 2000. *The Daily*. Online at www.statcan.ca/Daily/English/020123/d020123a.htm.

Statistics Canada. (2003a). "Education in Canada: Raising the standard. Data from the 2001 Census." Online at www.statcan.ca/bsolc/english/bsolc?catno=96F0030XIE2001012.

Statistics Canada. (2003b, September 24). "Aboriginal peoples survey: Well-being of the non-reserve Aboriginal population 2001." *The Daily*. Online at www.statcan.ca/Daily/English/030924/d030924b.htm.

Statistics Canada. (2003c, October 31). "Factors related to adolescents' self-perceived health: 2000/01." *The Daily*. Online at www.statcan.ca/Daily/English/031031/d031031b.htm.

Statistics Canada. (2006, June, 28). "The risk of first and second marriage dissolution." *The Daily*. Online at www.statcan.ca/Daily/English/060628/d060628b.htm.

Statistics Canada. (2007, September 12). "Family portrait: Continuity and change in Canadian families and households in 2006." *The Daily.* Online at www12.statcan.ca/english/census06/analysis/famhouse/index.cfm.

Third International Mathematics and Science Study. (1999). Online at nces.ed.gov/timss/results.asp.

Tremblay, R.E. (2000). "The origins of youth violence." *ISUMA, 1*(2), 19–24. Online at www.isuma.net/v01n02/tremblay/tremblay_e.pdf.

Chapter 12

American Medical Association Ad Hoc Committee on Health Literacy. (1999). "Health literacy: Report of the council on scientific affairs." *JAMA, 281*(6), 553–557.

Anderson, A. (2003). *Better health, better schools, better futures*. Toronto: OISE/UT.

Annan, K. (1997). Message on International Literacy Day, September 8.

Antone, E.M. (2003). "Aboriginal peoples: Literacy and learning." *Literacies, 1*(Spring), 9–12.

Antone E. (2004). Presentation at National Workshop on Literacy and Health research priorities, October 27–28, 2004.

Baker, D.W., Gazmararian, J.A., Williams, M.V., Scott, T., Parker, R.M., Green, D., Ren, J. & Peel, J. (2002). "Functional health literacy and the risk of hospital admission among medicare managed care enrolees." *American Journal of Public Health, 92*(8), 1278–1283.

Baker, D.W., Parker, R.M., Williams, M.V., Clark, W.S. & Nurss, J. (1997). "The relationship of patient reading ability to self-reported health and use of health services." *American Journal of Public Health, 87*(6), 1027–1030.

Battiste, M. (1984). "Micmac literacy and cognitive assimilation." Paper presented at the International Conference of the Mokakit Indian Education Research Association, London, Ontario, July 26.

Begley, S. (1996). "Your child's brain." *Newsweek* (February 19), 55–61.

Boyd, M. (1991). "Gender, nativity, and literacy: Proficiency and training issues." In K.C. Barker (Ed.), *Adult literacy in Canada: Results of national study* (pp. 86–94). Ottawa: Statistics Canada.

Breen, M.J. (1998). "Promoting literacy, improving health." In *Canada health action: Building on the legacy: V2 adults and seniors* (pp. 43–88). Ottawa: National Forum on Health.

Calamai, P. (1987). *Broken words: Why five million Canadians are illiterate: A special Southam survey.* Online at www.nald.ca/fulltext/Brokword/cover.htm.

Calamai, P. (1999). *Literacy matters report.* Toronto: ABC CANADA Literacy Foundation. Online at www.abc–canada.org/public_awareness/literacy_matters_report.asp.

Calamai, P. (2000). "The three L's: Literacy and life-long learning." An address to the Westnet 2000 conference, Calgary, November 2. Online at www.nald.ca/fulltext/3ls.

Canadian Business Task Force on Literacy. (1987). *The cost of illiteracy to Canadian business.* Toronto: Westmount Research Consultants.

Canadian Council on Learning. (2007a). *State of learning in Canada, 2007.* Ottawa: Canadian Council on Learning.

Canadian Council on Learning. (2007b). *Health literacy in Canada: Initial results from the International Adult Literacy and Skills Survey.* Ottawa: Canadian Council on Learning.

Canadian Council on Learning. (2008). *A healthy understanding: Health literacy in Canada.*

Canadian Public Health Association. (2000). *What the HEALTH! A literacy and health resource for youth.* Ottawa: Canadian Public Health Association. Online at www.worlded.org/us/health/docs/ culture/ materials/curricula_009. html.

Canadian Public Health Association. (2003). *Literacy and health research workshop: Setting priorities in Canada.* Online at www.nlhp.cpha.ca/clhrp/index_e.htm#workshop.

Charette, M.F. & Meng, R. (1998). "The determinants of literacy and numeracy and the effect of literacy and numeracy on our market outcomes." *Canadian Journal of Economics/Revue canadienne d'economique, 13*(3), 495–517. Online at www.nald.ca/fulltext/pat/Charette/page1.htm.

Clarkson, A. (2004). "Re-visioning literacy across a re-cultured curriculum: A review essay." York University, unpublished paper.

Daniels, S., Kennedy, B. & Kawachi, I. (2000). "Justice is good for our health: How greater economic equality would promote public health." *Boston Review, 25*(1), 4–19. Online at www.bostonreview.net/BR25.1/daniels.html.

Darville, R. (1992). *Adult literacy work in Canada.* Toronto: Canadian Association for Adult Education.

Davies, R. (1995). "Men for change." Halifax: Private correspondence.

Davis, T.C., Meldrum, H., Tippy, P.K.P., et al. (1996). "How poor literacy leads to poor health care." *Patient Care, 30*(16), 94–124.

Department for International Development. (2005). *Reducing poverty by tackling social exclusion.* London: DFID.

DeWit, D.J., Akst, L., Braun, K., Jelley, J., Lefebver, L., McKee, C., et al. (2002). *Sense of school membership: A mediating mechanism linking student perceptions of school culture with academic and behavioural functioning: Baseline data report of the school culture project.* Toronto: Centre for Addiction and Mental Health.

Drolet, M. (2005). *Participation in post-secondary education in Canada: Has the role of parental income and education changed over the 1990s?* Ottawa: Statistics Canada. Online at www.statcan.ca/english/research/11F0019MIE/11F0019MIE2005243.pdf.,

Edwards, C. (1995). "Due diligence: The challenge of language and literacy." *Accident Prevention, 42*(6), 18–21.

Education Quality and Accountability Office. (2003). *Ontario secondary school literacy test report of provincial results.* Online at www.eqao.com.

Federal, Provincial, and Territorial Advisory Committee on Population Health. (1999). *Toward a healthy future.* Ottawa: Health Canada.

Friedland, R. (1998). "New estimates of the high costs of inadequate health literacy." In Pfizer Inc. (Ed.), *Promoting health literacy: A call to action* (pp. 6–10). Proceedings of the Pfizer Conference, October 7–8, 1998. Washington: Pfizer Inc.

Frontier College. (1989). *Learning in the workplace.* Toronto: Frontier College. Online at www. frontiercollege. ca/english/programs/wkplace.htm.

Galabuzi, G. (2004). "Social exclusion." In D. Raphael (Ed.), *Social determinants of health: Canadian perspectives* (pp. 235–252). Toronto: Canadian Scholars' Press, Inc.

Gazmararian, J.A., Baker, D.W., Williams, M.V., Parker, R.M., Scott, T.L., Green, D.C., Fehrenbach, S.N., Ren, J. & Koplan, J.P. (1999). "Health literacy among medicare enrollees in a managed care organization." Comment in *JAMA, 282*(6), 527.

Grossman, M. & Joyce, T.J. "Socioeconomic status and health: a personal research perspective." Paper presented at a conference on Socioeconomic Status and Health, sponsored by the Henry J. Kaiser Family Foundation in Menlo Park, California, March 26–27.

Grossman, M. & Kaestner, R. (1997). "The effects of education on health." In R. Behermann & N. Stacey (Eds.), *The social benefits of education* (pp. 69–123). Ann Arbor: University of Michigan Press.

Grotsky, R. (1989). *Workplace literacy and health and safety: A research report.* Prepared for the Industrial Accident Prevention Association by Learning Communications Inc., Toronto.

Guerra, C.E. & Shea, J.A. (2003). "Functional health literacy: Comorbidity and health status." *Journal of General Internal Medicine, 18*(1), 174.

Halfon, N., Shulman E. & Hochstein M. (2001). "Brain development in early childhood." In N. Halfon, E. Shulman & M. Hochstein (Eds.), *Building community systems for young children* (pp. 1–27). Los Angeles: UCLA Center for Healthier Children, Families, and Communities.

Hawthorne, G. (1997). "Preteenage drug use in Australia: Key predictors and school-based drug education." *Journal of Adolescent Health, 20*(5), 384–395.

Health Canada. (2003). *How does literacy affect the health of Canadians?* Online at www.hc–sc.gc.ca/hppb/phdd/literacy/literacy.html.

HRSDC and Statistics Canada (2005). *Challenges of the knowledge-based society and economy.* On line at www.hrsdc.gc.ca/en/hip/lld/nls/Resources/10_fact.shtml.

Jadad, A.R. (1999). "Promoting partnerships: Challenges for the Internet age." *British Medical Journal, 318*(September 18), 761–764.

Kalichman, S.C., Ramachandran, B. & Catz, S. (1999). "Adherence to combination antiretroviral therapies in HIV patients of low health literacy." *Journal of General Internal Medicine, 5,* 267–273.

Karp, A., Kareholt, I., Qiu, C., Bellander, T., Winblad, B., Fratiglioni, L. (2004). "Relation of education and occupation-based socioeconomic status to incident of Alzheimer's disease." *American Journal of Epidemiology, 159,* 175–183.

Kirsch, I.S., Jungeblut, A., Jenkins, L. & Kolstad, A. (1993). *Adult literacy in America: A first look at the results of the National Adult Literacy Survey (NALS).* Washington: National Center for Educational Statistics, US Department of Education.

Kohn, A. (2004) *What does it mean to be well educated? And more essays on standards, grading, and other follies.* Boston: Beacon Press.

Koller, T. & Hertzman, C. (2006, February 10). Interview with Clyde Hertzman, director, Human Early Learning Partnership, University of British Columbia. Online at www.salute.toscara.it/promozione/hbsc/Hertzman.pdf.

Mustard, F. & McCain, M.N. (1999). *Early years study.* Toronto: Queen's Printer for Ontario.

OECD & Statistics Canada. (2000). *Literacy in the information age: Final report of the international adult literacy survey.* Online at www.statcan.ca/english/freepub/89-588-XIE/about.htm.

Parker, R.M., Ratzan, S.C. & Lurie, N. (2003). "Health literacy: A policy challenge for advancing high quality health care." *Health Affairs, 22*(4), 147.

Parkland Regional College. (1998). *Reaching the rainbow: Aboriginal literacy in Canada.* Melville: Parkland Regional College.

Perrin, B. (1989). *Literacy and health: Making the connection: The research report of the literacy and health project phase one: Making the world healthier and safer for people who can't read.* Ontario Public Health Association and Frontier College. Online at www.opha.on.ca/resources/ literacy1research.pdf.

Poureslami, I., Murphy, D., Balka, E., Nicol, A. & Rootman, I. (2007). "Assessing the effectiveness of informational video clips on Iranian immigrants attitudes toward and intention to use the BC HealthGuide Program in the Greater Vancouver area." *Medscape General Medicine, 9*, 12.

Puchner, L.D. (1993). *Early childhood, family, and health issues in literacy: International perspectives.* Philadelphia: NCAL International Paper IP93-2.

Ratzan, S.C. & Parker, R.M. (2000). "Introduction." In *National Library of Medicine Current Bibliographies in Medicine: Health Literacy.* NLM Pub. No. CBM 2000-1. C.R. Selden et al (Eds.). Bethesda, MD: National Institutes of Health, US Department of Health and Human Services.

Roberts, P. & Fawcett, G. (1998). *At risk: A socio-economic analysis of health and literacy among seniors.* Statistics Canada Cat. no. 89–552–MPE, no. 5. Ottawa: Statistics Canada.

Rootman, I. (1991). "Literacy and health in Canada: Contribution of the LSUDA survey." In Statistics Canada, *Adult literacy in Canada: Results of a national study* (pp. 65–66). Ottawa: Minister of Industry, Science, and Technology.

Rootman, I. & Gordon-El-Bihbety, D. (2006). "Staying the course. The captain's log continues. Literacy and health in Canada: Perspectives from the Second Canadian Conference on Literacy and Health." *Canadian Journal of Public Health, 97*(Supplement 2), S5–9.

Rootman, I. & Gordon-El-Bihbety, D. (2008). *A vision for a health literate Canada: Report of the Expert Panel on Health Literacy.* Ottawa: Canadian Public Health Association.

Rootman, I., Gordon-El-Bihbety, D., Frankish, J., Hemming, H., Kaszap, M., Langille, L., Quantz, D. & Ronson, B. (2003). *National literacy and health research program, needs assessment, and environmental scan.* Online at www.nlhp.cpha.ca/clhrp/index_e.htm.

Rootman, I. & Ronson, B. (2003). *Literacy and health research in Canada: Where have we been and where should we go?* Research paper. Ottawa: International Think Tank on Reducing Health Disparities and Promoting Equity for Vulnerable Populations.

Rudd, R.E., Moeykens, B.A. & Colton, T. (1999). "Health and literacy: A review of medical and public health literature." In NCSALL: *The annual review of adult learning and literacy,* vol. 1 (pp. 158–199). San Francisco: Jossey Bass.

Sarginson, R.J. (1997). *Literacy and health: A Manitoba perspective.* Winnipeg: Literacy Partners of Manitoba. Online at www.mb.literacy.ca/publications/lithealth/ack.htm.

Schillinger, D., Grumbach, K., Piette, J., Wang, F., Osmond, D., Daher, C., Palacios, J., Sullivan, G.D. & Bindman, A.B. (2002). "Association of health literacy with diabetes outcomes." *Journal of the American Medical Association, 288*(4), 475–482.

Schweinhart, L.J., Barnes, H.V., Weikart, D.P., Barnett, W.S. & Epstein, A.S. (1993). *Significant benefits: The High/ Scope Perry preschool study through age 27*. Ypsilanti: High/Scope Press.

Scott, T.L., Gazmararian, J.A., Williams, M.V. & Baker, D.W. (2002). "Health literacy and preventive health care use among medicare enrollees in a managed care organization." *Medical Care, 40*(5), 395–404.

Shohet, L. (1997). "Canadian budget shines spotlight on family literacy." Online at www.nald.ca/ naldnews/97spring/ budget.htm.

Shohet, L. (2002). *Health and literacy: Perspectives in 2002*. Montreal: The Centre for Literacy of Quebec. Online at www.staff.vu.edu.au/alnarc/onlineforum/AL_pap_shohet.htm.

Slater, C. & Carlton, B. (1985). "Behaviour, lifestyle, and socio-economic variables as determinants of health status: implications for health policy development." *American Journal of Preventative Medicine, 1*(5), 25–33.

Statistics Canada. (1996). *Reading the future: A portrait of literacy in Canada*. Online at www.nald. ca/nls/ials/ ialsreps/high1.htm.

Statistics Canada. (2005, May 11). "Adult literacy and life skills survey." *The Daily.* Online at www.statcan.ca/Daily/ English/0505111/d050511b.htm.

Statistics Canada & OECD. (2005). *Learning a living: First results of the Adult Literacy and Life Skills Survey, 2003.* Ottawa: Statistics Canada.

Totten, M. & Quigley, P. (2003). "Bullying, school exclusion, and literacy." Unpublished discussion paper sponsored by the Canadian Public Health Association.

Weiss, B.D. (2001). "Health literacy: An important issue for communicating health information to patients." *Chinese Medical Journal, 64*(11), 603–608.

Weiss, B.D., Blanchard, J.S., McGee, D.L., Hart, G., Warren, B., Burgoon, M. & Smith, K.J. (1994). "Illiteracy among Medicaid recipients and its relationship to health care costs." *Journal of Health Care for the Poor and Underserved, 5*(2), 99–111.

WHO. (2003). *The World Health Organization's health promoting school: Creating an environment for emotional and social well-being.* Geneva: Information Series on School Health, Document 10.

WHO, UNESCO, World Bank & UNICEF. (2000). *Focusing resources on effective school health: A FRESH start to enhancing the quality and equity of education.* World Education Forum 2000, Final Report. Online at www. freshschools.org/whatisfresh.htm.

Young, D.E. & Smith, L.L. (1992). *The involvement of Canadian Native communities in their health care programs: A review of the literature since the 1970's.* Edmonton: Canadian Circumpolar Institute and Centre for the Cross-Cultural Study of Health and Healing.

Zhong-Cheng, L., Wilkins, R., Wilkins, M. & Kramer, M. (2006). "Effect of neighbourhood income and maternal education on birth outcomes: A population-based study." *Canadian Medical Association Journal, 174*(10), 1415–1420.

Chapter 13

Alberta Provincial Community Nutritionist's Group. (2005). *The cost of eating in Alberta*. Online at www. foodsecurityalberta.ca/content.asp?Catid=4&rootid=4.

Antonishak, D., Bennewith, E., Lutz, H., Macdonald, J., Raja, S. & Sheppard, F. (2004). *The cost of eating in BC: Impact of a low-income on food security and health.* Vancouver: Dietitians of Canada, BC Region, and the Community Nutritionists Council of BC. On line at www.dietitians.ca.

Broughton, M.A., Janssen, P.S., Hertzman, C., Innis, S.M. & Frankish, C.J. (2006). "Predictors and outcomes of household food insecurity among inner city families with preschool children in Vancouver." *Canadian Journal of Public Health, 97*, 214–216.

Canadian Association of Food Banks. (2004). *HungerCount 2004*. Online at www.cafb-acba.ca/english/ EducationandResearch-ResearchStudies.html.

Canadian Association of Food Banks. (2006). *HungerCount 2006*. Online at www.cafb-acba.ca/english/EducationandResearch-ResearchStudies.html.

Canadian Association of Food Banks. (2007). *HungerCount 2007*. Toronto: CAFB. Online at www.cafb-acba.ca/english.

Che, J. & Chen, J. (2001). "Food insecurity in Canadian households." *Health Reports, 12*, 11–22.

Commission on Social Determinants of Health. (2007). *Achieving health equity: From root causes to fair outcomes.* Interim statement. Geneva: World Health Organization.

Dachner, N. & Tarasuk, V. (2002). "Homeless 'squeegee kids': Food insecurity and daily survival." *Social Science and Medicine, 54*, 1039–1049.

Dietitians of Canada. (2005). *Individual and household food insecurity in Canada: Position of Dietitians of Canada.* Online at www.dietitians.ca.

Engler-Stringer, R. & Berenbaum, S. (2007). "Exploring food security with collective kitchens participants in three Canadian cities." *Qualitative Health Research, 17*, 75–84.

Ewtushik, M. (2004). *The cost of eating in Newfoundland and Labrador—2003.* St. John's: Dietitians of Newfoundland and Labrador, Newfoundland and Labrador Public Health Association, Newfoundland and Labrador Association of Social Workers. Online at www.dietitians.ca.

Fano, T.J., Tyminski, S.M. & Flynn, M.A.T. (2004). "Evaluation of a collective kitchens program using the population health promotion model." *Canadian Journal of Dietetic Practice and Research, 65*(2), 72–80.

Food and Agriculture Association of the United Nations. (2006). *The state of food insecurity in the world 2006.* Online at www.fao.org/docrep/009/a0750e/a0750e00.htm.

Glanville, N.T. & McIntyre, L. (2006). "Diet quality of Atlantic families headed by single mothers." *Canadian Journal of Dietetic Practice and Research, 67*, 28–35.

Hamelin, A.M., Beaudry, M. & Habicht, J.-P. (2002). "Characterization of household food insecurity in Quebec: Food and feelings." *Social Science & Medicine, 54*, 119–132.

Health Canada. (2007). *Canadian Community Health Survey, cycle 2.2, Nutrition (2004)—Income-related household food security in Canada.* Ottawa: Office of Nutrition Policy and Promotion, Health Products and Food Branch.

Heimann, C. (2004). *Hunger in Canada: Perceptions of a problem.* Toronto: Totum Research Inc.

Ledrou, I. & Gervais, J. (2005) "Food insecurity." *Health Reports, 16*, 47–50.

McIntyre, L., Connor, S.K. & Warren, J. (2000). "Child hunger in Canada: Results of the 1994 National Longitudinal Survey of Children and Youth." *Canadian Medical Association Journal, 163*, 961–965.

McIntyre, L., Glanville, N.T., Officer, S., Anderson, B., Raine, K.D. & Dayle, J.B. (2002). "Food insecurity of low-income lone mothers and their children in Atlantic Canada." *Canadian Journal of Public Health, 93*, 411–415.

McIntyre, L., Glanville, N.T., Raine, K.D., Dayle, J.B., Anderson, B. & Battaglia, N. (2003). "Do low-income lone mothers compromise their nutrition to feed their children?" *Canadian Medical Association Journal, 168*, 686–691.

McIntyre, L., Officer, S. & Robinson, L. (2003). "Feeling poor: The felt experience of low-income lone mothers." *Affilia, 18*, 316–331.

McIntyre, L., Tarasuk, C. & Li, T.J. (2007). "Improving the nutritional status of food-insecure women: First, let them eat what they like." *Public Health Nutrition, 10*, 1288–1298.

McIntyre, L., Walsh, G. & Connor, S.K. (2001). *A follow-up study of child hunger in Canada.* Working Paper W-01-1-2E, Applied Research Branch, Strategic Policy. Ottawa: Human Resources Development Canada.

McIntyre, L., Williams, P. & Glanville, N.T. (2007). "Milk as metaphor: Low-income lone mothers' characterization of their challenges acquiring milk for their families." *Ecology of Food and Nutrition, 46*, 263–279.

McLaughlin, C., Tarasuk, V. & Kreiger, N. (2003). "An examination of at-home food preparation activity among low-income, food-insecure women." *Journal of the American Dietetic Association, 103*, 1506–1512.

Nord, M., Hooper, M. & Hopwood, H. (2007). "Food insecurity in Canada and the United States: An international comparison." Presented at the 19th IUHPE World Conference on Health Promotion & Health Education, Vancouver, BC, June 10–15.

Ostry, A.S. (2006). *Nutrition policy in Canada, 1870–1939*. Vancouver: UBC Press.

Power, E.M. (2005). "Determinants of healthy eating among low-income Canadians." *Canadian Journal of Public Health, 96*(Supplement 3), S37–S42.

Raine, K., McIntyre, L. & Dayle, J.B. (2003). "The failure of charitable school- and community-based nutrition programmes to feed hungry children." *Critical Public Health, 13*, 155–169.

Rainville, B. & Brink, S. (2001). *Food insecurity in Canada, 1998–1999.* Research paper R-01-2E. Ottawa: Applied Research Branch, Human Resources Development Canada.

Riches, G. (2002). "Food banks and food security: Welfare reform, human rights, and social policy. Lessons from Canada?" *Social Policy and Administration, 36*, 648–663.

Rideout, K., Riches, G., Ostry, A., Buckingham, D. & MacRae, R. (2007). "Bringing home the right to food in Canada: Challenges and possibilities for achieving food security." *Public Health Nutrition, 10*, 566–573.

Tarasuk, V. (2001). "Household food insecurity with hunger is associated with women's food intakes, health, and household circumstances." *Journal of Nutrition, 131*, 2670–2676.

Tarasuk, V. (2005). "Household food insecurity in Canada." *Topics in Clinical Nutrition, 20*, 299–312.

Tarasuk, V.S. & Beaton, G.H. (1999). "Household food insecurity and hunger among families using food banks." *Canadian Journal of Public Health 90,* 109–113.

Tarasuk, V., Dachner, N. & Li, J. (2005). "Homeless youth in Toronto are nutritionally vulnerable." *Journal of Nutrition, 135,* 1926–1933.

Tarasuk, V. & Eakin, J.M. (2003). "Charitable food assistance as symbolic gesture: An ethnographic study of food banks in Ontario." *Social Science & Medicine, 56*(7), 1505–1515.

Tarasuk, V. & Eakin, J.M. (2005). "Food assistance through 'surplus' food: Insights from an ethnographic study of food bank work." *Agriculture and Human Values, V22*(2), 177–186.

Tarasuk, V., McIntyre, L. & Li, J. (2007). "Low-income women's dietary intakes are sensitive to the depletion of household resources in one month." *Journal of Nutrition, 137*, 1980–1987.

United Nations. (1996). *International Covenant on Economic, Social and Cultural Rights*. Geneva: The Office of the High Commissioner for Human Rights. Online at www.unhchr.ch/html/menu3/b/a_cescr.htm.

United Nations Human Development Report Office. (2008). *Human development reports*. On line at hdr.undp.org/en/.

United Nations Office at Geneva. (2006, 8 May). *Committee on economic, social, and cultural rights reviews fourth and fifth periodic reports of Canada.* Online at: www.unog.ch/unog/website/news_media.nsf/(httpNewsByYear_en)/BE76C080E5463A74C12571650046E954?OpenDocument.

United States Department of Agriculture. (2006). *Food security in the United States: Hunger and food security.* Online at www.ers.usda.gov/Briefing/FoodSecurity/labels.htm.

United States Department of Agriculture. (2007). *Healthy eating index*. Online at www.cnpp.usda.gov/HealthyEatingIndex.htm.

Vozoris, N. & Tarasuk, V. (2003). "Prenatal and child nutrition programs in relation to food insecurity." *Canadian Review of Social Policy, 51* (Spring/Summer), 67–86.

Williams, P.L., Johnson, C.P., Kratzmann, M.L.V., Johnson, C.S.J., Anderson, B.J. & Chenhall, C. (2006). "Can households earning minimum wage in Nova Scotia afford a nutritious diet?" *Canadian Journal of Public Health, 97*, 430–434.

Wilson, B. & Tsoa, E. (2002). *HungerCount 2002. Eating their words: Government failure on food security*. Toronto: Canadian Association of Food Banks.

World Food Summit. (1995). *Declaration on World Food Security*. Rome: Food and Agriculture Organization of the United Nations.

Chapter 14

Adams, E.J., Grummer-Strawn, L. & Chavez, G. (2003). "Food insecurity is associated with increased risk of obesity in California women." *Journal of Nutrition, 133,* 1070–1074.

Agriculture and Agri-Food Canada. (1998). *Canada's action plan for food security: A response to the World Food Summit* (Rep. no. 1987E). Ottawa: Agriculture and Agri-Food Canada.

Alaimo, K., Olson, C.M. & Frongillo, E.A. (2002). "Family food insufficiency, but not low family income, is positively associated with dysthymia and suicide symptoms in adolescents." *Journal of Nutrition, 132,* 719–725.

Alaimo, K., Olson, C.M., Frongillo, E.A. & Briefel, R. (2001). "Food insufficiency, family income, and health of US preschool and school-aged children." *American Journal of Public Health, 91,* 781–786.

Badun, C., Evers, S. & Hooper, M. (1995). "Food security and nutritional concerns of parents in an economically disadvantaged community." *Journal of the Canadian Dietary Association, 56,* 75–80.

Bhattacharya, J., Currie, J. & Haider, S. (2004). "Poverty, food insecurity, and nutritional outcomes in children and adults." *Journal of Health Economics, 23,* 839–862.

Bronte-Tinkew, J., Zaslow, M., Capps, R., Horowitz, A. & McNamara, M. (2007). "Food insecurity works through depression, parenting, and infant feeding to influence overweight and health in toddlers." *Journal of Nutrition, 137,* 2160–2165.

Broughton, M.A., Janssen, P.S., Hertzman, C., Innis, S.M. & Frankish, C.J. (2006). "Predictors and outcomes of household food insecurity among inner city families with preschool children in Vancouver." *Canadian Journal of Public Health, 97,* 214–216.

Campbell, C.C. & Desjardins, E. (1989). "A model and research approach for studying the management of limited food resources by low income families." *Journal of Nutrition Education, 21,* 162–171.

Carmichael, S.L., Yang, W., Herring, A., Abrams, B. & Shaw, G.M. (2007). "Maternal food insecurity is associated with increased risk of certain birth defects." *Journal of Nutrition, 137,* 2087–2092.

Che, J. & Chen, J. (2001). "Food insecurity in Canadian households." *Health Reports, 12,* 11–22.

Cristofar, S.P. & Basiotis, P.P. (1992). "Dietary intakes and selected characteristics of women ages 19–50 years and their children ages 1–5 years by reported perception of food sufficiency." *Journal of Nutrition Education, 24,* 53–58.

Dietz, W.H. (1995). "Does hunger cause obesity?" *Pediatrics, 95,* 766–767.

Dixon, L.B., Winkleby, M.A. & Radimer, K.L. (2001). "Dietary intakes and serum nutrients differ between adults from food-insufficient and food-sufficient families: Third National Health and Nutrition Examination Survey, 1988–1994." *Journal of Nutrition, 131,* 1232–1246.

Dowler, E. & Calvert, C. (1995). *Nutrition and diet in lone-parent families in London*. London: Family Policy Studies Centre.

Drewnowski, A. & Specter, S. (2004). "Poverty and obesity: The role of energy density and energy costs." *American Journal of Clinical Nutrition, 79,* 6–16.

Dubois, L., Farmer, A., Girard, M. & Porcherie, M. (2006). "Family food insufficiency is related to overweight among preschoolers." *Social Science & Medicine, 63,* 1503–1516.

Hagan, J. & McCarthy, B. (1997). *Mean streets: Youth crime and homelessness*. Cambridge: Cambridge University Press.

Hamelin, A.M., Beaudry, M. & Habicht, J.-P. (2002). "Characterization of household food insecurity in Quebec: Food and feelings." *Social Science & Medicine, 54,* 119–132.

Hamelin, A.M., Habicht, J.P. & Beaudry, M. (1999). "Food insecurity: Consequences for the household and broader social implications." *Journal of Nutrition, 129,* 525S–528S.

Harrison, G.G., Manalo-LeClair, G., Ramirez, A., Chia, J.Y., Kurata, J., McGarvey, N., et al. (2005). *More than 2.9 million Californians now food insecure—one in three low-income, an increase in just two years.* Los Angeles: UCLA Center for Health Policy Research.

Health Canada. (2007a). *Canadian Community Health Survey Cycle 2.2, Nutrition (2004)—Income-related household food security in Canada. Supplementary data tables.* Ottawa: Office of Nutrition Policy and Promotion, Health Products and Food Branch, Health Canada.

Health Canada. (2007b). *Canadian Community Health Survey, Cycle 2.2, Nutrition (2004)—Income-related household food security in Canada.* Rep. no. 4696. Ottawa: Office of Nutrition Policy and Promotion, Health Products and Food Branch, Health Canada.

Health Canada. (2007c). *Eating well with Canada's Food Guide.* (2007). Rep. no. H164-38/1-2007E. Ottawa: Health Canada.

Heflin, C.M., Siefert, K. & Williams, D.R. (2005). "Food insufficiency and women's mental health: Findings from a 3-year panel of welfare recipients." *Social Science & Medicine, 61,* 1971–1982.

Jacobs Starkey, L., Gray-Donald, K. & Kuhnlein, H.V. (1999). "Nutrient intake of food bank users is related to frequency of food bank use, household size, smoking, education, and country of birth." *Journal of Nutrition, 129,* 883–889.

Jacobs Starkey, L. & Kuhnlein, H.V. (2000). "Montreal food bank users' intakes compared with recommendations of Canada's Food Guide to Healthy Eating." *Canadian Journal of Dietetic Practice and Research, 61,* 73–75.

Jacobs Starkey, L., Kuhnlein, H. & Gray-Donald, K. (1998). "Food bank users: Sociodemographic and nutritional characteristics." *Canadian Medical Association Journal, 158,* 1143–1149.

Joint Steering Committee. (1996). *Nutrition for health: An agenda for action.* Ottawa: Minister of Supply and Services Canada.

Jones, S.J. & Frongillo, E.A. (2007). "Food insecurity and subsequent weight gain in women." *Public Health Nutrition, 10,* 145–151.

Kaiser, L.L., Townsend, M.S., Melgar-Quinonez, H.R., Fujii, M.J. & Crawford, P.B. (2004). "Choice of instrument influences relations between food insecurity and obesity in Latino women." *American Journal of Clinical Nutrition, 80,* 1372–1378.

Kempson, K.M., Keenan, D.P., Sadani, P.S., Ridlen, S. & Rosato, N.S. (2002). "Food management practices used by people with limited resources to maintain food sufficiency as reported by nutrition educators." *Journal of the American Dietetic Association, 102,* 1795–1799.

Kendall, A., Olson, C.M. & Frongillo, E.A. (1996). "Relationship of hunger and food insecurity to food availability and consumption." *Journal of the American Dietetic Association, 96,* 1019–1024.

Kerstetter, S. & Goldberg, M. (2007). *A review of policy options for increasing food security and income security in British Columbia—a discussion paper.* Vancouver: Provincial Health Services Authority.

Khandor, E. & Mason, K. (2007). *The Street Health Report 2007.* Toronto: Street Health.

Kim, K. & Frongillo, E.A. (2007). "Participation in food assistance programs modifies the relation of food insecurity with weight and depression in elders." *Journal of Nutrition, 137,* 1005–1010.

Kirkpatrick, S. & Tarasuk, V. (2008). "Food insecurity is associated with nutrient inadequacies among Canadian adults and adolescents." *Journal of Nutrition, 138,* 604–612.

Kleinman, R.E., Murphy, J.M., Little, M., Pagano, M., Wehler, C.A., Regal, K., et al. (1998). "Hunger in children in the United States: Potential behavioral and emotional correlates." *Pediatrics, 101,* 1–6.

Klesges, L.M., Pahor, M., Shorr, R.I. & Wan, J.Y. (2001). "Financial difficult in acquiring food among elderly disabled women: Results from the women's health and aging study." *American Journal of Public Health, 91,* 68–75.

Knol, L.L., Haughton, B. & Fitzhugh, E.C. (2004). "Food insufficiency is not related to overall variety of foods consumed by young children in low-income families." *Journal of the American Dietetic Association, 104,* 640–644.

Laraia, B.A., Siega-Riz, A.M. & Evenson, K.R. (2004). "Self-reported overweight and obesity are not associated with concern about enough food among adults in New York and Louisiana." *Preventive Medicine, 38,* 175–181.

Lawn, J. & Harvey, D. (2003). *Nutrition and food security in Kugaaruk, Nunavut.* Rep. no. R2-265/2003E. Ottawa: Minister of Indian Affairs and Northern Development.

Lawn, J. & Harvey, D. (2004a). *Nutrition and food security in Fort Severn, Ontario.* Rep. no. R2-350/2004E. Ottawa: Minister of Indian Affairs and Northern Development.

Lawn, J. & Harvey, D. (2004b). *Nutrition and food security in Kangiqsujuaq, Nunavik.* Rep. no. R2-341/2004E. Ottawa: Minister of Indian Affairs and Northern Development.

Ledrou, I. & Gervais, J. (2005). "Food insecurity." *Health Reports, 16,* 47–50.

Lyons, A.-A., Park, J. & Nelson, C.H. (2008). "Food insecurity and obesity: A comparison of self-reported and measured height and weight." *American Journal of Public Health, 98,* 751–757.

Matheson, D.M., Varady, J., Varady, A. & Killen, J.D. (2002). "Household food security and nutritional status of Hispanic children in the fifth grade." *American Journal of Clinical Nutrition, 76,* 210–217.

McIntyre, L., Connor, S. & Warren, J. (1998). *A glimpse of child hunger in Canada.* Rep. no. W-98-26E. Ottawa: Human Resources Development Canada.

McIntyre, L., Connor, S.K. & Warren, J. (2000). "Child hunger in Canada: Results of the 1994 National Longitudinal Survey of Children and Youth." *Canadian Medical Association Journal, 163,* 961–965.

McIntyre, L., Glanville, T., Officer, S., Anderson, B., Raine, K.D. & Dayle, J.B. (2002). "Food insecurity of low-income lone mothers and their children in Atlantic Canada." *Canadian Journal of Public Health/Revue Canadienne de Sante Publique, 93,* 411–415.

McIntyre, L., Glanville, T., Raine, K.D., Dayle, J.B., Anderson, B. & Battaglia, N. (2003). "Do low-income lone mothers compromise their nutrition to feed their children?" *Canadian Medical Association Journal, 168,* 686–691.

McIntyre, L., Raine, K., Glanville, T. & Dayle, J.B. (2001). *Hungry mothers of barely fed children.* Rep. no. NHRDP no. 6603-1550-002. Halifax: CIHR/NHRDP.

McIntyre, L., Tarasuk, V. & Li, T.J. (2007). "Improving the nutritional status of food insecure women: First, let them eat what they like." *Public Health Nutrition, 10,* 1288–1298.

McLaughlin, C., Tarasuk, V. & Krieger, N. (2003). "An examination of at-home food preparation activity among low-income, food-insecure women." *Journal of the American Dietetic Association, 103,* 1506–1512.

Murphy, J.M., Wehler, C.A., Pagano, M.E., Little, M., Kleinman, R.E. & Jellinek, M.S. (1998). "Relationship between hunger and psychosocial functioning in low-income American children." *Journal of the American Academy of Child and Adolescent Psychiatry, 37,* 163–170.

National Council of Welfare. (2006). *Welfare incomes 2005.* Rep. no. 125. Ottawa: Minister of Public Works and Government Services.

Nelson, K., Brown, M.E. & Lurie, N. (1998). "Hunger in an adult patient population." *Journal of the American Medical Association, 279,* 1211–1214.

Nelson, K., Cunningham, W., Andersen, R., Harrison, G. & Gelberg, L. (2001). "Is food insufficiency associated with health status and health care utilization among adults with diabetes?" *Journal of General Internal Medicine, 16,* 404–411.

Olson, C.M. (1999). "Nutrition and health outcomes associated with food insecurity and hunger." *Journal of Nutrition, 129,* 521S–524S.

Olson, C.M., Bove, C.F. & Miller, E.O. (2007). "Growing up poor: Long-term implications for eating patterns and body weight." *Appetite, 49,* 198–207.

Power, E. (2005). *Individual and household food insecurity in Canada: Position of the Dietitians of Canada.* Ottawa: Dietitians of Canada.

Power, E.M. (2006). "Economic abuse and intra-household inequities in food security." *Canadian Journal of Public Health, 97,* 258–260.

Radimer, K.L., Olson, C.M., Greene, J.C., Campbell, C.C. & Habicht, J.-P. (1992). "Understanding hunger and developing indicators to assess it in women and children." *Journal of Nutrition Education, 24,* 36S–45S.

Ricciuto, L. & Tarasuk, V. (2007). "An examination of income-related disparities in the nutritional quality of food selections among Canadian households from 1986–2001." *Journal of Nutrition, 64,* 186–198.

Ricciuto, L., Tarasuk, V. & Yatchew, A. (2006). "Sociodemographic influences on food purchasing among Canadian households." *European Journal of Clinical Nutrition, 13,* 1–13.

Riches, G. (1997a). "Hunger, food security, and welfare policies: Issues and debates in First World societies." *Proceedings of the Nutrition Society, 56,* 63–74.

Riches, G. (1997b). "Hunger in Canada: Abandoning the right to food." In G. Riches (Ed.), *First World hunger, food security, and welfare politics* (pp. 46–77). London: Macmillan Press Ltd.

Riches, G. (2002). "Food banks and food security: Welfare reform, human rights, and social policy. Lessons from Canada?" *Social Policy & Administration, 36,* 648–663.

Rideout, K., Riches, G., Ostry, A., Buckingham, D. & MacRae, R. (2007). "Bringing home the right to food in Canada: Challenges and possibilities for achieving food security." *Public Health Nutrition, 10,* 566–573.

Rose, D. (1999). "Economic determinants and dietary consequences of food insecurity in the United States." *Journal of Nutrition, 129,* 517S–520S.

Rose, D. & Bodor, N. (2006). "Household food insecurity and overweight status in young school children: Results from the Early Childhood Longitudinal Study." *Pediatrics, 117,* 464–473.

Rose, D. & Oliveira, V. (1997a). "Nutrient intakes of individuals from food-insufficient households in the United States." *American Journal of Public Health, 87,* 1956–1961.

Rose, D. & Oliveira, V. (1997b). *Validation of a self-reported measure of household food insufficiency with nutrient intake data.* Rep. no. TB-1863. Washington: United States Department of Agriculture.

Sarlio-Lahteenkorva, S. & Lahelma, E. (2001). "Food insecurity is associated with past and present economic disadvantage and body mass index." *Journal of Nutrition, 131,* 2880–2884.

Seligman, H.K., Bindman, A.B., Vittinghoff, E., Kanaya, A.M. & Kushel, M.B. (2007). "Food insecurity is associated with diabetes mellitus: Results from the National Health Examination and Nutrition Examination Survey (NHANES) 1999–2002." *Journal of General Internal Medicine, 22,* 1018–1023.

Siefert, K., Heflin, C.M., Corcoran, M.E. & Williams, D.R. (2001). "Food insufficiency and the physical and mental health of low-income women." *Women & Health, 32,* 159–177.

Tarasuk, V.S. (2001). "Household food insecurity with hunger is associated with women's food intakes, health, and household circumstances." *Journal of Nutrition, 131,* 2670–2676.

Tarasuk, V. (2005). "Household food insecurity in Canada." *Topics in Clinical Nutrition, 20,* 299–312.

Tarasuk, V.S. & Beaton, G.H. (1999a). "Women's dietary intakes in the context of household food insecurity." *Journal of Nutrition, 129,* 672–679.

Tarasuk, V.S. & Beaton, G.H. (1999b). "Household food insecurity and hunger among families using food banks." *Canadian Journal of Public Health, 90,* 109–113.

Tarasuk, V., Dachner, N. & Li, J. (2005). "Homeless youth in Toronto are nutritionally vulnerable." *Journal of Nutrition, 135,* 1926–1933.

Tarasuk, V., McIntyre, L. & Li, J. (2007). "Low-income women's dietary intakes are sensitive to the depletion of household resources in one month." *Journal of Nutrition, 137,* 1980–1987.

Townsend, M.S., Peerson, J., Love, B., Achterberg, C. & Murphy, S.P. (2001). "Food insecurity is positively related to overweight in women." *Journal of Nutrition, 131,* 1738–1745.

Travers, K.D. (1995). "'Do you teach them how to budget?': Professional discourse in the construction of nutritional inequities." In D. Maurer & J. Sobal (Eds.), *Eating agendas* (pp. 213–240). Hawthorne: Aldine DeGruyter.

Vozoris, N. & Tarasuk, V. (2003). "Household food insufficiency is associated with poorer health." *Journal of Nutrition, 133,* 120–126.

Wehler, C.A., Scott, R.I. & Anderson, J.J. (1992). "The community childhood hunger identification project: A model of domestic hunger-demonstration project in Seattle, Washington." *Journal of Nutrition Education, 24,* 29S–35S.

Whitaker, R.C., Phillips, S.M. & Orzol, S.M. (2006). "Food insecurity and the risks of depression and anxiety in mothers and behavior problems in their preschool-aged children." *Pediatrics, 118,* e859–e868.

Whitaker, R.C. & Sarin, A. (2007). "Change in food security status and change in weight are not associated in urban women with preschool children." *Journal of Nutrition, 137,* 2134–2139.

Wilde, P.E. & Peterman, J.N. (2006). "Individual weight change is associated with household food security status." *Journal of Nutrition, 136,* 1395–1400.

Willows, N. (2005). "Determinants of healthy eating in Aboriginal peoples in Canada." *Canadian Journal of Public Health, 96,* S32–S36.

Chapter 15

Canada Mortgage and Housing Corporation. (2007). *Canadian housing observer.* Ottawa: CMHC. Available online, including extensive data tables. Online at www.cmhc-schl.gc.ca/.

Canadian Housing and Renewal Association. (2003). *Expiry of operating agreements: Findings on the big picture.* Quebec/Ontario regional meeting document, June 11. Online at www.chra-achru.ca.

Carter, T. (2000). *Canadian housing policy: Is the glass half empty or half full?* Ottawa: Canadian Housing and Renewal Association Research Paper. Online at www.chra-achru.ca.

Carver, Humphrey. (1948). *Houses for Canadians: A study of housing problems in the Toronto area.* Toronto: University of Toronto Press.

Cooper, M. (2001). *Housing affordability: A children's issue.* Research report. Ottawa: Canadian Policy Research Networks.

Federation of Canadian Municipalities. (2002). *Is this really an affordable rental housing program?* Affordability assessment, November 2001. Ottawa: Federation of Canadian Municipalities.

Federation of Canadian Municipalities. (2008a). *Quality of life in Canadian communities: Trends and issues in affordable housing and homelessness.* Ottawa: Federation of Canadian Municipalities. Online at www.fcm.ca.

Federation of Canadian Municipalities. (2008b). *Sustaining the momentum: Recommendations for a national action plan on housing and homelessness.* Ottawa: Federation of Canadian Municipalities. Online at www.fcm.ca.

Hulchanski, D. (2001). *A tale of two Canadas: Homeowners getting richer, renters getting poorer.* Research Bulletin no. 2. Toronto: Centre for Urban and Community Studies.

Hulchanski, D. (2007). *The three cities within Toronto: Income polarization among Toronto's neighbourhoods, 1970–2000.* Research Bulletin no. 41. Toronto: Centre for Urban and Community Studies.

Kothari, Miloon. (2007). *Preliminary observations of a fact-finding mission to Canada.* Geneva: United Nations Office of the High Commissioner for Human Rights. Online at www.ohchr.org.

Maclennan, D. (2008). *Trunks, tails, and elephants: The economic case for a modern housing policy* (draft). Ottawa: Canadian Housing and Renewal Association. Online at www.chra-achru.ca.

Martin, P. & Fontana, J. (1990). *Finding room.* National Liberal Task Force on Housing. Online at www.housingagain.web.net/pmartin.html.

National Housing and Homelessness Network. (2001). *State of the crisis 2001: A report on housing and homelessness in Canada.* Online at www.tdrc.net/2report3.htm.

National Housing and Homelessness Network. (2002). *Housing for all Canadians: More federal money required, more federal leadership required.* Pre-budget submission to the House of Commons Standing Committee on Finance, September 3..

National Housing and Homelessness Network. (2003). *NHHN housing report card*. Online at www.povnet.org/ downloads/nhhnreportcardnov2003.pdf.

Ontario Housing Supply Working Group. (2001). *Affordable rental housing supply: The dynamics of the market and recommendations for encouraging new supply*. Online at www.mah.gov. on.ca/userfiles/HTML/nts_1_3369_ 1.html.

Reitsma-Street, M., Schofield, J., Lund, B. & Kasting, C. (2001). *Housing policy options for women living in urban poverty: An action research project in three Canadian cities*. Online at www.swc-cfc.gc.ca/pubs/0660613417/ index_e.html.

Shapcott, Michael. (2007). *Ten things you should know about housing and homelessness*. Toronto: Wellesley Institute. Online at www.wellesleyinstitute.com.

Shapcott, Michael. (2008). *National housing report card*. Toronto: Wellesley Institute. Online at www.wellesleyinstitute. com.

TD Economics. (2003). *Affordable housing in Canada: In search of a new paradigm*. Online at www.action.web. ca/home/housing/alerts.shtml.

Toronto Disaster Relief Committee. (1998). *State of emergency declaration: An urgent call for emergency humanitarian relief and prevention measures*. Toronto: Toronto Disaster Relief Committee.

Toronto Disaster Relief Committee. (2000). *State of the crisis*. Toronto: Toronto Disaster Relief Committee.

Chapter 16

Ambrosio, E., Baker, D., Crowe, C. & Hardill, K. (1992). *The Street Health Report: A study of the health status and barriers to health care of homeless women and men in the city of Toronto*. Toronto: Street Health.

Bines, W. (1994). *The health of single homeless people*. York, UK: University of York, Centre for Health Policy. Online at www.york.ac.uk/inst/chp/bines.pdf.

Brunner, E. & Marmot, M. (1999). "Social organization, stress, and health." In M. Marmot & R. Wilkinson (Eds.), *Social determinants of health* (pp. 17–43). Oxford: Oxford University Press.

Bryant, T. (2002). "The role of knowledge in progressive social policy development and implementation." *Canadian Review of Social Policy, 49*(50), 5–24.

Bryant, T. (2003). "A critical examination of the hospital restructuring process in Ontario, Canada." *Health Policy, 64*, 193–205.

Bryant, T. (2004). "How knowledge and political ideology affect rental housing policy in Ontario: Application of a knowledge paradigms framework of policy change." *Housing Studies, 19*(4), 635–651.

Canada Mortgage and Housing Corporation. (2000). *Housing market survey: Statistics Canada small area data: Special tabulations calculations*. Ottawa: The Advocate Institute.

Canada Mortgage and Housing Corporation. (2001). *Welfare income versus current average market rent, Toronto CMA*. Ottawa: Canada Mortgage and Housing Corporation.

Cheung, A. & Hwang, S. (2004). "Risk of death among homeless women: A cohort study and review of the literature." *Canadian Medical Asociation Journal, 170*(8), 1243–1247.

City of Calgary. (2002). *The 2002 count of homeless persons, 2002 May 15*. Calgary: City of Calgary Planning and Policy Department.

City of Toronto. (2003). *The Toronto report card on housing and homelessness*. Toronto: City of Toronto.

City of Toronto Planning Policy & Research. (2006). *Profile Toronto: Rental housing supply and demand indicators*. Toronto: City of Toronto.

Coburn, D. (2000). "Income inequality, lowered social cohesion, and the poorer health status of populations: The role of neo-liberalism." *Social Science & Medicine, 51*, 135–146.

Coleman, W.D., Skogstad, G.D. & Atkinson, M.M. (1997). "Paradigm shifts and policy networks: Cumulative change in agriculture." *Journal of Public Policy, 16*(3), 273–301.

Daily Bread Food Bank. (2002). *Fact sheet: Turning our backs on our children: Hunger + decrepit housing = unhealthy, unsafe children.* Toronto: Daily Bread Food Bank.

Davey Smith, G. (2003). *Inequalities in health.* Bristol: Policy Press.

Dedman, D.J., Gunnell, D., Davey Smith, G. & Frankel, S. (2001). "Childhood housing conditions and later mortality in the Boyd Orr cohort." *Journal of Epidemiology and Community Health, 55,* 10–15.

Dunn, J.R. (2000). "Housing and health inequalities: Review and prospects for research." *Housing Studies, 15*(3), 341–366.

Dunn, J.R. (2002). *A population health approach to housing: A framework for research.* Ottawa: National Housing Research Committee and CMHC. Online at www.hpclearinghouse.ca/hcn/download/ A_Population_Health_Approach_to_Housing_FINAL.pdf.

Dunn, J. & Hayes, M. (1999). "Identifying Social Pathways for Health Inequalities: The Role of Housing." *Annals of the New York Academy of Sciences, 896,* 399–402.

Dunn, J., Hayes, M., Hulchanski, D., Hwang, S. & Potvin, L. (2006). "Housing as a socio-economic determinant of health: Findings of a national needs, gaps, and opportunities assessment." *Canadian Journal of Public Health, 97*(Supplement 3), S11–S15.

Dunning, W. (2007). *Dimensions of core housing need in Canada.* Ottawa: Co-operative Housing Federation of Canada.

Engeland, J., Lewis, R., Ehrlich, S., & Che, J. (2005). *Evolving housing conditions in Canada's census metropolitan areas, 1991–2001.* Ottawa: Statistics Canada.

Esping-Andersen, G. (1990). *The three worlds of welfare capitalism.* Princeton: Princeton University Press.

Freeman, A.J.M., Holmans, A.E. & Whitehead, C.M.E. (1996). "Is the UK different? International comparisons of tenure patterns." A study carried out by the Property Research Unit of Cambridge University. London: Council of Mortgage Lenders.

Homelessness Action Group. (2007). *Take action on homelessness: Facts and figures.* Toronto: Homelessness Action Group.

Howlett, M. & Ramesh, M. (1995). *Studying public policy: Policy cycles and policy subsystems.* Toronto: Oxford University Press.

Hulchanski, J.D. (2001). *A tale of two Canadas: Homeowners getting richer, renters getting poorer.* Toronto: Centre for Urban and Community Studies, University of Toronto.

Hulchanski, J.D. (2002). *Housing policy for tomorrow's cities.* Discussion Paper F/27 Family Network. Ottawa: Canadian Policy Research Networks.

Hwang, S. (2001). "Homelessness and health." *Canadian Medical Association Journal, 164*(2), 229–233.

Hwang, S., Orav, E., O'Connell, J.M., Lebow, J. & Brennan, T. (1997). "Causes of death in homeless adults in Boston." *Annals of Internal Medicine, 126,* 625–628.

Hwang, S., Fuller-Thomson, E., Hulchanski, J.D., Bryant, T., Habib, Y. & Regoeczi, W. (1999). *Housing and population health: A review of the literature.* Toronto: Faculty of Social Work, University of Toronto.

Innocenti Research Centre. (2001). *A league table of child deaths by injury in rich nations.* Florence: Innocenti Research Centre.

Jackson, A. (2005). *Work and labour in Canada: Critical issues.* Toronto: Canadian Scholars' Press Inc.

Jenkins, R. (1982). *Hightown rules: Growing up in a Belfast housing estate.* Leicester: National Youth Bureau.

Kirby, M. (2002). *The study of the state of the health care system in Canada.* Ottawa: Senate of Canada. Online at www.albertadoctors.org/advocacy/sustainability.

Kushner, C. (1998). *Better access, better care: A research paper on health services and homelessness in Toronto.* Toronto: Toronto Mayor's Homelessness Action Task Force.

Layton, J. (2000). *Homelessness: The making and unmaking of a crisis.* Toronto: Penguin.

Layton, J. & Shapcott, M. (2008). *Homelessness: How to end the national crisis.* Toronto: Penguin.

Marmot, M. & Wilkinson, R. (Eds.). (1999). *Social determinants of health.* Oxford: Oxford University Press.

Marsh, A., Gordon, D., Pantazis, C. & Heslop, P. (1999). *Home sweet home?: The impact of poor housing on health.* Bristol: Policy.

Mazankowski, D. (2001). *A framework for reform.* Edmonton: Premier's Advisory Council on Health. Online at www.albertadoctors.org/advocacy/sustainability/.

National Council of Welfare. (2006). *Welfare incomes: 2005.* Ottawa: National Council of Welfare.

National Housing and Homelessness Network. (2002). *More than half provinces betray commitments: NHHN "report card" on anniversary of Affordable Housing Framework Agreement.* Online at www.tdrc.net/2replst.htm.

Nordentoft, M. & Wandall-Holm, N. (2003). "10-year follow-up study of mortality among users of hostels for homeless people in Copenhagen." *British Medical Journal, 327,* 1–4.

Platt, S., Martin, C., Hunt, S. & Lewis, C. (1989). "Damp housing, mould growth, and symptomatic health state." *British Medical Journal, 298,* 1673–1678.

Ramsden, S.S., Bauer, S., el Kabir, D.J. (1988). "Tuberculosis among the central London single homeless: A four-year retrospective study." *Journal of the Royal College of Physicians of London, 22,* 16–17.

Romanow, R. (2002). *Building on values: The future of health care in Canada. Final report.* Saskatoon: Commission on the Future of Health Care in Canada.

Sandeman, G., Lyon, C., Lyons, G., Jackson. M., McKeen, M., Murray, J. & Robinson, K. (2002). *Community plan to address homelessness and housing insecurity in Peterborough city and county.* Peterborough: City of Peterborough.

Savage, A. (1988). *Warmth in winter: Evaluation of an information pack for elderly people.* Cardiff: University of Wales College of Medicine Research Team for the Care of the Elderly.

Shaw, M. (2001). "Health and housing: A lasting relationship." *Journal of Epidemiology and Community Health, 55,* 291.

Shaw, M. (2004). "Housing and public health." *Annual Review of Public Health, 25,* 397–418.

Shaw, M., Dorling, D. & Brimblecombe, N. (1999). "Life chances in Britain by housing wealth and for the homeless and vulnerably housed." *Environment and Planning A, 31*(12), 2239–2248.

Shaw, M., Dorling, D. & Davey Smith, G. (1999). "Poverty, social exclusion, and minorities." In M. Marmot & R. Wilkinson (Eds.), *Social determinants of health* (pp. 211–239). New York: Oxford University Press.

Shaw, M., Dorling, D., Gordon, D. & Davey Smith, G. (1999). *The widening gap: Health inequalities and policy in Britain.* Bristol: Policy.

Standing Senate Committee on Social Affairs, Science, and Technology. (2002). *The health of Canadians: The federal role.* Ottawa: Senate of Canada.

Statistics Canada. (1984, 1999). *Survey of financial security.* Ottawa: Statistics Canada.

Statistics Canada. (1995). *General social surveys.* Ottawa: Statistics Canada.

Statistics Canada. (2002). *2001 census: Collective dwellings.* Ottawa: Statistics Canada. Online at www12.statcan.ca/english/census01/Products/Analytic/companion/coll/pdf/96F0030XIE2001004.pdf www.statcan.ca/english/Pgdb/famil65a.htm.

Statistics Canada. (2004). *Owner households and tenant households by major payments and gross rent as a percentage of 2000 household income, provinces and territories.* Online at www40.statcan.ca/l01/cst01/famil65a.htm.

Strachan, D. (1988). "Damp housing and childhood asthma: Validation of reporting of symptoms." *British Medical Journal, 297,* 1223–1226.

Toronto Disaster Relief Committee. (1998). *The one per cent solution.* Toronto: TDRC. Online at www. tdrc.ca.

Watt, J. (2003). *Adequate and affordable housing: A child health issue.* Ottawa: Child and Youth Health Network for Eastern Ontario.

Wilkinson, D. (1999). *Poor housing and ill health: A summary of research evidence.* Edinburgh: The Scottish Office. Online at. www.scotland.gov.uk/Resource/Doc/156479/0042008.pdf.

World Health Organization. (1986). *Ottawa charter on health promotion.* Geneva: WHO.

Chapter 17

Across Boundaries. (1999). *Healing journey: Mental health of people of colour project.* Toronto: Across Boundaries.

Adams, D. (1995). *Health issues of women of colour: A cultural diversity perspective.* Thousand Oaks & London: Sage Books.

Agnew, V. (2002). *Gender, migration, and citizenship resources project: Part II: A literature review and bibliography on health.* Toronto: Centre for Feminist Research, York University.

Alliance for South Asian AIDS Prevention (ASAP). (1999). *Discrimination & HIV/AIDS in South Asian Communities: Legal, ethical, and human rights challenges, an ethno-cultural perspective.* Toronto: ASAP/Health Canada.

Anderson, J. (1987). "Migration and health: Perspectives on immigrant women." *Sociology of Health and Illness, 94*(4), 410–438.

Anderson, J. (1991). "Health care in a multicultural society: Future directions." Manitoba Council for Multicultural Health Conference, Building Bridges to Improve Access to Health Care. *Conference Proceedings Newsletter, 2*(1), 7–16.

Anderson, J.M. (2000). "Gender, race, poverty, health, and discourses of health reform in the context of globalization: A post-colonial feminist perspective in policy research." *Nursing Inquiry, 7*(4), 220–229.

Anderson, J., Blue, C., Holbrook, A. & Ng, M. (1993). "On chronic illness: Immigrant women in Canada's workforce: A feminist perspective." *Canadian Journal of Nursing Research, 25*(2), 7–22.

Anderson, J. & Kirkham, R. (1998). "Constructing nation: The gendering and racializing of the Canada health care system." In Veronica Strong-Boag et al., *Painting the maple: Essays on race, gender, and the construction of Canada* (pp. 242–261). Vancouver: UBC Press.

Beiser, M. (1988). *After the door has been opened: Mental health issues affecting immigrants and refugees in Canada. Report of the Canadian taskforce on mental health issues affecting immigrants and refugees.* Ottawa: Health and Welfare Canada.

Beiser, M., Gill, K. & Edwards, G. (1993). "Mental health care in Canada: Is it accessible and equal?" *Canada's Mental Health, 41*, 2–7.

Bloom, M. & Grant, M. (2001). *Brain gain: The economic benefits of recognizing learning and learning credentials in Canada.* Ottawa: Conference Board of Canada.

Bolaria, B. & Bolaria, R. (1994). "Immigrant status and health status: Women and racial minority immigrant workers." In B.S. Bolaria & R. Bolaria (Eds.), *Racial minorities, medicine, and health* (pp. 149–168). Halifax: Fernwood Press.

Byrne, D. (1999). *Social exclusion.* Buckingham: Open University Press.

Canadian Institute of Health Research. (2002). *Charting the course: Canadian Population Health Initiative—A Pan-Canadian consultation on population and public health priorities.* Ottawa: Canadian Institute for Health Research.

Chard, J., Badets, J. & Howatson-Lee, L. (2000). *Immigrant women: Women in Canada, 2000, a gender-based statistical report.* Ottawa: Statistic Canada.

Chen, Jiajian, Wilkins, Russell & Ng, Edward. (1996). "Life expectancy of Canada's immigrants from 1986 to 1991." *Health Report, 8*(3), 29–38.

Citizenship and Immigration Canada. (2002). *Facts and figures 2001.* Ottawa: CIC.

De Wolff, A. (2000). *Breaking the myth of flexible work.* Toronto: Contingent Workers Project.

Dibbs, R. & Leesti, T. (1995). *Survey of labour and income dynamics: Visible minorities and Aboriginal peoples.* Ottawa: Statistics Canada.

Dossa, P. (1999). *The narrative representation of mental health: Iranian women in Canada.* Vancouver: RIIM.

Dunn, J., & Dyck I. (1998). *Social determinants of health in Canada's immigrant population: Results from the national population health survey, #98-20.* Vancouver: The Metropolis Project.

Evans, R.G., Barer, M.L. & Marmor, T.R. (Eds.). (1994). *Why are some people healthy and others not? The determinants of health of populations.* New York: Aldine DeGruyter, 1994.

Fernando, S. (1991). *Mental health, race, and culture.* London: Macmillan/Mind.

Fong, E. (2000). "Spatial separation of the poor in Canadian cities." *Demography, 37*(4), 449–459.

Fowler, N. (1998). "Providing healthcare to immigrants. and refugees: the North Hamilton experience." *Canadian Medical Association 159*(4), 388–391.

Frank, J. (1995). "Why population health?" *Canadian Journal of Public Health, 86,* 162–164.

Galabuzi, G. (2001). *Canada's creeping economic apartheid: The economic segregation and social marginisation of racialised groups.* Toronto: CSJ Foundation for Research & Education.

Galabuzi, G. (2006). *Canada's economic apartheid: The social exclusion of racialized groups in the new century.* Toronto: Canadian Scholars' Press Inc.

Gill S. (1995) "Globalisation, market civilisation, and disciplinary neoliberalism." *Millennium: Journal of International Studies, 24(*3), 399–423.

Globerman, S. (1998). *Immigration and health care utilization patterns in Canada.* Vancouver: Research on Immigration and Integration in the Metropolis (RIIM).

Government of Canada. (1984). *The Canada Health Act.* Ottawa: Government of Canada.

Guildford, J. (2000). *Making the case for economic and social inclusion.* Ottawa: Health Canada.

Hayes, M.V. & Dunn, J.R. (1998). *Population health in Canada: A systematic review.* Ottawa: Canadian Policy Research Networks.

Health Canada. (1998). *Metropolis health domain seminar, final report.* Ottawa: Health Canada.

Henry, F. & Tator, C. (2000). "The theory and practice of democratic racism in Canada." In M.A. Kalbach & W.E. Kalbach (Eds.), *Perspectives on ethnicity in Canada* (pp. 285–302). Toronto: Harcourt Canada.

Hou, F. & Balakrishnan, T. (1996). "The integration of visible minorities in contemporary Canadian society." *Canadian Journal of Sociology, 21*(3), 307–326.

Human Resources Development Canada (HRDC). (2001). "Recent immigrants have experienced unusual economic difficulties." *Applied Research Bulletin, 7*(1), 7–9

Human Resources Development Canada (HRDC). (2002). *Knowledge matters: Skills and learning for Canadians—Canada's innovation strategy.* Ottawa: HRDC. Online at www.hrdc-drhc.gc.ca/sp-ps/sl-ca/doc/summary.shtml.

Hutchinson, J. (2000). "Urban policy and social exclusion." In Janie Percy-Smith (Ed.), *Policy responses to social exclusion: Towards inclusion?* (pp. 164–183). Buckingham: Open University Press.

Hyman, I. (2001). *Immigration and health.* Health Canada Working Paper No. 01-05. Ottawa: Queen's Printer, 2001.

Jackson, A. (2001). "Poverty and racism." *Perception, 24*(4), 4–6.

Jenson, J. (2002). *Citizenship: Its relationship to the Canadian diversity model.* Canadian Policy Research Networks (CPRN). Online at www.cprn.org.

Jenson, J. & Papillon, M. (2001). *The changing boundaries of citizenship: A review and a research agenda.* Canadian Policy Research Networks (CPRN). Online at www.cprn.org.

Kawachi, I.R. & Kennedy, B. (2002). *The health of nations: Why inequality is harmful to your health.* New York: The New Press.

Kawachi, I. Wilkinson, R. & Kennedy, B. (1999). "Introduction." In I. Kawachi, B. Kennedy & R. Wilkinson (Eds.), *The society and population health reader*, vol. 1 (pp. xi–xxxiv). New York: The New Press.

Kazemipur, A. & Halli, S. (1997). "Plight of immigrants: The spatial concentration of poverty in Canada." *Canadian Journal of Regional Sciences* Special Issue, *XX* (1, 2), 11–28.

Kazemipur, A. & Halli, S. (2000). *The new poverty in Canada*. Toronto: Thompson Educational Publishing.

Kilbride, K.M, Anisef, P., Baichman-Anisef, E. & Khattar, R. (2000). *Between two worlds: The experiences and concerns of immigrant youth in Ontario*. Toronto: CERIS and CIC-OASIS. Online at www.settlement.org.

Kunz, J.L., Milan, A. & Schetagne, S. (2001). *Unequal access: A Canadian profile of racial differences in education, employment, and income*. Toronto: Canadian Race Relations Foundation.

Kymlicka, W. & Norman, W. (1995). "Return of the citizen: A survey of recent work on citizenship theory." In Ronald Beiner (Ed.), *Theorizing citizenship* (pp. 283–322). Albany: State University of New York Press.

Lee, K. (2000). *Urban poverty in Canada: A statistical profile*. Ottawa: Canadian Council on Social Development.

Lee, Y. (1999). "Social cohesion in Canada: The role of the immigrant service sector." *OCASI Newsletter*, Issue 73(Summer/Autumn).

Ley, D. & Smith, H. (1997). "Immigration and poverty in Canadian cities, 1971–1991." Canadian *Journal of Regional Science 20*(1–2), 29–48.

Littlewood, P. (1999). *Social exclusion in Europe: Problems and paradigms*. Aldershot: Ashgate.

Lo, L. & Wang, S. (2000). "Economic impacts of immigrants in the Toronto CMA: A tax-benefit analysis." *Journal of International Migration and Integration 1*(3), 273–303.

Lynch, J. (2000). "Income inequality and health: Expanding the debate." *Social Science & Medicine, 51*, 1001–1005.

Madanipour, A. (1998). "Social exclusion and space." In A. Madanipour, G. Cars & J. Allen (Eds.), *Social exclusion in European cities* (pp. 75–94). London: Jessica Kingley.

Marmot, M. (1993). *Explaining socioeconomic differences in sickness absence: The Whitehall II study*. Toronto: Canadian Institute for Advanced Research.

Marmot, M. & Wilkinson, R. (Eds.). (1999). *Social determinants of health*. Oxford: Oxford University Press.

Marx, K. (1977) *Capital, Vol. I*. New York: Vintage Books.

Noh, S., Beiser, M., Kaspar, V., Hou, F. & Rummens, J. (1999). "Perceived racial discrimination, discrimination, and coping: A study of South East Asian refugees in Canada." *Journal of Health and Social Behaviour, 40*, 193–207.

Ontario Advisory Council on Women's Issues. (1990). *Women and mental health in Ontario: Immigrant and visible minority women*. Ottawa: Ministry of Health.

Ornstein, M. (2000). *Ethno-racial inequality in the City of Toronto: An analysis of the 1996 census*. Toronto: City of Toronto. Online at ceris.metropolis.net.

Ornstein, M. (2006). *Ethno-racial groups in Toronto, 1971–2001: A demographic and social-economic profile*. Toronto: City of Toronto.

Peel Region. (2000). *Report of the Peel regional taskforce on homelessness*. Mississauga: Region of Peel.

Pendakur, R. (2000). *Immigrants and the labour force: Policy, regulation, and impact*. Montreal: McGill-Queen's University Press.

Picot, G. & Hou, F. (2003). *The rise in low-income rates among immigrants in Canada*. Analytical Studies Branch Research Paper Series. Catalogue no. 11F0019MIE2003198. Ottawa: Statistics Canada.

Pon, G. (2000). "Beamers, cells, malls, and cantopop: Thinking through the geographies of Chineseness." In C.E. James (Ed.), *Experiencing difference* (pp. 222–234). Halifax: Fernwood.

Preston, V. & Man, G. (1999). "Employment experiences of Chinese immigrant women: An exploration of diversity." *Canadian Woman Studies/Cahiers de la femme, 19*, 115–122.

Quinn, J. (2002). "Food bank clients often well-educated immigrants." *The Toronto Star* (March 31), A12.

Randall, V. R. (1993). "Racist health care: reforming an unjust health care system to meet the needs of African-Americans." *Health Matrix, 3,* 127–194.

Raphael, D. (1999). "Health effects of economic inequality." *Canadian Review of Social Policy, 44,* 25–40.

Raphael, D. (2001). "From increasing poverty to societal disintegration: How economic inequality affects the health of individuals and communities." In H. Armstrong, P. Armstrong & D. Coburn (Eds.), *Unhealthy times: The political economy of health and care in Canada* (pp. 223–246). Toronto: Oxford University Press.

Reitz, J.G. (1988). "The institutional structure of immigration as a determinant of inter-racial competition: a comparison of Britain and Canada." *International Migration Review 22,* 117–146.

Reitz, J.G. (2001). "Immigrant skill utilization in the Canadian labour market: Implications of human capital research." *Journal of International Migration and Integration, 2*(3), 347–378.

Room, G. (1995). "Conclusions." In G. Room (Ed.), *Beyond the threshold: The measurement and analysis of social exclusion* (pp. 233–247). Bristol: The Polity Press.

Saloojee, A. (2002). *Social inclusion, citizenship, and diversity: Moving beyond the limits of multiculturalism.* Toronto: The Laidlaw Foundation.

Shaw, M., Dorling, D. & Smith, G.D. (1999). "Poverty, social exclusion, and minorities." In M. Marmot & R. Wilkinson (Eds.), *Social determinants of health* (pp. 211–239). Oxford: Oxford University Press.

Shields, J. (2002). "No safe haven: Markets, welfare, and migrants." Paper presented to the Canadian Sociology and Anthropology Association, Congress of the Social Sciences and Humanities, Toronto, June 1.

Siemiatycki, M. & Isin, E. (1997). "Immigration, ethno-racial diversity, and urban citizenship in Toronto." *Canadian Journal of Regional Sciences*, Special Issue *XX*(1, 2), 73–102.

Statistics Canada (2003, January 21). "Census of population: Immigration, birthplace and birthplace of parents, citizenship, ethnic origin, visible minorities and Aboriginal peoples." *The Daily*.

Tharoa, E. & Massaquoi, N. (2001). "Black Women and HIV/AIDS: Contextualizing their realities, their silence and proposing solutions." *Canadian Woman Studies, 21*(2), 2001, 72–80.

Vosco, L. (2000). *Temporary work: The gendered rise of a precarious employment relationship.* Toronto: University of Toronto Press.

White, P. (1998). "Ideologies, social exclusion and spatial segregation in Paris." In S. Musterd & W. Ostendorf (Eds.), *Urban segregation and the welfare state: Inequality and exclusion in western cities* (pp. 148–167). London: Routledge.

Wilkinson, R. (1996). *Unhealthy societies: The afflictions of inequality.* New York: Routledge.

Wilkinson, R. & Marmot, M. (1998). *Social determinants of health: The solid facts.* Copenhagen: World Health Organization. Online at www.who.dk/healthy-cities.

Wilson, W.J. (1987). *The truly disadvantaged: Inner city, the underclass, and public policy.* Chicago: University of Chicago Press.

Yalnizyan, A. (1998). *The growing gap: A report on growing inequality between the rich and poor in Canada.* Toronto: Centre for Social Justice Foundation for Research and Education.

Yalnizyan, A. (2007). *The rich and the rest of us: The changing face of Canada's growing gap.* Ottawa: Canadian Centre for Policy Alternatives.

Yanz, L., Jeffcoat, B., Ladd, D. & Atlin, J. (1999). *Policy options to improve standards for women garment workers in Canada and internationally.* Toronto: Maquila Solidarity Network/Status of Women Canada.

Yépez del Castillo, I. (1994). "A comparative approach to social exclusion: Lesson from France and Belgium." *International Labour Review, 133*(5–6), 613–633.

Chapter 18

Bach, M. (2002). *Social inclusion as solidarity: Rethinking the child rights agenda.* Toronto: Laidlaw Foundation.

Barata, P. (2000). *Social exclusion in Europe: Survey of literature.* Unpublished mimeo. Toronto: Laidlaw Foundation.

Bloor, M. & McIntosh, J. (1990). "Surveillance and concealment." In S.L. Cunningham-Burley & N.L. McKeganey (Eds.), *Readings in medical sociology* (pp. 159–181). New York: Tavistock/Routledge.

Dahrendorf, R. (1959). *Class and class conflict in industrial society.* Stanford: Stanford University Press.

Durning, A. (1989). "Mobilizing at the grassroots." In L. Brown et al. (Eds.), *State of the world 1989* (pp. 156–173). New York: Norton.

Foucault, M. (1979). *Discipline and punish: The birth of the prison.* Middlesex: Peregrine Books.

Foucault, M. (1980). *Power/knowledge: Selected interviews and other writings.* C. Gordon. (Ed.). New York: Pantheon.

Friedmann, J. (1992). *Empowerment: The politics of alternative development.* Oxford: Blackwell.

Galeano, E. (1973). *Open veins of Latin America: Five centuries of the pillage of a continent.* New York: Monthly Review Press.

Guildford, J. (2000). *Making the case for social and economic inclusion.* Halifax: Health Canada, Population and Public Health Branch, Atlantic Region.

Gyebi, J., Brykczynska, G. & Lister, G. (2002). *Globalisation: Economics and women's health.* London: UK Global Health Forum. Online at www.ukglobalhealth.org.

Hochschild, A.R. (2000). "Global care chains and emotional surplus value." In W. Hutton & A. Giddens (Eds.), *Global capitalism* (pp. 130–146). New York: New Press.

Hunter, A. & Staggenborg, S. (1988). "Local communities and organized action." In C. Milofsky (Ed.), *Community organization: Studies in resource mobilization and exchange* (pp. 243–276). Oxford: Oxford University Press.

Kelsey, J. (2002). *At the crossroads: Three essays.* Wellington: Bridget Williams Books.

Labonte, R. (1999). "Social capital and community development: Practitioner emptor." *Australian and New Zealand Journal of Public Health, 23*(4), 93–96.

Labonte, R. (2003). "Globalization, trade, and health: Unpacking the linkages, defining the healthy public policy options." In R. Hofrichter (Ed.), *Health and social justice: Politics, ideology, and inequity in the distribution of disease* (pp. 469–500). San Francisco: Jossey-Bass.

Labonte, R., Edwards, R., Green, C., Hershfield, L., Thompson, P., Sushnigg, C. & Sykes, R. (1994). *Equity in action: Analyses of 33 locality equity projects.* Toronto: Ontario Premier's Council on Health, Wellbeing and Social Justice.

Lister, R. (2000). *Strategies for social inclusion: Promoting social inclusion or social justice?* New York: St. Martin's Press.

Lyon, L. (1989). *The community in urban society.* Toronto: Lexington.

Milanovic, B. (1993). "The two faces of globalization: Against globalization as we know it." *World Development, 31,* 667–683.

Milanovic, B. (2003). *Can we discern the effect of globalization on income distribution? Evidence from Household Budget Surveys.* Washington: World Bank. Online at http://ideas.repec.org/p/wpa/wuwpit/0303004.html.

Sen, A. (2000). *Development as freedom.* New York: Knopf.

Taylor, S. & Ashworth, C. (1987). "Durkheim and social realism: An approach to health and illness." In G. Scambler (Ed.), *Sociological theory and medical sociology* (pp. 37–58). New York: Methuen.

Unsworth, B. (1993). *A sacred hunger.* New York: Norton.

Weisbrot, M., Kraev, E. & Chen, J. (2001). *The scorecard on globalization 1980–2000: 20 years of diminished progress.* Washington: Center for Economic and Policy Research.

Chapter 19

Aboriginal Healing and Wellness Strategy. (2006). *What is the Aboriginal healing and wellness strategy?* Online at www.ahwsontario.ca/about/strategy.html.

Aboriginal Healing and Wellness Strategy. (2007). *Strategy-wide performance measures findings.* Online at www.ahwsontario.ca/policies/pdf/Final%205005_006PerformanceMeasuresFindings2.pdf.

Adelson, N. (2005). "The embodiment of inequity: Health disparities in Aboriginal Canada." *Canadian Journal of Public Health, 96*(Supplement 2), S45–S61.

Assembly of First Nations. (2006). *Assembly of First Nations calls for urgent action to end First Nations poverty on World Diabetes Day.* Online at www.afn.ca/article.asp?id=3111.

Assembly of First Nations. (2007). *Resolution of claims 2006–2007 Annual Report.* Ottawa: AFN. Online at www.afn.ca/article.asp?id=127.

Canadian Broadcasting Corporation. (2007). *Harper promises bill to "revolutionize" lands claim process.* Online at www.cbc.ca/canada/story/2007/06/12/claims.html.

Canadian Encyclopedia. (2007). *Hudsons Bay Company.* Online at www.thecanadianencyclopedia.com/index.cfm?PgNm=TCE&Params=A1SEC822150.

Canadian Institute for Health Information. (2004). *Improving the health of Canadians.* Ottawa: Health Canada. Online at www.cihi.ca/cihiweb/dispPage.jsp?cw_page=PG_39_E&cw_topic=39&cw_rel=AR_322_E.

Chandler, M.J. & Lalonde, C. (1998). "Cultural continuity as a hedge against suicide in Canada's First Nations." *Transcultural Psychiatry, 35*(2), 191–219.

CTV. (2007). *Court dismisses Métis land claims worth billions.* Online at www.ctv.ca/servlet/ArticleNews/story/CTVNews/20071207/winnipeg_treaty_071207/20071207?hub=Canada.

Dean, H.J. (1998). "NIDDM-Y in First Nations children in Canada." *Clinical Pediatrics, 37,* 898–896.

Dean, H.J., Mundy, R.L. & Moffatt, M. (1992). "Non-insulin-dependent diabetes mellitus in Indian children in Manitoba." *Canadian Medical Association Journal, 147*(1), 52–57.

Dewailly, E., Ryan, J., Laliberte, C., Bruneau, S., Weber, J., Gingras, S. & Carrier, G. (1994). "Exposure of remote Maritime populations to coplanar PCBs." *Environmental Health Perspectives, 102*(11), 205–210.

Dickason, O.P. (1992). *Canada's First Nations: A history of founding peoples from the earliest times.* Toronto: McClelland & Stewart.

First Nations and Inuit Health Branch. (2005). *Ten years of health transfer First Nation and Inuit control.* Ottawa: Health Canada. Online at www.hc-sc.gc.ca/fnih-spni/pubs/agree-accord/10_years_ans_trans/11_future-avenir_e.html#New_Models.

First Nations and Inuit Health Branch. (2007a). *Transfer status as of June 2007.* Ottawa: Health Canada. Online at www.hc-sc.gc.ca/fnih-spni/finance/agree-accord/trans_rpt_stats_e.html.

First Nations and Inuit Health Branch. (2007b). *Contribution agreement.* Ottawa: Health Canada. Online at www.hc-sc.gc.ca/fnih-spni/finance/agree-accord/index_e.html.

First Nations and Inuit Regional Health Survey Steering Committee. (1999). *First Nations and Inuit Regional Health Survey national report, 1999.* St. Regis: First Nations and Inuit Regional Health Survey Steering Committee.

First Nations Centre, National Aboriginal Health Organization. (2005). *First Nations Regional Longitudinal Health Survey (RHS) 2002/03: Results for adults, youth, and children living in First Nations communities.* Ottawa: First Nations Centre. Online at www.naho.ca/firstnations/english/documents/RHS2002-03TechnicalReport_001.pdf.

Goddard, I. (1999). *Native languages and language families of North America.* Lincoln, NE: University of Nebraska Press.

Government of Ontario. (1994). *Aboriginal health policy—executive summary.* Toronto: Government of Ontario. Online at www.ahwsontario.ca/about/healthpolicy.html.

Harris, S., Gittelsohn, J., Hanley, A., Barnie, A., Wolever, T., Gao, J., et al. (1997). "The prevalence of NIDDM and associated risk factors in Native Canadians." *Diabetes Care, 20,* 185–187.

Harris, S., Perkins, B. & Whalen-Brough, E. (1996). "Non-insulin-dependent diabetes mellitus among First Nations children: A new entity among First Nations people of northwestern Ontario." *Canadian Family Physician, 42,* 869–876.

Health Canada. (2005). *Statistical profile on the health of First Nations in Canada.* Ottawa: Health Canada. Online at www.hc-sc.gc.ca/fnih-spni/pubs/gen/stats_profil_e.html.

Health Canada. (2007). *Canadian Community Health Survey, Cycle 2.2, Nutrition (2004)—income-related household food security in Canada.* Catalogue no. H164-42/2007E. Ottawa: Minister of Health, Office of Nutrition Policy and Promotion, Health Products and Food Branch.

Health Council of Canada. (2005). *The health status of Canada's First Nations, Métis, and Inuit people: A background paper to accompany health care renewal in Canada: Accelerating change.* Ottawa: Health Council of Canada. Online at healthcouncilcanada.ca/docs/papers/2005/BkgrdHealthyCdnsENG.pdf.

Hoekstra, P., Letcher, R., O'Hara, T., Backus, S., Solomon, K. & Muir, D. (2003). "Hydroxylated and methylsulfone-containing metabolites of polychlorinated biphenyls in the plasma and blubber of bowhead whales." *Environmental Toxicology and Chemistry, 11,* 2650–2658.

Horton, R. (2006). "Indigenous peoples: Time to act now for equity and health." *Lancet, 367,* 1705–1707.

Hull, J. (2006). *Aboriginal women: A profile from the 2001 census.* Prepared for Women's Issues and Gender Equality Directorate, Indian and Northern Affairs Canada. Online at www.ainc-inac.gc.ca/pr/pub/abw/index_e.html.

Hurley, M. (1999). *The Indian Act.* Ottawa: Parliamentary Research Branch. Online at dsp-psd.pwgsc.gc.ca/Collection-R/LoPBdP/EB/prb9923-e.htm.

Hurley, M. & Wherrett, J. (2000). *The report of the Royal Commission on Aboriginal Peoples.* Ottawa: Parliamentary Research Branch. Online at www.parl.gc.ca/information/library/PRBpubs/prb9924-e.htm.

International Symposium on the Social Determinants of Indigenous Health. (2007). *Social determinants and Indigenous health: The international experience and its policy implications.* In report on specially prepared document, presentations, and discussion at the International Symposium on the Social Determinants of Indigenous Health, Adelaide, Australia. Online at www.who.int/social_determinants/resources/indigenous_health_adelaide_report_07.pdf.

Inuit Tapirisat of Canada (2000). *We are the Inuit* (brochure). Ottawa: Inuit Tapirisat of Canada.

Inuit Tapirit Kanatami. (2007). *Backgrounder: Inuit suicide prevention.* Ottawa: Inuit Tapirit Kanatami. Online at www.itk.ca/media/backgrounder-suicide_prevention.php.

Inuit Tapirit Kanatami & Inuit Circumpolar Council (Canada). (2007). *Building Inuit Nunaat: The Inuit action plan.* Ottawa: ITK. Online at www.itk.ca/publications/20070129-en-inuit-action-plan_Web.pdf.

Kinghorn, A., Solomon, P. & Chan, H. (2007). "Temporal and spatial trends of mercury in fish collected in the English-Wabigoon river system in Ontario, Canada." *Science of the Total Environment, 372*(2–3), 615–623.

Kirmayer, L., Brass, G. & Tait, C. (2000). "The mental health of Aboriginal peoples: Transformations of identity and community." *The Canadian Journal of Psychiatry, 45*(7), 607–616.

Kovesi, T., Gilbert, N., Stocco, C., Fugler, D., Dales, R., Guay, M. & Miller, D. (2007). "Indoor air quality and the risk of lower respiratory tract infections in young Canadian Inuit children." *Canadian Medical Association Journal, 177*(2), 155–160.

Lawn, J. & Harvey, D. (2001). *Change in nutrition and food security in two Inuit communities, 1992 to 1997.* Catalogue no. R2-177/1997E. Ottawa: Minister of Indian Affairs and Northern Development.

Lawn, J. & Harvey, D. (2004). *Nutrition and food security in Fort Severn, Ontario Baseline survey for the Food Mail Pilot Project.* Catalogue no. R2-350/2004E-PDF. Ottawa: Minister of Indian Affairs and Northern Development.

Lawrence, B. (1999). "Real Indians and others mixed-race urban Native people, the Indian Act, and the rebuilding of Indigenous nations." PhD dissertation, University of Toronto.

Locust, C. (1999). "Overview of health programs for Canadian Aboriginal Peoples." In J. Galloway, B. Goldberg & J. Alpert (Eds.), *Primary care of Native American patients* (pp. 17–21). Woburn: Butterworth.

Luo, Z.C., Kierans, W.J., Wilkins, R., Liston, R.M., Uh, S. & Kramer, M. (2004). "Infant mortality among First Nations versus non-First Nations in British Columbia: Temporal trends in rural versus urban areas, 1981–2000." *International Journal of Epidemiology, 33*(6), 1252–1259.

Luo, Z.C., Wilkins, R., Platt, R. & Kramer, S. (2004). "Risk of adverse pregnancy outcomes among Inuit and North American Indian women in Quebec, 1985–97." *Paediatric & Perinatal Epidemiology, 18*(1), 40–50.

Lutz, H., Hamilton, M. & Heimbecker, D. (Eds.). (2005). *Howard Adams: Otapaway! The life of a Métis leader in his own words and in those of his contemporaries.* Saskatoon: Gabriel Dumont Institute.

MacMillan, H., MacMillan, A., Offord, D. & Dingle, J. (1996). "Aboriginal health." *Canadian Medical Association Journal, 155*(11), 1569–1578.

Marmot, M. (2007). "Achieving health equity: From root causes to fair outcomes." *Lancet, 370,* 1153–1163.

McIntyre, L., Walsh, G. & Connor, S. (2001). *A follow-up study of child hunger in Canada.* Working Paper W-01-1-2E. Applied Research Branch, Strategic Policy. Ottawa: Human Resources Development Canada.

Morris, A. (1880). *The treaties of Canada with the Indians of Manitoba and the North-West Territories, including negotiations on which they were based, and other information relating thereto.* Totonto: Belford & Clarke. Online at www.saskatchewanfiles.com/Treaty6.html.

Office of the Auditor General of Canada. (2005). *Report of the Commissioner of the Environment and Sustainable Development to the House of Commons—Chapter 5—First Nations drinking water.* Ottawa: Minister of Public Works and Government Services Canada.

Office of the High Commissioner for Human Rights. (1995). *The Rights of Indigenous Peoples.* Fact Sheet no. 9 (Rev. 1). Geneva: United Nations. Online at www.unhchr.ch/html/menu6/2/fs9.htm.

Ontario Ministry of Health. (1994). *New directions: Aboriginal health policy for Ontario.* Toronto: Ontario Ministry of Health.

Orr, P., Mcdonald, S., Milley, D. & Brown, R. (2001). "Bronchiolitis in Inuit children from a Canadian central Arctic community, 1995–1996." *International Journal of Circumpolar Health, 60*(4), 649–658.

Parliament of Canada. (1876). "Indian Act, 1876." In *Report of the Royal Commission on Aboriginal Affairs.* Indian and Northern Affairs CanadaOnline at www.ainc-inac.gc.ca/ch/rcap/sg/sg17_e.html.

Power, E. (2007). *Food security for First Nations and Inuit in Canada.* Background Paper. Ottawa: First Nations and Inuit Health Branch, Health Canada.

Public Health Agency of Canada. (2006). *HIV and AIDS in Canada: Surveillance report to June 30th 2006.* Ottawa: Surveillance and Risk Assessment Division, Centre for Infectious Disease Prevention and Control, Public Health Agency of Canada.

Public Health Agency of Canada. (2007). *Life and breath: Respiratory disease in Canada.* Ottawa: Ministry of Health.

Royal Commission on Aboriginal Peoples. (1996a). *People to people, nation to nation: Highlights from the Report of the Royal Commission on Aboriginal Peoples.* Ottawa: Ministry of Supply and Services Canada.

Royal Commission on Aboriginal Peoples. (1996b). *Report of the Royal Commission on Aboriginal Peoples.* Ottawa: Indian and Northern Affairs Canada.

Smylie, J. (2000). "A guide for health professionals working with Aboriginal peoples: The sociocultural context of Aboriginal peoples in Canada." *Journal of Society of Obstetricians and Gynecologists of Canada, 22*(12), 1070–1081.

Smylie, J. & Anderson, M. (2006). "Understanding the health of Indigenous peoples in Canada: Key methodologic and conceptual challenges." *Canadian Medical Association Journal, 175*(6), 602–605.

Smylie, J., Anderson, I., Ratima, M., Crengle, S. & Anderson, M. (2006). "Who is measuring and why? Indigenous health performance measurement systems in Canada, Australia, and New Zealand." The Lancet, 367, 2029–2031.

Statistics Canada. (2003a). *Aboriginal peoples of Canada, 2001 census-selected income characteristics (35), Aboriginal origin (14), age groups (6), and sex (3) for population for Canada, provinces, territories, and census metropolitan areas, 2001 census—20% sample data.* Catalogue no. 97F0011XCB2001055. Ottawa: Statistics Canada. Online at www.statcan.ca.

Statistics Canada. (2003b). *Aboriginal peoples of Canada, 2001 census-selected labour force characteristics (50), Aboriginal origin (14), age groups (5A), sex (3), and area or residence (7) for population 15 years and over, for Canada, provinces, and territories, 2001 census—20% sample data.* Catalogue no. 97F0011XCB2001052. Ottawa: Statistics Canada. Online at www.statcan.ca.

Statistics Canada. (2003c). *Aboriginal peoples of Canada, 2001 census-selected educational characteristics (29), Aboriginal origin (14), age groups (5A), sex (3), and area of residence (7) for population 15 years and over, for Canada provinces and territories, 2001 census—20% sample data.* Catalogue no. 97F0011XCB2001050. Online at www.statcan.ca.

Statistics Canada. (2003d). *Aboriginal peoples survey 2001—Initial findings: Well-being of the non-reserve Aboriginal population.* Catalogue no. 89-589-XIE. Ottawa: Statistics Canada.

Statistics Canada. (2008). *Aboriginal peoples in Canada in 2006: Inuit, Métis, and First Nations, 2006 census.* Catalogue no. 7-558-XIE. Ottawa: Ministry of Industry.

Trovato, F. (2000). "Canadian Indian mortality during the 1980s." *Social Biology, 47*(1), 135–145.

United Nations General Assembly. (2007). *United Nations declaration on the rights of Indigenous peoples.* Geneva: United Nations. Online at www.iwgia.org/graphics/Synkron-Library/Documents/InternationalProcesses/DraftDeclaration/07-09-13ResolutiontextDeclaration.pdf.

Wieman, C.A. (1999). "Return to Native roots: Aboriginal health building informed partnerships." Paper presented at The Society of Obstetricians and Gynaecologists of Canada 55th Annual Clinical Meeting, Montreal, June 25–29.

Wilkins, R., Uppal, S., Finès, P., Senécal, S., Guimond, E. & Dion, R. (2008). *Life expectancy in the Inuit-inhabited areas of Canada, 1989 to 2003.* Ottawa: Statistics Canada. Online at www.statcan.ca/english/freepub/82-003-XIE/2008001/article/10463-en.htm.

World Health Organization. (2007). *Commission on the Social Determinants of Health- Achieving Health Equity: From root causes to fair outcomes. Interim statement.* Geneva: World Health Organization.

Young, T. (1996). "Obesity among Aboriginal peoples in North America: Epidemiological patterns, risk factors, and metabolic consequences." In A. Angel, H. Anderson, C. Bouchard, D. Lau, L. Leiter & R. Mendelson (Eds.), *Progress in obesity research 7* (pp. 332–342). London: John Libby.

Young, T., Reading, J., Elias, B. & O'Neil, J. (2000). "Type 2 diabetes mellitus in Canada's First Nations: Status of an epidemic in progress." *CMAJ, 163*(5), 561–566.

Chapter 20

Adams, M. (2003). *Fire and ice: The United States, Canada, and the myth of converging values.* Toronto: Penguin Books Canada.

Albo, G., Langille, D. & Panitch, L. (1993). *A different kind of state: Popular power and democratic administration.* Toronto: Oxford University Press.

Broadbent, E. (Ed.). (2001). *Democratic equality: What went wrong?* Toronto: University of Toronto Press.

Brodie, J. & Jenson, J. (1988). *Crisis, challenge, and change: Party and class in Canada revisited.* Ottawa: Carleton University Press.

Campbell, B. (2007). *20 years later: Has free trade delivered on its promise?* Ottawa: Canadian Centre for Policy Alternatives.

Canada, Department of Finance. (2003). *Fiscal reference tables, October 2003.* Online at www.fin.gc.ca/frt/2003/frt03_e.pdf.

Centre for the Study of Living Standards. (2007). *Aggregate income and production trends.* Online at csls.ca/data/iptjue2007.pdf (based on Statistics Canada data).

Clarkson, S. (2002). *Uncle Sam and us: Globalization, neoconservatism, and the Canadian state.* Toronto: University of Toronto Press.

Crozier, M.J., Huntington, S.P. & Watanuki, J. (1975). *The crisis of democracy: Report on the governability of democracies to the Trilateral Commission.* New York: New York University Press.

Court, J. (2003). *Corporateering: How corporate power steals you personal freedom ... and what you can do about it.* New York: Tarcher/Putnam.

D'Aquino, T. & Dillon, J. (2008, February 6). *Building a Canadian environmental superpower: Strategic elements—testimony before the Standing Committee of Parliament on Environment and Sustainable Development regarding Bill C-377.* Ottawa: House of Commons.

D'Aquino, T.P. & Stewart- Patterson, D. (2001). *Northern edge: How Canadians can triumph in the global economy.* Toronto: Stoddart.

Dobbin, M. (2003a). *Paul Martin: CEO for Canada?* Toronto: Lorimer.

Dobbin, M. (2003b, November 9). "Paul Martin's mea culpa." *Winnipeg Free Press*, B4.

Frank, T. (2000). *One market under God: Extreme capitalism, market populism, and the end of economic democracy.* New York: Doubleday.

Glasbeek, H. (2002). *Wealth by stealth: Corporate crime, corporate law, and perversion of democracy.* Toronto: Between the Lines.

Grinspun, R. & Shamsie, Y. (2007). *Whose Canada? Continental integration, fortress North America, and the corporate agenda.* Ottawa: Canadian Centre for Policy Alternatives.

Harvey, D. (2005). *A brief history of neoliberalism.* Oxford & New York: Oxford University Press.

Hofrichter, R. (Ed.). (2003). *Health and social justice: Politics, ideology, and inequity in the distribution of disease.* San Francisco: Jossey-Bass.

Hurtig, M. (2003). *The vanishing country: Is it too late to save Canada?* Toronto: McClelland & Stewart.

Klein, N. (2007). *The shock doctrine: The rise of disaster capitalism.* Toronto: Alfred A. Knopf Canada.

Langille, D. (1987). "The Business Council on National Issues and the Canadian state." *Studies in Political Economy, 24*, 41–85.

Laxer, J. (1998). *The undeclared war: Class conflict in the age of cyber capitalism.* Toronto: Viking.

Mackenzie, H. (2007) *The great CEO pay race: Over before it begins.* Toronto: Canadian Centre for Policy Alternatives.

Marchak, P. (1991). *The integrated circus: The new right and the restructuring of global markets.* Montreal & Kingston: McGill-Queen's University Press.

McBride, S. (2001). *Paradigm shift: Globalization and the Canadian state.* Halifax: Fernwood.

McBride, S. & Shields, J. (1997). *Dismantling a nation: The transition to corporate rule in Canada.* Halifax: Fernwood.

McCann, T.C. (1986). *Taking reform seriously: Perspectives on public interest liberalism.* Ithaca: Cornell University Press.

McQuaig, L. (2002). *All you can eat: Greed, lust, and the new capitalism.* Toronto: Penguin Viking.

Model, D. (2003). *Corporate rule: Understanding and challenging the new world order.* Montreal: Black Rose.

Montbiot, G. (2000). *Captive state: The corporate takeover of Britain*. London: Macmillan.

Moscovitch, A. & Albert, J. (Eds.). (1987). *The benevolent state: The growth of welfare in Canada*. Toronto: Garamond.

Navarro, V. & Shi, L. (2003). "The political context of social inequalities and health." In Richard Hofrichter (Ed.), *Health and social justice: Politics, ideology, and inequity in the distribution of disease* (pp. 195–216). San Francisco: Jossey-Bass.

Panitch, L. & Leys, C. (2003). *The new imperial challenge*. Halifax: Fernwood.

Phillips, K. (2002). *Wealth and democracy: A political history of the American rich*. New York: Broadway.

Raphael, D. (2007). *Poverty and policy in Canada: Implications for health and quality of life*. Toronto: Canadian Scholars' Press Inc.

Stanford, J. (1999). *Paper boom: Why real prosperity requires a new approach to Canada's economy*. Toronto: Canadian Centre for Policy Alternatives and James Lorimer.

Teeple, G. (2000). *Globalization and the decline of social reform: Into the twenty-first century*. Aurora: Garamond Press.

Yalnizyan, A. (2007). *The rich and the rest of us: The changing face of Canada's growing gap*. Toronto: Canadian Centre for Policy Alternatives.

Chapter 21

Ali, A., Massaquoi, N. & Brown, M. (2003). "Racial discrimination as a health risk for female youth: Implications for policy and health care delivery in Canada." *Directions: Research Reviews from the Canadian Race Relations Foundation, 1*(2), 12–21.

American Psychiatric Association. (2004). *Diagnostic and statistical manual of mental disorders, Fourth Edition, Text Revision (DSM-IV-TR)*. Arlington, VA: American Psychiatric Association.

Ball, J. & Elixhauser, A. (1996). "Treatment differences between Blacks and Whites with colorectal cancer." *Medical Care, 34*, 970–984.

Bella, L. & Yetman, L. (2000). *Challenging heterosexism: Towards non-heterosexist policy and regulation in health and social security agencies*. Halifax: Maritime Center for Excellence in Women's Health.

Bonde, J. P. (2008). "Psychosocial factors at work and risk of depression: A systematic review of the epidemiological evidence." *Occupational and Environmental Medicine, 65*, 438–445.

Breen, N., Wesley, M., Merril, R. & Johnson, K. (1999). "The relationship of socioeconomic status and access to minimum expected therapy among female breast cancer patients in the Black-White Cancer Survival Study." *Ethnicity and Disease, 9*, 111–125.

Brooks, S.E., Chen, T.T., Ghosh, A., Mullen, C.D., Gardner, J.F. & Bacquet, C.R. (2000). "Cervical cancer outcomes analysis: Impact of age, race, and co-morbid illness on hospitalizations for co-morbid cancer of the cervix." *Gynecologic Oncology, 79*, 107–115.

Brown, D.R., Keith, V.M., Jackson, J.S. & Gary, L. (2003). "(Dis)respected and (dis)regarded: Experiences of racism and psychological distress." In D.R. Brown & V.M. Keith (Eds.), *In and out of our right minds: The mental health of African-American women* (pp. 83–98). New York: Columbia University Press.

Canadian Council on Social Development. (2007). *Poverty statistics*. Ottawa: Canadian Council on Social Development.

Canadian Health Services Research Foundation (CHSRF). (2007). *Networks*. Online at www.chsrf.ca/knowledge_transfer/networks_e.php.

Canadian Institute for Health Information. (2004). *Improving the health of Canadians*. Ottawa: Canadian Institute for Health Information.

Canadian Institute for Health Information. (2006). *How healthy are rural Canadians? An assessment of their health status and health determinants*. Ottawa: . Canadian Institute for Health Information.

Canadian Medical Association. (2007). "Responding to the Globe." *Canadian Medical Association Journal, 177*(6), 685.

Canadian Nurses Association. (2006). *Social justice: A means to an end and an end in itself.* Online at cna-aiic. ca/CNA/documents/pdf/publications/Social_Justice_e.pdf.

Canadian Population Health Institute. (2004). *Improving the health of Canadians: Aboriginal peoples health.* Ottawa: Canadian Population Health Institute. Online at secure.cihi.ca/cihiweb/dispPage.jsp?cw_page=media_ 25feb2004_2_e#report.

Canadian Population Health Institute. (2006). *How healthy are rural Canadians? An assessment of their health status and determinants of health.* Ottawa: Canadian Population Health Institute. Online at secure.cihi.ca/cihiweb/ products/summary_rural_canadians_2006_e.pdf.

Clancy, C., Adshead, F., Laurell, A.C. & Carlson, I.N. (2005). "Spreading the health: Government's role in addressing health disparities." In M. Drexler, *Health disparities and the body politic* (pp. 11–23). Boston: Harvard School of Public Health.

Cole, L. & Foster, S. (2000). *From the ground up: Environmental racism and the rise of the environmental justice movement.* New York: New York University Press.

Cooper, G., Yuan, Z. & Rimm, A. (2000). "Patterns of endoscopic follow-up after surgery for non-metastatic colorectal cancer." *Gastrointestinal Endoscopy, 52*, 33–38.

Curtis, L.J. & MacMinn, W.J. (2007). *Health care utilization in Canada: 25 years of evidence.* Social and Economic Dimensions of an Aging Population (SEDAP) Research Paper no. 190. Hamilton: McMaster University.

Davies, H.T.O, Washington, A.E. & Bindman, A.B. (2002). "Health care report cards: Implications for vulnerable patient groups and the organizations providing them care." *Journal of Health Politics, Policy, & Law, 27*(3), 379–399.

Dei, S.G. & Calliste, A. (2000). "Mapping the terrain: Power, knowledge, and anti-racism education." In George Dei & Agnes Calliste (Eds.), *Anti-racist feminism: Critical race and gender studies* (pp. 11–40). Halifax: Fernwood Publishing.

Earle, C., Venditti, L., Neuman, P., Gelber, R., Weinstein, M., Potosky, A., et al. (2000). "Who gets chemotherapy for metastatic lung cancer?" *Chest, 117*, 1239–1246.

Edwards, J.M. & Buescher, P.A. (2002). *Cervical cancer disparities between African American women and White women in North Carolina 1995–1998.* Raleigh, NC: State Center for Health Statistics, North Carolina Deprtment of Health and Human Services.

Edwards, M. (2004). *Civil society.* Cambridge: Polity Press.

Enang [Etowa], J. (2001). *Black women's health: A synthesis of health research relevant to Black Nova Scotians.* Online at www.acewh.dal.ca/eng/reports/BWHNFinal.pdf.

Etowa, J., Keddy, B., Egbeyemi, J. & Eghan, F. (2007). "Depression: The 'invisible grey fog': Influencing the mental health of African-Canadian women." *International Journal of Mental Health Nursing, 16*, 213–223.

Etowa, J., Weins, J., Bernard. W.T. & Clow, B. (2007). "Determinants of Black women's health in rural and remote communities." *Canadian Journal of Nursing Research, 39*(3), 56–76

Galabuzi, G.E. (2006). *Canada's economic apartheid: The social exclusion of racialized groups in the new century.* Canadian Scholars' Press Inc.

Gilson, L., Doherty, J., Loewenson, R. & Francis, V. (2007). *Challenging inequity through health systems: Final report, knowledge network on health systems.* Geneva: The World Health Organization Commission on the Social Determinants of Health.

Graham, H. & Kelly, M. (2006). *Mapping the public policy landscape: Developing the evidence base for tackling health inequalities and differential effects.* London: Economic and Social Research Council.

Gruskin, S., Mills, E.J. & Tarantala, D. (2007). "Health and human rights I: History, principles, and practice of health and human rights." *Lancet, 370*, 449–455.

Hall, J.J. & Taylor, R. (2003). "Health for all beyond 2000: The demise of the Alma-Ata Declaration and primary health care in developing countries." *Medical Journal of Australia, 178*, 17–20.

Hayward, K. & Colman, R. (2003). *The tides of change: Addressing inequality and chronic disease in Atlantic Canada*. Halifax: Population and Public Health Branch, Health Canada.

Health Canada. (2003). *A statistical profile of the health of First Nations in Canada*. Ottawa: Health Canada.

Health Canada. (2005). *Canada's health care system*. Ottawa: Health Canada.

Health Canada. (2008). *Health care system delivery*. Ottawa: Health Canada. Online at www.hc-sc.gc.ca/hcs-sss/delivery-prestation/index-eng.php.

Holley, H.L. (1998). "Geography and mental health: A review." *Social Psychiatry and Psychiatric Epidemiology, 33*, 535–542.

Illich, I. (1976). *Limits to medicine, medical nemesis: The expropriation of health*. Middlesex: Penguin Books.

Isaacs, S., Keogh, S., Menard, C., & Hockin, J. (2000). "Suicide in the Northwest Territories: A descriptive review." *Chronic Diseases in Canada, 19*(4). Online at www.phac-aspc.gc.ca/publicat/cdic-mcc/19-4/index.html

James, C. (2003). *Seeing ourselves: Exploring race, ethnicity and culture*. Toronto: Thompson Educational Publishing.

Kisley, S., Smith, M., Laurence, D. & Maaten, S. (2005). "Mortality in individuals who have had psychiatric treatment: Population-based study in Nova Scotia." *The British Journal of Psychiatry, 187*, 552–558.

Krieger, N. (2005). "Introduction." In M. Drexler (Ed.), Health disparities and the body politic (pp. 5–10). Cambridge: Harvard School of Public Health.

Krieger, N., Chen, J., Waterman, P., Soobader, M., Subramanian, S. & Carson, R. (2003). "Choosing area based socioeconomic measures to monitor social inequalities in low birth weight and childhood lead poisoning: The Public Health Disparities Geocoding Project." *Journal of Epidemiology Community Health, 57*(3), 186–199.

Labonte, R., Schrecker, T & Gupta, A.S. (2005). *Health for some: Death, disease, and disparity in a globalizing era*. Toronto: Centre for Social Justice.

McDaniel, S.A. & Chappell, N.L. (1999). "Health care in regression: Contradictions, tensions, and implications for Canadian seniors." *Canadian Public Policy, 25*(1), 1223–1232.

McGibbon, E. (2000). "The situated knowledge of helpers." In C. James (Ed.), *Experiencing difference* (pp. 185–200). Halifax: Fernwood Publishing.

McGibbon, E. & McPherson, C. (2006). "An application of interpretative pedagogy: The St. Francis Xavier University violence and health workshop." *Journal of Nursing Education, 45(*2), 81–85.

McIntosh, P. (1988). *White privilege: Unpacking the invisible knapsack*. Working Paper 189. Wellesley: Wellesley College Centre for Research on Women.

McIntyre, L., Wien, F., Rudderham, S., Etter, L., Moore, C., MacDonald, N. & Johnson, S. (2001). *An exploration of the stress experience of Mi'kmaq on-reserve female youth in Nova Scotia*. Halifax: Maritime Center of Excellence for Women's Health.

McPherson, C., Popp, J. & Lindstrom, R. (2006). "Re-examining the paradox of structure: A Child Health Network perspective." *Healthcare Papers, 7*(2), 46–52.

Medeiros, D.M., Seehaus, M., Elliot, J. & Melaney, A. (2004). "Providing mental health services for LGBT teens in a community adolescent health clinic." *Journal of Gay and Lesbian Psychotherapy, 8*(3/4), 83–95.

Mettlin, C., Murphy, G., Cunningham, M., & Menck, H. (1997). "The National Cancer Database Report on race, age, and region variations in prostate cancer treatment." *Cancer, 80*(7), 1261–1266.

Ministerial Advisory Council on Rural Health. (2002). *Rural health in rural hands: Strategic directions for rural, remote, northern, and Aboriginal communities*. Ottawa: Health Canada.

Morgan, S. (2006). "Pharmaceutical research and policy." *Research Spotlight* (August), 1. CIHR Institute of Health Services and Policy Research.

Morrison, L. & L'Heureux, J. (2001). "Suicide and gay/lesbian/bisexual youth: Implications for clinicians." *Journal of Adolescence, 24*, 39–49.

Mettlin, C., Murphy, G., Cunningham, M. & Menck, H. (1997). "The National Cancer Database Report on race, age, and region variations in prostate cancer treatment." *Cancer, 80*, 1261–1266.

Navarro, V. (2002). "Health and equity in the world in an era of globalization." In V. Navarro (Ed.). *The political economy of social inequalities: Consequences for health and quality of life.* (pp. 109–120). New York: Baywood Publishing Company Inc.

New Brunswick Human Development Council (NBHDC). (2007). *Child and family poverty report card: New Brunswick.* Saint John: NBHDC.

Nova Scotia Department of Health. (2005). *Cultural competence guide for primary health care professionals.* Halifax: Department of Health.

Ocean, C. (2005). *Policies of exclusion, poverty, and health: Stories from the front.* Duncan: WISE.

Oliver, M.N. & Muntaner, C. (2005). "Researching health inequities among African Americans: The imperative to understand social class." *International Journal of Health Services, 35*(3), 485–498.

Pratt, L., Fred, D., Crum, R., Armenan, H., Gallo, J. & Eaton, W. (1999). "Depression, psychotropic medications, and risk of myocardial infarction." *Circulation, 94*, 3123–3129.

Public Health Agency of Canada. (2006). *Backgrounder: Improving the health of Canada's Aboriginal people.* Ottawa: Health Canada.

Rachlis, M. (2004). *Prescription for excellence: How innovation is saving Canada's health care system.* Toronto: Harper Collins Publishers Ltd.

Raphael, D. & Bryant, T. (2006). "Public health concerns in Canada, the US, the UK, and Sweden." In D. Raphael, T. Bryant & M. Rioux (Eds.), *Staying alive: Critical perspectives on health, illness, and health care* (pp. 347–372). Toronto: Canadian Scholars' Press Inc.

Shaw, M., Dorling, D., Gordon, D. & Smith, G.D. (1999). *The widening gap: Health inequalities and policy in Britain.* Bristol: The Policy Press.

Schrag, D., Cramer, L., Bach, P. & Begg, C. (2001). "Age and adjuvant chemotherapy use after surgery for Stage III colon cancer." *Journal of the National Cancer Institute, 93*, 850–857.

Shelby, P. (1999). "Isolated and invisible: Gay, lesbian, and bisexual youth." *The Canadian Nurse, 95*(4), 34.

Skocpol, T. (2003). *Diminished democracy: From membership to management in America life.* Oklahoma City: University of Oklahoma Press.

Smith, D.B. (1998). "Addressing racial inequalities in health care: Civil rights monitoring and reports cards." *Journal of Health Politics, Policy, and Law, 23*(1), 75–105.

Smith, D.B. (2005a). "Racial and ethnic health disparities and the unfinished civil rights agenda." *Health Affairs, 24*(2), 317–325.

Smith, D.B. (2005b). *Eliminating disparities in treatment and the struggle to end segregation.* New York: The Commonwealth Fund. Online at www.commonwealthfund.org/.

Smith, R.A., Cokkinides, V. & Harmon, J. (2005). "American Cancer Society guidelines for the early detection of cancer." *Cancer Journal Clinics, 55*, 31–44.

Statistics Canada. (2001). *Aboriginal Peoples' Survey, Canadian Community Health Survey,* 2000/2001. Ottawa: Statistics Canada.

Statistics Canada. (2005). *Women in Canada: A gender-based statistical report* (5th ed.). Ottawa: The Minister of Industry.

Statistics Canada. (2006). *Immigrant labour market outcomes, selected age-sex groups.* Online at www.statcan. ca/english/freepub/71-606-XIE/2007001/findings/age-en.htm.

Stoppard, J.M. (2000). *Understanding depression: Feminist social constructionist approaches.* London: Routledge.

Stout, M.D. & Kipling, G.D. (1998). *Aboriginal women in Canada: Strategic directions for policy development.* Ottawa: Status of Women Policy Research Fund.

UNICEF. (2005). *Child poverty in rich countries*. Florence: UNICEF Innocenti Research Center.

United Nations Committee on the Rights of the Child (CRC). (2003). *Convention on the rights of the child*, 33rd Session, May 19–June 6, General Comment 4. UN Document. CRC/GC/2003/4.

United Nations General Assembly. (1979). *Convention on the elimination of all forms of discrimination against women,* December 18, resolution 34/80.

United Nations General Assembly. (1989). *International covenant on the rights of the child*, December 12, UN Doc. A/RES/44/25.

United Nations General Assembly. (1996). *International covenant on economic, social, and cultural rights,* 21st Session, resolution 2200A/21, UN Doc. A/6316.

Vilshanskaya, O. & Stride, V. (2003). *Four steps towards equity: A tool for health promotion practice.* Online at mhcs.health.nsw.gov.au/pubs/f/pdf/4-steps-towards-equity.pdf.

Walks, R.A. & Bourne, L.S. (2006). "Ghettos in Canada's cities? Racial segregation, ethnic enclaves, and poverty concentration in Canadian urban areas." *The Canadian Geographer, 50*(3), 273–297.

Wilkinson, R., & Marmot, M. (Eds.). (2003). *Social determinants of health: The solid facts.* Copenhagen: World Health Organization.

Williams, R.F.G. & Collins, P. (2001). "Racial residential segregation: A fundamental cause of racial disparities in health." *Public Health Reports, 116*, 404–416.

Williams, R.F.G. & Doessel, D.P. (2006). "Measuring inequality: Tools and illustration." *International Journal for Health Equity, 5*(5). Online at www.equityhealthj.com/content/5/1/5.

World Health Organization. (2005). *Commission on the social determinants of health meeting report*, August. Geneva: World Health Organization.

World Health Organization. (2006a). *Gender and women's mental health.* Geneva: WHO.

World Health Organization. (2006b). *Meeting report: The first meeting of the commission on the social determinants of health regional civil society facilitators.* Geneva: WHO.

Zola, E. (1974). "Medicine as an institution of social control." In J. Ehrenreich (Ed.), *The cultural crisis of modern medicine* (pp. 80–89). New York: Monthly Review Press.

Chapter 22

Baker, M. (1997). *The restructuring of the Canadian welfare state: Ideology and policy.* SPRC Discussion Paper no. 77. Sydney, Australia: Social Policy Research Centre.

Baldwin, D.A. (Ed.). (1993). *Neorealism and neoliberalism: The contemporary debate.* New York: Columbia University Press.

Banting, K. (1987). *The welfare state and Canadian federalism* (2nd ed.). Montreal: McGill-Queen's University Press.

Banting, K. (2005). "Canada: Nation-building in a federal welfare state." In Herbert Obinger, Stephan Liebfried & Francis G. Castles (Eds.), *Federalism and the welfare state: New world and European experiences* (pp. 89–137). Cambridge: Cambridge University Press.

Barber, B. (1984). *Strong democracy: Participatory politics for a new age.* Boston: Little & Brown.

Barrow, C.W. (1993). *Critical theories of the state: Marxist, neo-Marxist, post-Marxist.* Madison: University of Wisconsin Press.

Bernstein, R.J. (1983). *Beyond objectivism and relativism: Science, hermeneutics, and praxis.* Philadelphia: University of Pennsylvania Press.

Bobrow, D.B. & Dryzek, J.S. (1987). *Policy analysis by design.* Pittsburgh: University of Pittsburgh Press.

Bremmer, I. & Taras, R. (Eds.). (1997). *New states, new politics: Building the post-Soviet nations.* Cambridge: Cambridge University Press.

Brooks, S. & Miljan, L. (2003). *Public policy in Canada: An Introduction* (4th ed.). Oxford: Oxford University Press.

Buonanno, L., Zablotney, S. & Keefer, R. (2001). *Politics versus science in the making of new regulatory regime for food in Europe.* Online at eiop.or.at/eiop/texte/2001-012a.htm.

Caldwell, L.K. (1990). *Between two worlds: Science, the environmental movement, and policy choice.* New York: Cambridge University Press.

Castaneda, J.G. (1994). *Utopia unarmed: The Latin American left after the Cold War.* New York: Vintage Books.

Commission on the Future of Health Care (2002). *Interim report.* Ottawa: Commission on the Future of Health Care.

Cook, T.E. & Morgan, P.M. (Eds.). (1971). *Participatory democracy.* San Francisco: Canfield Press.

Dahl, R.A. (1961). *Who governs? Democracy and power in an American city.* Yale Studies in Political Science, 4. New Haven: Yale University Press.

Dye, T.R. (1972). *Understanding public policy.* Upper Saddle River, NJ: Prentice-Hall, Inc.

Eckersley, R. (2004). *The green state: Rethinking democracy and sovereignty.* Cambridge: MIT University Press.

Ehrenfeld, D. (1981). *The arrogance of humanism* (2nd ed.). Oxford: Oxford University Press.

ESRC Global Environmental Change Program. (1999). *The politics of GM food: Risk, science, and public trust.* Special Briefing no. 5 ed. London: ESRC.

Fernandez Kilberto, A.E. (1993). "Chile: The laboratory experiment of international neo-Liberalism." In Henk Overbeek (Ed.), *Restructuring hegemony in the global political economy* (pp. 58–75). London: Routledge.

Fisher, Frank. (1990). *Technocracy and the politics of expertise.* London: Sage Publications.

Fisher, F. (1998). "Beyond empiricism: Policy inquiry in postpositivist perspective." *Policy Studies Journal, 26*(1), 129–146.

Fisher, F. & Forester, J. (Eds.). (1993). *The argumentative turn in policy analysis and planning.* Durham & London: Duke University Press.

Foucault, M. (1972). *The archeology of knowledge.* London: Tavistock.

Foucault, M. (1995). *Discipline and punish: The birth of the prison.* New York: Vintage Books.

Fukuyama, F. (1992). *The end of history and the last man.* London: Avon Books.

Gamble, A. (1988). *The free economy and the strong state: The politics of Thatcherism.* London: MacMillan.

Gill, S.R. (1993). "Neo-liberalism and the shift towards a US-centered transnational hegemony." In Henk Overbeek (Ed.), *Restructuring hegemony in the global political economy* (pp. 246–282). London: Routledge.

Hampson, F. O., with Daudelin, J., Hay, J. B., Martin, T. & Reid, H. (2002). *Madness in the multitude: Human security and world disorder.* Oxford: Oxford University Press.

Harnisch, A. (2002). "Multi-level governance beyond the nation state: The end of legitimate democratic politics." *The Bologna Center Journal of International Affairs* (Spring). Online at www.jhubc.it/bcjournal/archive/print/2002/globaldemocracy.pdf.

Held, D. (1989). *Political theory and the modern state: Essays on state, power, and democracy.* Stanford: Stanford University Press.

Hill, M. (2006). *Social policy in the modern world: A comparative text.* Malden: Blackwell Publishing.

Hooghe, L. & Marks, G. (2001). "Types of multi-level governance." *European Integration Online Papers, 5*(11). Online at papers.ssrn.com/sol3/papers.cfm?abstract_id=302786.

Howlett, M. & Ramesh, M. (2003). *Studying public policy: Policy cycles and policy Subsystems.* Oxford: Oxford University Press.

Jervis, R. (1999). "Realism, neoliberalism, and cooperation." *International Security, 24*(1) (Summer), 42–63.

Kramer, D.C. (1982). *Participatory democracy: Developing ideals of the political left.* Cambridge: Schenkman Publishing Co.

Kuehls, T. (1996). *Beyond sovereign territory.* Minneapolis: University of Minnesota Press.

Lasswell, H.D. (1951). "The policy orientation." In Daniel Lerner & Harold D. Lasswell (Eds.), *The policy sciences* (pp. 3–16). Stanford: Stanford University Press.

Lasswell, H. (1970). "The emerging conception of the policy sciences." *Policy Sciences, 1,* 3–14.

Laumann, E.O. (1987). *The organizational state: Social choice in national policy domains.* Madison: University of Wisconsin Press.

Mitchell, T. (1991). "The limits of the state: Beyond statist approaches and their critics." *American Political Science Review, 85,* 77–96.

Nederveen Pieterse, J. (2001). "Participatory democracy reconceived." *Futures, 33,* 407–422.

Neiman, M. & Stambough, S. (1998). "Rational choice theory and the evaluation of public policy." *Policy Studies Journal, 26*(3), 449–465.

Obinger, H., Leibfried, S. & Castles, F. (Eds) (2005). *Federalism and the welfare state: New world and European experiences.* Cambridge: Cambridge University Press.

Organisation for Economic Co-operation and Development. (2002). *OECD Health Data 2002.* Online at www.oecd.org/document/22/0,3343,en_2649_34487_1935190_119690_1_1_1,00.html.

Overbeek, H. & van der Pijl, K. (1993). "Restructuring capital and restructuring hegemony: Neo-liberalism and the unmaking of the post-war order." In Henk Overbeek & Kees van der Pijl (Eds.), *Restructuring hegemony in the global political economy* (pp. 1–27). London: Routledge.

Page, B. (1996). "The mass media as political actors." *PS: Political Science and Politics, 29,* 20–24.

Pal, L.A. (1997). *Beyond policy analysis: Public issue management in turbulent times.* Scarborough: ITP Nelson.

Parenti, M. (1993). *Inventing reality: The politics of news media.* New York: St. Martin's Press.

Pateman, C. (1980). "The civic culture: A philosophic critique." In Gabriel A. Almond & Sidney Verba (Eds.), *The civic culture revisited* (pp. 57–102). Boston: Little, Brown.

Peters, G.B. & Pierre, J. (2002). *Multi-level governance: A view from the garbage can.* Manchester Papers in Politics: EPRU Series.

Pontusson, J. (1995). "From comparative public policy to political economy: Putting political institutions in their place and taking interests seriously." *Comparative Political Studies, 28*(April), 117–147.

Powell, W. & DiMaggio, Pl. (Eds.). (1991). *The new institutionalism in organizational analysis.* Chicago: University of Press Chicago.

Radin, B. (2000). *Beyond Machiavelli: Policy analysis comes of age.* Washington, DC: Georgetown University Press.

Robertson, A. (1998). "Shifting discourses on health in Canada: From health promotion to population health." *Health Promotion International, 13*(2), 155–166.

Skocpol, T. (1985). "Bringing the state back in." In P. Evans et al. (Eds.), *Bringing the state back in* (pp. 3–43). Cambridge: Cambridge University Press.

Skocpol, T. (1989). "A society without a 'state'? Political organization, social conflict, and welfare provision in the United States." *Journal of Public Policy, 7*(4), 349–371.

Smith, A. (1776). *An inquiry into the nature and causes of the wealth of nations.* Edinburgh: Germain Gernier.

Stone, D. (1997). *Policy paradox: The art of political decision making* (2nd ed.). New York: W.W. Norton.

Strange, S. (1996). *The retreat of the state.* Cambridge: Cambridge University Press.

Telo, M. (Ed.). (2001). *European Union and new regionalism.* Aldershot: Ashgate.

Torgerson, D. (1986). "Between knowledge and politics: Three faces of policy analysis." *Policy Sciences, 19,* 33–59.

Vaillancourt, Y. (1988). *L'Evolution des politiques sociales au Québec, 1940–1960.* Montreal: Presses de l'Université de Montréal.

Weber, C. (1995). *Simulating sovereignty: Intervention, the state, and symbolic exchange.* Cambridge: Cambridge University Press.

Chapter 23

Anderson, R.A., et al. (1999). "7a-Merhyl-19Notestosterone (MENT) maintains sexual behavior and more in hypogonad men." *Journal of Clinical Endocrinology and Metabolism, 78*, 711–716.

Armstrong, P. & Jansen, I. (2003). *Assessing the impact of restructuring and work reorganization in long-term care.* Toronto: National Network on Environments and Women's Health.

Avison, W.R. (1998). "The health consequences of unemployment." In *Determinants of health: Adults and seniors*, vol. 2. of Papers commissioned by the National Forum on Health. Sainte-Foy, QC: Éditions MultiMondes.

Basen, G., Eichler, M. & Lippman, A. (Eds.). (1993). *Misconceptions: The social construction of choice and the new reproductive and genetic technologies.* Quebec: Voyageur.

Breen, M.J. (1998). "Promoting literacy, improving health." In National Forum on Health, *Determinants of health adults and seniors*, vol. 2. Ottawa: Éditions MultiMondes.

Canadian Institutes for Health Research. (CIHR). (2007). *Gender and sex-based analysis in health research: A guide for CIHR researchers and reviewers.* Online at www.cihr-irsc.gc.ca/e/32919.html.downloaded 30/12/2007.

Carver, V. & Ponée, C. (Eds.). (1995). *Women, work, and wellness.* Toronto: Addiction Research Foundation.

Cochrane, J. (1995). "Stress and the working woman." In Virginia Carver & Charles Ponée (Eds.), *Women, work, and wellness* (pp. 127–140). Toronto: Addiction Research Foundation.

Cohen, R. (2000). "'Mon is a stranger': The negative impact of immigration policies on the family life of Filipina domestic workers." *Canadian Ethnic Studies, 32*(3), 76–89.

Creese, G., Dyck, I. & McLaren, A. (2006). *The "flexible" immigrant: Household strategies and the labour market.* RIIM, Working Paper Series no. 06-19. Vancouver: Centre of Excellence.

Das Gupta, T. (1996). "Anti-Black racism in nursing in Ontario." *Studies in Political Economy, 51*(Fall), 97–116.

DesMeules, M. et al (2003). *Women's health surveillance report.* Ottawa: Public Health Agency of Canada. Online at www.phac-aspc.gc.ca/publicat/whsr-rssf/intro-eng.php.

Dion Stout, M., Kipling, G. & Stout, R. (2001). *Aboriginal women's health research synthesis project.* Online at www.cwhn.ca.

Doyal, L. (1995). *What makes women sick gender and the political economy of health.* New Brunswick: Rutgers University Press.

Doyal, L., Payne, S. & Cameron, A. (2003). *Promoting gender equality in health.* Manchester: Equal Opportunities Commission.

European Agency for Safety and Health at Work. (2003). *Gender issues in safety and health at work.* Luxembourg: European Agency for Safety and Health at Work.

Fausto-Sterling, A. (1985). *Myths of gender.* New York: Basic Books.

Fausto-Sterling, A. (2000). *Sexing the body: Gender, politics, and the construction of the body.* New York: Basic Books.

Foucault, M. (1978). *The history of sexuality, vol. 1: An introduction.* New York: Vintage.

Fowler, R.A., Sabur, N., Li, P., Juurlii, D.N., Pinto, R., Hladunewich, M.A., Adhikari, N.K.J., Sibbald, W.J. & Martin, C.M. (2007). "Sex-and age-based differences in the delivery and outcomes of critical care." *Canadian Medical Association Journal, 177*(December), 1513–1519.

Greaves, L. et al. (1999). *CIHR 2000: Sex, gender, and women's health.* Vancouver: BC Centre of Excellence for Women's Health, British Columbia Women's Hospital and Health Centre.

Greaves, L. & Richardson, L. A. (2007). "Tobacco use, women, gender, and chronic obstructive pulmonary disease: Are the connections being adequately made?" *The Proceedings of the American Thoracic Society, 4*, 675–679.

Guruge, S., Donner, G.L. & Morrison, L. (2000). "The impact of Canadian health care reform on recent immigrants and refugees." In D.L. Gustafson (Ed.), *Care and consequences: The impact of health care reform* (pp. 222–242). Halifax: Fernwood.

Doyal, L., Payne, S. & Cameron, A. (2003). *Promoting gender equality in health.* Manchester: Equal Opportunities Commission.

Health Canada. (1999). *Health Canada's women's health strategy.* Ottawa: Minister of Public Works and Government Services.

Health Canada. (2000). *Health Canada's gender-based analysis policy.* Ottawa: Minister of Health.

Health Canada. (2003). *Exploring concepts of gender and health.* Ottawa: Women's Health Bureau, Health Canada.

Hennessy, T. (2006). "CCPA launches major project to promote equality in Canada." *The CCPA Monitor, 13*(7) (December/January), 1, 6, 7.

Jackson, B., Pederson, A. & Boscoe, M. (2006). *Gender-based analysis and wait times: New questions, new knowledge.* Online at www.cwhn.ca.

Karasek, R.A. (1979). "Job demands, job decision latitude, and mental strain: Implications for job design." *Administrative Science Quarterly, 24*, 285–308.

Karasek, R.A. & Theorell, T. (1990). *Healthy work: Stress, productivity, and the reconstruction of working life.* New York: Basic Books.

Lakeman, L. (2006). "Linking violence and poverty in CASAC report." In A. Medovarski & B. Cranney (Eds.), *Canadian women's studies introductory reader* (pp. 380–389). Toronto: INANNA Publications.

Laroche, M. (2000). "Health status and health services utilization of Canadian immigrant and non-immigrant populations." *Canadian Public Policy, 26*(1), 51–75.

Lewis, S. (2005). *Race against time.* Toronto: House of Anansi.

Lips, H. (2007). *Sex and gender.* New York: McGraw-Hill.

Lock, M. (1998). "Menopause: Lessons from anthropology." *Psychosomatic Medicine, 60*, 410–419.

Marmot, M.G. (1986). "Social inequalities in mortality: The social environment." In R.G. Wilkinson (Ed.), *Class and health: Research and longitudinal data* (pp. 21–33). London: Tavistock.

Messing, K. (1998). *One-eyed science: Occupational health and women workers.* Philadelphia: University of Philadelphia Press.

Messing, K., Lippel, K., Demers, D. & Mergler, D. 2000. "Equality and difference in the workplace: Physical job demands , occupational illnesses, and sex differences." *National Women's Studies Association Journal, 12*(3), 21–49.

Mulvihill, M., Mailloux, L. & Atkin, W. (2002). *Advancing policy and research responses to immigrant women and refugee women's health in Canada.* Ottawa: Centres of Excellence for Women's Health.

National Forum on Health. (1998). *Determinants of health: Children and youth*, vol. 1 of Papers commissioned by the National Forum on Health. Sainte-Foy, QC: Éditions MultiMondes.

Neufeld, A., Harrison, M.J., Hughes, K., & Stewart, M. (2007). "Non-supportive interactions in the experience of women family caregivers." *Health and Social Care in the Community, 15*(6), 530–541.

Rose, S., Kamin, L. & Lewontin, R.C. (1984). *Not in our genes: Biology, ideology, and human nature.* New York: Penguin.

Rosenberg, H. (1990). "The home is the workplace." In Meg Luxton, Harriet Rosenberg & S. Arat-Kroc (Eds.), *Through the kitchen window* (pp. 37–61). Toronto: Garamond.

Sherwin, S. et al (1998). *The politics of women's health: Exploring agency and autonomy.* Philadelphia: Temple University Press.

Shields, M. (2006). "Stress, health, and the benefit of social support." *Health Reports, 15*(1) (January), 9–38.

Statistics Canada. (2006). *Women in Canada* (5th ed.). Ottawa: Ministry of Industry.

Status of Women Canada. (1995). *Setting the stage for the next century: The federal plan for gender equality.* Ottawa: Status of Women Canada.

Stellman, J.M. (1977). *Women's work, women's health.* New York: Pantheon.

Stellman, J.M. & Daum, S.M. (1973). *Work is dangerous to your health.* New York: Vintage.

United Nations (1995). *Fourth world conference on women action for equality, development and peace.* New York: United Nations.

Vosko, L. (2006). *Precarious employment: Understanding labour market insecurity in Canada.* Kingston: McGill-Queen's University Press.

Wilkinson, R.G. (1992). "Income distribution and life expectancy." *British Medical Journal, 304,* 165–168.

Wilkinson, R. (2005). *The impact of inequality.* London: New Press.

World Health Organization (2008). *Gender, sexual orientation, and behavioural genetics.* Online at www.who.int/genomics/gender/en/index2.html.

Chapter 24

Alesina, A. & Glaeser, E.L. (2004). *Fighting poverty in the US and Europe: A world of difference.* Toronto: Oxford University Press.

Atlantic Centre of Excellence for Women's Health. (2000). *Social and Economic Inclusion in Atlantic Canada.* Online at www.travelhealth.gc.ca/ph-sp/case_studies-etudes_cas/cs_atl-ec_atl/index-eng.php.

Bezruchka, S. (2006). "Epidemiological approaches." In D. Raphael, T. Bryant & M. Rioux (Eds.), *Staying alive: Critical perspectives on health, illness, and health care* (pp. 13–34). Toronto: Canadian Scholars' Press Inc.

Black, J. & Shillington, E.R. (2005). *Employment insurance: Research summary for the Task Force for Modernizing Income Security for Working Age Adults.* Toronto: Toronto City Summit Alliance.

Brooks, S. & Miljan, L. (2003). "Theories of public policy." In S. Brooks & L. Miljan (Eds.), *Public policy in Canada: An introduction* (pp. 22–49). Toronto: Oxford University Press.

Canadian Labour Congress. (2003). "Economy." *Economic Review and Outlook, 14*(2).

Canadian Population Health Initiative. (2002). *Canadian Population Health Initiative brief to the Commission on the Future of Health Care in Canada.* Online at secure.cihi.ca/cihiweb/en/downloads/cphi_policy_romanowbrief_e.pdf.

Coburn, D. (2000). "Income inequality, social cohesion, and the health status of populations: The role of neo-liberalism." *Social Science & Medicine, 51*(1), 135–146.

Coburn, D. (2004). "Beyond the income inequality hypothesis: Globalization, neo-liberalism, and health inequalities." *Social Science & Medicine, 58,* 41–56.

Coburn, D. (2006). "Health and health care: A political economy perspective." In D. Raphael, T. Bryant & M. Rioux (Eds.), *Staying alive: Critical perspectives on health, illness, and health care* (pp. 59–84). Toronto: Canadian Scholars' Press Inc.

Curry-Stevens, A. (2003). *When markets fail people.* Toronto: Centre for Social Justice Foundation for Research and Education.

Curry-Stevens, A. (2004). "Arrogant capitalism: Changing futures, changing lives." *Canadian Review of Social Policy, 52,* 158–164.

Curry-Stevens, A. (in press). "Building the case for the study of the middle class: Shifting our gaze from margins to center." *International Journal of Social Welfare.*

Ehrenreich, B. (2001). *Nickel and dimed: On (not) getting by in America.* New York: Metropolitan/Owl.

EKOS Research Associates. (2002). *Trust and confidence in federal government.* Online at www.cbc.ca/sunday/polls/oct27.pdf.

Esping-Andersen, G. (1985). *Politics against markets: The social democratic road to power.* Princeton: Princeton University Press.

Esping-Andersen, G. (1990). *The three worlds of welfare capitalism.* Princeton: Princeton University Press.

Esping-Andersen, G. (1999). *Social foundations of post-industrial economies.* New York: Oxford University Press.

Finnish Ministry of Social Affairs and Health. (1999). *Poverty and social exclusion.* Helsinki: Ministry of Social Affairs and Health.

Finnish Ministry of Social Affairs and Health. (2001). *National action plan against poverty and social exclusion.* Helsinki: Ministry of Social Affairs and Health.

Finnish Ministry of Social Affairs and Health. (2002). *Trends in social protection in Finland, 2002.* Helsinki: Ministry of Social Affairs in Finland.

Government of Sweden. (2005). *Sweden's report on measures to prevent poverty and social exclusion.* Stockholm: Government Offices of Sweden.

Hatfield, J. (2002). *Fortunate son: George W. Bush and the making of an American president.* New York: Soft Skull Press.

Hobgood, M. (2000). *Dismantling privilege: An ethics of accountability.* Cleveland: Pilgrim.

Hofrichter, R. (2003). "The politics of health inequities: Contested terrain." In R. Hofrichter (Ed.), *Health and social justice: A reader on ideology, and inequity in the distribution of disease* (pp. 1–56). San Francisco: Jossey Bass.

Hulchanski, D.J. (2002). *Can Canada afford to help cities, provide social housing, and end homelessness? Why are provincial governments doing so little?* Online at www.tdrc.net/2rept29.htm.

Lincoln, Y. & Guba, E. (1985). *Naturalist inquiry.* Newbury Park: Sage.

Mackenbach, J. & Bakker, M. (Eds.). (2002). *Reducing inequalities in health: A European perspective.* London: Routledge.

Mackenbach, J. & Bakker, M. (2003). "Tackling socioeconomic inequalities in health: Analysis of European experiences." *Lancet, 362,* 1409–1414.

McLaren, P. (2003). "Critical pedagogy: A look at the major concepts." In A. Darder (Ed.), *The critical pedagogy reader* (pp. 69–96). New York: Routledge Falmer.

McQuaig, L. (1987). *Behind closed doors: How the rich won control of Canada's tax system—and ended up richer.* Toronto: Viking.

McQuaig, L. (1993). *The wealthy banker's wife: The assault of equality in Canada.* Toronto: Penguin.

Moore, M. (2003). *Dude, where's my country?* New York: Warner.

Muntaner, C. (1999). "Teaching social inequalities in health: Barriers and opportunities." *Scandinavian Journal of Public Health, 27,* 161–165.

Murphy, B., Roberts, P. & Wolfson, M. (2007). "High-income Canadians." *Perspectives on Labour and Income, 8,* 1–13.

Myles, J. & Pierson, P. (1997). *Friedman's revenge: The reform of "liberal" welfare states in Canada and the United States.* Ottawa: Caledon Institute.

Navarro, V., Borrell, C., Benach, J., Muntaner, C., Quiroga, A., Rodrigues-Sanz, M., et al. (2004). "The importance of the political and the social in explaining mortality differentials among the countries of the OECD, 1950–1998." In V. Navarro (Ed.), *The political and social contexts of health.* Amityville: Baywood Press.

Nettleton, S. (1997). "Surveillance, health promotion, and the formation of a risk identity." In M. Sidell, L. Jones, J. Katz & A. Peberdy (Eds.), *Debates and dilemmas in promoting health* (pp. 314–324). London: Open University Press.

O'Neill, M., Pederson, A., Dupere, S. & Rootman, I. (Eds.). (2007). *Health promotion in Canada: Critical perspectives.* Toronto: Canadian Scholars' Press Inc.

Raphael, D. (1998). "Public health responses to health inequalities." *Canadian Journal of Public Health, 89,* 380–381.

Raphael, D. (2002). "Addressing health inequalities in Canada." *Leadership in Health Services, 15*(3), 1–8.

Raphael, D. (2003). "Barriers to addressing the determinants of health: Public health units and poverty in Ontario, Canada." *Health Promotion International, 18,* 397–405.

Raphael, D. (2006). "Social determinants of health: Present status, unresolved questions, and future directions." *International Journal of Health Services, 36*(4), 651–677.

Raphael, D. (2007a). "Poverty and the future of the Canadian welfare state." In D. Raphael (Ed.), *Poverty and policy in Canada: Implications for health and quality of life* (pp. 365–398). Toronto: Canadian Scholars' Press Inc.

Raphael, D. (2007b). "The politics of poverty." In D. Raphael (Ed.), *Poverty and policy in Canada: Implications for health and quality of life* (pp. 303–334). Toronto: Canadian Scholars' Press Inc.

Raphael, D. & Bryant, T. (2002). "The limitations of population health as a model for a new public health." *Health Promotion International, 17,* 189–199.

Raphael, D. & Bryant, T. (2006a). "Maintaining population health in a period of welfare state decline: Political economy as the missing dimension in health promotion theory and practice." *Promotion and Education, 13*(4), 236–242.

Raphael, D. & Bryant, T. (2006b). "The state's role in promoting population health: Public health concerns in Canada, USA, UK, and Sweden." *Health Policy, 78,* 39–55.

Raphael, D., Bryant, T. & Curry-Stevens, A. (2004). "Toronto Charter outlines future health policy directions for Canada and elsewhere." *Health Promotion International, 19,* 269–273.

Readers Digest Canada. (2003). *So, whom do we trust?* Online at www.readersdigest.ca/advertising/media-january03. html.

Saint-Arnaud, S. & Bernard, P. (2003). "Convergence or resilience? A hierarchial cluster analysis of the welfare regimes in advanced countries." *Current Sociology, 51*(5), 499–527.

Shaw, M., Dorling, D., Gordon, D., & Smith, G.D. (1999). *The widening gap: health inequalities and policy in Britain.* Bristol: The Policy Press.

Sauve, R. (2002). *The dreams and the reality: Assets, debts, and the net worth of Canadian households.* Ottawa: Vanier Institute for the Family.

Scarth, T. (Ed.). (2004). *Hell and high water: An assessment of Paul Martin's record and implications for the future.* Ottawa: Canadian Centre for Policy Alternatives.

Stanford, J. (2004). "Paul Martin, the deficit, and the debt: Taking another look." In T. Scarth (Ed.), *Hell and high water: An assessment of Paul Martin's record and implications for the future* (pp. 31–54). Ottawa: Canadian Centre for Policy Alternatives.

Statistics Canada. (2001). *The assets and debts of Canadians: An overview of the results of the survey of financial security.* Ottawa: Statistics Canada.

Swedish National Institute for Public Health. (2003). *Sweden's new public health policy.* Stockholm: Swedish National Institute for Public Health.

Tal, B. & Preston, L. (2005). *The end of home-made savings.* Toronto: CIBC World Markets.

Teeple, G. (2000). *Globalization and the decline of social reform: Into the twenty-first century.* Aurora: Garamond Press.

Tesh, S. (1990). *Hidden arguments: Political ideology and disease prevention policy.* New Brunswick: Rutgers University Press.

Travers, K.D. (1997). "Reducing inequities through participatory research and community empowerment." *Health Education and Behaviour, 24*(3), 344–356.

Vandenbroucke, F. (2002). "Foreword." In G. Esping-Andersen (Ed.), *Why we need a new welfare state* (pp. viii–xxvi). New York: Oxford University Press.

Wilson, J. (1983). "Positivism." In D. Wilson (Ed.), *Social theory* (pp. 11–18). Englewood Cliffs: Prentice Hall.

World Health Organization Regional Office for Europe. (1997). *Twenty steps for developing a Healthy Cities project.* Copenhagen: World Health Organization Regional Office for Europe.

World Health Organization Regional Office for Europe. (2003). *Healthy cities: Books and published technical documents.* Copenhagen: World Health Organization.

Wright, E.O. (1994). "The class analysis of poverty." In E.O. Wright (Ed.), *Interrogating inequality* (pp. 32–50). New York: Verso.

Zweig, M. (2000). *The working class majority: America's best-kept secret.* Ithaca: Cornell University Press.

Contributors' Biographies

Carolyne Alix is a MSc-educated demographer and researcher at the Quebec Public Health Institute. Her research covers general population health, particularly social inequalities in health.

Pat Armstrong is a professor in Sociology and Women's Studies at York University. She holds a CHSRF/CIHR chair in Health Services and chairs Women and Health Care Reform, a group funded under Health Canada's Women's Health Contribution Programme.

Nathalie Auger is a physician-epidemiologist specializing in community medicine at the Quebec Public Health Institute and is affiliated with the Department of Social and Preventive Medicine, University of Montreal. Dr. Auger's research focuses on perinatal health epidemiology, gender equity, social inequalities in health, neighbourhood influences on health, and tobacco marketing to youth.

Toba Bryant is an assistant professor of Sociology at York University. Dr. Bryant's PhD from the University of Toronto examined the policy change process through case studies of health care and housing policy development during the Common Sense Revolution in Ontario. She is the co-editor of *Staying Alive: Critical Perspectives on Health, Illness, and Health Care* and author of *Introduction to Health Policy*, both published by Canadian Scholars' Press Inc. She is currently a co-investigator of a CIHR-funded study of globalization and health and a SSHRC-funded study of the incidence and management of type 2 diabetes among vulnerable populations.

Tracey Burns is a research and policy analyst in the Education Directorate of the Organisation for Economic Co-operation and Development in Paris. She works on issues of knowledge management, evidence-based policy research in education, and social inclusion. She holds a PhD (Northeastern University) in Experimental Psychology with a specialty in early language acquisition.

Fernando Cartwright is principal research scientist for the Canadian Council on Learning in Ottawa. He is the architect of the Composite Learning Index, an index of the state of learning in Canada, which draws upon a variety of data sources and methodologies, including geographic information systems and multivariate modelling.

Ann Curry-Stevens is an assistant professor in the Graduate School of Social Work at Portland State University in Oregon. She was co-director of management and research at the Centre for Social Justice from 1999–2001 and lead researcher and author of the Centre for Social Justice's third annual update on inequality in Canada, *When Markets Fail People*. Ann's work with the social determinants of health began at the start of her career in social work in 1983 as she began to connect the dots regarding inequality, racism, and poverty and troubling youth behaviour. Her speciality became transformative education, helping others to see through the status quo and into the asymmetries of power and privilege that so define life experiences and outcomes. In 2003, Ann published a collection of her best work in *An Educator's Guide for Changing the World,* available for downloading or ordering at www.socialjustice.org.

Janice Foley is an associate professor in the Faculty of Business Administration at the University of Regina. She earned a PhD in Organizational Behaviour (minor in Industrial Relations) from the Sauder School of Business at UBC. She assumed her first academic position at the University of Winnipeg in 1998 and moved to the University of Regina in 2000. Her research interests are concerned with globalization's impacts on organizations, including unions and employees; healthy workplaces; and quality of work life. Her current research interests include organized labour's response to globalization and changing workplace practices and their impact on employee health and work-life quality.

Martha Friendly is executive director of the Toronto-based Childcare Resource and Research Unit (CRRU). She has worked on early childhood education and care research since participating in one of the first evaluations of the American Head Start program in the 1960s. Established by Martha at the University of Toronto in the early 1980s, CRRU specializes in early childhood education and child-care policy and research. Martha has written many scholarly and popular publications on early childhood education and care and works closely with community and advocacy groups, other researchers and government policy-makers, supporting formation of a universal system of early childhood education and child care. Born in New York City, Martha immigrated to Canada in 1971.

Grace-Edward Galabuzi is an associate professor at Ryerson University in the Department of Politics and Public Administration, and a research associate at the Centre for Social Justice in Toronto. He is the author of *Canada's Economic Apartheid: The Social Exclusion of Racialized Groups in the New Century,* published by Canadian Scholars' Press Inc. Dr. Galabuzi has worked in the Ontario government as a senior policy analyst on justice issues and is a former provincial coordinator of the Ontario Alliance for Employment Equity. He has been involved in many community campaigns regarding social justice issues such as anti-racism, anti-poverty, community development, human rights, education reform, anti-poverty, and police reform.

Lars K. Hallstrom is Canada research chair in Public Policy and Governance at St. Francis Xavier University, and an associate professor in the Department of Political Science. From 2005 to 2008 he served as principal investigator and acting director of the National Collaborating Centre for Determinants of Health hosted by St. Francis Xavier University. He is involved in a number of research and policy-relevant initiatives seeking to link the social, environmental, and health sciences closer together. A graduate of both the University of Calgary and Purdue University, he has published on topics ranging from political humour to environmental theory to European politics, but his current research focuses primarily on environmental risk and political participation in the public policy process.

Andrew Jackson is national director of Social and Economic Policy with the Canadian Labour Congress, where he has worked since 1989. He is also a research professor in the Institute of Political Economy at Carleton University, a research associate with the Canadian Centre for Policy Alternatives, and a fellow with the School of Policy Studies at Queen's University. Mr. Jackson's areas of interest include the labour market and the quality of jobs, income distribution and poverty, macroeconomic policy, social policy, and the impacts of globalization on workers. He has written numerous articles for popular and academic publications, and is the author of *Work and Labour in Canada: Critical Issues,* published by Canadian Scholars' Press Inc. in 2005. Andrew Jackson was educated at the London School of Economics (BSc [Econ]; MSc [Econ]), and at the University of British Columbia. Prior to joining the CLC, he worked for the then leader of the New Democratic Party, Ed Broadbent, and for the Canadian Labour and Business Centre.

Ronald Labonte is Canada research chair in Globalization and Health Equity, Institute of Population Health, and professor, Department of Epidemiology and Community Medicine, University of Ottawa. Recent books include:

From Local to Global Empowerment: Health Promotion in Action (with Glenn Laverack) (Palgrave-Macmillan, 2008); *Critical Public Health: A Reader* (with Judith Green) (Routledge, 2007); *Health for Some: Death, Disease, and Disparity in a Globalizing Era* (with Ted Schrecker and Amit Sen Gupta) (Centre for Social Justice, 2005); and *Fatal Indifference: The G8, Africa, and Global Health* (with Ted Schrecker, David Sanders, and Wilma Meeus) (University of Cape Town Press/IDRC Books, 2004).

David Langille teaches Health Policy at the University of Toronto. A political economist by training, his research and writing deals with the influence of transnational corporations on the Canadian state and the role of social movements in maintaining democracy. He is writing a book about the politics of global capitalism and the search for alternatives, and helping to produce a documentary about poverty reduction in Canada and in Europe. Founding director of the Centre for Social Justice, he is currently co-chair of the Ontario Coalition for Social Justice.

Elizabeth McGibbon is an associate professor at St. Francis Xavier University. She received her master's and doctoral degrees in Nursing Science at Dalhousie University (1999) and the University of Toronto (2004). Dr. McGibbon's research program focuses on critical social science applications to health issues and her paper presentations and publications focus on bringing a critical perspective to conventional health field knowledge. Her research grants include CIHR, CSHRF, and NHSRF-funded studies in the area of inequities in access to health services, gender and health, and racism and health. Her knowledge of health inequity and its impact on health outcomes of racialized and marginalized peoples is based on over 20 years of mental health clinical practice and working for change in large institutions and in the community. She is a founding member of the International Association for Qualitative Research, and currently sits as Canada's representative on the International Advisory Board. She was one of the lead authors in the successful proposal for the Public Health Agency of Canada's National Collaborating Center: Determinants of Health, 2006.

Lynn McIntyre is a professor in the Department of Community Health Sciences at the University of Calgary. She previously held an academic appointment at Dalhousie University in Nova Scotia. She holds both a medical degree and a master's degree in Community Health and Epidemiology and is a fellow of the Royal College of Physicians and Surgeons of Canada in Community Medicine. The focus of her research is hunger and food insecurity and she conducts studies both domestically and globally. Much of her research deals with how women and children experience food insecurity.

Michael Polanyi coordinates research, education, and advocacy on Canadian poverty and social justice issues at KAIROS: Canadian Ecumenical Justice Initiatives, based in Toronto. He has a PhD in Environmental Studies from York University. He was a researcher at the Institute for Work & Health in Toronto from 1995–2002, after which he joined the University of Regina as a faculty researcher with the Saskatchewan Population Health Research and Evaluation Unit and an assistant professor in the Faculty of Kinesiology and Health Studies. Over the past 15 years, he has coordinated community-based research and social action projects with students, low-income people, immigrants, refugees, injured workers, and people of faith.

Dennis Raphael is a professor in the School of Health Policy and Management at York University. His research is concerned with public policy and population health, income inequality and health, and the political economy of health. He is the author of *Poverty and Policy in Canada: Implications for Health and Quality of Life* and co-editor of *Staying Alive: Critical Perspectives on Health, Illness, and Health Care,* both published by Canadian Scholars' Press Inc. Dr. Raphael served on the Advisory Committee of the Public Health Agency's National Coordinating Centre on the Determinants of Health at St. Francis Xavier University in Antigonish, Nova Scotia, from 2006 to 2008.

Krista Rondeau holds the position of research associate in the Department of Community Health Sciences at the University of Calgary. She is a registered dietician, and is currently conducting research on food insecurity among post-secondary students for a master's degree in Health Promotion Studies.

Barbara Ronson, a former high school teacher and graduate of the doctoral program at OISE/UT, is an independent researcher, teacher, and consultant in health promotion and education. Since graduating from OISE/UT she has worked at the Centre for Health Promotion, Department of Public Health Sciences, University of Toronto, for seven years, Acadia University for two years, and Quantum Solutions Canada for four years. She is currently conducting research on Aboriginal health literacy at University of Toronto. At the Centre for Health Promotion where she was consultant and fellow, she handled special programs in literacy and health, child and youth health, and school and workplace health. She was also founding co-chair of the Ontario Healthy Schools Coalition, an active work group of the Ontario Public Health Association and the Centre for Health Promotion. The coalition now has over 200 members and has been playing an important role in education reform across the province.

Irving Rootman is the executive director of the Health and Learning Knowledge Centre at the University of Victoria and co-chair of the CPHA Expert Panel on Health Literacy. Most recently (2002–2007), he was a Michael Smith Foundation for Health Research distinguished scholar and professor in the Faculty of Human and Social Development at the University of Victoria. From 1990–2001, he was the first director of the Centre for Health Promotion at the University of Toronto. From 1973–1990, he was a researcher, research manager, and program manager for Health and Welfare Canada. He has been a technical adviser, consultant, and senior scientist for the World Health Organization and a former member of the Health Promotion and Disease Prevention Advisory Board and the Health Literacy Committee of the US Institute of Medicine and of the Canadian Minister of Health's Science Advisory Board. He has published widely in health promotion and co-authored and edited several books in health promotion, including the second edition of *Health Promotion in Canada*, published by Canadian Scholars' Press Inc. He is a recipient of R.F. Defries Award, the highest award of the Canadian Public Health Association. He received his PhD in Sociology from Yale University in 1970. His areas of expertise are literacy and health, health promotion, school health, evaluation, and participatory research.

Michael Shapcott is director of Community Engagement at the Wellesley Institute. Previously, he worked at the University of Toronto's Centre for Urban and Community Studies. He is co-editor, with Dr. David Hulchanski, of *Finding Room: Policy Options for a Canadian Rental Housing Strategy*. He has worked at the local, provincial, national, and international levels. He attended the Faculty of General Studies at the University of Calgary and the Faculty of Law at the University of Toronto, where he completed the Intensive Program in Poverty Law. In 2007, he completed studies on the Political Economy of Public Policy at the London School of Economics.

Peter Smith is a researcher at the Institute for Work & Health in Toronto. He has a PhD from the Institute of Medical Science at the University of Toronto. His major research interests are in the changing nature of work in Canada and other developed countries and their impact on the health of workers. In particular he is interested in how these changes affect particular subgroups of labour force participants (e.g., particular occupational groups, women, and recent immigrants).

Brenda L. Smith-Chant is an associate professor with the department of Psychology at Trent University. Her research interests include exploring the influence of social factors, such as language and education, on children's cognitive development. She teaches courses in the area of child development, the development of individuals with exceptionalities, and cognition and instruction (i.e., examining the interaction between instructional techniques and how information is processed by the brain). Currently, Brenda is working as a senior researcher with the Ministry of Children and Youth Services for the evaluation of Best Start, Ontario's initiative to support families and children in the early years.

Janet Smylie is a physician and research scientist at the Centre for Research on Inner City Health and associate professor in the Department of Public Health Sciences at the University of Toronto. Dr. Smylie completed her master's of Public Health at Johns Hopkins University. She has practised and taught family medicine in a variety of Aboriginal communities both urban and rural. She is a member of the Métis nation of Ontario, with Métis roots in Saskatchewan. She is the immediate past vice-president of the Indigenous Physicians Association in Canada. Her current research interests are focused in the area of Aboriginal health and include: health indicators of relevance to Aboriginal communities; interfacing Indigenous knowledge and Western science; and the health of young Aboriginal families.

Valerie Tarasuk is a professor in the Department of Nutritional Sciences at the University of Toronto. Much of her research focuses on problems of domestic food insecurity, considering their origins and nutrition implications, and examining current policy and program responses.

Emile Tompa holds a PhD in Economics from McMaster University. He is a labour and health economist with a background in aging and retirement issues. Dr. Tompa is a scientist at the Institute for Work & Health in Toronto, an adjunct assistant professor in the Department of Economics at McMaster University in Hamilton, and an adjunct assistant professor in the Department of Public Health Sciences at the University of Toronto. His current research agenda is centred on labour-market experiences and their health and human development consequences; insurance and regulatory mechanisms for occupational health and safety; and workplace interventions directed at improving the health of workers.

Diane-Gabrielle Tremblay is the Canada research chair the Socio-Organizational Challenges of the Knowledge Economy. She is professor and director of research at the Télé-université of the Université du Quebec à Montréal. She is president of the Committee on Sociology of Work of the International Sociological Association, member of the Executive Council of the Society for the Advancement of Socio-Economics. She is also president of the Political Economy Association of Quebec and editor of the electronic journal *Interventions économiques.* She has been invited professor at the University of Lille I, the University of Paris I, the Lyon Business School, the European School of Management, and the Université of Louvain-la-Neuve, in Belgium. Also co-chair of the Bell Canada Research Chair on Technology and work organization, she has published many articles and books on employment and types of employment, job training, innovation in the workplace and work organization, as well as work-life balance. See www.teluq.uquebec.ca/chaireecosavoir/cvdgt.

Charles Ungerleider, professor of the Sociology of Education at the University of British Columbia, is the director of research and knowledge mobilization for the Canadian Council on Learning. His most recent book, *Failing Our Kids: How We Are Ruining Our Public Schools*, was published by McClelland & Stewart in 2003.

COPYRIGHT ACKNOWLEDGEMENTS

Part 1 opening photo: © iStockphoto.com/Caitlin Cahill ist2_2885436_in_the_kitchen

Part 2 opening photo: © iStockphoto.com/Amanda Rohde ist2_1943264_right_for_the_position

Part 3 opening photo: © iStockphoto.com/Sean Locke ist2_3933447_off_to_school

Part 4 opening photo: © iStockphoto.com/Millanovic ist2_1897569_child_eating_3

Part 5 opening photo: © iStockphoto.com/Loretta Hostettler 2_4854842_motherly_love

Part 6 opening photo: © iStockphoto.com/Rosemarie Gearhart ist2_3600453_together

Figure 1.1: "Percentages of premature years of life lost (0–74 yrs) to Canadians in urban Canada due to various causes, 1996," adapted from the Statistics Canada publication *Health Reports—Supplement*, Catalogue 82-003, volume 13, *2002 Annual Report*, Chart 9, p. 54.

Table 1.1: M. Shields and S. Tremblay, "The Health of Canada's Communities," *Health Reports—Supplement* 13 (July 2002), p. 13.

Figure 1.2: "Percentage of income-related premature years of life lost (0–74 yrs) caused by specific diseases in urban Canada, 1996," adapted from the Statistics Canada publication *Health Reports—Supplement*, Catalogue 82-003, volume 13, *2002 Annual Report*, Chart 10, p. 54.

Table 1.2: D. Raphael, "A Society in Decline: The Social, Economic, and Political Determinants of Health Inequalities in the USA," in *Health and Social Justice: A Reader on Politics, Ideology, and Inequality in the Distribution of Disease*, ed. R. Hofrichter (San Francisco: Jossey Bass/Wiley, 2003), pp. 59–88. Reprinted with permission of the author.

Figure 2.1: M.G. Marmot and R.G. Wilkinson, *Social Determinants of Health*, 2nd edition. Copyright © 2005. By permission of Oxford University Press, Inc.

Figure 2.2: From M. Benzeval, A. Dilnot, K. Judge, and J. Taylor, "Income and Health over the Lifecourse: Evidence and Policy Implications," in *Understanding Health Inequalities*, ed. H. Graham (Berkshire, UK: Open University Press, 2001), p. 98. Reproduced with the kind permission of the Open University Press Publishing Company.

Figure 2.3: A. Steptoe, "Psychophysiological Bases of Disease," *Comprehensive Clinical Psychology*, vol. 8, *Health Psychology*, ed. D.W. Johnston and M. Johnston (1969): 39–78. Used by permission of Elsevier Books.

Figure 2.4: From E. Graham, M. MacLeod, D. Johnston, C. Dibben, I. Morgan, and S. Briscoe, "Individual Deprivation, Neighbourhood, and Recovery from Illness," in *Understanding Health Inequalities*, ed. H. Graham (Berkshire, UK: Open University Press, 2001), p. 177. Reproduced with the kind permission of the Open University Press Publishing Company.

Figure 2.5: From J. Lynch, "Income Inequality and Health: Expanding the Debate," *Social Science and Medicine* 51 (2000), p. 1003.

Figure 2.6: From D. Coburn, "Beyond the Income Inequality Hypothesis: Globalization, Neo-Liberalism, and Health Inequalities," *Social Science and Medicine* 58 (2004), p. 44.

Figure 3.1: Author's calculations based on data from Statistics Canada, "Survey of Labour & Income Dynamics and Survey on Consumer Finances Market," CANSIM Table # 202-0703.

Table 3.1: Data drawn from A. Yalnizyan, *The Growing Gap: A Report on Growing Inequality between the Rich and Poor in Canada* (Toronto: Centre for Social Justice, 1998), and A. Yalnizyan, *Canada's Great Divide: The Politics of the Growing Gap between Rich and Poor in the 1990s* (Toronto: Centre for Social Justice, 2000). Used with permission.

Table 3.2: A. Curry-Stevens, *When Markets Fail People: Exploring the Widening Gap between Rich and Poor in Canada* (Toronto: CSJ Foundation for Research and Education, 2001). Used with permission.

Figure 3.2: A. Yalnizyan, *The Growing Gap: A Report on Growing Inequality between the Rich and Poor in Canada* (Toronto: Centre for Social Justice, 1998). Used with permission.

Table 3.3: A. Curry-Stevens, *When Markets Fail People: Exploring the Widening Gap between Rich and Poor in Canada* (Toronto: CSJ Foundation for Research and Education, 2001). Used with permission.

Figure 3.3: Athor's calculations based on data from Statistics Canada, "Survey of Labour & Income Dynamics and Survey on Consumer Finances," CANSIM Table 202-0201.

Figure 3.4: A. Curry-Stevens, *When Markets Fail People: Exploring the Widening Gap between Rich and Poor in Canada* (Toronto: CSJ Foundation for Research and Education, 2001). Used with permission.

Table 3.4: A. Curry-Stevens, "Arrogant Capitalism: Changing Futures, Changing Lives," *Canadian Review of Social Policy* 51 (June 2003), pp. 137–142. Used with permission.

Table 3.5: K. Scott, "A Lost Decade: Income Inequality and the Health of Canadians," paper presented to the Social Determinants of Health across the Lifespan Conference, Toronto, November 2002. Additional source: Author's analysis of Statistics Canada, "Survey of Labour & Income Dynamics and Survey on Consumer Finances." Used with permission of the author.

Figure 3.5: B. Murphy, R. Roberts, and M. Wolfson, "High Income Canadians," *Perspectives on Labour and Income* 8, no. 9 (2007), pp. 5–17.

Table 3.6: Adapted from C. Lindsay and M. Almey, "Income and Earnings," in *Women in Candaa: A Gender-based Statistical Report* (2006), pp. 133–158. Ottawa: Statistics Canada.

Figure 3.6: Author's analysis of data presented in R. Morisette and X. Zhang, "Revisiting Wealth Inequality," *Perspectives on Labor and Income* 7, no. 12 (2006), 5–16.

Figure 3.7: Author's analysis of data presented in R. Morisette and X. Zhang, "Revisiting Wealth Inequality," *Perspectives on Labor and Income* 7, no. 12 (2006), 5–16.

Figure 4.1: Statistics Canada and Canadian Institute for Health Information, Health Indicators, Volume 2005, no. 1 (82-221-X1E). www.statscan.ca:8096/bsolc/english/bsole?catno=82-221-X1E.

Table 4.1: Minister of Health and Social Services, Birth and Death Registry, Quebec, 1981–2004. Copy authorized by Les Publications du Québec.

Figure 4.2: Statistics Canada and Canadian Institute for Health Information, Health Indicators, Volume 2005, no. 1 (82-221-X1E). www.statscan.ca:8096/bsolc/english/bsole?catno=82-221-X1E.

Table 4.2: Canadian Community Health Survey, cycle 3.1, 2005.

Figure 4.3: Minister of Health and Social Services, Birth and Death Registry, Quebec, 1981–2004. Copy authorized by Les Publications du Québec.

Figure 4.4: Minister of Health and Social Services, Birth and Death Registry, Quebec, 1981–2004. Copy authorized by Les Publications du Québec.

Figure 4.5: Minister of Health and Social Services, Birth and Death Registry, Quebec, 1981–2004. Copy authorized by Les Publications du Québec.

Figure 4.6: Minister of Health and Social Services, Quebec Public Health Insitute, Third Report on the National Health of the Population of Quebec (in press). Copy authorized by Les Publications du Québec. Copy authorized by Les Publications du Québec.

Table 5.1: Suzanne Asselin, "Conditions de travail et remuneration," *Données Sociales du Québec* (Institut de la Statistique du Québec, 2005), p. 129. Copy authorized by Les Publications du Québec.

Figure 5.1: Statistics Canada, *Enquete sur la population active*. Special calculations of the Statistical Institute of Quebec (2005), p. 129.

Figure 5.2: L. Vosko, N. Zukewich ,and C. Cranford, "Le travail précaire: une nouvelle typologie de l'emploie," *L'emploi et le revenue en perspective*. Statistics Canada, 2003, Graph C, p. 23.

Table 5.2: Statistics Canada (2001), *Femmes au Canada: une mise à jour du chapitre sur le travail*. Ottawa: Publication No. 89F0133XIF.

Table 6.1: W. Lewchuk, A. de Wolff, A. King, and M. Polanyi, "The Hidden Costs of Precarious Employment: Health and the Employment Relationship," in L.F. Vosko, ed., *Precarious Employment: Understanding Labour Market Insecurity in Canada* (Montreal: McGill-Queen's University Press, 2006). Used with permission of the publisher.

Figure 6.1: From W. Lewchuk, A. de Wolff, A. King, and M. Polanyi, "Beyond Jog Strain: Employment Strain and the Health Effects of Precarious Employment," Work in a Global Society Working Paper 2005-1. Hamilton: Labour Studies Programme, McMaster University. Used with permission.

Box 6.1: www.statcan.ca/english/indepth/75-001/online/01003/hi-fs_200310_02_a.html

Figure 6.2: From E. Tompa, R. Dolinschi, S. Trevithick, H. Scott, and S. Bhattacharyy, "Work-related Precariousness: Canadian Trends and Policy Implications." Working Paper #281 (Toronto: Institute for Work & Health, 2005). Used with permission.

Figure 6.3: From E. Tompa, R. Dolinschi, S. Trevithick, H. Scott, and S. Bhattacharyya, "Work-related Precariousness: Canadian Trends and Policy Implications." Working Paper #281 (Toronto: Institute for Work & Health, 2005). Used with permission.

Figure 9.1: M. Friendly, J. Beach, C. Ferns, and M. Turiano, *Trends and Analysis 2007* (Toronto: Childcare Resource and Research Unit, 2007). Reprinted with permission.

Box 9.2: Maureen McTeer, "Mr. Harper, Leave the Child-care Program Alone," *The Globe and Mail*, February 6, 2006. Reprinted with permission of the author.

Figure 9.2: M. Friendly, J. Beach, C. Ferns, and M. Turiano, *Trends and Analysis 2007* (Toronto: Childcare Resource and Research Unit, 2007). Reprinted with permission.

Figure 9.3: M. Friendly, J. Beach, C. Ferns, and M. Turiano, *Trends and Analysis 2007* (Toronto: Childcare Resource and Research Unit, 2007). Reprinted with permission.

Table 10.1: H.M. Skeels, "Adult Status of Children with Constraining Early Life Experiences," *Monographs of the Society for Research in Child Development* 31 (105) (1966): 1–65. Permission to reprint from Blackwell Publishing.

Table 10.2: New Zealand Ministry of Education (n.d.). Reference for ECE review of early childhood education: Consultation document. © Ministry of Education, New Zealand. Retrieved 30 November 2007 from www.minedu.govt.nz/web/downloadable/d19677_v1/references.doc. Used with permission.

Box 11.1: Marie Drolet (2005), *Participation in Post-secondary Education in Canada: Has the Role of Parental Income and Education Changed over the 1990s?* Catalogue 11F0019MIE, no. 243. Ottawa: Statistics Canada. Data from the Survey of Labour and Income Dynamics (SLID), 1993–2001.

Box 11.2: Statistics Canada, *The Daily*, October 31, 2003.

Figure 12.2: "Average Personal Income, by Level of Prose Literacy and Sex," from *The Value of Words: Literacy and Economic Security in Canada, 2001.* www.statcan.ca/english/freepub/89F0100XIE/value.htm.

Figure 12.3: OECD and Statistics Canada (1995), Literacy, Economy and Society: Results of the First International Literacy Survey.

Box 12.2: BC Teachers' Federation, "School Libraries Are Threatened, Despite Powerful Evidence They're Key to Student Achievement." News Release, October 27, 2003. Reprinted with permission of BCTF.

Box 13.2: From M. Rock, L. McIntyre, and K. Rondeau, "Discomforting Comfort Foods: Stirring the Pot on Kraft Dinner in Canada," *Agriculture and Human Values (forthcoming). Reprinted by permission.*

Figure 13.2: *Canadian Coummunity Health Survey, Cycle 2.2, Nutrition (2004)—Income-related Household Food Insecurity in Canada. Health Canada (2007). Reproduced with the permission of the Minister of Public Works and Government Services Canada, 2008.*

Figure 13.3: Adapted from L. McIntyre, N.T. Glanville, K.D. Raine, J.B. Dayle, and N. Battaglia, "Do Low-income Lone Mothers Compromise Their Nutrition to Feed Their Children?" Reprinted from *Canadian Medical Association Journal* 168 (18 March 2003), pp. 686–691, by permission of the publisher. © 2003 Canadian Medical Association.

Box 14.1: Carol Goar, "The Best Medicine Money Can Buy," *The Toronto Star,* October 17, 2007. Available online from www.thestar.article/267732. Reprinted with permission of Torstar Syndication Services.

Table 14.1: *Canadian Community Health Survey, Cycle 2.2, Nutrition (2004)—Income-related Household Food Insecurity in Canada. Health Canada (2007). Reproduced with the permission of the Minister of Public Works and Government Services Canada, 2008.*

Figures 14.1 to 14.4: *Adapted from S. Kirkpatrick, V. Tarasuk, "Food Insecurity Is Associated with Nutrient Inadequacies among Canadian Adults and Adolescents," Journal of Nutrition 138 (2008), pp. 604–612.*

Figure 14.5: N. Vozoris and V. Tarasuk, "Household Food Insufficiency is Associated with Poorer Health," *Journal of Nutrition* 133 (2003), pp. 120–126. Used with permission.

Figure 15.1: Statistics Canada, Survey of Government Revenues and Expenditures, CANSIM Table 3850002.

Box 16.1: Executive Summary, *Women and Housing in Canada: Barriers to Equality* (2002). Ottawa: Centre for Equality Rights in Accommodation (Women's Program). Online at www. equalityrights.org /cera /barriers.htm. Used with permission.

Figure 16.1: From *Highlights Report 2004: Quality of Life in Canadian Municipalities* (Chart 27, p. 27), by the Federation of Canadian Municipalities, 2004. Ottawa: Federation of Canadian Municipalities.

Table 16.1: W. Bines, *The Health of Single Homeless People* (York, UK: University of York, Centre for Housing Policy, 1994). Used with permission.

Table 17.1: Statistics Canada, 2001 Census Analysis Series, *The Changing Profile of Canada's Labour Force, 2001 Census*, Catalogue No. 96F0030XIE2001009, February 2003.

Table 17.2: Statistics Canada, 2001 Census Analysis Series, *The Changing Profile of Canada's Labour Force, 2001 Census*, Catalogue No. 96F0030XIE2001009, February 2003.

Table 17.3: Statistics Canada, 2001 Census Analysis Series, *The Changing Profile of Canada's Labour Force, 2001 Census*, Catalogue No. 96F0030XIE2001009, February 2003.

Table 17.4: Statistics Canada, 2001 Census Analysis Series, *The Changing Profile of Canada's Labour Force, 2001 Census*, Catalogue No. 96F0030XIE2001009, February 2003.

Table 17.5: Statistics Canada, 2001 Census Analysis Series, *The Changing Profile of Canada's Labour Force, 2001 Census*, Catalogue No. 96F0030XIE2001009, February 2003.

Table 17.6: Statistics Canada, 2001 Census Analysis Series, *The Changing Profile of Canada's Labour Force, 2001 Census*, Catalogue No. 96F0030XIE2001009, February 2003.

Box 19.1: Summary of Outcomes" (pp. 2–3), from *Social Determinants and Indigenous Health: The International Experience and Its Policy Implications*. Report on specially prepared documents, presentations and discussion at the International Symposium on the Social Determinants of Indigenous Health Adelaide, 29–30 April 2007 for the Commission on Social Determinants of Health. Reprinted with permission of the CSDH.

Figure 19.1A: From J. Smylie, "A Guide for Health Professionals Working with Aboriginal Peoples: The Sociocultural Context of Aboriginal Peoples in Canada," *Journal of the Society of Obstetricians and Gynecologists of Canada* 22, no. 12 (2000), pp. 1070–1081. Reprinted courtesy of the Society of Obstetricians and Gynecologists of Canada.

INDEX